The APRN's Complete Guide to Prescribing Pediatric Drug Therapy

2018

Mari J. Wirfs, PhD, MN, RN, ANP-BC, FNP-BC, CNE, is a nationally certified adult nurse practitioner (ANCC since 1997) and family nurse practitioner (AANP since 1998) and certified nurse educator (NLN since 2008). Her career spans 45 years in collegiate undergraduate and graduate nursing education and clinical practice in critical care, pediatrics, psychiatric–mental health nursing, and advanced practice primary care nursing. Her PhD is in higher education administration and leadership. During her academic career, she has achieved the rank of professor with tenure in two university systems. She is a frequent guest lecturer on a variety of advanced practice topics to professional groups and general health care topics to community groups.

Dr. Wirfs was a member of the original medical staff in the establishment of Baptist Community Health Services, a community-based nonprofit primary care clinic founded post-hurricane Katrina in the New Orleans Lower Ninth Ward. Since 2002, Dr. Wirfs has served as clinical director and primary care provider at the Family Health Care Clinic, serving faculty, staff, students, and their families at New Orleans Baptist Theological Seminary (NOBTS). She is also adjunct graduate faculty, teaching Neuropsychology and Psychopharmacology, in the NOBTS Guidance and Counseling program. She is a long-time member of the National Organization of Nurse Practitioner Faculties (NONPF), Sigma Theta Tau National Honor Society of Nursing, and several other academic honor societies.

Dr. Wirfs has completed, published, and presented six quantitative research studies focusing on academic leadership, nursing education, and clinical practice issues, including one for the Army Medical Department conducted during her 8 years reserve service in the Army Nurse Corps. Dr. Wirfs has co-authored family primary care certification review books and study materials. Her first prescribing guide, *Clinical Guide to Pharmacotherapeutics for the Primary Care Provider,* was published by Advanced Practice Education Associates (APEA) from 1999 to 2014. *The APRN's Complete Guide to Prescribing Drug Therapy 2018* (launched in 2016), *The APRN's Complete Guide to Prescribing Pediatric Drug Therapy 2018* (launched in 2017), and *The PA's Complete Guide to Prescribing Drug Therapy 2018* (launched in 2017) are Springer Publishing Company's handbook editions accompanied by the free e-book version with quarterly electronic updates.

The APRN's Complete Guide to Prescribing Pediatric Drug Therapy

2018

Mari J. Wirfs, PhD, MN, RN, ANP-BC, FNP-BC, CNE

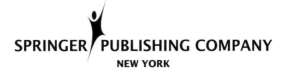

SPRINGER PUBLISHING COMPANY
NEW YORK

Springer Publishing Company, LLC
11 West 42nd Street
New York, NY 10036
www.springerpub.com

Acquisitions Editor: Margaret Zuccarini
Composition: Exeter Premedia Services Private Ltd.

ISBN: 978-0-8261-6668-5
e-book ISBN: 978-0-8261-6669-2

17 18 19 / 5 4 3 2 1

This book is a quick reference for health care providers practicing in primary care settings. The information has been extrapolated from a variety of professional sources and is presented in condensed and summary form. It is not intended to replace or substitute for complete and current manufacturer prescribing information, current research, or knowledge and experience of the user. For complete prescribing information, including toxicities, drug interactions, contraindications, and precautions, the reader is directed to the manufacturer's package insert and the published literature. The inclusion of a particular brand name neither implies nor suggests that the author or publisher advises or recommends the use of that particular product or considers it superior to similar products available by other brand names. Neither the author nor the publisher makes any warranty, expressed or implied, with respect to the information, including any errors or omissions, herein.

Library of Congress Cataloging-in-Publication Data

Names: Wirfs, Mari J., author.
Title: The APRN's complete guide to prescribing pediatric drug therapy, 2018 / Mari J. Wirfs.
Other titles: Complete guide to prescribing pediatric drug therapy, 2018
Description: New York, NY: Springer Publishing Company, LLC, [2017] | Includes bibliographical references and index.
Identifiers: LCCN 2017002668| ISBN 9780826166685 | ISBN 9780826166692 (e-book)
Subjects: | MESH: Drug Therapy—nursing | Pediatric Nursing | Advanced Practice Nursing—methods | Handbooks
Classification: LCC RM170 | NLM WY 49 | DDC 615.5/8—dc23
LC record available at https://lccn.loc.gov/2017002668

Printed in the United States of America by McNaughton & Gunn.

CONTENTS

SECTION I: PEDIATRIC DRUG THERAPY BY CLINICAL DIAGNOSIS

SECTION II: APPENDICES

Kelley M. Anderson, PhD, FNP
Assistant Professor of Nursing, Georgetown University School of Nursing & Health Studies, Washington, DC

Kathleen Bradbury-Golas, DNP, RN, FNP-C, ACNS-BC
Associate Clinical Professor, Drexel University, Philadelphia, Pennsylvania, Family Nurse Practitioner, Virtua Medical Group, Hammonton and Linwood, New Jersey

Lori Brien, MS, ACNP-BC
Instructor, AG-ACNP Program, Georgetown University School of Nursing & Health Studies, Washington, DC

Jill C. Cash, MSN, APN
Nurse Practitioner, Logan Primary Care, West Frankfort, Illinois

Catherine M. Concert, DNP, RN, FNP-BC, AOCNP, NE-BC, CNL, CGRN
Nurse Practitioner—Radiation Oncology, Laura and Isaac Perlmutter Cancer Center, New York University Langone Medical Center; Clinical Assistant Professor, Pace University Lienhard School of Nursing, New York, New York

Aileen Fitzpatrick, DNP, RN, FNP-BC
Clinical Assistant Professor, Pace University Lienhard School of Nursing, New York, New York

Tracy P. George, DNP, APRN-BC, CNE
Assistant Professor of Nursing, Amy V. Cockroft Fellow 2016–2017, Francis Marion University, Florence, South Carolina

Norma Stephens Hannigan, DNP, MPH, FNP-BC, DCC, FAANP
Clinical Professor of Nursing, Coordinator, Accelerated Second Degree (A2D) Program/Sophomore Honors Program, Hunter College, CUNY Hunter-Bellevue School of Nursing, New York, New York

Ella T. Heitzler, PhD, WHNP-BC, FNP-BC, RNC-OB
Assistant Professor, Georgetown University School of Nursing & Health Studies, Washington, DC

Melissa H. King, DNP, FNP-BC, ENP-BC
Director of Advanced Practice Providers, Director of TelEmergency, Department of
Emergency Medicine, University of Mississippi Medical Center, Jackson, Mississippi

Jan Stockton, MSN, RN, ACNS-BC
Infectious Disease Clinical Nurse Specialist, The Christ Hospital Health Network,
Cincinnati, Ohio

Michael Watson, DNP, APRN, FNP-BC
Lead Family Nurse Practitioner, Wadley Regional Medical Center, Emergency
Department, Texarkana, Texas

*	single-scored tablet
**	cross-scored tablet
(II), (III), (IV), (V)	Drug Enforcement Agency (DEA) controlled substance schedule
(A), (B), (C), (D), (X)	Food and Drug Administration (FDA) pregnancy category
ABSSSI	acute bacterial skin and skin structure infection
ac	before meal
ACEI	angiotensin converting enzyme inhibitor
ALT	liver enzyme; alanine transaminase (ALT)
AM	ante meridiem, morning
AMD	age-related macular degeneration
Amp	ampule
APAP	acetaminophen
AST	liver enzyme, aspartate transaminase
Apo-B	apolipoprotein B
ARB	angiotensin receptor blocker
ART	antiretroviral treatment
ASE	adverse side effect
AVB	atrioventricular heart block
BCG vaccine	*Bacillus Calmette-Guerin* vaccine; tuberculosis vaccine
bid	bis in die, twice a day
BP	blood pressure
CAD	coronary artery disease
calib applicator	calibrated applicator
cap	capsule
CAP	community acquired pneumonia

CCB	calcium channel blocker
CFC	chlorofluorocarbon, inhaler propellant
chew tab	chewable tablet
Child-Pugh A	mild liver disease/dysfunction
Child-Pugh B	moderate liver disease/dysfunction
Child-Pugh C	severe liver disease/dysfunction
CHF	congestive heart failure
CKD	chronic kidney disease
clnsr	cleanser
conc	concentrate, concentration
conj estra	conjugated estrogen
cont-rel	controlled-release, continuous release
COPD	chronic obstructive pulmonary disease
cplt	caplet
Cr	creatinine
CR	controlled-release
CrCl	creatinine clearance measured in mL/min
CRI	chronic renal insufficiency
CRF	chronic renal failure
crm	cream
CVD	cardiovascular disease
CYP	cytochrome p
DAA	direct-acting antiviral
DDAVP	desmopressin acetate
dL	deciliter
DM	diabetes mellitus
DME	diabetic macular edema
DMARDs	disease modifying antirheumatoid drugs
DR	diabetic retinopathy

DVT	deep vein thrombosis
ec, ent-coat	enteric-coated
EDTA	edetate calcium disodium
EE	ethinyl estradiol
EKG	electrocardiogram
EIA	exercise-induced asthma
EIAED	enzyme-inducing antiepileptic drug
EIB	exercise-induced bronchospasm
elix	elixir
emol, emolcrm	emollient, emollient cream
ER	extended-release
ESA	erythropoiesis stimulating agent
ESR	erythrocyte sedimentation rate
ESRD	end stage renal disease
est	estradiol
EX, ext-rel	extended-release
film-coat	film-coated
(G)	generic, generic availability
GABHS	group a beta-hemolytic streptococcus
GAD	generalized anxiety disorder
GFR	glomerular filtration rate
GI	gastrointestinal
GLP-1	glucagon peptide-1
gm	gram
gtt, gtts	drop, drops
GU	genitourinary
H_2O_2	hydrogen peroxide
HAART	highly active antiretroviral treatment
HAV	hepatitis A virus

HBV	hepatitis C virus
HCT	hematocrit
HCT, HCTZ	hydrochlorothiazide
HCV	hepatitis C virus
HDL, HDL-C	high density lipoprotein cholesterol
HeFH	heterozygous familial hypercholesterolemia
HFA	hydrofluoroalkane (inhaler propellant phasing in)
Hgb	hemoglobin
HgbA1c	hemoglobin A1c, the standard POC diagnostic test for diabetes
hgc	hard-gel capsule
HoFH	homozygous familial hypercholesterolemia
HPV	human papillomavirus
HR	heart rate in beats per minute
HRT	hormone replacement therapy
HS	hour of sleep, bedtime
IBS-C	irritable bowel syndrome with constipation
IBS-D	irritable bowel syndrome with diarrhea
ID	intradermal
IM	intramuscular
immed-rel	immediate-release
inhal	inhalation
inj	injection
IU	international unit
IUD	intrauterine device
IV	intravenous
JRA	juvenile rheumatoid arthritis
K^+	potassium
kg	kilogram
L	liter, 1,000 ml

LAA	long-acting anticholinergic
LABA	long-acting beta agonist
LAR	long-acting release
LDL, LDL-C	low density lipoprotein cholesterol
LFTs	liver function tests
Liq	liquid
lotn	lotion
LR	lactated ringers IV solution
MAOI	monoamine oxidase inhibitor
mcg	microgram
mCNY	myopic choroidal neovascularization
MDD	major depressive disorder
MDI	metered dose inhaler
mfr pkg insert	manufacturer package insert
mg	milligram
mg/dL	milligrams per deciliter
mg/kg/day	milligram per kilogram per day
ml, mL	milliliter
MRSA	methicillin-resistant staphylococcus aureus
MS	multiple sclerosis
MTX	methotrexate
Na^+	sodium
NaCl	sodium chloride
NaHCO3	sodium bicarbonate
NAT	nucleic acid testing
NE	not established
NGU	non-gonococcal urethritis
NMDA	n-methyl-d-aspartate receptor antagonist
NNRTI	non-nucleoside reverse transcriptase inhibitor
NOH	neurogenic orthostatic hypotension

non-HDL-C	non-high density lipoprotein cholesterol
nPEP	non-occupational postexposure prophylaxis
NR	not rated, pregnancy category not assigned
NRTI	nucleoside reverse transcriptase inhibitor
NS	nasal spray; normal saline
NSAID	non-steroidal anti-inflammatory drug
OA	osteoarthritis
OCD	obsessive-compulsive disorder
OCP	oral contraceptive pill
ODT	orally disintegrating tablet
oint	ointment
ophth	ophthalmic, pertaining to the eye
orally-disint	orally disintegrating
OSAHS	obstructive sleep apnea hypopnea syndrome
OTC	over-the-counter
otic	pertaining to the ear
oz	ounce, 30 ml
pc	after meals
PCOS	polycystic ovarian syndrome; Stein-Leventhal disease
Pediatric	newborn to ≤18 years-of-age
PEG	polyethylene glycol
PEP	postexposure prophylaxis
PDE5	phosphodiesterase type 5 inhibitor
PJIA	polyarticular juvenile idiopathic arthritis
PLLR	FDA pregnancy and lactation labeling final rule
PM	post meridiem, evening
PMDD	premenstrual dysphoric disorder
PMHx	past medical history
PPI	proton pump inhibitor
PO	per oral, by mouth

PO4³⁻	phosphate
POC	point of care
Post-op	post-operative
PR	per rectum
PRN	as needed
PTSD	post-traumatic stress disorder
PUD	peptic ulcer disease
pwdr	powder
pwdr w. diluent	powder with diluent
q	per
qd	once daily
qHS	per hour of sleep, bedtime
qid	quarter in die, four times-a-day
RA	rheumatoid arthritis
RAI	reversible anticholinesterase inhibitor
RBC	red blood cell
RVO	retinal vein occlusion
SC	subcutaneous
SCII	subcutaneous insulin infusion
sgc	soft-gel capsule
SGOT	serum glutamic-oxaloacetic transaminase
SGPT	serum glutamic-pyruvic transaminase
SL	sublingual, under the tongue
SNRI	selective serotonin and norepinephrine reuptake inhibitor
Soln	solution
SR	sustained-release
SSRI	selective serotonin reuptake inhibitor
STD	sexually transmitted disease
Supp	suppository

susp	suspension
sust-rel	sustained-release
SWSD	shift work sleep disorder
syr	syrup
T1DM	type 1 diabetes mellitus
T2DM	type 2 diabetes mellitus
T3	liothyronine
T4	levothyroxine
tab	tablet
TCA	tricyclic antidepressant
TG	triglyceride
tid	ter in die, three times-a-day
TMP/SMX	trimethoprim-sulfamethoxazole
trans-sys	transdermal system
TRD	treatment-resistant depression
TSH	thyroid stimulating hormone
tsp	teaspoon, 4-5 ml
TSSRI	thienobenzodiazepine-selective serotonin reuptake inhibitor
ULN	upper limit of normal
VVC	vulvovaginal candidiasis
WBC	white blood cell
w.	with
XL	extra long-acting
XOI	xanthine oxidase inhibitor
XR	extended-release

The APRN's Complete Guide to Prescribing Pediatric Drug Therapy is a prescribing reference intended for use by health care providers in all clinical practice settings who are involved in the primary care management of pediatric patients (defined herein as newborn to age 21 years) with acute, episodic, and chronic health problems. If pediatric indications for a drug have not been established *or* if a drug is not recommended for an age subgroup, this information is noted accordingly. Where a manufacturer's package insert refers to "children," the term refers to patients under 12 years of age. For quick reference weight-based dosing of a drug, the user is directed to the dose by weight table for that drug in the appendices. Comments are interspersed throughout, including such clinically useful information as laboratory values to be monitored, patient teaching points, and safety information.

This reference is divided into two major sections that are organized in a concise and easy-to-read format, **Section I** presents drug treatment regimens for over 500 clinical diagnoses. Each drug is listed alphabetically by generic name, whether the drug is available over the counter (OTC), DEA schedule (I, II, III, IV, V), generic availability (G), dosing regimens from birth to ≥18 years, available dose forms, whether tablets, caplets, or chew tabs are scored (*) or cross-scored (**), flavors of chewable, sublingual, buccal, and liquid forms, and information regarding additives (e.g., dye-free, sugar-free, preservative-free <u>or</u> preservative type, and alcohol-free <u>or</u> alcohol content). For a prescription drug that was FDA-approved *prior to June 30, 2015*, the former 5-letter pregnancy category still applies and are so noted as A, B, C, D, X. *See page* 459 for descriptions of these FDA pregnancy categories. For drugs FDA-approved *after June 30, 2015*, the 5-letter categories are no longer used and there is no replacement (categorical nomenclature) at this time. Rather, information regarding special populations, including pregnant and breastfeeding females, is addressed in a structured narrative format. Prescribers should refer to the drug's FDA labeling (https://www.fda.gov/Drugs/default.htm) <u>or</u> the manufacturer's package insert for this information. Prescription drugs submitted for FDA approval after June 30, 2015 use the new format immediately, while labeling for prescription drugs approved on or after June 30, 2015 are phased in gradually. Although drugs approved prior to June 29, 2015 are not subject to the FDA's **Pregnancy and Lactation Labeling Final Rule (PLLR)**, the *pregnancy letter category must be removed by June 29, 2018*. Labeling for over-the-counter (OTC) medicines will not change, as OTC drugs are not affected by the new FDA pregnancy labeling. For a more detailed explanation of the final rule and new narrative format, visit https://www.drugs.com/pregnancy-categories.html

Section II presents clinically useful information in a convenient table format, including: the JNC-8 recommendations for hypertension management, the U.S. schedule of controlled substances and the FDA pregnancy categories, measurement conversions, childhood immunization recommendations, brand-name drugs (with contents) for the management of common respiratory symptoms, anti-infectives by classification, pediatric dosing by weight for liquid forms, glucocorticosteroids by potency and route of administration, and contraceptives by route of administration and estrogen and/or progesterone content. An alphabetical cross-reference index of drugs by generic and brand name, with FDA 5-letter pregnancy category and controlled drug schedule, facilitates quick identification of drugs by alternate names, relative safety during pregnancy, and DEA schedule.

Selected diagnoses (e.g., HIV, ADHD, growth failure, multiple sclerosis, cystic fibrosis, hepatitis, seizure disorders) and selected drugs (e.g., anti-neoplastics, antipsychotics, antiarrhythmics, anti-HIV drugs, contraceptives) are included as pediatric patients treated by specialists are also followed and treated by primary care providers for total (holistic) care of the patient.

Safe, efficacious, prescribing and monitoring of drug therapy regimens for children and adolescents requires adequate knowledge about (a) the pharmacodynamics and pharmacokinetics of drugs, (b) concomitant therapies, and (c) individual characteristics of the patient (e.g., age, weight, current and past medical history, physical examination findings, hepatic and renal function, co-morbidities, and risk factors). Users of this clinical guide are encouraged to utilize the manufacturer's package insert, recommendations and guidance of specialists, standard of practice protocols, and the current research literature for more comprehensive information about specific drugs (e.g., special precautions, drug-drug and drug-food interactions, risk versus benefit, age-related considerations, adverse reactions) and appropriate use with individual patients.

ACKNOWLEDGMENTS

This publication, which we consider to be a "must have" for students, academicians, and practicing clinicians with prescriptive authority, represents the culmination of Springer Publishing Company's collaborative team effort. Margaret Zuccarini, Publisher, Emerita, Nursing, Joanne Jay, Vice President, Production and Manufacturing, and the Editorial Committee, shared my vision for a handy pocket prescribing reference for new and experienced prescribers in primary care. Joanne Jay designed the contents for ease and efficiency of user navigation. The production team at Exeter Premedia Services, on behalf of Springer Publishing Company, understood the critical nature of exactness in this prescribing resource, and faithfully managed the complex files as content was updated and cross-paginated for the final product. The work of the reviewers from academia and clinical practice was essential to the process and their contributions are greatly appreciated. I am proud of my association with these dedicated professionals and I thank them on behalf of the medical and advanced practice nursing community worldwide, for supporting the end goal of quality health care for all.

ACE-Is and **ARBS** are contraindicated in the 2nd and 3rd trimesters of pregnancy. Addition of a daily ACE-I or ARB is strongly recommended for renal protection in patients with hypertension and/or diabetes. The "ACE inhibitor cough," a dry cough, is an adverse side effect produced by an accumulation of bradykinins that occurs in 5-10% of the population and resolves within days of discontinuing the drug.

Alcohol is contraindicated with concomitant *narcotic analgesics*, *benzodiazepines*, *SSRIs*, *antihistamines*, *TCAs*, and other sedating agents due to risk of over-sedation.

Alpha-1 blockers have a potential adverse side effect of sudden hypotension, especially with first dose. Alert the patient regarding this "first-dose effect" and recommend the patient sit or lie down to take the first dose. Usually start at lowest dose and titrate upward.

Aspirin is contraindicated in children and adolescents with *Varicella* or other viral illness, and 3rd trimester of pregnancy.

Beta-blockers, by all routes of administration, are generally contraindicated in severe COPD, history of <u>or</u> current bronchial asthma, sinus bradycardia, and 2nd <u>or</u> 3rd degree AV block. Use a cardio-specific beta blocker where appropriate in these cases.

Calcium channel blockers may cause the adverse side effect of pedal edema (feet, ankles, lower legs) that resolves with discontinuation of the drug.

Codeine is known to be excreted in breast milk. <12 years: not recommended; 12-<18: use extreme caution; not recommended for children and adolescents with asthma or other chronic breathing problem. The FDA and the European Medicines Agency (EMA) are investigating the safety of using *codeine*-containing medications to treat pain, cough, and colds in children 12-<18 years because of the potential for serious side effects, including slowed or difficult breathing.

Corticosteroids increases blood sugar in patients with diabetes and decreases immunity; therefore, consider risk *vs* benefit in susceptible patients, use lowest effective dose, and taper gradually to discontinue.

Erythromycin may increase INR with concomitant *warfarin*, as well as increase serum level of *digoxin*, *benzodiazepines*, and *statins*.

Estrogen-progesterone and **progesterone-only contraceptives** are contraindicated in pregnancy (pregnancy category X)

Finasteride, a 5-alpha reductase inhibitor, is associated with low but increased risk of high-grade prostate cancer. Pregnant females should not touch broken tablets.

Fluoroquinolones and **quinolones** are contraindicated <18 years-of-age, pregnancy, and breastfeeding. *Exception:* in the case of anthrax, *ciprofloxacin* is indicated for patients <18 years-of-age and dosed based on mg/kg body weight. Risk of tendonitis or tendon rupture (ex: *ciprofloxacin, gemifloxacin, levofloxacin, moxifloxacin, norfloxacin, ofloxacin*).

The U.S. Preventive Services Task Force (USPSTF) recommends *against* using hormone replacement therapy (**HRT**) for primary prevention of chronic conditions among postmenopausal women. The harms associated with combined use of estrogen and a progestin, such as increased risks of invasive breast cancer, venous thromboembolism, and coronary heart disease, far outweigh the benefits.

Ibuprofen is contraindicated in children <6 months of age and in the 3rd trimester of pregnancy.

Metronidazole and **tinidazole** are contraindicated in the 1st trimester of pregnancy. Alcohol is contraindicated during treatment with oral forms and for 72 hours after therapy due to a possible *disulfiram*-like reaction (nausea, vomiting, flushing, headache).

Oral **PDE5 inhibitors** are contraindicated in patients taking nitrates due to risk of hypotension or syncope (ex: *avanafil, sildenafil, tadalafil, vardenafil*).

Statins are strongly recommended as adjunctive therapy for patients with diabetes, with <u>or</u> without abnormal lipids.

Sulfonamides are not recommended in pregnancy or lactation. *CrCl 15-30 mL/min:* reduce dose by 1/2; *CrCl <15 mL/min:* not recommended (ex: *sulfamethoxazole, trimethoprim*). Contraindicated with G6PD deficiency. A high fluid intake is indicated during sulfonamide therapy to avoid crystallization in the kidneys.

Tetracyclines are contraindicated in children <8 years-of-age, pregnancy, and breastfeeding (discolors developing tooth enamel). A side effect may be photo-sensitivity (photophobia). Do not take with antacids, calcium supplements, milk or other dairy, or 2 hours of taking another drug (ex: *doxycycline, minocycline, tetracycline*).

Tramadol is known to be excreted in breast milk. The FDA and the European Medicines Agency (EMA) are investigating the safety of using *tramadol*-containing medications to treat pain in children 12-18 years because of the potential for serious side effects, including slowed or difficult breathing.

The **Transmucosal Immediate Release Fentanyl (TIRF) Risk Evaluation and Mitigation Strategy (REMS)** program is an FDA-required program designed to ensure informed risk-benefit decisions before initiating treatment, and while patients are treated to ensure appropriate use of TIRF medicines. The purpose of the TIRF REMS Access program is to mitigate the risk of misuse, abuse, addiction, overdose, and serious complications due to medication errors with the use of TIRF medicines. You must enroll in the TIRF REMS Access program to prescribe, dispense, or distribute TIRF medicines. To register, call the TIRF REMS Access program at 1-866-822-1483 or register online at https://www.tirfremsaccess.com/TirfUI/rems/home.action

Live vaccines are contraindicated in patients who are immunosuppressed or receiving immunosuppressive therapy, including immunosuppressive levels of corticosteroid therapy.

PEDIATRIC DRUG THERAPY BY CLINICAL DIAGNOSIS

ACETAMINOPHEN OVERDOSE

ANTIDOTE/CHELATING AGENT

➤ *acetylcysteine* (B)(G) *Loading dose:* 150 mg/kg administered over 15 minutes; *Maintenance:* 50 mg/kg administered over 4 hours; then 100 mg/kg administered over 16 hours

Acetadote *Vial: soln for IV infusion after dilution:* 200 mg/ml (30 ml; dilute in D$_5$W) (preservative-free)

Comment: *acetaminophen* overdose is a medical emergency due to the risk of irreversible hepatic injury. An IV infusion of *acetylcysteine* should be started as soon as possible and within 24 hours if the exact time of ingestion is unknown. Use a serum *acetaminophen* nomogram to determine need for treatment. Extreme caution is needed if used with concomitant hepatotoxic drugs.

ACNE ROSACEA

Comment: All acne rosacea products should be applied sparingly to clean, dry skin as directed. Avoid use of topical corticosteroids.

➤ *ivermectin* (C) apply bid

Soolantra *Crm:* 1% (30 gm)

Comment: **Soolantra** is a macrocyclic lactone. Exactly how it works to treat acne rosacea is unknown.

TOPICAL ALPHA-1A ADRENOCEPTOR AGONIST

➤ *oxymetazoline hcl* (B) <18 years: not recommended; ≥18 years: apply a pea-sized amount once daily in a thin layer covering the entire face (forehead, nose, cheeks, and chin) avoiding the eyes and lips; wash hands immediately

Rhofade *Crm* 1% (30 g tube)

Comment: **Rhofade** acts as a vasoconstrictor. Use with caution in patients with cerebral or coronary insufficiency, Raynaud's phenomenon, thromboangiitis obliterans, scleroderma, or Sjögren's syndrome. **Rhofade** may increase the risk of angle closure glaucoma in patients with narrow-angle glaucoma. Advise patients to seek immediate medical care if signs and symptoms of potentiation of vascular insufficiency or acute angle closure glaucoma develop.

TOPICAL ALPHA2A-AGONIST

➤ *brimonidine* (B) <18 years: not recommended; ≥18 years: apply to affected area once daily

Mirvaso *Gel:* 0.33% (30, 45 gm tube; 30 gm pump)

Comment: For persistent erythema; constricts dilated facial blood vessels to reduce redness.

TOPICAL ANTIMICROBIALS

➤ *azelaic acid* (B) apply affected area bid

Azelex *Crm:* 20% (30, 50 gm)

Finacea *Gel:* 15% (30 gm); *Foam:* 15% (50 gm)

➤ *metronidazole* (B) apply affected area bid
    MetroCream apply bid
        Emol crm: 0.75% (45 gm)
    MetroGel apply once daily
        Gel: 1% (60 gm tube; 55 gm pump)
    MetroLotion apply bid
        Lotn: 0.75% (2 oz)
➤ *sodium sulfacetamide* (C)(G) apply 1-3 x daily
    Klaron *Lotn:* 10% (2 oz)
➤ *sodium sulfacetamide/sulfur* (C)
    Clenia Emollient Cream apply 1-3 x daily
        Wash: sod sulfa 10%/*sulfur* 5% (10 oz)
    Clenia Foaming Wash wash affected area once <u>or</u> twice daily
        Wash: sod sulfa 10%/*sulfur* 5% (6, 12 oz)
    Rosula Gel apply 1-3 x daily
        Gel: sod sulfa 10%/*sulfur* 5% (45 ml)
    Rosula Lotion apply tid
        Lotn: sod sulfa 10%/*sulfur* 5% (45 ml) (alcohol-free)
    Rosula Wash wash bid
        Clnsr: sod sulfa 10%/*sulfur* 5% (335 ml)

ORAL ANTIMICROBIALS

➤ *doxycycline* (D)(G) <8 years: not recommended; ≥8 years, ≤100 lb: 2 mg/lb on first day in 2 divided doses, followed by 1 mg/lb/day in 1-2 divided doses; ≥8 years, >100 lb: 40-100 mg bid; *see page* 561 *for dose by weight table*
    Acticlate *Tab:* 75, 150** mg
    Adoxa *Tab:* 50, 75, 100, 150 mg ent-coat
    Doryx *Tab:* 50, 75, 100, 150, 200 mg del-rel
    Monodox *Cap:* 50, 75, 100 mg
    Oracea *Cap:* 40 mg del-rel
    Vibramycin *Tab:* 100 mg; *Cap:* 50, 100 mg; *Syr:* 50 mg/5 ml (raspberry-apple) (sulfites); *Oral susp:* 25 mg/5 ml (raspberry)
    Vibra-Tab *Tab:* 100 mg film-coat
➤ *minocycline* (D)(G) <8 years: not recommended; ≥8 years, ≤100 lb: 2 mg/lb on first day in 2 divided doses, followed by 1 mg/lb q 12 hours x 9 more days; ≥8 years, >100 lb: 200 mg on first day; then 100 mg q 12 hours x 9 more days
    Dynacin *Cap:* 50, 100 mg
    Minocin *Cap:* 50, 75, 100 mg; *Oral susp:* 50 mg/5 ml (60 ml) (custard) (sulfites, alcohol 5%)

ACNE VULGARIS

TOPICAL ANTIMICROBIALS

Comment: All topical antimicrobials should be applied sparingly to clean, dry skin.
➤ *azelaic acid* (B) apply to affected area bid
    Azelex *Crm:* 20% (30, 50 gm)
    Finacea *Gel:* 15% (30 gm); *Foam:* 15% (50 g)

▷ *benzoyl peroxide* (C)(G) may discolor clothing and linens.
    Benzac-W initially apply to affected area once daily; increase to bid-tid as tolerated
        Gel: 2.5, 5, 10% (60 gm)
    Benzac-W Wash wash affected area bid
        Wash: 5% (4, 8 oz); 10% (8 oz)
    Benzagel apply to affected area one or more times/day
        Gel: 5, 10% (1.5, 3 oz) (alcohol 14%)
    Benzagel Wash wash affected area bid
        Gel: 10% (6 oz)
    Desquam X₅ wash affected area bid
        Wash: 5% (5 oz)
    Desquam X₁₀ wash affected area bid
        Wash: 10% (5 oz)
    Triaz apply to affected area daily bid
        Lotn: 3, 6, 9% (bottle), 3% (tube); *Pads:* 3, 6, 9% (jar)
    ZoDerm apply once or twice daily
        Gel: 4.5, 6.5, 8.5% (125 ml); *Crm:* 4.5, 6.5, 8.5% (125 ml); *Clnsr:* 4.5, 6.5, 8.5% (400 ml)
▷ *clindamycin* topical (B) <12 years: not recommended; ≥12 years: apply once daily
    Cleocin T (G) *Pad:* 1% (60/pck; alcohol 50%); *Lotn:* 1% (60 ml); *Gel:* 1% (30, 60 gm); *Soln w. applicator:* 1% (30, 60 ml) (alcohol 50%)
    Clindagel *Gel:* 1% (42, 77 gm)
    Evoclin Foam: 1% (50, 100 gm) (alcohol)
▷ *clindamycin/benzoyl peroxide* topical (C) <12 years: not recommended; ≥12 years: apply once daily; *benzoyl peroxide* may discolor clothing and linens
    Acanya (G) apply qd-bid
        Gel: clin 1.2%/*benz* 2.5% (50 gm)
    BenzaClin (G) apply bid
        Gel: clin 1%/*benz* 5% (25, 50 gm)
    Duac *Gel:* apply daily in the evening
        clin 1%/*benz* 5% (45 gm)
    Onexton Gel apply once daily
        Gel: clin 1.2%/*benz* 3.75% (50 gm pump) (alcohol-free)m(preservative-free)
▷ *dapsone* topical (C) <12 years: not recommended; ≥12 years: apply to affected area bid
    Aczone *Gel:* 5, 7.5% (30, 60, 90 gm pump)
▷ *erythromycin/benzoyl peroxide* (C) initially apply once daily; increase to bid as tolerated; *benzoyl peroxide* may discolor clothing and linens
    Benzamycin Topical Gel *Gel: eryth* 3%/*benz* 5% (46.6 gm/jar)
▷ *sodium sulfacetamide* (C)(G) apply tid
    Klaron *Lotn:* 10% (2 oz)

ORAL ANTIMICROBIALS

▷ *doxycycline* (D)(G) <8 years: not recommended; ≥8 years, ≤100 lb: 2 mg/lb on first day in 2 divided doses, followed by 1 mg/lb/day in 1-2 divided doses; ≥8 years, >100 lb: 100 mg bid; *see page 561 for dose by weight table*
    Acticlate *Tab:* 75, 150** mg
    Adoxa *Tab:* 50, 75, 100, 150 mg ent-coat

Doryx *Tab:* 50, 75, 100, 150, 200 mg del-rel
Monodox *Cap:* 50, 75, 100 mg
Oracea *Cap:* 40 mg del-rel
Vibramycin *Tab:* 100 mg; *Cap:* 50, 100 mg; *Syr:* 50 mg/5 ml (raspberry-apple) (sulfites); *Oral susp:* 25 mg/5 ml (raspberry)
Vibra-Tab *Tab:* 100 mg film-coat

▶ **erythromycin base (B)(G)** <45 kg: 30-50 mg in 2-4 divided doses x 7-10 days; ≥45 kg: 250 mg qid, 333 mg tid <u>or</u> 500 mg bid x 7-10 days; then taper to lowest effective dose
Ery-Tab *Tab:* 250, 333, 500 mg ent-coat
PCE *Tab:* 333, 500 mg

▶ **erythromycin ethylsuccinate (B)(G)** 30-50 mg/kg/day in 4 divided doses x 7-10 days; may double dose with severe infection; max 100 mg/kg/day <u>or</u> 400 mg qid; *see page 563 for dose by weight table*
EryPed *Oral susp:* 200 mg/5 ml (100, 200 ml) (fruit); 400 mg/5 ml (60, 100, 200 ml) (banana); *Oral drops:* 200, 400 mg/5 ml (50 ml) (fruit); *Chew tab:* 200 mg wafer (fruit)
E.E.S. *Oral susp:* 200, 400 mg/5 ml (100 ml) (fruit)
E.E.S. Granules *Oral susp:* 200 mg/5 ml (100, 200 ml) (cherry)
E.E.S. 400 Tablets *Tab:* 400 mg

▶ **minocycline (D)(G)** <8 years: not recommended; ≥8 years: initially 50-100 mg once daily; reduce dose after improvement
Dynacin *Cap:* 50, 100 mg
Minocin *Cap:* 50, 75, 100 mg; *Oral susp:* 50 mg/5 ml (60 ml) (custard) (sulfites, alcohol 5%)

▶ **tetracycline (D)(G)** <8 years: not recommended; ≥8 years, ≤100 lb: 25-50 mg/kg/day in 2-4 divided doses; *see page 574 for dose by weight table*; ≥8 years, >100 lb: initially 1 gm/day in 2-4 divided doses; after improvement, 125-500 mg once daily
Achromycin V *Cap:* 250, 500 mg
Sumycin *Tab:* 250, 500 mg; *Cap:* 250, 500 mg; *Oral susp:* 125 mg/5 ml (100, 200 ml) (fruit) (sulfites)

Comment: *tetracycline* is contraindicated <8 years-of-age, in pregnancy, and lactation (discolors developing tooth enamel). A side effect may be photosensitivity (photophobia). Do not give with antacids, calcium supplements, milk <u>or</u> other dairy, <u>or</u> within two hours of taking another drug.

TOPICAL RETINOIDS

Comment: Wash affected area with a soap-free cleanser; pat dry and wait 20 to 30 minutes; then apply sparingly to affected area; use only once daily in the evening. Avoid applying to eyes, ears, nostrils, and mouth.

▶ **adapalene (C)** <12 years: not recommended; ≥12 years: apply once daily at HS
Differin *Crm:* 0.1% (45 gm); *Gel:* 0.1, 0.3% (45 gm) (alcohol-free); *Pad:* 0.1% 30/pck) (alcohol 30%); *Lotn:* 0.1% (2, 4 oz)

▶ **tazarotene (X)** <12 years: not recommended; ≥12 years: apply once daily at HS
Avage Cream *Crm:* 0.1% (30 gm)
Tazorac Cream *Crm:* 0.05, 0.1% (15, 30, 60 gm)
Tazorac Gel *Gel:* 0.05, 0.1% (30, 100 gm)

▶ **tretinoin (C)** <12 years: not recommended; ≥12 years: apply to affected area once daily at HS
Atralin Gel *Gel:* 0.05% (45 gm)

Avita *Crm:* 0.025% (20, 45 gm); *Gel:* 0.025% (20, 45 gm)
Renova *Crm:* 0.02% (40 gm); 0.05% (40, 60 gm)
Retin-A Cream *Crm:* 0.025, 0.05, 0.1% (20, 45 gm)
Retin-A Gel *Gel:* 0.01, 0.025% (15, 45 gm) (alcohol 90%)
Retin-A Liquid *Soln:* 0.05% (alcohol 55%)
Retin-A Micro Gel *Gel:* 0.04, 0.08, 0.1% (20, 45 gm)
Tretin-X Cream *Crm:* 0.075% (35 gm) (paraben-free, alcohol-free, propylene-glycol-free)

TOPICAL RETINOID/ANTIMICROBIAL COMBINATIONS

Comment: Wash affected area with a soap-free cleanser; pat dry and wait 20-30 minutes; then apply sparingly to affected area; use only once daily in the evening. Avoid eyes, ears, nostrils, and mouth.
▷ *adapalene/benzoyl peroxide* (C) <18 years: not recommended; ≥18 years: apply a thin film to the affected area once daily; *benzoyl peroxide* may discolor clothing and linens
    Epiduo Gel *Gel: adap* 0.1%/*benz* 2.5% (45 gm)
▷ *tretinoin/clindamycin* (C) <18 years: not recommended; ≥18 years: apply a thin film to the affected area once daily
    Ziana *Gel: tret* 0.025%/*clin* 1.2% (30, 60 gm)

ORAL RETINOID

Comment: Oral retinoids are indicated only for severe recalcitrant nodular acne unresponsive to conventional therapy including systemic antibiotics.
▷ *isotretinoin* (X) <12 years: not recommended; ≥12 years: initially 0.5-1 mg/kg/day in 2 divided doses; maintenance 0.5-2 mg/kg/day in 2 divided doses x 4-5 months; repeat only if necessary 2 months following cessation of first treatment course
    Accutane *Cap:* 10, 20, 40 mg (parabens)
    Amnesteem *Cap:* 10, 20, 40 mg (soy)
Comment: *isotretinoin* is *highly teratogenic* and, therefore, female patients should be counseled prior to initiation of treatment as follows: Two negative pregnancy tests are required prior to initiation of treatment and monthly thereafter. Not for use in females who are <u>or</u> who may become pregnant <u>or</u> who are breastfeeding. Two effective methods of contraception should be used for 1 month prior to, during, and continuing for 1 month following completion of treatment. Low-dose *progestin* (mini-pill) may be an *inadequate* form of contraception. No refills; a new prescription is required every 30 days and prescriptions must be filled within 7 days. Serum lipids should be monitored until response is established (usually initially and again after 4 weeks). Bone growth, serum glucose, ESR, RBCs, WBCs, and liver enzymes should be monitored. Blood should not be donated during, <u>or</u> for 1 month after, completion of treatment. Avoid the sun and artificial UV light. *Isotretinoin* should be discontinued if any of the following occurs: visual disturbances, tinnitus, hearing impairment, rectal bleeding, pancreatitis, hepatitis, significant decrease in CBC, hyperlipidemia (particularly hypertriglyceridemia).

ORAL CONTRACEPTIVES

see **Combined Oral Contraceptives** *page* 476
see **Progesterone-Only Contraceptives ("Mini-Pill")** *page* 485

ACROMEGALY

GROWTH HORMONE RECEPTOR ANTAGONIST

▶ *pegvisomant* (B) <12 years: not recommended; ≥12 years: *Loading dose:* 40 mg SC;
Maintenance: 10 mg SC daily; titrate by 5 mg (increments or decrements, based on
IGF-1 levels) every 4 to 6 weeks; max 30 mg/day
   Somavert *Inj:* 10, 15, 20 mg
   Comment: Prior to initiation of *pegvisomant*, patients should have baseline fasting
   serum glucose, HgbA1c, serum potassium and magnesium, liver function tests
   (LFTs), EKG, and gall bladder ultrasound.

Cyclohexapeptide Somatostatin

▶ *pasireotide* (C) <12 years: not recommended; ≥12 years: administer SC in the thigh
or abdomen; initial dose is 0.6 mg or 0.9 mg bid. Titrate dose based on response
and tolerability; for patients with moderate hepatic impairment (Child-Pugh B), the
recommended initial dosage is 0.3 mg twice daily and max dose 0.6 mg twice daily;
avoid use in patients with severe hepatic impairment (Child-Pugh C)
   Signifor LAR *Amp:* 0.3, 0.6, 0.9 mg/ml, single-dose, long-act rel (LAR) susp for inj

ACTINIC KERATOSIS

Comment: *pasireotide* is also indicated for destroying superficial basal cell carcinoma
(sBCC) lesions.
▶ *diclofenac sodium* (C; D ≥30 wks)(G) <18 years: not established; ≥18 years:
   Solaraze Gel *Gel:* 3% (50 gm) (benzyl alcohol)
   Comment: Contraindicated with *aspirin* allergy. As with other NSAIDs,
   Solaraze Gel should be avoided in late pregnancy (≥30 weeks) because it may
   cause premature closure of the ductus arteriosus.
   Voltaren Gel <12 years: not recommended; ≥12 years: apply qid; avoid non-
   intact skin
   Gel: 1% (100 gm)
▶ *diclofenac sodium* 3% (C; D ≥30 wks)(G) <12 years: not recommended; ≥12 years:
apply to lesions bid x 60-90 days
▶ *fluorouracil* (X)(G) <12 years: not recommended; ≥12 years: apply to lesion(s)
daily-bid until erosion occurs, usually 2-4 weeks
   Carac *Crm:* 0.5% (30 gm)
   Efudex (G) *Crm:* 5% (25 gm); *Soln:* 2, 5% (10 ml w. dropper)
   Fluoroplex *Crm:* 1% (30 gm); *Soln:* 1% (30 ml w. dropper)
▶ *imiquimod* (B)
   Aldara (G) <18 years: not recommended; ≥18 years: rub into lesions before
   bedtime and remove with soap and water 8 hours later; treat 2 times per week;
   max 16 weeks
   Crm: 5% (single-use pkts/carton)
   Zyclara <12 years: not recommended; ≥12 years: rub into lesions before
   bedtime and remove with soap and water 8 hours later; treat for 2-week cycles
   separated by a 2-week no-treatment cycle; max 2 packs per application; max
   one treatment course per area
   Crm: 3.75% (single-use pkts; 28/carton) (parabens)

▷ *ingenol mebutate* (C) <18 years: not recommended; ≥18 years: limit application to one contiguous skin area of about 25 cm² using one unit dose tube; allow treated area to dry for 15 minutes; wash hands immediately after application; may remove with soapy water after 6 hours; *Face and Scalp*: apply 0.015% gel to lesions daily x 3 days; *Trunk and Extremities*: apply 0.05% gel to lesions daily x 2 days

    Picato *Gel*: 0.015% (3 single-use tubes), 0.05% (2 single-use tubes)

 # ALCOHOL DEPENDENCE/ALCOHOL WITHDRAWAL SYNDROME

ALCOHOL WITHDRAWAL SYNDROME

Comment: Total length of time of a given detoxification regimen and/or length of time of treatment at any dose reduction level may be extended based on patient-specific factors, including potential or actual seizure, hallucinosis, increased sympathetic nervous system activity (severe anxiety, unwanted elevation in vital signs). If any of these symptoms are anticipated or occur, revert to an earlier step in the dosing regimen to stabilize the patient, extend the detoxification timeline and consider appropriate adjunctive drug treatments (e.g., anticonvulsants, antipsychotic agents, antihypertensive agents, sedative hypnotic agents).

▷ *clorazepate* (D)(IV)(G) <18 years: not recommended; ≥18 years: *De-escalating dosage schedule: Day 1:* 30 mg initially, followed by 30-60 mg in divided doses; *Day 2:* 45-90 mg in divided doses; *Day 3:* 22.5-45 mg in divided doses; *Day 4:* 15-30 mg in divided doses; Thereafter, gradually reduce the daily dose to 7.5-15 mg; then discontinue when patient's condition is stable; max dose 90 mg/day

    Tranxene *Tab*: 3.75, 7.5, 15 mg
    Tranxene T-Tab *Tab*: 3.75*, 7.5*, 15*mg

▷ *chlordiazepoxide* (D)(IV)(G)
    Librium <18 years: not recommended; ≥18 years: 50-100 mg q 6 hours x 24-72 hours; then q 8 hours x 24-72 hours; then q 12 hours x 24-72 hours; then daily x 24-72 hours

      Cap: 5, 10, 25 mg
    Librium Injectable <12 years: not recommended; ≥12 years: 50-100 mg IM or IV; then 25-50 mg IM tid-qid prn; max 300 mg/day

      Inj: 100 mg
▷ *diazepam* (D)(IV)(G) <18 years: not recommended; ≥18 years: 2-10 mg q 6 hours x 24-72 hours; then q 8 hours x 24-72 hours; then q 12 hours x 24-72 hours; then daily x 24-72 hours

    Diastat *Rectal gel delivery system*: 2.5 mg
    Diastat AcuDial *Rectal gel delivery system*: 10, 20 mg
    Valium *Tab*: 2*, 5*, 10*mg
    Valium Injectable *Vial*: 5 mg/ml (10 ml); *Amp*: 5 mg/ml (2 ml); *Prefilled syringe*: 5 mg/ml (5 ml)
    Valium Intensol Oral Solution *Conc oral soln*: 5 mg/ml (30 ml w. dropper) (alcohol 19%)
    Valium Oral Solution *Oral soln*: 5 mg/5 ml (500 ml) (wintergreen spice)
▷ *oxazepam* (C) <18 years: not recommended; ≥18 years: 500 mg once daily x 1-2 weeks; then 250 mg once daily 10-15 mg tid-qid x 24-72 hours; decrease dose and/or frequency every 24-72 hours; total length of therapy 5-14 days; max 120 mg/day

    Cap: 10, 15, 30 mg

ABSTINENCE THERAPY

GABA Taurine Analog

➤ *acamprosate* (C)(G) <18 years: not recommended; ≥18 years: 666 mg tid; begin therapy during abstinence; continue during relapse; *CrCl 30-50 mL/min:* max 333 mg tid; *CrCl <30 mL/min:* contraindicated
  Campral *Tab:* 333 mg ext-rel
  Comment: **Campral** does not eliminate <u>or</u> diminish alcohol withdrawal symptoms.

AVERSION THERAPY

➤ *disulfiram* (X)(G) <18 years: not recommended; ≥18 years: 500 mg once daily x 1-2 weeks; then 250 mg once daily
  Antabuse *Tab:* 250, 500 mg; *Chew tab:* 200, 500 mg
  Comment: *disulfiram* use requires informed consent. Contraindications: severe cardiac disease, psychosis, concomitant use of *isoniazid, phenytoin, paraldehyde,* and topical and systemic alcohol-containing products. Approximately 20% remains in the system for 1 week after discontinuation.

Nutritional Support

➤ *thiamine* (A)(G) <18 years: not recommended; ≥18 years: 500 mg once daily x 1-2 weeks; then 250 mg once daily injectable 50-100 mg IM/IV daily (<u>or</u> tid if severely deficient)
  Vial: 100 mg/1 ml (1 ml)

ALLERGIC REACTION: GENERAL

PARENTERAL ANTIHISTAMINE

➤ *diphenhydramine* injectable (B)(G)
  Benadryl Injectable <12 years: *See mfr pkg insert:* 1.25 mg/kg up to 25 mg IM x 1 dose; then q 6 hours prn; ≥12 years: 25-50 mg IM immediately; then q 6 hours prn
  Vial: 50 mg/ml (1 ml single use); 50 mg/ml (10 ml multi-dose); *Amp:* 10 mg/ml (1 ml); *Prefilled syringe:* 50 mg/ml (1 ml)
Oral Prescription Drugs for the Management of Allergy, Cough, and Cold Symptoms *see page* 523
Topical Corticosteroids *see page* 494
Parenteral Corticosteroids *see page* 499
Oral Corticosteroids *see page* 498

AMEBIASIS

AMEBIASIS (INTESTINAL)

➤ *diiodohydroxyquin (iodoquinol)* (C)(G) <6 years: 40 mg/kg/day in 3 divided doses pc x 20 days; max 1.95 g; 6-<12 years: 420 mg tid pc x 20 days; ≥12 years: 650 mg tid pc x 20 days
  Tab: 210, 650 mg

▷ *metronidazole* (not for use in 1st; B in 2nd, 3rd)(G) <12 years: 35-50 mg/kg/day in
3 divided doses x 10 days; ≥12 years: 750 mg tid x 5-10 days
Flagyl *Tab:* 250*, 500*mg
Flagyl 375 *Cap:* 375 mg
Flagyl ER *Tab:* 750 mg ext-rel
Comment: Alcohol is contraindicated during treatment with oral *metronidazole*
and for 72 hours after therapy due to a possible *disulfiram*-like reaction (nausea,
vomiting, flushing, headache).
▷ *tinidazole* (not for use in 1st; B in 2nd, 3rd) <3 years: not recommended; 3-12
years: 50 mg/kg daily x 3 days; take with food; max 2 gm/day; ≥12 years: 2 gm daily
x 3 days; take with food
Tindamax *Tab:* 250*, 500*mg
▷ *paromomycin* 25-35 mg/kg/day in 3 divided doses x 5-10 days
Humatin *Cap:* 250 mg

AMEBIASIS (EXTRAINTESTINAL)

▷ *chloroquine phosphate* (C)(G) <12 years: *see mfr pkg insert;* ≥12 years: 1 gm PO
daily x 2 days; then 500 mg daily x 2 to 3 weeks or 200-250 mg IM daily x 10-12
days (when oral therapy is impossible); use with intestinal amebicide
Aralen *Tab:* 500 mg; *Amp:* 50 mg/ml (5 ml)

AMEBIC LIVER ABSCESS

ANTI-INFECTIVES

▷ *metronidazole* (not for use in 1st; B in 2nd, 3rd)(G) <12 years: not recommended;
≥12 years: 250 mg tid or 500 mg bid or 750 mg daily x 7 days
Flagyl *Tab:* 250*, 500*mg
Flagyl 375 *Cap:* 375 mg
Flagyl ER *Tab:* 750 mg ext-rel
Comment: Alcohol is contraindicated during treatment with oral *metronidazole*
and for 72 hours after therapy due to a possible *disulfiram*-like reaction (nausea,
vomiting, flushing, headache).
▷ *tinidazole* (not for use in 1st; B in 2nd, 3rd) <3 years: not recommended; 3-12
years: 50 mg/kg once daily x 3-5 days; take with food; max 2 gm/day; ≥12 years: 2
gm once daily x 3-5 days; take with food
Tindamax *Tab:* 250*, 500*mg

AMENORRHEA: SECONDARY

▷ *estrogen/progesterone* (X)
Premarin (*estrogen*) 0.625 mg daily x 25 days; then 5 days off; repeat monthly
Provera (*progesterone*) 5-10 mg last 10 days of cycle; repeat monthly
▷ *human chorionic gonadotropin* 5,000-10,000 units IM x 1 dose following last dose
of menotropins
Pregnyl *Vial:* 10,000 units (10 ml) w. diluent (10 ml)

➤ **medroxyprogesterone** (X) *Monthly:* 5-10 mg last 5-10 days of cycle; begin on the
16th or 21st day of cycle; repeat monthly; *One-time only:* 10 mg once daily x 10 days
    Amen *Tab:* 10 mg
    Provera *Tab:* 2.5, 5, 10 mg
➤ **norethindrone** (X) 2.5-10 mg daily x 5-10 days
    Aygestin *Tab:* 5 mg
➤ **progesterone, micronized** (X)(G) 400 mg q HS x 10 days
    Prometrium *Cap:* 100, 200 mg
    Comment: Administration of **progesterone** induces optimum secretory transformation
of the **estrogen**-primed endometrium. Administration of **progesterone** is
contraindicated with breast cancer, undiagnosed vaginal bleeding, genital
cancer, severe liver dysfunction or disease, missed abortion, thrombophlebitis,
thromboembolic disorders, cerebral apoplexy, and pregnancy.

ANAPHYLAXIS

➤ **epinephrine** (C)(G) <2 years: 0.05-0.1 ml; 2-6 years: 0.1 ml; ≥6-12 years: 0.2 ml;
All: q 20-30 minutes as needed up to 3 doses; ≥12 years: 0.3-0.5 mg (0.3-0.5 ml of a
1:1000 soln) SC q 20-30 minutes as needed up to 3 doses
Parenteral Corticosteroids *see page* 499
Oral Corticosteroids *see page* 498

ANAPHYLAXIS EMERGENCY TREATMENT KITS

➤ **epinephrine** (C) <15 kg: 0.01 mg/kg SC or IM in thigh; may repeat if needed; 15-30
kg: 0.15 mg; ≥12 years. ≥30 kg: 0.3 ml IM or SC in thigh; may repeat if needed
    Adrenaclick *Autoinjector:* 0.15, 0.3 mg (1 mg/ml; 1, 2/carton) (sulfites)
    Auvi-Q *Autoinjector:* 0.15, 0.3 mg (1 mg/ml; 1/pck w. 1 non-active training
device) (sulfites)
    EpiPen *Autoinjector 0.3 mg* (*epi* 1:1000, 0.3 ml (1, 2/carton) (sulfites)
    EpiPen Jr *Autoinjector 0.15 mg* (*epi* 1:2000, 0.3 ml) (1, 2/carton) (sulfites)
    Twinject *Autoinjector:* 0.15, 0.3 mg (epi 1:1000) (1, 2/carton) (sulfites)
➤ **epinephrine/chlorpheniramine** (C) infants-2 years: 0.05-0.1 ml SC or IM; 2-<6
years: 0.15 ml SC or IM plus 1 PO tab **chlorpheniramine**; 6-<12 years: 0.2 ml SC or
IM plus 2 chewable **chlorpheniramine** tabs; ≥12 years: **epinephrine** 0.3 ml SC or IM
plus 4 chewable **chlorpheniramine** tabs
    Ana-Kit: 0.3 ml syringes of *epi* 1:1000 (2/carton) for self-injection plus 4 *chlor* 2
mg chew tabs

ANEMIA OF CHRONIC KIDNEY DISEASE (CKD) AND CHRONIC RENAL FAILURE (CRF)

ERYTHROPOIESIS STIMULATING AGENTS (ESAS)

➤ **darbepoetin alpha** (erythropoiesis stimulating protein) (C) <12 years: not recommended; ≥12 years: administer IV or SC q 1-2 weeks; do not increase more
frequently than once per month; *Not currently receiving epoetin alpha:* initially 0.75
mcg/kg once weekly; adjust based on Hgb levels (target not to exceed 12 gm/dL);

reduce dose if Hgb increases more than 1 gm/dL in any 2-week period; suspend therapy if polycythemia occurs; *Converting from epoetin alpha and for dose titration:* see mfr pkg insert

> **Aranesp** *Vial:* 25, 40, 60, 100, 150, 200, 300, 500 mcg/ml (single dose) for IV or SC administration (preservative-free, albumin [human] or polysorbate 80)
>
> **Aranesp Singleject, Aranesp Sureclick Singleject** *Prefilled syringe:* 25, 40, 60, 100, 150, 200, 300, 500 mcg (single dose) for IV or SC administration (preservative-free, albumin [human] or polysorbate 80)

▶ *peginesatide* **(C)** <12 years: not established; ≥12 years: use lowest effective dose; initiate when Hgb <10 gm/dL; do not increase dose more often than every 4 weeks; if Hgb rises rapidly (i.e., >1 gm/dL in 2 weeks or >2 gm/dL in 4 weeks), reduce dose by 25% or more; if Hgb approaches or exceeds 11 gm/dL, reduce or interrupt dose and then when Hgb decreases, resume dose at approximately 25% below previous dose; if Hgb does not increase by >1 g/dL after 4 weeks, increase dose by 25%; if response inadequate after a 12-week escalation period, use lowest dose that will maintain Hgb sufficient to reduce need for RBC transfusion; discontinue if response does not improve; *Not currently on ESA:* initially 0.04 mg/kg as a single IV or SC dose once monthly; *Converting from epoetin alfa:* administer first dose 1 week after last epoetin alfa; *Converting from darbepoetin alfa:* administer first dose at next scheduled dose of darbepoetin alfa

> **Omontys** *Vial, single use:* 2, 3, 4, 5, 6 mg (0.5 ml) (preservative-free); *Vial, multi-use:* 10, 20 mg (2 ml) (preservatives); *Prefilled syringe:* 2, 3, 4, 5, 6 mg (0.5 ml) (preservative-free)

ERYTHROPOIETIN HUMAN, RECOMBINANT

▶ *epoetin alpha* **(C)** <1 month: not recommended; ≥1 month-12 years: individualize; *Dialysis:* initially 50 units/kg 3 x/week IV or SC; target Hct 30-36%; ≥12 years: individualize; initially 50-100 units/kg 3 x/week; IV (dialysis or non-dialysis) or SC (non-dialysis); usual max 200 units/kg 3 x/week (dialysis) or 150 units/kg 3 x/week (non-dialysis); target Hct 30-36%

> **Epogen** *Vial:* 2,000, 3,000, 4,000, 10,000, 40,000 units/ml (1 ml) single use for IV or SC administration (albumin [human]; preservative-free)
>
> **Epogen Multidose** *Vial:* 10,000 units/ml (2 ml); 20,000 units/ml (1 ml) for IV or SC administration (albumin [human]; benzoyl alcohol)
>
> **Procrit** *Vial:* 2,000, 3,000, 4,000, 10,000, 40,000 units/ml (1 ml) single use for IV or SC administration (albumin [human]) (preservative-free)
>
> **Procrit Multidose** *Vial:* 10,000 units/ml (2 ml); 20,000 units/ml, (1 ml) for IV or SC administration (albumin [human]; benzoyl alcohol)

ANEMIA: FOLIC ACID DEFICIENCY

▶ *folic acid* **(A)(OTC)** 0.4-1 mg once daily

Comment: *folic acid (vitamin B₉)* 400 mcg daily is recommended during pregnancy to prevent neural tube defects. Females who have had a baby with a neural tube defect should take 400 mcg every day, even when not planning to become pregnant, and if planning to become pregnant should take 4 mg daily during the month before becoming pregnant until at least the 12th week of pregnancy.

ANEMIA: IRON DEFICIENCY

Comment: Hemochromatosis and hemosiderosis are contraindications to iron therapy. *Iron* supplements are best absorbed when taken between meals and with *vitamin C*-rich foods. Excessive *iron* may be extremely hazardous to infants and young children. All vitamin and mineral supplements should be kept out of the reach of children.

IRON PREPARATIONS

▷ *ferrous gluconate* (A)(G) <12 years: not recommended: ≥12 years: 1 tab once daily
  Fergon (OTC) *Tab:* iron 27 mg (240 mg as gluconate)
▷ *ferrous sulfate* (A)(G)
  Feosol Tablets (OTC) <6 years: use elixir; ≥6-12 years: 1 tab tid pc; ≥12 years: 1 tab tid-qid pc and HS
    Tab: iron 65 mg (200 mg as sulfate)
  Feosol Capsules (OTC) <12 years: not recommended; ≥12 years: 1-2 caps daily
    Cap: iron 50 mg (169 mg as sulfate) sust-rel
  Feosol Elixir (OTC) <1 year: not recommended; >1-11 years: 2.5-5 ml tid between meals; ≥12 years: 5-10 ml tid between meals
  Fer-In-Sol (OTC) <4 years, use drops; ≥4 years: 5 ml once daily
    Syr: iron 18 mg (90 mg as sulfate) per 5 ml (480 ml)
  Fer-In-Sol Drops (OTC) <4 years: 0.6 ml daily; ≥4 years: use syrup
    Oral drops: iron 15 mg (75 mg as sulfate) per 5 ml (50 ml)

ANEMIA: MEGALOBLASTIC/ANEMIA: PERNICIOUS

Comment: Signs of *vitamin B12* deficiency include megaloblastic anemia, glossitis, paresthesias, ataxia, spastic motor weakness, and reduced mentation.
▷ *vitamin B12 (cyanocobalamin)* (A)(G) 500 mcg intranasally once a week; may increase dose if serum B12 levels decline; adjust dose in 500 mcg increments
  Nascobal Nasal Spray *Intranasal gel:* 500 mcg/0.1 ml (1.3 ml, 4 doses) (citric acid, benzalkonium chloride)

Comment: Nascobal Nasal Spray is indicated for maintenance of hematologic remission following IM B12 therapy without nervous system involvement. Must be primed before each use.

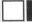

ANGINA PECTORIS: STABLE

CALCIUM ANTAGONISTS

Comment: Calcium antagonists are contraindicated with history of ventricular arrhythmias, sick sinus syndrome, 2nd <u>or</u> 3rd degree heart block, cardiogenic shock, acute myocardial infarction, and pulmonary congestion.
▷ *amlodipine* (C)(G) <12 years: not recommended; ≥12 years: 5-10 mg daily
  Norvasc *Tab:* 2.5, 5, 10 mg
▷ *diltiazem* (C)(G)
  Cardizem <12 years: not recommended; ≥12 years: initially 30 mg qid; may increase gradually every 1-2 days; max 360 mg/day in divided doses

  Tab: 30, 60, 90, 120 mg
 Cardizem CD <12 years: not recommended; ≥12 years: initially 120-180 mg daily; adjust at 1- to 2-week intervals; max 480 mg/day
  Cap: 120, 180, 240, 300, 360 mg ext-rel
 Cardizem LA <12 years: not recommended; ≥12 years: initially 180-240 mg daily; titrate at 2 week intervals; max 540 mg/day
  Tab: 120, 180, 240, 300, 360, 420 mg ext-rel
 Cartia XT <12 years: not recommended; ≥12 years: initially 180 mg or 240 mg once daily; max 540 mg once daily
  Cap: 120, 180, 240, 300 mg ext-rel
 Dilacor XR <12 years: not recommended; ≥12 years: initially 180 mg or 240 mg once daily; max 540 mg once daily
  Cap: 180, 240 mg ext-rel
 Tiazac <12 years: not recommended; ≥12 years: initially 120-180 mg daily; max 540 mg/day
  Cap: 120, 180, 240, 300, 360, 420 mg ext-rel

➢ *nicardipine* (C)(G) <12 years: not recommended; ≥12 years: initially 20 mg tid; adjust q 3 days; max 120 mg/day
 Cardene *Cap:* 20, 30 mg

➢ *nifedipine* (C)(G)
 Adalat CC <12 years: not recommended; ≥12 years: initially 30 mg once daily; usual range 30-60 mg tid; max 90 mg/day
  Tab: 30, 60, 90 mg ext-rel
 Procardia <12 years: not recommended; ≥12 years: initially 10 mg tid; titrate over 7-14 days: max 30 mg/dose and 180 mg/day in divided doses
  Cap: 10, 20 mg
 Procardia XL <12 years: not recommended; ≥12 years: initially 30-60 mg daily; titrate over 7-14 days; max dose 90 mg/day
  Tab: 30, 60, 90 mg ext-rel

➢ *verapamil* (C)(G)
 Calan <12 years: not recommended; ≥12 years: 80-120 mg tid; increase daily or weekly if needed
  Tab: 40, 80*, 120*mg
 Calan SR <12 years: not recommended; ≥12 years: initially 120 mg once daily; increase weekly if needed
  Tab: 120, 180, 240 mg
 Covera HS <12 years: not recommended; ≥12 years: initially 180 mg q HS; titrate in steps to 240 mg; then to 360 mg; then to 480 mg if needed
  Tab: 180, 240 mg ext-rel
 Isoptin SR <12 years: not recommended; ≥12 years: initially 120-180 mg in the AM; may increase to 240 mg in the AM; then 180 mg q 12 hours or 240 mg in the AM and 120 mg in the PM; then 240 mg q 12 hours
  Tab: 120, 180*, 240*mg sust-rel

BETA-BLOCKERS

Comment: Beta-blockers are contraindicated with history of sick sinus syndrome (SSS), 2nd or 3rd degree heart block, cardiogenic shock, pulmonary congestion, asthma, moderate to severe COPD with FEV1 <50% predicted, patients with chronic bronchodilator treatment.

▷ *atenolol* (D)(G) <12 years: not recommended; ≥12 years: initially 25-50 mg daily; increase weekly if needed; max 200 mg daily
    Tenormin *Tab:* 25, 50, 100 mg

▷ *metoprolol succinate* (C)(G) <12 years: not recommended; ≥12 years: initially 12.5-25 mg in a single dose daily; increase weekly if needed; reduce if symptomatic bradycardia occurs; max 400 mg/day
    Toprol-XL *Tab:* 25*, 50*, 100*, 200*mg ext-rel

▷ *metoprolol tartrate* (C)(G) <12 years: not recommended; ≥12 years: initially 25-50 mg bid; increase weekly if needed; max 400 mg/day
    Lopressor *Tab:* 25, 37.5, 50, 75, 100 mg

▷ *nadolol* (C)(G) <12 years: not recommended; ≥12 years: initially 40 mg daily; increase q 3-7 days; max 240 mg/day
    Corgard *Tab:* 20*, 40*, 80*, 120*, 160*mg

▷ *propranolol* (C)(G)
    Inderal <12 years: not recommended; ≥12 years: initially 10 mg bid; usual range 160-320 mg/day in divided doses
        Tab: 10*, 20*, 40*, 60*, 80*mg
    Inderal LA <12 years: not recommended; ≥12 years: initially 80 mg daily in a single dose; increase q 3-7 days; usual range 120-160 mg/day; max 320 mg/day in a single dose
        Cap: 60, 80, 120, 160 mg sust-rel
    InnoPran XL <12 years: not recommended; ≥12 years: initially 80 mg q HS; max 120 mg/day
        Cap: 80, 120 mg ext-rel

NITRATES

Comment: Use a daily nitrate dosing schedule that provides a dose-free period of 14 hours <u>or</u> more to prevent tolerance. *Aspirin* and *acetaminophen* may relieve nitrate-induced headache. *Isosorbide* is not recommended for use in MI <u>and/or</u> CHF. Nitrate use is a contraindication for using phosphodiesterase type 5 inhibitors: *sildenafil* (**Viagra**), *tadalafil* (**Cialis**), *vardenafil* (**Levitra**).

▷ *isosorbide dinitrate* (C)
    Dilatrate-SR 40 <12 years: not recommended; ≥12 years: mg once daily; max 160 mg/day
        Cap: 40 mg sust-rel
    Isordil Titradose initially <12 years: not recommended; ≥12 years: 5-20 mg q 6 hours; maintenance 10-40 mg q 6 hours
        Tab: 5, 10, 20, 30, 40 mg

▷ *isosorbide mononitrate* (C)
    Imdur <12 years: not recommended; ≥12 years: initially 30-60 mg q AM; may increase to 120 mg daily; max 240 mg/day
        Tab: 30*, 60*, 120 mg ext-rel
    Ismo <12 years: not recommended; ≥12 years: 20 mg upon awakening; then 20 mg 7 hours later
        Tab: 20*mg

▷ *nitroglycerin* (C)(G)
    Nitro-Bid Ointment <12 years: not recommended; ≥12 years: initially 1/2 inch q 8 hours; titrate in 1/2 inch increments
        Oint: 2% (20, 60 gm)

Nitrodisc <12 years: not recommended; ≥12 years: initially one 0.2-0.4 mg/hour patch for 12-14 hours/day
> *Transdermal disc:* 0.2, 0.3, 0.4 mg/hour (30, 100/carton)

Nitrolingual Pump Spray <12 years: not recommended; ≥12 years: 1-2 sprays on <u>or</u> under tongue; max 3 sprays/15 minutes
> *Spray:* 0.4 mg/dose (14.5 g, 200 doses)

Nitromist <12 years: not recommended; ≥12 years: 1-2 sprays at onset of attack, on <u>or</u> under the tongue while sitting; may repeat q 5 minutes as needed; max 3 sprays/15 minutes; may use prophylactically 5-10 minutes prior to exertion; do not inhale spray; do not rinse mouth for 5-10 minutes after use
> *Lingual aerosol spray:* 0.4 mg/actuation (230 metered sprays)

Nitrostat <12 years: not recommended; ≥12 years: 1 tab SL; may repeat q 5 minutes x 3
> *SL tab:* 0.3 (1/100 gr), 0.4 (1/150 gr), 0.6 (1/4 gr) mg

Transderm-Nitro <12 years: not recommended; ≥12 years: initially one 0.2 mg/hour <u>or</u> 0.4 mg/hour patch for 12-14 hours/day
> *Transdermal patch:* 0.1, 0.2, 0.4, 0.6, 0.8 mg/hour

NON-NITRATE PERIPHERAL VASODILATOR

▷ *hydralazine* (C)(G) <12 years: not recommended; ≥12 years: initially 10 mg qid x 2-4 days; then increase to 25 mg qid for remainder of first week; then increase to 50 mg qid; max 300 mg/day
> *Tab:* 10, 25, 50, 100 mg

NITRATE/PERIPHERAL VASODILATOR COMBINATION

▷ *isosorbide/hydralazine HCl* (C) <12 years: not established; ≥12 years: initially 1 tab tid; max 2 tabs tid
> **Bodily** *Tab:* isosorb 20 mg/hydral 37.5 mg

NON-NITRATE ANTIANGINAL

▷ *ranolazine* (C) <12 years: not recommended; ≥12 years: initially 500 mg bid; may increase to max 1 gm bid
> **Ranexa** *Tab:* 500, 1000 mg ext-rel
> **Comment:** **Ranexa** is indicated for the treatment of chronic angina that is inadequately controlled with other antianginals. Use with amlodipine, beta-blocker, <u>or</u> nitrate.

ANOREXIA/CACHEXIA

APPETITE STIMULANTS

▷ *cyproheptadine* (B)(G) <2 years: not recommended; ≥2-6 years: 2 mg bid-tid prn; max 12 mg/day; 7-14 years: 4 mg bid-tid prn; max 16 mg/day; >14 years: initially 4 mg tid prn; then adjust as needed; usual range 12-16 mg/day; max 32 mg/day
> **Periactin** *Tab:* cypro 4*mg; *Syr:* cypro 2 mg/5 ml

▷ *dronabinol* (cannabinoid) (B)(III) <12 years: not recommended; ≥12 years: initially 2.5 mg bid before lunch and dinner; may reduce to 2.5 mg q HS <u>or</u> increase to 2.5 mg before lunch and 5 mg before dinner; max 20 mg/day in divided doses
> **Marinol** *Cap:* 2.5, 5, 10 mg (sesame oil)

▷ *megestrol* (progestin) **(X)(G)** <12 years: not recommended; ≥12 years: 40 mg qid
    Megace *Tab:* 20*, 40*mg
    Megace ES *Oral susp (concentrate):* 125 mg/ml; 625 mg/5 ml (5 oz)
    (lemon-lime)
    Megace Oral Suspension *Oral susp:* 40 mg/ml (8 oz); 820 mg/20 ml)
    (lemon-lime)
    Megestrol Acetate Oral Suspension (G) 125 mg/ml
  Comment: *megestrol* is indicated for the treatment of anorexia, cachexia, or an
unexplained, significant weight loss in patients with a diagnosis of AIDS.

ANTHRAX (*BACILLUS ANTHRACIS*)

POSTEXPOSURE PROPHYLAXIS OF INHALATIONAL ANTHRAX AND TREATMENT OF INHALED AND CUTANEOUS ANTHRAX INFECTION

Immune Globulin

▷ *bacillus anthracis immune globulin intravenous (human)* **(NE)** <16 years: not
established; 5-<10 kg: 1 vial; 10-<18 kg: 2 vials; 18-<25 kg: 3 vials; 25-<35 kg: 4
vials; 35-<50 kg: 5 vials; 50-<60 kg: 6 vials; ≥60 kg: 7 vials; ≥16 years: administer
via IV infusion at a maximum rate of 2 ml/min; dose is weight-based as follows, but
may be doubled in severe cases if weight >5 kg
    Anthrasil *Vial:* (60 units) sterile solution of purified human immune globulin G
    (IgG) containing polyclonal antibodies that target the anthrax toxins of *Bacillus
    anthracis* for IV infusion
    Comment: **Anthrasil** is indicated for the emergent treatment of inhaled anthrax
    in combination with appropriate antibacterial agents
▷ *ciprofloxacin* **(C)** <18 years: 20-40 mg/kg/day divided q 12 hours; ≥18 years: 500
mg or 10-15 mg/kg/day) q 12 hours for 60 days; max 1.5 gm/day; start as soon as
possible after exposure
    Cipro (G) *Tab:* 250, 500, 750 mg; *Oral susp:* 250, 500 mg/5 ml (100 ml)
    (strawberry)
    Cipro XR *Tab:* 500, 1000 mg ext-rel
    ProQuin XR *Tab:* 500 mg ext-rel
▷ *doxycycline* **(D)(G)** <8 years: not recommended; ≥8 years, ≤100 lb: 2 mg/lb on first
day in 2 divided doses, followed by 1 mg/lb/day in 1-2 divided doses; ≥8 years, >100
lb: 100 mg bid; *see page* 561 *for dose by weight table*
    Acticlate *Tab:* 75, 150** mg
    Adoxa *Tab:* 50, 75, 100, 150 mg ent-coat
    Doryx *Tab:* 50, 75, 100, 150, 200 mg del-rel
    Monodox *Cap:* 50, 75, 100 mg
    Oracea *Cap:* 40 mg del-rel
    Vibramycin *Tab:* 100 mg; *Cap:* 50, 100 mg; *Syr:* 50 mg/5 ml (raspberry-apple)
    (sulfites); *Oral susp:* 25 mg/5 ml (raspberry)
    Vibra-Tab *Tab:* 100 mg film-coat
  Comment: *doxycycline* is contraindicated <8 years-of-age, in pregnancy, and
lactation (discolors developing tooth enamel). A side effect may be photo-
sensitivity (photophobia). Do not take with antacids, calcium supplements, milk or
other dairy, or within 2 hours of taking another drug.

▷ *minocycline* (D)(G) <8 years: not recommended; ≥8 years, ≤100 lb: 2 mg/lb on first day in 2 divided doses, followed by 1 mg/lb q 12 hours x 9 more days; ≥8 years, >100 mg: 100 mg q 12 hours

  Dynacin *Cap:* 50, 100 mg
  Minocin *Cap:* 50, 75, 100 mg; *Oral susp:* 50 mg/5 ml (60 ml) (custard) (sulfites, alcohol 5%)

Comment: *minocycline* is contraindicated <8 years-of-age, in pregnancy, and lactation (discolors developing tooth enamel). A side effect may be photo-sensitivity (photophobia). Do not give with antacids, calcium supplements, milk or other dairy, or within two hours of taking another drug.

TREATMENT OF INHALATIONAL, GI, AND OROPHARYNGEAL ANTHRAX

▷ *ciprofloxacin* (C) <18 years: 10-15 mg/kg IV q 12 hours (start as soon as possible); then switch to 10-15 mg/kg PO q 12 hours for 60 days; ≥18 years: 400 mg IV q 12 hours (start as soon as possible); then, switch to 500 mg PO q 12 hours for total 60 days max 1.5 gm/day;

  Cipro (G) *Tab:* 250, 500, 750 mg; *Oral susp:* 250, 500 mg/5 ml (100 ml) (strawberry); *IV conc:* 10 mg/ml after dilution (20, 40 ml); *IV premix:* 2 mg/ml (100, 200 ml)
  Cipro XR *Tab:* 500, 1,000 mg ext-rel
  ProQuin XR *Tab:* 500 mg ext-rel

Comment: *ciprofloxacin* is contraindicated <18 years-of-age, and during pregnancy and lactation. Risk of tendonitis or tendon rupture. Infuse IV *ciprofloxacin* over 60 minutes.

▷ *doxycycline* (D)(G) <8 years: not recommended; ≥8 years, ≤100 lb: 2 mg/lb on first day in 2 divided doses, followed by 1 mg/lb/day in 1-2 divided doses for 10 days; ≥8 years, >100 lb: 100 mg bid day 1; then 100 mg daily x 10 days; *see page 561 for dose by weight table*

  Acticlate *Tab:* 75, 150** mg
  Adoxa *Tab:* 50, 75, 100, 150 mg ent-coat
  Doryx *Tab:* 50, 75, 100, 150, 200 mg del-rel
  Monodox *Cap:* 50, 75, 100 mg
  Oracea *Cap:* 40 mg del-rel
  Vibramycin *Tab:* 100 mg; *Cap:* 50, 100 mg; *Syr:* 50 mg/5 ml (raspberry-apple) (sulfites); *Oral susp:* 25 mg/5 ml (raspberry)
  Vibra-Tab *Tab:* 100 mg film-coat

Comment: *doxycycline* is contraindicated <8 years-of-age, in pregnancy, and lactation (discolors developing tooth enamel). A side effect may be photo-sensitivity (photophobia). Do not take with antacids, calcium supplements, milk or other dairy, or within 2 hours of taking another drug.

▷ *minocycline* (D)(G) <8 years: not recommended; ≥8 years, ≤100 lb: 2 mg/lb on first day in 2 divided doses, followed by 1 mg/lb q 12 hours x 9 more days; ≥8 years, >100 lb: 100 mg q 12 hours

  Dynacin *Cap:* 50, 100 mg
  Minocin *Cap:* 50, 75, 100 mg; *Oral susp:* 50 mg/5 ml (60 ml) (custard) (sulfites, alcohol 5%)

Comment: *minocycline* is contraindicated <8 years-of-age, in pregnancy, and lactation (discolors developing tooth enamel). A side effect may be photo-sensitivity (photophobia). Do not give with antacids, calcium supplements, milk or other dairy, or within two hours of taking another drug.

ANXIETY DISORDER: GENERALIZED (GAD)/ANXIETY DISORDER: SOCIAL (SAD)

1ST GENERATION ANTIHISTAMINE

▷ *diphenhydramine* (B)(G)
  Benadryl (OTC) <2 years: not recommended; 2-6 years: 6.25 mg q 4-6 hours; max 37.5 mg/day; >6-12 years: 12.5-25 mg q 4-6 hours; max 150 mg/day; >12 years: 25-50 mg q 6-8 hours; max 100 mg/day
  Chew tab: 12.5 mg (grape) (phenylalanine); *Liq:* 12.5 mg/5 ml (4, 8 oz); *Cap:* 25 mg; *Tab:* 25 mg; *Dye-free soft gel:* 25 mg;
  Dye-free liq: 12.5 mg/5 ml (4, 8 oz)

▷ *diphenhydramine* injectable (B)(G)
  Benadryl Injectable <12 years: *See mfr pkg insert:* 1.25 mg/kg up to 25 mg IM x 1 dose; then q 6 hours prn; ≥12 years: 25-50 mg IM immediately; then q 6 hours prn
  Vial: 50 mg/ml (1 ml single use); 50 mg/ml (10 ml multi-dose); *Amp:* 10 mg/ml (1 ml); *Prefilled syringe:* 50 mg/ml (1 ml)

▷ *hydroxyzine* (C)(G) <6 years: 50 mg/day divided qid; ≥6-12 years: 50-100 mg/day divided qid; ≥12 years: 50-100 mg qid; max 600 mg/day
  Atarax *Tab:* 10, 25, 50, 100 mg; *Syr:* 10 mg/5 ml (alcohol 0.5%)
  Vistaril *Cap:* 25, 50, 100 mg; *Oral susp:* 25 mg/5 ml (4 oz) (lemon)

Comment: *hydroxyzine* is contraindicated in early pregnancy and in patients with a prolonged QT interval. It is not known whether this drug is excreted in human milk; therefore, *hydroxyzine* should not be given to nursing mothers.

AZAPIRONE

▷ *buspirone* (B) <6 years: not recommended; ≥6 years: initially 7.5 mg bid; may increase by 5 mg/day q 2-3 days; max 60 mg/day
  BuSpar *Tab:* 5, 10, 15*, 30* mg

BENZODIAZEPINES

Comment: If possible when considering a benzodiazepine to treat anxiety, a short-acting benzodiazepine should be used only prn to avert intense anxiety and panic and for the least time necessary while a different non-addictive antianxiety regimen (e.g., SSRI, SNRI, TCA, *buspirone*, beta-blocker) is established and effective treatment goals achieved. Benzodiazepines have a high addiction potential when they are chronically used and are common drugs of abuse. *Benzodiazepine withdrawal syndrome* may include restlessness, agitation, anxiety, insomnia, tachycardia, tachypnea, diaphoresis, and may be potentially life-threatening depending on the benzodiazepine and the length of use. Symptoms of withdrawal from short-acting benzodiazepines, such as *alprazolam* (Xanax), *oxazepam*, *lorazepam* (Ativan), *triazolam* (Halcion), usually appear within 6-8 hours after the last dose and may continue 10-14 days. Symptoms of withdrawal from long-acting benzodiazepines, such as *diazepam* (Valium), *clonazepam* (Klonopin), *chlordiazepoxide* (Librium), usually appear within 24-96 hours after the last dose and may continue from 3-4 weeks to 3 months. People who are heavily dependent on benzodiazepines may experience *protracted withdrawal syndrome* (PAWS), random periods of sharp withdrawal symptoms months after quitting. A closely monitored medical detoxification regimen may be required for a safe withdrawal and to prevent PAWS. Detoxification includes gradual tapering of the benzodiazepine along with other medications to manage the withdrawal symptoms.

Short Acting

▷ *alprazolam* (D)(IV)(G)

Niravam <18 years: not recommended; ≥18 years: initially 0.25-0.5 mg tid; may titrate every 3-4 days; max 4 mg/day

Tab: 0.25*, 0.5*, 1*, 2*mg orally-disint

Xanax <18 years: not recommended; ≥18 years: initially 0.25-0.5 mg tid; may titrate every 3-4 days; max 4 mg/day

Tab: 0.25*, 0.5*, 1*, 2*mg

Xanax XR <18 years: not recommended; ≥18 years: initially 0.5-1 mg once daily, preferably in the AM; increase at intervals of at least 3-4 days by up to 1 mg/day. Taper no faster than 0.5 mg every 3 days; max 10 mg/day. When switching from immediate-release *alprazolam*, give total daily dose of immediate-release once daily.

Tab: 0.5, 1, 2, 3 mg ext-rel

▷ *oxazepam* (C)(IV)(G) <12 years: not recommended; ≥12 years: 10-15 mg tid-qid for moderate symptoms; 15-30 mg tid-qid for severe symptoms

Cap: 10, 15, 30 mg

Intermediate Acting

▷ *lorazepam* (D)(IV)(G) <12 years: not recommended; ≥12 years: 1-10 mg/day in 2-3 divided doses

Ativan *Tab:* 0.5, 1*, 2*mg

Lorazepam Intensol *Oral conc:* 2 mg/ml (30 ml w. graduated dropper)

Long Acting

▷ *chlordiazepoxide* (D)(IV)(G)

Librium <6 years: not recommended; 6-12 years: 5 mg bid-qid; increase to 10 mg bid-tid; ≥12 years: 5-10 mg tid-qid for moderate symptoms; 20-25 mg tid-qid for severe symptoms

Cap: 5, 10, 25 mg

Librium Injectable <12 years: not recommended; ≥12 years: 50-100 mg IM <u>or</u> IV; then 25-50 mg IM tid-qid prn; max 300 mg/day

Inj: 100 mg

▷ *chlordiazepoxide/clidinium* (D)(IV) <12 years: not recommended; ≥12 years: 1-2 caps tid-qid: max 8 caps/day

Librax *Cap: chlor* 5 mg/*clid* 2.5 mg

▷ *clonazepam* (D)(IV)(G) <18 years: not recommended; ≥18 years: initially 0.25 mg bid; increase to 1 mg/day after 3 days

Klonopin *Tab:* 0.5*, 1, 2 mg

Klonopin Wafers dissolve in mouth with <u>or</u> without water

Wafer: 0.125, 0.25, 0.5, 1, 2 mg orally-disint

▷ *clorazepate* (D)(IV)(G) <9 years: not recommended; ≥9 years: 30 mg/day in divided doses; max 60 mg/day

Tranxene *Tab:* 3.75, 7.5, 15 mg

Tranxene SD do not use for initial therapy

Tab: 22.5 mg ext-rel

Tranxene SD Half Strength do not use for initial therapy
  Tab: 11.25 mg ext-rel
Tranxene T-Tab *Tab:* 3.75*, 7.5*, 15*mg
▷ *diazepam* (D)(IV)(G) <12 years: not recommended; ≥12 years: 2-10 mg bid to qid
  Diastat *Rectal gel delivery system:* 2.5 mg
  Diastat AcuDial *Rectal gel delivery system:* 10, 20 mg
  Valium *Tab:* 2*, 5*, 10*mg
  Valium Injectable *Vial:* 5 mg/ml (10 ml); *Amp:* 5 mg/ml (2 ml); *Prefilled syringe:* 5 mg/ml (5 ml)
  Valium Intensol Oral Solution *Conc oral soln:* 5 mg/ml (30 ml w. dropper) (alcohol 19%)
  Valium Oral Solution *Oral soln:* 5 mg/5 ml (500 ml) (wintergreen spice)

TRICYCLIC ANTIDEPRESSANTS (TCAs)

Comment: Co-administration of SSRIs and TCAs requires extreme caution.
▷ *amitriptyline* (C)(G) <12 years: not recommended; ≥12 years: 10-20 mg q HS *Tab:* 10, 25, 50, 75, 100, 150 mg
▷ *amoxapine* (C) <12 years: not recommended; ≥12 years: initially 50 mg bid-tid; after 1 week may increase to 100 mg bid-tid; usual effective dose 200-300 mg/day; if total dose exceeds 300 mg/day, give in divided doses (max 400 mg/day); may give as a single bedtime dose (max 300 mg q HS)
  Tab: 25, 50, 100, 150 mg
▷ *clomipramine* (C)(G) <10 years: not recommended; 10-<16 years: initially 25 mg daily in divided doses; gradually increase; max 3 mg/kg or 100 mg, whichever is smaller; >16 years: initially 25 mg daily in divided doses; gradually increase to 100 mg during first 2 weeks; max 250 mg/day; total maintenance dose may be given at HS
  Anafranil *Cap:* 25, 50, 75 mg
▷ *desipramine* (C)(G) <12 years: not recommended; ≥12 years: 100-200 mg/day in single or divided doses; max 300 mg/day
  Norpramin *Tab:* 10, 25, 50, 75, 100, 150 mg
▷ *doxepin* (C)(G) <12 years: not recommended; ≥12 years: 75 mg/day; max 150 mg/day
  Cap: 10, 25, 50, 75, 100, 150 mg; Oral conc: 10 mg/ml (4 oz w. dropper)
▷ *imipramine* (C)(G) <12 years: not recommended; ≥12 years:
  Tofranil initially 75 mg daily (max 200 mg); adolescents initially 30-40 mg daily (max 100 mg/day); if maintenance dose exceeds 75 mg daily, may switch to **Tofranil PM** for divided or bedtime dose
  Tab: 10, 25, 50 mg
  Tofranil PM initially 75 mg daily 1 hour before HS; max 200 mg
  Cap: 75, 100, 125, 150 mg
▷ *nortriptyline* (D)(G) <12 years: not recommended; ≥12 years: initially 25 mg tid-qid; max 150 mg/day
  Pamelor *Cap:* 10, 25, 50, 75 mg; *Oral soln:* 10 mg/5 ml (16 oz)
▷ *protriptyline* (C) <12 years: not recommended; ≥12 years: initially 5 mg tid; usual dose 15-40 mg/day in 3-4 divided doses; max 60 mg/day
  Vivactil *Tab:* 5, 10 mg
▷ *trimipramine* (C) <12 years: not recommended; ≥12 years: initially 75 mg/day in divided doses; max 200 mg/day
  Surmontil *Cap:* 25, 50, 100 mg

PHENOTHIAZINES

▷ *prochlorperazine* (C)(G)

    Compazine <12 years: not recommended; ≥12 years: 5 mg tid-qid
        Tab: 5 mg; *Syr:* 5 mg/5 ml (4 oz) (fruit); *Rectal supp:* 2.5, 5, 25 mg
    Compazine Spansule <12 years: not recommended; ≥12 years: 15 mg q AM <u>or</u> 10 mg q 12 hours
        Spansule: 10, 15 mg sust-rel

▷ *trifluoperazine* (C)(G) <12 years: not recommended; ≥12 years: 1-2 mg bid; max 6 mg/day; max 12 weeks

    Stelazine *Tab:* 1, 2, 5, 10 mg

SELECTIVE SEROTONIN REUPTAKE INHIBITORS (SSRIs)

Comment: Co-administration of SSRIs with TCAs requires extreme caution. Concomitant use of MAOIs and SSRIs is absolutely contraindicated. Avoid St. John's wort and other serotonergic agents. A potentially fatal adverse event is *serotonin syndrome*, caused by serotonin excess. Milder symptoms require HCP intervention to avert severe symptoms that can be rapidly fatal without urgent/emergent medical care. Symptoms include restlessness, agitation, confusion, tachycardia, hypertension, dilated pupils, muscle twitching, muscle rigidity, loss of muscle coordination, diaphoresis, diarrhea, headache, shivering, piloerection, hyperpyrexia, cardiac arrhythmias, seizures, loss of consciousness, coma, death. Common symptoms of the *serotonin discontinuation syndrome* include flu-like symptoms (nausea, vomiting, diarrhea, headaches, diaphoresis); sleep disturbances (insomnia, nightmares, constant sleepiness); mood disturbances (dysphoria, anxiety, agitation); cognitive disturbances (mental confusion, hyperarousal); and sensory and movement disturbances (imbalance, tremors, vertigo, dizziness, electric-shock-like sensations in the brain often described by sufferers as "brain zaps").

▷ *citalopram* (C)(G) <12 years: not recommended; ≥12 years: initially 20 mg once daily; may increase after one week to 40 mg once daily; max 40 mg

    Celexa *Tab:* 10, 20, 40 mg; *Oral soln:* 10 mg/5 ml (120 ml) (pepper mint)(sugar-free, alcohol-free, parabens)

▷ *escitalopram* (C)(G) <12 years: not recommended; 12-17 years: initially 10 mg daily; may increase to 20 mg daily after 3 weeks; ≥17 years: initially 10 mg daily; may increase to 20 mg daily after 1 week; *Hepatic impairment:* 10 mg once daily

    Lexapro *Tab:* 5, 10*, 20*mg
    Lexapro Oral Solution *Oral soln:* 1 mg/ml (240 ml) (peppermint) (parabens)

▷ *fluoxetine* (C)(G)

    Prozac <8 years: not recommended; 8-17 years: initially 10 mg/day; may increase after 1 week to 20 mg/day; range 20-60 mg/day; range for lower weight children, 20-30 mg/day; ≥17 years: initially 20 mg daily; may increase after 1 week; doses >20 mg/day should be divided into AM and noon doses; max 80 mg/day
        Cap: 10, 20, 40 mg; *Tab:* 30*, 60*mg; *Oral soln:* 20 mg/5 ml (4 oz) (mint)
    Prozac Weekly <12 years: not recommended; ≥12 years: following daily *fluoxetine* therapy at 20 mg/day for 13 weeks, may initiate **Prozac Weekly** 7 days after the last 20 mg *fluoxetine* dose
        Cap: 90 mg ent-coat del-rel pellets

▷ *levomilnacipran* (C) <12 years: not recommended; ≥12 years: swallow whole; initially 20 mg once daily for 2 days; then increase to 40 mg once daily; may increase dose in 40 mg increments at intervals of ≥2 days; max 120 mg once daily; *CrCl 30-59 mL/min:* max 80 mg once daily; *CrCl 15-29 mL/min:* max 40 mg once daily
  Fetzima *Cap:* 20, 40, 80, 120 mg ext-rel
▷ *paroxetine maleate* (D)(G)
  Paxil <12 years: not recommended; ≥12 years: initially 20 mg daily in AM; may increase by 10 mg/day at weekly intervals as needed; max 60 mg/day
    Tab: 10*, 20*, 30, 40 mg
  Paxil CR <12 years: not recommended; ≥12 years: initially 25 mg daily in AM; may increase by 12.5 mg at weekly intervals as needed; max 62.5 mg/day
    Tab: 12.5, 25, 37.5 mg cont-rel ent-coat
  Paxil Suspension <12 years: not recommended; ≥12 years: initially 20 mg daily in AM; may increase by 10 mg/day at weekly intervals as needed; max 60 mg/day
    Oral susp: 10 mg/5 ml (250 ml) (orange)
▷ *sertraline* (C)(G) <6 years: not recommended; 6-<12 years: initially 25 mg daily; max 200 mg/day; 12-17 years: initially 50 mg daily; max 200 mg/day ≥17 years: initially 50 mg daily; increase at 1 week intervals if needed; max 200 mg daily; dilute oral concentrate immediately prior to administration in 4 oz water, ginger ale, lemon/lime soda, lemonade, <u>or</u> orange juice
  Zoloft *Tab:* 25*, 50*, 100*mg; *Oral conc:* 20 mg per ml (60 ml) (alcohol 12%)

SEROTONIN AND NOREPINEPHRINE REUPTAKE INHIBITORS (SNRIs)

▷ *desvenlafaxine* (C)(G) <18 years: not recommended; ≥18 years: swallow whole; initially 50 mg once daily; max 120 mg/day
  Pristiq *Tab:* 50, 100 mg ext-rel
▷ *duloxetine* (C)(G) <12 years: not recommended; ≥12 years: swallow whole; initially 30 mg once daily x 1 week; then, increase to 60 mg once daily; max 120 mg/day
  Cymbalta *Cap:* 20, 30, 40, 60 mg del-rel
▷ *venlafaxine* (C)(G)
  Effexor initially <12 years: not recommended; ≥12 years: 75 mg/day in 2-3 divided doses; may increase at 4 day intervals in 75 mg increments to 150 mg/day; max 225 mg/day
    Tab: 37.5, 75, 150, 225 mg
  Effexor XR <18 years: not recommended; ≥18 years: initially 75 mg q AM; may start at 37.5 mg daily x 4-7 days, then increase by increments of up to 75 mg/day at intervals of at least 4 days; usual max 375 mg/day
    Tab/Cap: 37.5, 75, 150 mg ext-rel
▷ *vortioxetine* (C) <18 years: not established; ≥18 years: initially 10 mg once daily; max 30 mg/day
  Brintellix *Tab:* 5, 10, 15, 20 mg

COMBINATION AGENTS

▷ *chlordiazepoxide/amitriptyline* (D)(G)
  Limbitrol <12 years: not recommended; ≥12 years: 3-4 tabs/day in divided doses
    Tab: chlor 5 mg/*amit* 12.5 mg
  Limbitrol DS <12 years: not recommended; ≥12 years: 3-4 tabs/day in divided doses; max 6 tabs/day

Tab: chlor 10 mg/*amit* 25 mg
▷ *perphenazine/amitriptyline* **(C)(G)** <12 years: not recommended; ≥12 years: 1 tab bid-qid
Tab: **Etrafon 2-10:** *perph* 2 mg/*amit* 10 mg
Etrafon 2-25: *perph* 2 mg/*amit* 25 mg
Etrafon 4-25: *perph* 4 mg/*amit* 25 mg

APHTHOUS STOMATITIS (MOUTH ULCER, CANKER SORE)

ANTI-INFLAMMATORY AGENTS

▷ *dexamethasone* elixir **(B)** <12 years: not recommended; ≥12 years: 5 ml swish and spit q 12 hours
Elix: 0.5 mg/ml
▷ *triamcinolone acetonide* 0.1% dental paste **(NE)(G)** press (do not rub) thin film onto lesion at bedtime and, if needed, 2-3 x daily after meals; re-evaluate if no improvement in 7 days
Oralone *Dental paste:* 0.1% (5 gm)
▷ *triamcinolone* 1% in **Orabase (B)** <12 years: not recommended; ≥12 years: apply 1/4 inch to each ulcer bid-qid until ulcer heals
Kenalog in Orabase *Crm:* 1% (15, 60, 80 gm)

TOPICAL ANESTHETICS

▷ *benzocaine* topical gel **(C)(G)** apply tid-qid
▷ *benzocaine* topical spray **(C)(G)** 1 spray area every 2 hours as needed; retain for 15 seconds, then spit
Cepacol Spray (OTC), Chloraseptic Spray (OTC)
▷ *lidocaine* viscous soln **(B)(G)** <3-11 years: 1.25 ml; apply with cotton-tipped applicator; may repeat after 3 hours; max 8 doses/day; ≥12 years: 15 ml gargle <u>or</u> swish, then spit; repeat after 3 hours; max 8 doses/day
Xylocaine Viscous Solution *Viscous soln:* 2% (20, 100, 450 ml)
▷ *triamcinolone* **(Kenalog)** in **Orabase (C)** apply tid-qid

DEBRIDING AGENT/CLEANSER

▷ *carbamide peroxide 10%* **(NE)(OTC)** apply 10 drops to affected area; swish x 2-3 minutes, then spit; do not rinse; repeat treatment qid
Gly-Oxide *Liq:* 10% (50, 60 ml squeeze bottle w. applicator)

ANTI-INFECTIVES

▷ *minocycline* **(D)(G)** <8 years: not recommended; ≥8 years: swish and spit 10 ml susp (50 mg/5 ml) <u>or</u> 1 x 100 mg cap <u>or</u> 2 x 50 mg caps dissolved in 180 ml water, bid x 4-5 days
Dynacin *Cap:* 50, 100 mg
Minocin *Cap:* 50, 75, 100 mg; *Oral susp:* 50 mg/5 ml (60 ml) (custard) (sulfites, alcohol 5%)

Comment: *minocycline* is contraindicated <8 years-of-age, in pregnancy, and lactation (discolors developing tooth enamel). A side effect may be photo-sensitivity (photophobia). Do not give with antacids, calcium supplements, milk <u>or</u> other dairy, <u>or</u> within two hours of taking another drug.

▷ *tetracycline* (D)(G) <8 years: not recommended; ≥8 years: swish and spit 10 ml susp (125 mg/5 ml) <u>or</u> one 250 mg tab/cap dissolved in 180 ml water qid x 4-5 days

Achromycin V *Cap:* 250, 500 mg

Sumycin *Tab:* 250, 500 mg; *Cap:* 250, 500 mg; *Oral susp:* 125 mg/5 ml (100, 200 ml) (fruit) (sulfites)

Comment: *tetracycline* is contraindicated <8 years-of-age, in pregnancy, and lactation (discolors developing tooth enamel). A side effect may be photo-sensitivity (photophobia). Do not give with antacids, calcium supplements, milk <u>or</u> other dairy, <u>or</u> within two hours of taking another drug.

ASPERGILLOSIS (*SCEDOSPORIUM APIOSPERMUM, FUSARIUM* SPP.)

INVASIVE INFECTION

▷ *isavuconazonium* (C) <18 years: not established; ≥18 years: swallow cap whole; *Loading dose:* 372 mg q 8 hours x 6 doses (48 hours); *Maintenance:* 372 mg once daily starting 12-24 hours after last loading dose

Cresemba *Cap:* 186 mg; Vial: 372 mg pwdr for reconstitution (7/blister pck) (preservative-free)

Comment: **Cresemba** is indicated for the treatment of invasive aspergillus and mucormycosis in patients ≥18 years old who are at high risk to being severely compromised.

▷ *posaconazole* (D) <13 years: not recommended; ≥13 years: take with food; swallow tab whole; *Day 1:* 300 mg bid; then 300 mg once daily for duration of treatment (e.g., resolution of neutropenia <u>or</u> immunosuppression)

Noxafil *Tab:* 100 mg del-rel; *Oral susp:* 40 mg/ml (105 oz w. dosing spoon) (cherry)

Comment: **Noxafil** is indicated as prophylaxis for invasive aspergillus and candida infections in patients ≥13 years old who are at high risk due to being severely compromised.

▷ *voriconazole* (D)(G) <12 years: not recommended; ≥12 years: *PO:* <40 kg: 100 mg q 12 hours; may increase to 150 mg q 12 hours if inadequate response; ≥40 kg: 200 mg q 12 hours; may increase to 300 mg q 12 hours if inadequate; *IV:* 6 mg/kg q 12 hours x 2 doses; then 4 mg/kg q 12 hour; max rate 3 mg/kg/hour over 1-2 hours; response

Vfend *Tab:* 50, 200 mg

Vfend I.V. for Injection *Vial:* 200 mg pwdr for reconstitution (preservative-free)

Vfend *Oral susp:* 40 mg/ml pwdr for reconstitution (75 ml)(orange)

ASTHMA

Parenteral Corticosteroids *see page* 499
Oral Corticosteroids *see page* 498

LEUKOTRIENE RECEPTOR ANTAGONISTS (LRAs)

Comment: The LRAs are indicated for prophylaxis and chronic treatment, only. Not for primary (rescue) treatment of acute asthma attack.

➤ *montelukast* (B)(G) <12 months: not recommended; 12-23 months: one 4 mg granule pkt daily; 2-5 years: one 4 mg chew tab or granule pkt daily; >5-14 years: one 5 mg chew tab daily; >14 years: 10 mg once daily in the PM; for EIB, take at least 2 hours before exercise; max 1 dose/day

Singulair *Tab:* 10 mg

Singulair Chewable *Chew tab:* 4, 5 mg (cherry) (phenylalanine)

Singulair Oral Granules *Granules:* 4 mg/pkt; take within 15 minutes of opening pkt; may mix with applesauce, carrots, rice, or ice cream

➤ *zafirlukast* (B) <7 years: not recommended; 7-11 years: 10 mg bid 1 hour ac or 2 hours pc; >11 years: 20 mg bid, 1 hour ac or 2 hours pc

Accolate *Tab:* 10, 20 mg

➤ *zileuton* (C)(G) <12 years: not recommended; ≥12 years:

Zyflo 600 mg qid

Tab: 600 mg

Zyflo CR 1200 mg bid

Tab: 600 mg ext-rel

IGE BLOCKER (IGG1K MONOCLONAL ANTIBODY)

➤ *omalizumab* (B) <12 years: not recommended; ≥12 years: 150-375 mg SC every 2-4 weeks based on body weight and pretreatment serum total IgE level; max 150 mg/injection site; 30-90 kg + IgE >30-100 IU/ml 150 mg q 4 weeks; 90-150 kg + IgE >30-100 IU/ml or 30-90 kg + IgE >100-200 IU/ml or 30-60 kg + IgE >200-300 IU/ml 300 mg q 4 hours; >90-150 kg + IgE >100-200 IU/ml or >60-90 kg + IgE >200-300 IU/ml or 30-70 kg + IgE >300-400 IU/ml 225 mg q 2 weeks; >90-150 kg + IgE >200-300 IU/ml or >70-90 kg + IgE >300-400 IU/ml or 30-70 kg + IgE >400-500 IU/ml or 30-60 kg + IgE >500-600 IU/ml or 30-60 kg + IgE >600-700 IU/ml 375 mg q 2 weeks

Xolair *Vial:* 150 mg pwdr for SC injection after reconstitution (preservative-free)

INHALED ANTICHOLINERGICS

➤ *ipratropium bromide* (C)(G) <12 years: not established; ≥12 years:

Atrovent 2 inhalations qid; additional inhalations as required; max 12 inhalations/day

Inhaler: 18 mcg/actuation (14 g, 200 inh)

Atrovent Inhalation Solution 500 mcg tid-qid prn by nebulizer

Inhal soln: 0.02% (500 mcg in 2.5 ml; 25/carton)

Comment: *ipratropium bromide* is contraindicated with severe hypersensitivity to milk proteins.

INHALED CORTICOSTEROIDS

Comment: *Instruct patient to rinse mouth after using an inhaled steroid to reduce risk of oral candidiasis. Not for primary (rescue) treatment of acute asthma attack.*

▷ *beclomethasone dipropionate* (C)(G) <12 years: not established; ≥12 years:
Previously using only bronchodilators: initiate 40-80 mcg bid; max 320 mcg bid;
Previously using inhaled corticosteroid: initiate 40-160 mcg bid; max 320 mcg/day;
Previously taking a systemic corticosteroid: attempt to wean off the systemic drug
after approximately 1 week after initiating; rinse mouth after use
> **Quark**
>> *Inhal aerosol:* 40, 80 mcg/metered dose actuation (8.7 g, 120 inh) metered
>> dose inhaler (chlorofluorocarbon [CFC]-free)

▷ *budesonide* (B)
> **Pulmicort Flexhaler** <6 years: not recommended; 6-12 years: 1-2 inhalations bid;
> >12 years: initially 180-360 mcg bid; max 360 mcg bid; rinse mouth after use
>> *Flexhaler:* 90 mcg/actuation (60 inh); 180 mcg/actuation (120 inh)
> **Pulmicort Respules** (G) <12 months: not recommended; 12 months-8 years:
> *Previously using only bronchodilators:* initiate 0.5 mg/day once daily or in 2
> divided doses; may start at 0.25 mg daily; *Previously using inhaled corticoste-
> roids:* initiate 0.5 mg once daily or in 2 divided doses; max 1 mg/day; *Previously
> taking oral corticosteroids:* initiate 1 mg/day daily or in 2 divided doses; >8-12
> years: use flexhaler; rinse mouth after use; >12 years: use **Pulmicort Flexhaler**
>> *Inhal susp:* 0.25, 0.5, 1 mg/2 ml (30/carton)

▷ *ciclesonide* (C) <12 years: not recommended; ≥12 years: initially 80 mcg bid; max
320 mcg/day; rinse mouth after use; *Previously on inhaled corticosteroid:* initially 80
mcg bid; *Previously on oral steroid:* 320 mg bid
> **Alvesco** *Inhal aerosol:* 80, 160 mcg/actuation (6.1 g, 60 inh)

▷ *flunisolide* (C)
> **AeroBid, AeroBid-M** <6 years: not recommended; 6-15 years: 2 inhalations bid;
> >15 years: initially 2 inhalations bid; max 8 inhalations/day; rinse mouth after
> use
>> *Inhaler:* 250 mcg/actuation (7 g, 100 inh)
> **Aerospan HFA** <6 years: not recommended; 6-11 years: 80 mcg bid; max
> 160 mcg bid; >11 years: initially 160 mcg bid; max 320 mcg bid
>> *Inhaler:* 80 mcg (5.1 g, 60 doses; 80 mcg, 120 doses)

▷ *fluticasone furoate* (C) <12 years: not recommended; ≥12 years: *Currently not on
inhaled corticosteroid:* usually initiate at 100 mcg once daily at the same time each
day; may increase to 200 mcg once daily if inadequate response after 2 weeks; max
200 mcg/day; rinse mouth after use
> **Arnuity Ellipta** *Inhal:* 100, 200 mcg/dry pwdr per inhalation (30 doses)
> Comment: **Arnuity Ellipta** is not for primary treatment of status asthmaticus
> or acute asthma episodes. **Arnuity Ellipta** is contraindicated with severe
> hypersensitivity to milk proteins.

▷ *fluticasone propionate* (C)
> **Flovent HFA** <11 years: use **Flovent Diskus**; ≥12 years: initially 88 mcg bid; (C)
> *Previously using an inhaled corticosteroid:* initially 88-220 mcg bid; *Previously
> taking an oral corticosteroid:* 880 mcg bid; rinse mouth after use
>> *Inhaler:* 44 mcg/actuation (7.9 g, 60 inh; 13 g, 120 inh); 110 mcg/actuation
>> (13 g, 120 inh); 220 mcg/actuation (13 g, 120 inh) (CFC-free)
> **Flovent Diskus** <4 years: not recommended; 4-11 years: initially 50 mcg bid;
> max 100 mcg bid; rinse mouth after use; ≥11 years: may use **Flovent HFA**;
> initially 100 mcg bid; max 500 mcg bid; *Previously using an inhaled cortico-
> steroid:* initially 100-250 mcg bid; max 500 mcg bid; *Previously taking an oral
> corticosteroid:* 1000 mcg bid

Diskus: 50, 100, 250 mcg/inh dry pwdr (60 blisters w. diskus)
▷ *mometasone furoate* (C)
    Asmanex HFA <12 years: not recommended; ≥12 years: 220-440 mcg once daily <u>or</u> bid; max 880 mcg/day; rinse mouth after use
    Inhaler: 100, 200 mcg/actuation (13 g, 120 inh)
    Asmanex Twisthaler <4 years: not recommended; 4-11 years: 110 mcg once daily in the PM; ≥12 years: may use **Asmanex HFA**; rinse mouth after use
    Inhaler: 110 mcg/actuation (30 inh), 220 mcg/actuation (30, 60, 120 inh)
▷ *triamcinolone* (C)
    Azmacort <6 years: not recommended; 6-12 years: 1-2 inhalations tid <u>or</u> 2-4 inhalations bid; >12 years: 2 inhalations tid-qid <u>or</u> 4 inhalations bid; rinse mouth after use
    Inhaler: 100 mcg/actuation (20 g, 240 inh)

INHALED MAST CELL STABILIZERS (PROPHYLAXIS)

Comment: IMCSs are for prophylaxis and chronic treatment, only. Not for primary (rescue) treatment of acute asthma attack.
▷ *cromolyn sodium* (B)(G)
    Intal <2 years: not recommended; 2-5 years: use inhal soln via nebulizer; >5 years: 2 inhalations qid via inhaler
    Inhaler: 0.8 mg/actuation (8.1, 14.2 g; 112, 200 inh) 2 inhalations qid; 2 inhalations up to 10-60 minutes before precipitant as prophylaxis; rinse mouth after use
    Intal Inhalation Solution <2 years: not recommended; ≥2 years: 20 mg by nebulizer qid; 20 mg up to 10-60 minutes before precipitant as prophylaxis
    Inhal soln: 20 mg/2 ml (60, 120/carton)
▷ *nedocromil sodium* (B)
    Tilade <6 years: not recommended; ≥6 years: 2 sprays qid; rinse mouth after use
    Inhaler: 1.75 mg/spray (16.2 g; 104 sprays)
    Tilade Nebulizer Solution 0.5% <2 years: not recommended; ≥2 years: initially 1 amp qid by nebulizer; 2-5 years: initially 1 amp tid by nebulizer; ≥5 years: 1 amp qid by nebulizer
    Inhal soln: 11 mg/2.2 ml (2 ml; 60, 120/carton)

INHALED BETA AGONISTS (BRONCHODILATORS)

▷ *albuterol sulfate* (C)(G)
    AccuNeb Inhalation Solution <2 years: not recommended; 2-12 years: initially 0.63 mg <u>or</u> 1.25 mg tid-qid; 6-12 years: *Severe asthma <u>or</u> >40 kg <u>or</u> 11-12 years:* initially 1.25 mg tid-qid by nebulizer; >12 years: not recommended
    Inhal soln: 0.63, 1.25 mg/3 ml (3 ml, 25/carton) (preservative-free)
    Albuterol Inhalation Solution (G) <2 years: not recommended; ≥2 years: 1 vial via nebulizer q 4-6 hours prn
    Inhal soln: 0.63 mg/3 ml (0.021%); 1.25 mg/3 ml (0.042%) (25/carton)
    Albuterol Inhalation Solution 0.5% (G) <4 years: not recommended; ≥4 years: 1 vial via nebulizer q 4-6 hours prn
    Inhal soln: 0.083% (25/carton)
    Albuterol Nebules (G) <12 years: use other forms; ≥12 years: 2.5 mg (0.5 ml of 5% diluted to 3 ml with sterile NS <u>or</u> 3 ml of 0.083%) tid-qid via nebulizer

Inhal soln: 0.083% (25/carton)

Proair HFA Inhaler <4 years: not established; ≥4 years: 1-2 inhalations q 4-6 hours prn; 2 inhalations 15 minutes before exercise as prophylaxis for exercise-induced asthma (EIA)

Inhaler: 90 mcg/actuation (0.65 g, 200 inh) (CFC-free)

Proair RespiClick <12 years: not established; ≥12 years: 1-2 inhalations q 4-6 hours prn; 2 inhalations 15-30 minutes before exercise as prophylaxis for exercise-induced asthma (EIA)

Inhaler: 90 mcg/actuation (8.5 g, 200 inh)

Proventil HFA Inhaler <4 years: use syrup; ≥4 years: 1-2 inhalations q 4-6 hours prn; 2 inhalations 15 minutes before exercise as prophylaxis for exercise-induced asthma (EIA)

Inhaler: 90 mcg/actuation with a dose counter (6.7 g, 200 inh)

Proventil Inhalation Solution <12 years: use syrup; ≥12 years: 2.5 mg diluted to 3 ml with normal saline tid-qid prn by nebulizer

Inhal soln: 0.5% (20 ml w. dropper); 0.083% (3 ml; 25/carton)

Ventolin Inhaler <2 years: not recommended; 2-4 years: use syrup; >4 years: 2 inhalations q 4-6 hours prn; 2 inhalations 15 minutes before exercise as prophylaxis for exercise-induced asthma

Inhaler: 90 mcg/actuation (17 g, 220 inh)

Ventolin Rotacaps <4 years: not recommended; ≥4 years 1-2 caps q 4-6 hours prn; 2 inhalations 15 minutes before exercise as prophylaxis for exercise-induced asthma (EIA)

Rotacaps: 200 mcg/Rotacaps (100 doses/Rotacaps)

Ventolin 0.5% Inhalation Solution <2 years: not recommended; ≥2 years: initially 0.1-0.15 mg/kg/dose tid-qid prn; 10-15 kg: 0.25 ml diluted to 3 ml with normal saline by nebulizer tid-qid prn; >15 kg: 0.5 ml diluted to 3 ml with normal saline by nebulizer tid-qid prn

Inhal soln: 20 ml w. dropper

Ventolin Nebules <2 years: not recommended; ≥2 years: initially 0.1-0.15 mg/kg/dose tid-qid prn; 10-15 kg: 1.25 mg <u>or</u> 1/2 nebule tid-qid prn; >15 kg: 2.5 mg <u>or</u> 1 nebule tid-qid prn

Inhal soln: 0.083% (3 ml; 25/carton)

➤ *isoproterenol* (B) <12 years: not recommended; ≥12 years: *Rescue:* 1 inhalation prn; repeat if no relief in 2-5 minutes; *Maintenance:* 1-2 inhalations q 4-6 hours

Medihaler-ISO *Inhaler:* 80 mcg/actuation (15 ml, 30 inh)

➤ *levalbuterol* (C)(G) <12 years: not recommended; ≥12 years: initially 0.63 mg tid q 6-8 hours prn by nebulizer; may increase to 1.25 mg tid at 6-8 hour intervals as needed

Xopenex *Inhal soln:* 0.31, 0.63, 1.25 mg/3 ml (24/carton) (preservative-free)

Xopenex HFA *Inh:* 45 mg (15 g, 200 inh) (preservative-free)

Xopenex Concentrate *Vial:* 1.25 mg/0.5 ml (30/carton) (preservative-free)

➤ *metaproterenol* (C)(G)

Alupent <6 years: use syrup; 6-12 years: via nebulizer 0.1-0.2 ml diluted with normal saline to 3 ml, up to q 4 hours prn; >12 years: 2-3 inhalations tid-qid prn; max 12 inhalations/day

Inhaler: 0.65 mg/actuation (14 g, 200 doses)

Alupent Inhalation Solution <6 years: use syrup 6-12 years: via nebulizer 0.1-0.2 ml diluted with normal saline to 3 ml, up to q 4 hours prn; >12 years: 5-15 inhalations tid-qid prn <u>or</u> q 4 hours prn for acute attack

Inhal soln: 5% (10, 30 ml w. dropper)
➤ *pirbuterol* (C) <12 years: not recommended; ≥12 years: 1-2 inhalations q 4-6 hours prn; max 12 inhalations/day
    Maxair *Autohaler:* 200 mcg/actuation (14 g, 400 inh); *Inhaler:* 200 mcg/actuation (25.6 g, 300 inh)
➤ *terbutaline* (B) <12 years: not recommended; ≥12 years: 2 inhalations q 4-6 hours prn
    Inhaler: 0.2 mg/actuation (10.5 g, 300 inh)

INHALED RACEPINEPHRINE (BRONCHODILATOR)

➤ *racepinephrine* (C)(OTC)(G) <4 years: not recommended; ≥4 years: 1-3 inhalations not more than every 3 hours; max 12 inhalations/24 hours
    Asthmanefrin Inhaler *Starter kit:* 10 x 0.5 ml vials 2.25% solution for atomized inhalation w. EZ Breathe Atomizer; *Refills:* 30 x 0.5 ml vials 2.25% solution for atomized inhalation
Comment: Inhalational epinephrine is only recommended for use during pregnancy when there are no alternatives and benefit outweighs risk.

INHALED LONG-ACTING ANTICHOLINERGIC

➤ *tiotropium (as bromide monohydrate)* (C) <12 years: not recommended; ≥12 years: 2 inhalations once daily using inhalation device; do not swallow caps
    Spiriva HandiHaler *Inhal device:* 18 mcg/cap pwdr for inhalation (5, 30, 90 caps w. inhalation device)
    Spiriva Respimat *Inhal device:* 1.25, 2.5 mcg/actuation cartridge w. inhalation device (4 g, 60 metered actuations) (benzalkonium chloride)
Comment: *tiotropium* is for prophylaxis and chronic treatment, only. Not for primary (rescue) treatment of acute attack. Avoid getting powder in eyes. Caution with narrow-angle glaucoma, BPH, bladder neck obstruction, and pregnancy. Contraindicated with allergy to *atropine* or its derivatives (e.g., *ipratropium*).

INHALED ANTICHOLINERGIC/BETA AGONIST

➤ *ipratropium bromide/albuterol sulfate* (C)
    Combivent <12 years: not recommended; ≥12 years: 2 inhalations qid; additional inhalations as required; max 12 inhalations/day
    Inhaler: ipra 18 mcg/*albu* 90 mcg/actuation (14.7 g, 200 inh)
    Duoneb <18 years: not recommended; ≥18 years: 1 vial via nebulizer 4-6 times daily prn
    Inhal soln: ipra 0.5 mg (0.017%)/*albu* 2.5 mg (0.083%) per 3 ml (23/carton)
➤ *olodaterol* (C)
    Striverdi Respimat <12 years: not established; ≥12 years: 12 mcg q 12 hours
    Inhal soln: 2.5 mcg/cartridge (metered actuation) (40 g, 60 metered actuations) (benzalkonium chloride)
    Comment: Striverdi Respimat is contraindicated in persons with asthma without use of long-term control medication.
➤ *salmeterol* (C)(G) <4 years: not recommended; 4-12 years: 1 inhalation q 12 hours prn; 1 inhalation at least 30-60 minutes before exercise as prophylaxis for exercise-induced asthma; do not use extra doses for exercise-induced bronchospasm if

already using regular dose; >12 years: 2 inhalations q 12 hours prn; 2 inhalations at least 30-60 minutes before exercise as prophylaxis for exercise-induced asthma; do not use extra doses for exercise-induced bronchospasm if already using regular dose
Serevent Diskus
Diskus (pwdr): 50 mcg/actuation (60 doses/disk)

CORTICOSTEROID/INHALED LONG-ACTING BETA AGONIST (LABA)

▷ *budesonide/formoterol* (C) <12 years: not recommended; ≥12 years: 1 inhalation bid; rinse mouth after use
    Symbicort 80/4.5 *Inhaler: bud* 80 mcg/*for* 4.5 mcg
    Symbicort 160/4.5 *Inhaler: bud* 160 mcg/*for* 4.5 mcg

▷ *fluticasone propionate/salmeterol* (C)
    Advair HFA *Not previously using inhaled steroid:* start with 2 inh 45/21 <u>or</u> 115/21 bid; if insufficient response after 2 weeks, use next higher strength; max 2 inh 230/50 bid; allow 12 hours between doses; *Already using inhaled steroid;* see mfr pkg insert; rinse mouth after use
    Advair HFA 45/21 <12 years: not recommended
      Inhaler: flu pro 45 mcg/*sal* 21 mcg/actuation (CFC-free)
    Advair HFA 115/21 <12 years: not recommended
      Inhaler: flu pro 115 mcg/*sal* 21 mcg/actuation (CFC-free)
    Advair HFA 230/21 <12 years: not recommended
      Inhaler: flu pro 230 mcg/*sal* 21 mcg/actuation (CFC-free)
    Advair Diskus *Not previously using inhaled steroid:* start with 1 inh 100/50 bid; *Already using inhaled steroid:* see mfr pkg insert; rinse mouth after use
    Advair Diskus 100/50 <4 years: not recommended; ≥4 years: 1 inhalation bid; not a rescue inhaler; allow 12 hours between doses
      Diskus: flu pro 100 mcg/*sal* 50 mcg/actuation (60 blisters)
    Advair Diskus 250/50 4-12 years: use 100/50 strength; >12 years: 1 inhalation bid; rinse mouth after use; not a rescue inhaler; allow 12 hours between doses
      Diskus: flu pro 250 mcg/*sal* 50 mcg/actuation (60 blisters)
    Advair Diskus 500/50 4-12 years: use 100/50 strength; ≥12 years: 1 inhalation bid; rinse mouth after use; not a rescue inhaler; allow 12 hours between doses
      Diskus: flupro 500 mcg/*sal* 50 mcg/actuation (60 blisters)

▷ *fluticasone furoate/vilanterol* (C) <17 years: not established; ≥17 years: 1 inhalation 100/25 once daily at the same time each day
    Breo Ellipta 100/25 *Inhal pwdr: flu* 100 mcg/*vil* 25 mcg dry pwdr per inhal (30 doses)
    Breo Ellipta 200/25 *Inhal pwdr: flu* 200 mcg/*vil* 25 mcg dry pwdr per inhal (30 doses)
    Comment: Breo Ellipta is contraindicated with severe hypersensitivity to milk proteins.

▷ *mometasone furoate/formoterol fumarate* (C) <12 years: not established; ≥12 years: 2 inhalations bid; not a rescue inhaler; rinse mouth after use;
    Dulera 100/5 *Inhaler: mom* 100 mcg/*for* 5 mcg (HFA)
    Dulera 200/5 *Inhaler: mom* 200 mcg/*for* 5 mcg (HFA)

ANTICHOLINERGIC/INHALED LONG-ACTING BETA AGONIST (LABA)

▷ *glycopyrrolate/formoterol fumarate* (C) ≥18 years: not established: >18 years: 2 inhalations bid (AM & PM)

Bevespi Aerosphere *Metered dose inhaler:* **9/4.8** *Inhal pwdr: gly 9 mcg/for 4.8 mcg per inhal* (10.7 g, 120 inh)

ORAL BETA2-AGONISTS (BRONCHODILATORS)

▷ *albuterol* (C)

Albuterol Syrup (G) <2 years: not recommended; 2-6 years: 0.1 mg/kg tid; initially max 2 mg tid; may increase gradually to 0.2 mg/kg tid; max 4 mg tid; >6-12 years: 2 mg tid-qid; may increase gradually; max 6 mg qid; ≥12 years: 2-4 mg tid-qid; may increase gradually; max 8 mg qid

Syr: 2 mg/5 ml

Proventil <6 years: use syrup; ≥6 years: 2-4 mg tid-qid prn

Tab: 2, 4 mg

Proventil Repetabs 4-8 mg q 12 hours prn

Repetab: 4 mg sust-rel

Proventil Syrup <2 years: not recommended; 2-6 years: 0.1 mg/kg tid prn; max initially 5 ml tid prn; may increase gradually to 0.2 mg/kg tid prn; max 10 ml tid; >6-14 years: 5 ml tid-qid prn; may increase gradually; max 60 ml/day in divided doses; >14 years: 5-10 ml tid-qid prn; may increase gradually; max 20 ml qid prn

Syr: 2 mg/5 ml

Ventolin <2 years: not recommended; 2-6 years: 0.1 mg/kg tid prn; max initially 2 mg tid prn; may increase gradually to 0.2 mg/kg tid; max 4 mg tid; >6-14 years: 2 mg tid-qid prn; may increase gradually; max 6 mg tid; >14 years: 2-4 mg tid-qid prn; may increase gradually; max 8 mg qid

Tab: 2, 4 mg; *Syr:* 2 mg/5 ml (strawberry)

VoSpire ER <6 years: not recommended; 6-12 years: 4 mg q 12 hours; max 24 mg/day q 12 hours; >12 years: 4-8 mg q 12 hours prn; max 32 mg/day divided q 12 hours; swallow whole

Tab: 4, 8 mg ext-rel

▷ *metaproterenol* (C)

Alupent <6 years: not recommended (doses of 1.3-2.6 mg/kg/day have been used); ≥6-9 years (<60 lb): 10 mg tid-qid prn; >9-12 years (>60 lb): 20 mg tid-qid prn; >12 years: 20 mg tid-qid prn

Tab: 10, 20 mg; *Syr:* 10 mg/5 ml

METHYLXANTHINES

Comment: Check serum theophylline level just before 5th dose is administered. Therapeutic theophylline level: 10-20 mcg/ml.

▷ *theophylline* (C)(G)

Theo-24 <45 kg: initially 12-14 mg/kg/day; max 300 mg/day; increase after 3 days to 16 mg/kg/day to max 400 mg; after 3 more days increase to 30 mg/kg/day to max 600 mg/day; ≥45 kg: initially 300-400 mg once daily at HS; after 3 days, increase to 400-600 mg once daily at HS; max 600 mg/day

Cap: 100, 200, 300, 400 mg ext-rel

Theo-Dur <6 years: not recommended; 6-15 years: initially 12-14 mg/kg/day in 2 divided doses; max 300 mg/day; then increase to 16 mg/kg in 2 divided doses; max 400 mg/day; then to 20 mg/kg/day in 2 divided doses; max 600 mg/day; ≥15 years: initially 150 mg bid; increase to 200 mg bid after 3 days; then to 300 mg bid after 3 more days

      Tab: 100, 200, 300 ext-rel
    Theolair-SR <12 years: not recommended; ≥12 years: 200-500 once daily
      Tab: 200, 250, 300, 500 sust-rel
    Uniphyl <12 years: not recommended; ≥12 years: 400-600 mg once daily
      Tab: 400*, 600* mg cont-rel

METHYLXANTHINE/EXPECTORANT

▷ *dyphylline/guaifenesin* (C) <12 years: not recommended; ≥12 years: 1 tab qid
    Lufyllin GG *Tab: dyphy* 200 mg/*guaif* 200 mg; *Elix: dyphy* 100 mg/*guaif* 100 mg
    per 15 ml

HUMANIZED INTERLEUKIN-5 ANTAGONIST MONOCLONAL ANTIBODY

▷ *mepolizumab* (NE) <12 years: not recommended; ≥12 years: 100 mg SC once every
    4 weeks in upper arm, abdomen, or thigh
    Nucala *Vial:* 100 mg pwdr for reconstitution, single use (preservative-free)
    Comment: **Nucala** is an add-on maintenance treatment for severe asthma. There
    is a pregnancy exposure registry that monitors pregnancy outcomes in females
    exposed to **Nucala** during pregnancy. Health care providers can enroll patients
    or encourage patients to enroll themselves by calling 1-877-311-8972 or visiting
    www.mothertobaby.org/asthma.

ATTENTION DEFICIT HYPERACTIVITY DISORDER (ADHD)

SELECTIVE NOREPINEPHRINE REUPTAKE INHIBITOR (SNRI)

▷ *atomoxetine* (C) <6 years: not recommended; ≥6 years, <70 kg: initially 0.5 mg/kg/
    day: increase after at least 3 days to 1.2 mg/kg/day; max 1.4 mg/kg/day or 100 mg/
    day (whichever is less); ≥6 years, >70 kg: take one dose daily in the morning or in
    two divided doses in the morning and late afternoon or early evening; initially 40
    mg/kg; increase after at least 3 days to 80 mg/kg; then after 2-4 weeks may increase
    to max 100 mg/day
    Strattera *Cap:* 10, 18, 25, 40, 60, 80, 100 mg
Comment: *atomoxetine* is not associated with stimulant or euphoric effects. May
discontinue without tapering.

STIMULANTS

▷ *amphetamine sulfate* (C)(II)
    Adzenys XT-ODT <6 years: not recommended; ≥6 years: take with or without
    food; individualize the dosage according to the therapeutic needs and response;
    initially 6.3 mg once daily in the morning; increase in increments of 3.1 mg or
    6.3 mg at weekly intervals; max recommended dose 18.8 mg once daily (6-12
    years-of-age) and 12.5 mg once daily (≥13 years-of-age)
    Comment: Patients taking **Adderall XR** may be switched to **Adzenys XR-ODT**
    at the equivalent dose taken once daily; switching from any other amphetamine
    products (e.g., **Adderall** immediate-release), discontinue that treatment, and

titrate with **Adzenys XR-ODT** using the titration schedule (see mfr pkg insert). No dosage adjustments for renal or hepatic insufficiency are provided in the manufacturer's labeling.

ODT: 3.1, 6.3, 9.4, 12.5, 15.7, 18.8 mg orally-disint (orange) (fructose)

Dyanavel XR Oral Suspension <6 years: not recommended; ≥6 years: initially 2.5 mg or 5 mg once daily in the morning; may increase in increments of 2.5 mg to 5 mg per day every 4-7 days; max 20 mg per day; shake bottle prior to administration

Oral susp: 2.5 mg/ml (464 ml)

Evekeo <3 years: not recommended; ≥3-5 years: initially 2.5 mg once or twice daily at the same time(s) each day; may increase by 2.5 mg/day at weekly intervals; max 40 mg/day; >5 years: initially 5 mg once or twice daily at the same time(s) each day; may increase by 5 mg/day at weekly intervals; max 40 mg/day

Tab: 5, 10 mg

▷ *dextroamphetamine sulfate* (C)(II)(G) <3 years: not recommended; ≥3-5 years: 2.5 mg daily; may increase by 2.5 mg daily at weekly intervals if needed; >5-12 years: initially 5 mg daily or bid; may increase by 5 mg/day at weekly intervals; usual max 40 mg/day; >12 years: initially 10 mg daily; may increase by 10 mg/day at weekly intervals; max 40 mg/day; may switch to daily dose with sust-rel spansules when titrated

Dexedrine *Tab:* 5*mg (tartrazine)

Dexedrine Spansule *Cap:* 5, 10, 15 mg ext-rel

Dextrostat *Tab:* 5, 10 mg (tartrazine)

▷ *dextroamphetamine saccharate/dextroamphetamine sulfate/amphetamine aspartate/ amphetamine sulfate* (C)(II)(G)

Adderall <6 years: not indicated; ≥6-12 years: initially 5 mg daily; may increase by 5 mg/day at weekly intervals; >12 years: initially 10 mg daily; may increase weekly by 10 mg/day; usual max 60 mg/day in 2-3 divided doses; first dose on awakening; then q 4-6 hours prn

Tab: 5**, 7.5**, 10**, 12.5**, 15**mg, 3.75 mg, 20**, 30**mg

Adderall XR <6 years: not recommended; 6-12 years: initially 10 mg daily in the AM; may increase by 10 mg/day at weekly intervals; max 30 mg/day; 13-17 years: 10-20 mg by mouth daily in the AM; may increase by 10 mg/day at weekly intervals; max 40 mg/day; >12 years: initially 20 mg by mouth once daily in AM; may increase by 10 mg/day at weekly intervals; max: 60 mg/day; do not chew; may sprinkle on applesauce

Cap: 5, 10, 15, 20, 25, 30 mg ext-rel

▷ *dexmethylphenidate* (C)(II)(G)

Focalin <6 years: not established; ≥6 years: initially 2.5 mg bid; allow at least 4 hours between doses; may increase at 1 week intervals; max 20 mg/day

Tab: 2.5, 5, 10*mg (dye-free)

Focalin ER <6 years: not established; ≥6 years: initially 5 mg weekly; usual dose 10-30 mg/day

Cap: 15, 30 mg ext-rel

Focalin XR <6 years: not established; ≥6 years: initially 5 mg weekly; usual dose 10-30 mg/day

Cap: 5, 10, 15, 20, 25, 30, 35, 40 mg ext-rel

▷ *lisdexamfetamine dimesylate* (C)(II) <6 years: not recommended; ≥6 years: 30 mg once daily in the AM; may increase by 10-20 mg/day at weekly intervals; max 70 mg/day

Vyvanse *Cap:* 20, 30, 40, 50, 60, 70 mg

Comment: May dissolve **Vyvanse** capsule contents in water; take immediately.

▸ *methylphenidate (regular-acting)* (C)(II)(G)

Methylin, Methylin Chewable, Methylin Oral Solution <6 years: not recommended; 6-12 years: initially 5 mg bid ac (breakfast and lunch); may increase 5-10 mg/day at weekly intervals; max 60 mg/day; >12 years: usual dose 20-30 mg/day in 2-3 divided doses 30-45 minutes before a meal; max 60 mg/day

Tab: 5, 10*, 20*mg; *Chew tab:* 2.5, 5, 10 mg; (grape) (phenylalanine); *Oral soln:* 5, 10 mg/5 ml (grape)

Ritalin <6 years: not recommended; ≥6 years: initially 5 mg bid ac (breakfast and lunch); may increase by 5-10 mg at weekly intervals as needed; max 60 mg/day; 10-60 mg/day in 2-3 divided doses 30-45 minutes ac; max 60 mg/day

Tab: 5, 10*, 20*mg

▸ *methylphenidate (long-acting)* (C)(II)

Concerta <6 years: not recommended; ≥6-12 years: initially 18 mg daily; max 54 mg/day; >12-17 years: initially 18 mg daily; max 72 mg/day or 2 mg/kg, whichever is less; >17 years: initially 18 mg q AM; may increase in 18 mg increments as needed; max 54 mg/day; do not crush or chew

Tab: 18, 27, 36, 54 mg sust-rel

Metadate CD (G) <6 years: not recommended; ≥6 years: initially 20 mg daily; may gradually increase by 20 mg/day at weekly intervals as needed; max 60 mg/day; do not crush or chew

Cap: 10, 20, 30, 40, 50, 60 mg immed- and ext-rel beads

Metadate ER <6 years: not recommended; ≥6-<12 years: use in place of regular-acting *methylphenidate* when the 8-hour dose of **Metadate-ER** corresponds to the titrated 8-hour dose of regular-acting *methylphenidate*; ≥12 years: 1 tab daily in the AM; do not crush or chew

Tab: 10, 20 mg ext-rel (dye-free)

QuilliChew ER <6 years: not recommended; ≥6 years: initially 1 x 10 mg chew tab once daily in the AM; may gradually increase by 20 mg/day at weekly intervals as needed; max 60 mg/day

Chew tab: 20*, 30*, 40 mg ext-rel

Quillivant XR <6 years: not recommended; ≥6 years: initially 20 mg once daily in the AM, with or without food; may be titrated in increments of 10-20 mg/day at weekly intervals; daily doses above 60 mg have not been studied and are not recommended; shake the bottle vigorously for at least 10 seconds to ensure that the correct dose is administered

Bottle: 5 mg/ml, 25 mg/5 ml pwdr for reconstitution; 300 mg (60 ml), 600 mg (120 ml), 750 mg (150 ml), 900 mg (180 ml)

Comment: **Quillivant XR** must be reconstituted by a pharmacist, not by the patient or caregiver.

Ritalin LA (G) 1 cap daily in the AM; <6 years: not recommended; ≥6 years: use in place of regular-acting *methylphenidate* when the 8-hour dose of **Ritalin LA** corresponds to the titrated 8-hour dose of regular-acting *methylphenidate*; max 60 mg/day

Cap: 10, 20, 30, 40 mg ext-rel (immed- and ext-rel beads)

Ritalin SR 1 cap daily in the AM; <6 years: not recommended; ≥6 years: use in place of regular-acting *methylphenidate* when the 8-hour dose of **Ritalin SR** corresponds to the titrated 8-hour dose of regular-acting *methylphenidate*; max 60 mg/day

Tab: 20 mg sust-rel (dye-free)

▷ *methylphenidate* (transdermal patch) (C)(II)(G) <6 years: not recommended;
≥6-17 years: initially 10 mg patch applied to hip 2 hours before desired effect daily
in the AM; may increase by 5-10 mg at weekly intervals; max 60 mg/day; not
applicable >17 years
    Daytrana *Transdermal patch:* 10, 15, 20, 30 mg
▷ *pemoline* (B)(IV) <6 years: not recommended; ≥6 years: 18.75-112.5 mg/day;
usually start with 37.5 mg in AM; may increase 18.75 mg/day at weekly intervals;
max 112.5 gm/day
    Cylert *Tab:* 18.75*, 37.5*, 75*mg
    Cylert Chewable *Chew tab:* 37.5*mg
    Comment: Check baseline serum ALT and monitor every 2 weeks thereafter.

CENTRAL ALPHA2A-AGONIST

▷ *guanfacine* (B)(G) <6 years: not recommended; ≥6-17 years: initially 1 mg once
daily; may increase by 1 mg/day at weekly intervals; usual max 4 mg/day; not
applicable >17 years
    Intuniv *Tab:* 1, 2, 3, 4 mg ext-rel
    Comment: Take **Intuniv** with water, milk, or other liquid. Do not take with a
high-fat meal. Withdraw gradually by 1 mg every 3-7 days.

OTHER AGENTS

▷ *clonidine* (C)
    Catapres <12 years: not recommended; ≥12 years: initially 0.1 mg bid; usual
    range 0.2-0.6 mg/day in divided doses; max 2.4 mg/day
        Tab: 0.1*, 0.2*, 0.3*mg
    Catapres-TTS <12 years: not recommended; ≥12 years: initially 0.1 mg patch
    weekly; increase after 1-2 weeks if needed; max 0.6 mg/day
        Patch: 0.1, 0.2 mg/day (12/carton); 0.3 mg/day (4/carton)
    Kapvay (G) <12 years: not recommended; ≥12 years: initially 0.1 mg bid; usual
    range 0.2-0.6 mg/day in divided doses; max 2.4 mg/day
        Tab: 0.1, 0.2 mg
    Nexiclon XR <12 years: not recommended; ≥12 years: initially 0.18 mg (2 ml)
    suspension or 0.17 mg tab once daily; usual max 0.52 mg (6 ml suspension)
    once daily
        Tab: 0.17, 0.26 mg ext-rel; *Oral susp:* 0.09 mg/ml ext-rel (4 oz)

AMINOKETONES (FOR THE TREATMENT OF ADHD)

▷ *bupropion HCl* (B)(G)
    Wellbutrin <18 years: not recommended; ≥18 years: initially 100 mg bid for at
    least 3 days; may increase to 375 or 400 mg/day after several weeks; then after
    at least 3 more days, 450 mg in 4 divided doses; max 450 mg/day, 150 mg/single
    dose
        Tab: 75, 100 mg
    Wellbutrin SR <12 years: not recommended; ≥12 years: initially 150 mg in AM
    for at least 3 days; may increase to 150 mg bid if well tolerated; usual dose 300
    mg/day; max 400 mg/day
        Tab: 100, 150 mg sust-rel

Wellbutrin XL <12 years: not recommended; ≥12 years: initially 150 mg in AM for at least 3 days; increase to 150 mg bid if well tolerated; usual dose 300 mg/day; max 400 mg/day
  Tab: 150, 300 mg sust-rel

BACTERIAL ENDOCARDITIS: PROPHYLAXIS

Comment: Bacterial endocarditis prophylaxis is appropriate for persons with a history of previous infective endocarditis, persons with a prosthetic cardiac valve or prosthetic material used for valve repair, cardiac transplant patients who develop cardiac valvulopathy, congenital heart disease (CHD), unrepaired cyanotic CHD including palliative shunts and conduits, completely repaired congenital heart defect(s) with prosthetic material or device, whether placed by surgery or by catheter intervention, during the first 6 months after the procedure, repaired CHD with residual defects at the site or adjacent to the site of a prosthetic patch or prosthetic device (which may inhibit endothelialization), or any other condition deemed to place a patient at high risk.

DENTAL, ORAL, RESPIRATORY TRACT, OR ESOPHAGEAL PROCEDURES

▷ *amoxicillin* (B)(G) 50 mg/kg as a single dose or 50 mg/kg (max 3 gm) 1 hour before procedure and (max 1.5 gm) 25 mg/kg 6 hours later; *see page 543 for dose by weight table* ≥40 kg: 2 gm PO 30-60 minutes before procedure as a single dose or 3 gm 1 hour before procedure and 1.5 gm 6 hours later
  Amoxil *Cap:* 250, 500 mg; *Tab:* 875*mg; *Chew tab:* 125, 200, 250, 400 mg (cherry-banana-peppermint) (phenylalanine); *Oral susp:* 125, 250 mg/5 ml (80, 100, 150 ml) (strawberry); 200, 400 mg/5 ml (50, 75, 100 ml) (bubble gum); *Oral drops:* 50 mg/ml (30 ml) (bubble gum)
  Trimox *Tab:* 125, 250 mg; *Cap:* 250, 500 mg; *Oral susp:* 125, 250 mg/5 ml (80, 100, 150 ml) (raspberry-strawberry)
▷ *ampicillin* (B)(G) <12 years: 50 mg/kg PO/IM/IV 30-60 minutes before procedure; *see page 547 for oral dose by weight table;* ≥12 years: 2 gm PO/IM/IV 30-60 minutes before procedure
Omnipen, Principen *Cap:* 250, 500 mg; *Oral susp:* 125, 250 mg/5 ml (100, 150, 200 ml) (fruit)
▷ *ampicillin/sulbactam* (B)(G) <12 years: 50 mg/kg IV 30-60 minutes before procedure; ≥12 years: 2 gm IV 30-60 minutes before procedure
  Unasyn Vial: 1.5, 3 g
▷ *azithromycin* (B) <12 years: 15 mg/kg 30-60 minutes before procedure; max 500 mg; *see page 548 for dose by weight table;* ≥12 years: 500 mg 30-60 minutes before procedure
  Zithromax *Tab:* 250, 500, 600 mg; *Oral susp:* 100 mg/5 ml (15 ml); 200 mg/5 ml (15, 22.5, 30 ml) (cherry)
▷ *cefazolin* (B) <12 years: 25 mg/kg IM/IV 30-60 minutes before procedure; ≥12 years: 1 gm IM/IV 30-60 minutes before procedure
  Ancef *Vial:* 250, 500 mg; 1, 5 g
  Kefzol *Vial:* 500 mg; 1 g
▷ *ceftriaxone* (B)(G) <12 years: 50 mg/kg IM/IV as a single dose 30-60 minutes before procedure; ≥12 years: 1 gm IM/IV as a single dose 30-60 minutes before procedure

Rocephin Vial: 250, 500 mg; 1, 2 g

➤ *cephalexin* (B)(G) <12 years: 50 mg/kg as a single dose 30-60 minutes before procedure; *see page 557 for dose by weight table;* ≥12 years: 2 gm as a single dose 30-60 minutes before procedure

Keflex *Cap:* 250, 333, 500, 750 mg; *Oral susp:* 125, 250 mg/5 ml (100, 200 ml) (strawberry)

➤ *clarithromycin* (C)(G) <12 years: 15 mg/kg as a single dose 30-60 minutes before procedure; *see page 558 for dose by weight table;* ≥12 years: 500 mg or 500 mg ext-rel as a single dose 30-60 minutes before procedure

Biaxin *Tab:* 250, 500 mg

Biaxin Oral Suspension *Oral susp:* 125, 250 mg/5 ml (50, 100 ml) (fruit punch)

Biaxin XL *Tab:* 500 mg ext-rel

➤ *clindamycin* (B)(G) <12 years: 20 mg/kg (max 300 mg) 1 hour before procedure and 10 mg/kg (max 150 mg) 6 hours later; take with a full glass of water; *see page 559 for dose by weight table;* ≥12 years: 600 mg PO as a one time single dose or 300 mg 30-60 minutes before procedure and 150 mg 6 hours later; take with a full glass of water

Cleocin *Cap:* 75 (tartrazine), 150 (tartrazine), 300 mg

Cleocin Pediatric Granules *Oral susp:* 75 mg/ml (100 ml) (cherry)

➤ *erythromycin estolate* (B)(G) <12 years: 20 mg/kg 1 hour before procedure; then 10 mg/kg 6 hours later; *see page 562 for dose by weight table;* ≥12 years: 1 gm 1 hour before procedure; then 500 mg 6 hours later

Ilosone *Pulvule:* 250 mg; *Tab:* 500 mg; *Liq:* 125, 250 mg/5 ml (100 ml)

➤ *penicillin V potassium* (B)(G) <12 years: <60 lb: 1 gm 1 hour before procedure; then 500 mg 6 hours later or 1 gm 1 hour before procedure; then 500 mg q 6 hours x 8 doses; *see page 572 for dose by weight table;* ≥12 years: 2 gm 1 hour before procedure; then 1 gm 6 hours later or 2 gm 1 hour before procedure; then 1 gm q 6 hours x 8 doses

Pen-VK *Tab:* 250, 500 mg; *Oral soln:* 125 mg/5 ml (100, 200 ml); 250 mg/5 ml (100, 150, 200 ml)

BACTERIAL VAGINOSIS
(BV; *GARDNERELLA VAGINALIS*)

PROPHYLAXIS AND RESTORATION OF VAGINAL ACIDITY

➤ *acetic acid/oxyquinolone* (C) <12 years: not recommended; ≥12 years: one full applicator intravaginally bid for up to 30 days

Relagard *Gel: acet acid* 0.9%/*oxyq* 0.025% (50 gm tube w. applicator)

Comment: The following treatment regimens for *bacterial vaginosis* are published in the **2015 CDC Sexually Transmitted Diseases Treatment Guidelines**. Treatment regimens are presented by generic drug name first, followed by information about brands and dose forms. BV is associated with adverse pregnancy outcomes, including premature rupture of the membranes, preterm labor, preterm birth, intra-amniotic infection, and postpartum endometritis. Therefore, treatment is recommended for all pregnant females with symptoms or positive screen.

RECOMMENDED REGIMENS

Regimen 1
▷ *metronidazole* 500 mg bid x 7 days

Regimen 2
▷ *metronidazole* gel 0.75% one full applicatorful (5 gm) once daily x 5 days

Regimen 3
▷ *clindamycin* cream 2% one full applicatorful (5 gm) intravaginally once daily at bedtime x 5 days

CDC ALTERNATE REGIMENS

Regimen 1
▷ *tinidazole* 2 gm once daily x 2 days

Regimen 2
▷ *tinidazole* 1 gm once daily x 5 days

Regimen 3
▷ *clindamycin* 300 mg bid x 7 days

Regimen 4
▷ *clindamycin* ovules 100 mg intravaginally once daily at bedtime x 3 days

Drug Brands and Dose Forms

▷ *clindamycin* (B)
    Cleocin (G) *Cap:* 75 (tartrazine), 150 (tartrazine), 300 mg
    Cleocin Pediatric Granules (G) *Oral susp:* 75 mg/5 ml (100 ml) (cherry)
    Cleocin Vaginal Cream *Vag crm:* 2% (21, 40 gm tubes w. applicator)
    Cleocin Vaginal Ovules *Vag supp:* 100 mg
▷ *metronidazole* (not for use in 1st; B in 2nd, 3rd)
    Flagyl *Tab:* 250*, 500*mg
    Flagyl 375 *Cap:* 375 mg
    Flagyl ER *Tab:* 750 mg ext-rel
    MetroGel-Vaginal, Vandazole *Vag gel:* 0.75% (70 gm w. applicator) (parabens)
    Comment: Alcohol is contraindicated during treatment with oral *metronidazole* and for 72 hours after therapy due to a possible *disulfiram*-like reaction (nausea, vomiting, flushing, headache).
▷ *tinidazole* (not for use in 1st; B in 2nd, 3rd)
    Tindamax *Tab:* 250*, 500*mg

BELL'S PALSY

▷ *prednisone* (C)(G) <18 years: *see page* 498 for oral corticosteroid options; ≥18 years: 80 mg once daily x 3 days; then 60 mg daily x 3 days; then 40 mg daily x 3 days; then 20 mg x 1 dose; then discontinue

Deltasone *Tab:* 2.5*, 5*, 10*, 20*, 50*mg

BILE ACID DEFICIENCY

BILE ACID

▷ *ursodiol* (B) <12 years: not recommended; ≥12 years: *Dissolution* of radiolucent non-calcified gallstones <20 mm diameter: 8-10 mg/kg/day in 2-3 divided doses; *Prevention:* 13-15 mg/kg/day in 4 divided doses

Actigall *Cap:* 300 mg

Comment: *ursodiol* decreases the amount of cholesterol produced by the liver and absorbed by the intestines. It helps break down cholesterol that has formed into stones in the gallbladder. *ursodiol* increases bile flow in patients with primary biliary cirrhosis. It is used to treat small gallstones in people who cannot have cholecystectomy surgery and to prevent gallstones in overweight patients undergoing rapid weight loss. *ursodiol* is not used for treating gallstones that are calcified.

BINGE EATING DISORDER

CENTRAL NERVOUS SYSTEM (CNS) STIMULANT

▷ *lisdexamfetamine dimesylate* (C)(II) <18 years: not established; ≥18 years: swallow whole or may open and mix/dissolve contents of cap in yogurt, water, orange juice and take immediately; 30 mg once daily in the AM; may adjust in increments of 20 mg at weekly intervals; target dose 50-70 mg/day; max 70 mg/day; *GFR 15-<30 mL/ min:* max 50 mg/day; *GFR <15 mL/min, ESRD:* max 30 mg/day

Vyvanse *Cap:* 10, 20, 30, 40, 50, 60 70 mg

Comment: **Vyvanse** is not approved or recommended for weight loss treatment of obesity.

BIPOLAR I DISORDER: DEPRESSION

Comment: The cornerstone of treatment for bipolar I disorder: Depression is mood stabilizers (**lithium** and **valproate**). Common adjunctive agents include antiepileptics, antipsychotics, and combination agents. Mounting evidence suggests that antidepressants are not effective in the treatment of bipolar depression. A major study funded by the National Institute of Mental Health (NIMH) found that adding an antidepressant to a mood stabilizer was no more effective in treating bipolar I depression than using a mood stabilizer alone. Another NIMH study found that antidepressants work no better than placebo. If antidepressants are used at all, they should be combined with a mood stabilizer such as *lithium* or *valproic acid*. Taking an antidepressant without a mood stabilizer is likely to trigger a manic episode. Antidepressants can increase mood cycling. Many experts believe that over time, antidepressant use in people with bipolar disorder has a mood destabilizing effect, increasing the frequency of manic and depressive episodes. Other drugs and conditions that can mimic bipolar I disorder include thyroid disorders, corticosteroids, adrenal disorders (e.g., Addison's disease, Cushing's syndrome), antianxiety drugs, vitamin B_{12} deficiency, and neurological disorders (e.g., epilepsy, multiple sclerosis).

MOOD STABILIZERS

Lithium Salts Mood Stabilizer

▷ *lithium carbonate* (D)(G) <12 years: not recommended; ≥12 years: swallow whole; *Usual maintenance:* 900-1200 mg/day in 2-3 divided doses

    Lithobid *Tab:* 300 mg slow-rel

Comment: Toxic and therapeutic levels of lithium are close. Draw blood for serum levels 8-12 hours after previous dose. Signs and symptoms of *lithium* toxicity can occur below 2 mEq/L and include blurred vision, tinnitus, weakness, dizziness, nausea, abdominal pains, vomiting, diarrhea to (severe) hand tremors, ataxia, muscle twitches, nystagmus, seizures, slurred speech, decreased level of consciousness, coma, death. Other potential adverse reactions may include dry mouth, metallic taste, polydipsia, polyuria, arrhythmias, renal toxicity, hypotension, lethargy, pseudotumor cerebri, extrapyramidal symptoms.

Valproate Mood Stabilizer

▷ *divalproex sodium* (D)(G) <12 years: not recommended; ≥12 years: take once daily; swallow ext-rel form whole; initially 25 mg/kg/day in divided doses; max 60 mg/kg/day

    Depakene *Cap:* 250 mg; *Syr:* 250 mg/5 ml (16 oz)
    Depakote *Tab:* 125, 250 mg
    Depakote ER *Tab:* 250, 500 mg ext-rel
    Depakote Sprinkle *Cap:* 125 mg

ANTIEPILEPTICS

▷ *carbamazepine* (D) <12 years: not recommended; ≥12 years: ext-rel oral forms should be swallowed whole; may open caps and sprinkle on applesauce (do not crush or chew beads); initially 400 mg/day in 2 divided doses; adjust in increments of 200 mg/day; max 1.6 gm/day. *Elderly:* reduce initial dose and titrate slowly; oral doses are preferred; IV administration is recommended when the patient is unable to swallow an oral form (see **Carnexiv**)

    Carbatrol (G) *Cap:* 200, 300 mg ext-rel
    Carnexiv *Vial:* 10 mg/ml (20 ml)

Comment: The total daily dose of **Carnexiv** is 70% of the total daily oral *carbamazepine* dose (see mfr pkg insert for dosage conversion table). The total daily dose should be equally divided into four 30-minute infusions, separated by 6 hours. Must be diluted prior to administration. Patients should be switched back to oral *carbamazepine* at their previous total daily oral dose and frequency of administration as soon as clinically appropriate. The use of **Carnexiv** for more than 7 consecutive days has not been studied.

Equetro (G) *Cap:* 100, 200, 300 mg ext-rel
Tegretol *Tab:* 200*mg; *Chew tab:* 100*mg; *Oral susp:* 100 mg/5 ml (450 ml; citrus-vanilla)
Tegretol XR (G) *Tab:* 100, 200, 400 mg ext-rel
Comment: **carbamazepine** is indicated in mixed episodes in bipolar I disorder.

▷ **lamotrigine (C)(G)** <12 years: not recommended; ≥12 years: *Not taking an enzyme-inducing antiepileptic drug (EIAED) (e.g., phenytoin, carbamazepine, phenobarbital, primidone, valproic acid):* 25 mg once daily x 2 weeks; then 50 mg once daily x 2 weeks; then 100 mg once daily x 2 weeks; then target dose 200 mg once daily; *Concomitant valproic acid:* 25 mg every other day x 2 weeks; then 25 mg once daily x 2 weeks; then 50 mg once daily x 1 week; then target dose 100 mg once daily; *Concomitant EIAED, not valproic acid:* 50 mg once daily x 2 weeks; then 100 mg daily in divided doses; then increase weekly by 100 mg in divided doses to target dose 400 mg/day in divided doses daily
Lamictal *Tab:* 25*, 100*, 150*, 200*mg
Lamictal Chewable Dispersible Tab *Chew tab:* 2, 5, 25, 50 mg (black current)
Lamictal ODT *ODT:* 25, 50, 100, 200 mg
Lamictal XR *Tab:* 25, 50, 100, 200 mg ext-rel
Comment: **lamotrigine** is indicated for maintenance treatment of bipolar I disorder. See mfr pkg insert for drug interactions, interactions with contraceptives and hormone replacement therapy, and discontinuation protocol

ANTIPSYCHOTICS

Comment: Common side effects of antipsychotic drugs include drowsiness, weight gain, sexual dysfunction, dry mouth, constipation, blurred vision. *Neuroleptic Malignant Syndrome* (NMS) and *Tardive Dyskinesia* (TD) are adverse side effects (ASEs) most often associated with the older antipsychotic drugs. Risk is decreased with the newer "atypical" antipsychotic drugs. However, these syndromes can develop, although much less commonly, after relatively brief treatment periods at low doses. Given these considerations, antipsychotic drugs should be prescribed in a manner that is most likely to minimize the occurrence. NMS, a potentially fatal symptom complex, is characterized by hyperpyrexia, muscle rigidity, altered mental status and evidence of autonomic instability (irregular pulse or blood pressure, tachycardia, diaphoresis, and cardiac dysrhythmia). Additional signs may include elevated creatine phosphokinase (CPK), myoglobinuria (rhabdomyolysis), and acute renal failure (ARF). TD is a syndrome consisting of potentially irreversible, involuntary, dyskinetic movements that can develop in patients with antipsychotic drugs. Characteristics include repetitive involuntary movements, usually of the jaw, lips and tongue, such as grimacing, sticking out the tongue and smacking the lips. Some affected people also experience involuntary movement of the extremities or difficulty breathing. The syndrome may remit, partially or completely, if antipsychotic treatment is withdrawn. If signs and symptoms of NMS and/or TD appear in a patient, management should include immediate discontinuation of antipsychotic drugs and other drugs not essential to concurrent therapy, intensive symptomatic treatment, medical monitoring, and treatment of any concomitant serious medical problems. The risk of developing NMS and/or TD, and the likelihood that either syndrome will become irreversible, is believed to increase as the duration of treatment and the total cumulative dose of antipsychotic drugs administered to the patient increase. The first and only FDA-approved treatment for TD is **valbenazine (Ingrezza)** (*see page 395*)

▷ *aripiprazole* (C)(G) <10 years: not recommended; ≥10-17 years: initially 2 mg/day in a single dose for 2 days; then increase to 5 mg/day in a single dose for 2 days; then increase to target dose of 10 mg/day in a single dose; may increase by 5 mg/day at weekly intervals as needed to max 30 mg/day; >17 years: initially 15 mg once daily; may increase to max 30 mg/day

  Abilify *Tab:* 2, 5, 10, 15, 20, 30 mg

  Abilify Discmelt *Tab:* 15 mg orally-disint (vanilla) (phenylalanine)

  Abilify Maintena *Vial:* 300, 400 mg ext-rel pwdr for IM injection after reconstitution; 300, 400 mg single-dose prefilled dual-chamber syringes w. supplies

  Comment: **Abilify** is indicated for acute and maintenance treatment of mixed episodes in bipolar I disorder, as monotherapy *or* as adjunct to *lithium* or *valproic acid.*

▷ *asenapine* (C) <10 years: not established; 10-17 years: *Monotherapy:* initially 2.5 mg bid; may increase to 5 mg bid after 3 days; then to 10 mg bid after 3 more days; max 10 mg bid: >17 years: *Monotherapy:* 10 mg bid; *Adjunctive therapy:* 5 mg bid; may increase to max 10 mg bid; allow SL tab to dissolve on tongue; do not split, crush, chew, *or* swallow; do not eat *or* drink for 10 minutes after administration

  Saphris *SL tab:* 2, 5, 5, 10 mg (black cherry)

  Comment: **Saphris** is indicated for acute treatment of manic *or* mixed episodes in bipolar I disorder, as monotherapy *or* as adjunct to *lithium* or *valproic acid*.

▷ *cariprazine* (NE) <12 years: not established: ≥12 years: administer dose once daily; initially 1.5 mg once daily; Day 2: increase to 3 mg; may further increase by 1.5-3 mg increments on subsequent days based on patient response and tolerability; usual range 3-6 mg once daily; max 6 mg/day; *Initiating a strong CYP3A4 inhibitor while taking* **Vraylar**: decrease **Vraylar** dose by half; *Initiating* **Vraylar** *while taking a strong CYP3A4 inhibitor: Day 1:* 1.5 mg; *Day 2:* skip dose; *Day 3 and subsequent days:* 1.5 mg once daily; increase by 1.5-3 mg once daily; max 6 mg/day

  Vraylar

    Cap: 1.5, 3, 4.5, 6 mg; 7-count (1 x 1.5 mg, 6 x 3 mg) mixed blister pck

  Comment: **Vraylar** is an atypical antipsychotic with partial agonist activity at D2 and 5-HT1A receptors and antagonist activity at 5-HT2A receptors. It is indicated for acute treatment of mixed episodes in bipolar I disorder. There is a **Vraylar** pregnancy exposure registry that monitors pregnancy outcomes in females exposed to **Vraylar** during pregnancy. For more information, contact the National Pregnancy Registry for Atypical Antipsychotics at 866-961-2388 *or* visit https://womensmentalhealth.org/clinical-and-research-programs/pregnancyregistry.

▷ *lurasidone* (B) <18 years: not established; ≥18 years: initially 20 mg once daily; usual range 20 to max 120 mg/day; take with food; *CrCl <50 mL/min, moderate hepatic impairment (Child Pugh 7-9):* max 80 mg/day; *Child Pugh 10-15):* max 40 mg/day

  Latuda *Tab:* 20, 40, 60, 80, 120 mg

  Comment: **Latuda** is indicated for major depressive episodes associated with bipolar I disorder as monotherapy and as adjunctive therapy with *lithium* or *valproic* acid. Contraindicated with concomitant strong CYP3A4 inhibitors (e.g., *ketoconazole, voriconazole, clarithromycin, ritonavir*) and inducers (e.g., *phenytoin, carbamazepine, rifampin, St. John's wort*); see mfr pkg insert if patient taking moderate CYP3A4 inhibitors (e.g., *diltiazem, atazanavir, erythromycin, fluconazole, verapamil*). The efficacy of LATUDA in the treatment of mania associated with bipolar disorder has not been established.

➢ *quetiapine fumarate* (C)(G)

    SeroQUEL <10 years: not recommended; ≥10-17 years: initially 25 mg bid, titrate q 2nd or 3rd day in increments of 25-50 mg bid-tid; max 600 mg/day in 2-3 divided doses: >17 years: initially 25 mg bid, titrate q 2nd or 3rd day in increments of 25-50 mg bid-tid; usual maintenance 400-600 mg/day in 2-3 divided doses

      Tab: 25, 50, 100, 200, 300, 400 mg

    SeroQUEL XR <18 years: not recommended; ≥18 years: swallow whole; administer once daily in the PM; *Day 1:* 50 mg; *Day 2:* 100 mg; *Day 3:* 200 mg; *Day 4:* 300 mg; usual range 400-600 mg/day

      Tab: 50, 150, 200, 300, 400 mg ext-rel

➢ *risperidone* (C) *Tab:* initially 2-3 mg once daily; may adjust at 24 hour intervals by 1 mg/day; usual range 1-6 mg/day; max 6 mg/day; *Oral soln:* do not take with cola or tea; *M-tab:* dissolve on tongue with or without fluid; *Consta:* administer deep IM in the deltoid or gluteal; give with oral *respiridone* or other antipsychotic x 3 weeks; then stop oral form; 25 mg IM every 2 weeks; max 50 mg every 2 weeks

    Risperdal <5 years: not established; 5-10 years: initially 0.5 mg once daily at the same time each day adjust at 24 hour intervals by 0.5-1 mg to target dose 2.5 mg/day; usual range 1-6 mg/day; max 6 mg/day; >10 years: *See generic risperidone above for dosing ≥10 years*

      Tab: 0.25, 0.5, 1, 2, 3, 4 mg; *Oral soln:* 1 mg/ml (100 ml)

    Risperdal Consta <18 years: not established; *See generic risperidone above for dosing ≥18 years*

      Vial: 12.5, 25, 37.5, 50 mg pwdr for long-acting IM inj after reconstitution, single use w. diluent and supplies

    Risperdal M-Tab <10 years: not established; ≥10 years: *See generic risperidone above for dosing ≥10 years*

      Tab: 0.5, 1, 2, 3, 4 mg orally-disint (phenylalanine)

Comment: **Risperdal** tabs, oral solution, and M-tabs are indicated for the short-term monotherapy of acute mania or mixed episodes associated with bipolar I disorder, or in combination with *lithium* or *valproic acid* in patients >12 years-of-age. **Risperdol Consta** is indicated as monotherapy or adjunctive therapy to *lithium* or *valproic acid* for the maintenance treatment mania and mixed episodes in bipolar I disorder.

➢ *ziprasidone* (C)(G) <12 years: not recommended; ≥12 years: initially 40 mg bid; on day 2, may increase to 60-80 mg bid

    Geodon *Cap:* 20, 40, 60, 80 mg

    Comment: **Geodon** is indicated for acute and maintenance treatment of mixed episodes in bipolar I disorder, as monotherapy or as adjunct to *lithium* or *valproic acid.*

COMBINATION AGENTS

Thienobenzodiazepine/Selective Serotonin Reuptake Inhibitor Combinations

➢ *fluoxetine* (C)(G)

    Prozac <12 years: not recommended; ≥12 years: initially *olanzapine* 5 mg plus fluoxetine 20 mg daily in the PM; range *olanzapine* 5-12.5 mg plus *fluoxetine* 20-50 mg; risk of hypotension, or hepatic impairment, slow metabolizers, or sensitive to *olanzapine*, initially *olanzapine* 2.5-5 mg plus *fluoxetine* 20 mg daily in the PM; *fluoxetine* doses >20 mg/day may be divided into AM and noon doses

Cap: 10, 20, 40 mg; *Tab:* 30*, 60*mg; *Oral soln:* 20 mg/5 ml (4 oz) (mint)
Prozac Weekly <12 years: not recommended; ≥12 years: following daily *fluoxetine* therapy at 20 mg/day for 13 weeks, may initiate **Prozac Weekly** 7 days after the last 20 mg *fluoxetine* dose

▷ *olanzapine/fluoxetine* (C) <10 years: not recommended; 10-17 years: initially 1 x 3/25 cap once daily in the PM; max 1 x 12/50 cap once daily in the PM; >17 years: initially 1 x 6/25 cap once daily in the PM; titrate; max 1 x 12/50 cap once daily in the PM

Symbyax
Cap: **Symbyax 3/25:** *olan* 3 mg/*fluo* 25 mg
Symbyax 6/25: *olan* 6 mg/*fluo* 25 mg
Symbyax 6/50: *olan* 6 mg/*fluo* 50 mg
Symbyax 12/25: *olan* 12 mg/*fluo* 25 mg
Symbyax 12/50: *olan* 12 mg/*fluo* 50 mg

Comment: **Symbyax** is indicated for the treatment of depressive episodes associated with bipolar I disorder and treatment-resistant depression (TRD).

BIPOLAR I DISORDER: MANIA

Comment: The cornerstone of treatment for bipolar I disorder: Mania is mood stabilizers (*lithium* and *valproic acid*). Common adjunctive agents include antiepileptics and antipsychotics. Drugs and conditions that can mimic bipolar I disorder include thyroid disorders, corticosteroids, antidepressants, adrenal disorders (e.g., Addison's disease, Cushing's syndrome), antianxiety drugs, drugs for Parkinson's disease, vitamin B12 deficiency, neurological disorders (e.g., epilepsy, multiple sclerosis).

MOOD STABILIZERS

Lithium Salts Mood Stabilizer

▷ *lithium carbonate* (D)(G) <12 years: not recommended; ≥12 years: swallow whole; *Acute mania:* 1800 mg/day in 2-3 divided doses; *Usual maintenance:* 900-1200 mg/day in 2-3 divided doses
Lithobid *Tab:* 300 mg slow-rel
Comment: Signs and symptoms of *lithium* toxicity can occur below 2 mEq/L and include blurred vision, tinnitus, weakness, dizziness, nausea, abdominal pains, vomiting, diarrhea to (severe) hand tremors, ataxia, muscle twitches, nystagmus, seizures, slurred speech, decreased level of consciousness, coma, death.

Valproate Mood Stabilizer

▷ *divalproex sodium* (D)(G) <12 years: not recommended; ≥12 years: initially 25 mg/kg/day in divided doses; max 60 mg/kg/day; initially use immed-rel form and titrate; take ext-rel form once daily and swallow whole
Depakene *Cap:* 250 mg; *Syr:* 250 mg/5 ml (16 oz)
Depakote *Tab:* 125, 250 mg
Depakote ER *Tab:* 250, 500 mg ext-rel
Depakote Sprinkle *Cap:* 125 mg

ANTIEPILEPTICS

➤ *carbamazepine* (D) <12 years: not recommended; ≥12 years: initially 400 mg/day in 2 divided doses; adjust in increments of 200 mg/day; max 1.6 gm/day; take oral dose once daily; swallowed whole; may open caps and sprinkle on applesauce (do not crush or chew beads); oral doses are preferred; IV administration is recommended when the patient is unable to swallow an oral form (see **Carnexiv**)

Carbatrol (G) *Cap:* 200, 300 mg ext-rel
Carnexiv *Vial:* 10 mg/ml (20 ml)
Comment: The total daily dose of Carnexiv is 70% of the total daily oral *carbamazepine* dose. See mfr pkg insert for dosage conversion table. The total daily dose should be equally divided into four 30-minute infusions, separated by 6 hours. Must be diluted prior to administration. Patients should be switched back to oral *carbamazepine* at their previous total daily oral dose and frequency of administration as soon as clinically appropriate. The use of **Carnexiv** for more than 7 consecutive days has not been studied.
Equetro (G) *Cap:* 100, 200, 300 mg ext-rel
Tegretol(G) *Tab:* 200*mg; *Chew tab:* 100*mg; *Oral susp:* 100 mg/5 ml (450 ml; citrus-vanilla)
Tegretol XR (G) *Tab:* 100, 200, 400 mg ext-rel
Comment: *carbamazepine* is indicated in mixed episodes in bipolar I disorder.

➤ *lamotrigine* (C)(G) <12 years: not recommended; ≥12 years: *Not taking an enzyme-inducing antiepileptic drug (EIAED)* (*e.g., phenytoin, carbamazepine, phenobarbital, primidone, valproic acid*): 25 mg once daily x 2 weeks; then 50 mg once daily x 2 weeks; then 100 mg once daily x 2 weeks; then target dose 200 mg once daily; *Concomitant valproic acid:* 25 mg every other day x 2 weeks; then 25 mg once daily x 2 weeks; then 50 mg once daily x 1 week; then target dose 100 mg once daily; *Concomitant EIAED, not valproic acid:* 50 mg once daily x 2 weeks; then 100 mg daily in divided doses; then increase weekly by 100 mg in divided doses to target dose 400 mg/day in divided doses daily

Lamictal *Tab:* 25*, 100*, 150*, 200*mg
Lamictal Chewable Dispersible Tab *Chew tab:* 2, 5, 25, 50 mg (black current)
Lamictal ODT *ODT:* 25, 50, 100, 200 mg
Lamictal XR *Tab:* 25, 50, 100, 200 mg ext-rel
Comment: *lamotrigine* is indicated for maintenance treatment of bipolar I disorder. See mfr pkg insert for drug interactions, interactions with contraceptives and hormone replacement therapy, and discontinuation protocol

➤ *topiramate* (D)(G) <12 years: not recommended; ≥12 years: initially 25 mg daily in the PM; then 25 mg bid; then, 25 mg in the AM and 50 mg in the PM; then, 50 mg bid

Topamax *Tab:* 25, 50, 100, 200 mg
Topamax Sprinkle Caps *Cap:* 15, 25 mg
Trokendi XR *Cap:* 25, 50, 100, 200 mg ext-rel
Quedexy XR *Cap:* 25, 50, 100, 150, 200 mg ext-rel

ANTIPSYCHOTICS

Comment: Side effects of antipsychotics include drowsiness, weight gain, sexual dysfunction, dry mouth, constipation, blurred vision. Patients receiving an antipsychotic agent should be monitored closely for the following adverse side effects:

neuroleptic malignant syndrome, extrapyramidal reactions, tardive dyskinesia, blood dyscrasias, anticholinergic effects, drowsiness, hypotension, photo-sensitivity, retinopathy, and lowered seizure threshold. Use lower doses for elderly or debilitated patients. Prescriptions should be written for the smallest practical amount. Foods and beverages containing alcohol are contraindicated for patients receiving any psychotropic drug. *Neuroleptic Malignant Syndrome* (NMS) and *Tardive Dyskinesia* (TD) are adverse side effects (ASEs) most often associated with the older antipsychotic drugs. Risk is decreased with the newer "atypical" antipsychotic drugs. However, these syndromes can develop, although much less commonly, after relatively brief treatment periods at low doses. Given these considerations, antipsychotic drugs should be prescribed in a manner that is most likely to minimize the occurrence. NMS, a potentially fatal symptom complex, is characterized by hyperpyrexia, muscle rigidity, altered mental status and evidence of autonomic instability (irregular pulse or blood pressure, tachycardia, diaphoresis, and cardiac dysrhythmia). Additional signs may include elevated creatine phosphokinase (CPK), myoglobinuria (rhabdomyolysis), and acute renal failure (ARF). TD is a syndrome consisting of potentially irreversible, involuntary, dyskinetic movements that can develop in patients with antipsychotic drugs. Characteristics include repetitive involuntary movements, usually of the jaw, lips and tongue, such as grimacing, sticking out the tongue and smacking the lips. Some affected people also experience involuntary movement of the extremities or difficulty breathing. The syndrome may remit, partially or completely, if antipsychotic treatment is withdrawn. If signs and symptoms of NMS and/or TD appear in a patient, management should include immediate discontinuation of antipsychotic drugs and other drugs not essential to concurrent therapy, intensive symptomatic treatment, medical monitoring, and treatment of any concomitant serious medical problems. The risk of developing NMS and/or TD, and the likelihood that either syndrome will become irreversible, is believed to increase as the duration of treatment and the total cumulative dose of antipsychotic drugs administered to the patient increase. The first and only FDA-approved treatment for TD is *valbenazine* (**Ingrezza**) (*see page 395*).

▷ *aripiprazole* (**C**)(**G**) <10 years: not recommended; ≥10-17 years: initially 2 mg/day in a single dose for 2 days; then increase to 5 mg/day in a single dose for 2 days; then increase to target dose of 10 mg/day in a single dose; may increase by 5 mg/day at weekly intervals as needed to max 30 mg/day; >17 years: initially 15 mg once daily; may increase to max 30 mg/day

> **Abilify** *Tab:* 2, 5, 10, 15, 20, 30 mg
> **Abilify Discmelt** *Tab:* 15 mg orally-disint (vanilla) (phenylalanine)
> **Abilify Maintena** *Vial:* 300, 400 mg ext-rel pwdr for IM injection after reconstitution; 300, 400 mg single-dose prefilled dual-chamber syringes w. supplies
> Comment: **Abilify** is indicated for acute and maintenance treatment of mixed episodes in bipolar I disorder, as monotherapy or as adjunct to *lithium* or *valproic acid.*

▷ *asenapine* (**C**) <10 years: not established; 10-17 years: *Monotherapy:* initially 2.5 mg bid; may increase to 5 mg bid after 3 days; then to 10 mg bid after 3 more days; max 10 mg bid; >17 years: allow SL tab to dissolve on tongue; do not split, crush, chew, or swallow; do not eat or drink for 10 minutes after administration; *Monotherapy:* 10 mg bid; *Adjunctive therapy:* 5 mg bid; may increase to max 10 mg bid

> **Saphris** *SL tab:* 2, 5, 5, 10 mg (black cherry)
> Comment: **Saphris** is indicated for acute treatment of manic or mixed episodes in bipolar I disorder, as monotherapy or as adjunct to *lithium* or *valproic acid.*

▷ *cariprazine* (NE) <12 years: not established: ≥12 years: administer dose once daily; initially 1.5 mg once daily; Day 2: increase to 3 mg; may further increase by 1.5-3 mg increments on subsequent days based on patient response and tolerability; usual range 3-6 mg once daily; max 6 mg/day; *Initiating a strong CYP3A4 inhibitor while taking Vraylar:* decrease **Vraylar** dose by half; *Initiating* **Vraylar** *while taking a strong CYP3A4 inhibitor: Day 1:* 1.5 mg; *Day 2:* skip dose; *Day 3 and subsequent days:* 1.5 mg once daily; increase by 1.5-3 mg once daily; max 6 mg/day

Vraylar *Cap:* 1.5, 3, 4.5, 6 mg; 7-count (1 x 1.5 mg, 6 x 3 mg) mixed blister pck

Comment: **Vraylar** is an atypical antipsychotic with partial agonist activity at D2 and 5-HT1A receptors and antagonist activity at 5-HT2A receptors. It is indicated for acute treatment of mixed episodes in bipolar I disorder. There is a **Vraylar** pregnancy exposure registry that monitors pregnancy outcomes in females exposed to **Vraylar** during pregnancy. For more information, contact the National Pregnancy Registry for Atypical Antipsychotics at 866-961-2388 or visit https://womensmentalhealth.org/clinical-and-research-programs/pregnancyregistry. Safety and effectiveness in pediatric patients have not been established.

▷ *chlorpromazine* (C)(G) ≥6 months-12 years: initially 0.25 mg/lb every 4-6 hours prn or 0.5 mg/lb rectally q 6-8 hours prn; >12 years: initially 10 mg tid-qid; may increase semi-weekly by 25-50 mg/day

Thorazine *Tab:* 10, 25, 50, 100, 200 mg; *Spansule:* 30, 75, 150 mg sust-rel; *Syr:* 10 mg/5 ml (4 oz) (orange custard); *Oral conc:* 30 mg/ml (4 oz); 100 mg/ml (2, 8 oz); *Supp:* 25, 100 mg

Comment: *chlorpromazine* is indicated for rapid control of severe psychotic symptoms.

▷ *quetiapine fumarate* (C)(G)

SeroQUEL <10 years: not recommended; ≥10-17 years: initially 25 mg bid, titrate q 2nd or 3rd day in increments of 25-50 mg bid-tid; max 600 mg/day in 2-3 divided doses; >17 years: initially 25 mg bid, titrate q 2nd or 3rd day in increments of 25-50 mg bid-tid; usual maintenance 400-600 mg/day in 2-3 divided doses

Tab: 25, 50, 100, 200, 300, 400 mg

SeroQUEL XR <18 years: not recommended; ≥18 years: swallow whole; administer once daily in the PM; *Day 1:* 50 mg; *Day 2:* 100 mg; *Day 3:* 200 mg; *Day 4:* 300 mg; usual range 400-600 mg/day

Tab: 50, 150, 200, 300, 400 mg ext-rel

▷ *risperidone* (C) *Tab:* initially 2-3 mg once daily; may adjust at 24 hour intervals by 1 mg/day; usual range 1-6 mg/day; max 6 mg/day; *Oral soln:* do not take with cola or tea; *M-tab:* dissolve on tongue with or without fluid; *Consta:* administer deep IM in the deltoid or gluteal; give with oral ***respiridone*** or other antipsychotic x 3 weeks; then stop oral form; 25 mg IM every 2 weeks; max 50 mg every 2 weeks

Risperdal <5 years: not established; 5-10 years: initially 0.5 mg once daily at the same time each day adjust at 24 hour intervals by 0.5-1 mg to target dose 2.5 mg/day; usual range 1-6 mg/day; max 6 mg/day; >10 years: *See generic* **risperidone** *above for dosing* ≥ *10 years*

Tab: 0.25, 0.5, 1, 2, 3, 4 mg; *Oral soln:* 1 mg/ml (100 ml)

Risperdal Consta <18 years: not established; *See generic* **risperidone** *above for dosing* ≥ *18 years*

Vial: 12.5, 25, 37.5, 50 mg pwdr for long-acting IM inj after reconstitution, single use w. diluent and supplies

Risperdal M-Tab <10 years: not established; ≥10 years: *See generic* **risperidone** *above for dosing ≥ 10 years*

Tab: 0.5, 1, 2, 3, 4 mg orally-disint (phenylalanine)

Comment: **Risperdal** tabs, oral solution, and M-tabs are indicated for the short term monotherapy of acute mania or mixed episodes associated with bipolar I disorder, or in combination with *lithium* or *valproic acid* in patients >12 years-of-age. **Risperdol Consta** is indicated as monotherapy or adjunctive therapy to *lithium* or *valproic acid* for the maintenance treatment mania and mixed episodes in bipolar I disorder.

▷ *ziprasidone* (C)(G) <12 years: not recommended; ≥12 years: initially 40 mg bid; on day 2, may increase to 60-80 mg bid

Geodon *Cap:* 20, 40, 60, 80 mg

Comment: **Geodon** is indicated for acute and maintenance treatment of mixed episodes in bipolar I disorder, as monotherapy or as adjunct to *lithium* or *valproic acid*.

BITE: CAT

TETANUS PROPHYLAXIS

▷ *tetanus toxoid* vaccine (C) 0.5 ml IM x 1 dose if previously immunized

Vial: 5 Lf units/0.5 ml (0.5, 5 ml); *Prefilled syringe:* 5 Lf units/0.5 ml (0.5 ml)

see Tetanus page 398 for patients not previously immunized

ANTI-INFECTIVES

▷ *amoxicillin/clavulanate* (B)(G)

Augmentin <40 kg: 40-45 mg/kg/day divided tid x 10 days or 90 mg/kg/day divided bid x 10 days; *see page 545 for dose by weight table;* ≥40 kg: 500 mg tid or 875 mg bid x 10 days

Tab: 250, 500, 875 mg; *Chew tab:* 125, 250 mg (lemon-lime); 200, 400 mg (cherry-banana) (phenylalanine); *Oral susp:* 125 mg/5 ml (banana), 250 mg/5 ml (75, 100, 150 ml) (orange); 200, 400 mg/5 ml (50, 75, 100 ml) (orange) (phenylalanine)

Augmentin ES-600 <3 months: not recommended; ≥3 months, <40 kg: 90 mg/kg/day divided q 12 hours x 10 days; *see page 546 for dose by weight table;* ≥40 kg: not recommended

Oral susp: 600 mg/5 ml (50, 75, 100, 125, 150, 200 ml) (strawberry cream) (phenylalanine)

Augmentin XR <16 years: use other forms; ≥16 years: 2 tabs q 12 hours x 7-10 days

Tab: 1000*mg ext-rel

▷ *cefuroxime axetil* (B)(G) <3 months: not recommended; 3 months-12 years: 30 mg/kg/day in 2 divided doses x 10 days; *see page 556 for dose by weight table;* ≥12 years: 500 mg bid x 10 days

Ceftin *Tab:* 250, 500 mg; *Oral susp:* 125, 250 mg/5 ml (50, 100 ml) (tutti-frutti)

▷ *doxycycline* (D)(G) <8 years: not recommended; ≥8 years, ≤100 lb: 2 mg/lb on first day in 2 divided doses, followed by 1 mg/lb/day in 1-2 divided doses x 10 days; ≥8 years, >100 lb: 100 mg bid x 10 days; *see page 561 for dose by weight table*

Acticlate *Tab:* 75, 150** mg

Adoxa *Tab:* 50, 75, 100, 150 mg ent-coat
Doryx *Tab:* 50, 75, 100, 150, 200 mg del-rel
Monodox *Cap:* 50, 75, 100 mg
Oracea *Cap:* 40 mg del-rel
Vibramycin *Tab:* 100 mg; *Cap:* 50, 100 mg; *Syr:* 50 mg/5 ml (raspberry-apple)
(sulfites); *Oral susp:* 25 mg/5 ml (raspberry)
Vibra-Tab *Tab:* 100 mg film-coat

Comment: *doxycycline* is contraindicated <8 years-of-age, in pregnancy, and
lactation (discolors developing tooth enamel). A side effect may be photo-
sensitivity (photophobia). Do not take with antacids, calcium supplements, milk <u>or</u>
other dairy, <u>or</u> within 2 hours of taking another drug.

▷ *penicillin V potassium* (B)(G) <12 years: 25-75 mg/kg day divided q 6-8 hours x 3
days; *see page 572 for dose by weight table;* ≥12 years: 500 mg PO qid x 3 days
Pen-VK *Tab:* 250, 500 mg; *Oral soln:* 125 mg/5 ml (100, 200 ml); 250 mg/5 ml
(100, 150, 200 ml)

BITE: DOG

TETANUS PROPHYLAXIS

▷ *tetanus toxoid* vaccine (C) 0.5 ml IM x 1 dose if previously immunized
Vial: 5 Lf units/0.5 ml (0.5, 5 ml)
Prefilled syringe: 5 Lf units/0.5 ml (0.5 ml)
see *Tetanus page 398* for patients not previously immunized

ANTI-INFECTIVES

▷ *amoxicillin/clavulanate* (B)(G)
Augmentin <40 kg: 40-45 mg/kg/day divided tid x 10 days <u>or</u> 90 mg/kg/day
divided bid x 10 days; *see page 545 for dose by weight table;* ≥40 kg: 500 mg tid
<u>or</u> 875 mg bid x 10 days
Tab: 250, 500, 875 mg; *Chew tab:* 125, 250 mg (lemon-lime); 200, 400 mg
(cherry-banana) (phenylalanine); *Oral susp:* 125 mg/5 ml (banana), 250
mg/5 ml (75, 100, 150 ml) (orange); 200, 400 mg/5 ml (50, 75, 100 ml)
(orange) (phenylalanine)
Augmentin ES-600 <3 months: not recommended; ≥3 months, <40 kg: 90 mg/
kg/day divided q 12 hours x 10 days; *see page 546 for dose by weight table;* ≥40
kg: not recommended
Oral susp: 600 mg/5 ml (50, 75, 100, 125, 150, 200 ml) (strawberry cream)
(phenylalanine)
Augmentin XR <16 years: use other forms; ≥16 years: 2 tabs q 12 hours x 7-10
days
Tab: 1000*mg 8-16 mg/kg/day in 3-4 divided doses x 10 days; *see page 545
for dose by weight table;* administer with TMP-SMX; ≥12 years: 300 mg qid x
10 days; administer with fluoroquinolone
Cleocin (G) *Cap:* 75 (tartrazine), 150 (tartrazine), 300 mg
Cleocin Pediatric Granules (G) *Oral susp:* 75 mg/5 ml (100 ml)(cherry)
▷ *doxycycline* (D)(G) <8 years: not recommended; ≥8 years, ≤100 lb: 2 mg/lb on first
day in 2 divided doses, followed by 1 mg/lb/day in 1-2 divided doses x 5-10 days; ≥8
years, >100 lb: 100 mg bid x 5-10 days; *see page 561 for dose by weight table*

Acticlate *Tab:* 75, 150** mg
Adoxa *Tab:* 50, 75, 100, 150 mg ent-coat
Doryx *Tab:* 50, 75, 100, 150, 200 mg del-rel
Monodox *Cap:* 50, 75, 100 mg
Oracea *Cap:* 40 mg del-rel
Vibramycin *Tab:* 100 mg; *Cap:* 50, 100 mg; *Syr:* 50 mg/5 ml (raspberry-apple) (sulfites); *Oral susp:* 25 mg/5 ml (raspberry)
Vibra-Tab *Tab:* 100 mg film-coat

Comment: *doxycycline* is contraindicated <8 years-of-age, in pregnancy, and lactation (discolors developing tooth enamel). A side effect may be photo-sensitivity (photophobia). Do not take with antacids, calcium supplements, milk or other dairy, or within 2 hours of taking another drug.

▷ *penicillin V potassium* (B)(G) <12 years: 50 mg/kg/day in 4 divided doses x 3 days; see *page 572 for dose by weight table;* ≥12 years: 500 mg PO qid x 3 days
Pen-VK *Tab:* 250, 500 mg; *Oral soln:* 125 mg/5 ml (100, 200 ml); 250 mg/5 ml (100, 150, 200 ml)

BITE: HUMAN

TETANUS PROPHYLAXIS

▷ *tetanus toxoid* vaccine (C) 0.5 ml IM x 1 dose if previously immunized
Vial: 5 Lf units/0.5 ml (0.5, 5 ml)
Prefilled syringe: 5 Lf units/0.5 ml (0.5 ml)
see **Tetanus** *page* 398 for patients not previously immunized

ANTI-INFECTIVES

▷ *amoxicillin/clavulanate* (B)(G)
Augmentin <40 kg: 40-45 mg/kg/day divided tid x 10 days or 90 mg/kg/day divided bid x 10 days; see *page 545 for dose by weight table;* ≥40 kg: 500 mg tid or 875 mg bid x 10 days
Tab: 250, 500, 875 mg; *Chew tab:* 125, 250 mg (lemon-lime); 200, 400 mg (cherry-banana) (phenylalanine); *Oral susp:* 125 mg/5 ml (banana), 250 mg/5 ml (75, 100, 150 ml) (orange); 200, 400 mg/5 ml (50, 75, 100 ml) (orange) (phenylalanine)
Augmentin ES-600 <3 months: not recommended; ≥3 months, <40 kg: 90 mg/kg/day divided q 12 hours x 10 days; see *page 546 for dose by weight table;* ≥40 kg: not recommended
Oral susp: 600 mg/5 ml (50, 75, 100, 125, 150, 200 ml) (strawberry cream) (phenylalanine)
Augmentin XR <16 years: use other forms; ≥16 years: 2 tabs q 12 hours x 7-10 days
Tab: 1000*mg ext-rel
▷ *cefoxitin* (B) <3 months: not recommended; ≥3 months: 80-160 mg/kg/day IM in 3-4 divided doses x 10 days; max 12 gm/day
Mefoxin Injectable *Vial:* 1, 2 g
▷ *ciprofloxacin* (C) <18 years: not recommended; ≥18 years: 500 mg bid x 10 days; max 1.5 gm/day

Cipro (G) *Tab:* 250, 500, 750 mg; *Oral susp:* 250, 500 mg/5 ml (100 ml) (strawberry)
Cipro XR *Tab:* 500, 1000 mg ext-rel
ProQuin XR *Tab:* 500 mg ext-rel
Comment: *ciprofloxacin* is contraindicated <18 years-of-age, and during pregnancy and lactation. Risk of tendonitis or tendon rupture.

➤ *erythromycin base* (B)(G) <45 kg: 30-40 mg/kg/day in 4 divided doses x 10 days; ≥45 kg: 250 mg qid x 10 days
Ery-Tab *Tab:* 250, 333, 500 mg ent-coat
PCE *Tab:* 333, 500 mg

➤ *erythromycin ethylsuccinate* (B)(G) 30-50 mg/kg/day in 4 divided doses x 10 days; may double dose with severe infection; *see page 563 for dose by weight table;* max 100 mg/kg/day or 400 mg qid
EryPed *Oral susp:* 200 mg/5 ml (100, 200 ml) (fruit); 400 mg/5 ml (60, 100, 200 ml) (banana); *Oral drops:* 200, 400 mg/5 ml (50 ml) (fruit); *Chew tab:* 200 mg wafer (fruit)
E.E.S. *Oral susp:* 200, 400 mg/5 ml (100 ml) (fruit)
E.E.S. Granules *Oral susp:* 200 mg/5 ml (100, 200 ml) (cherry)
E.E.S. 400 Tablets *Tab:* 400 mg

➤ *trimethoprim/sulfamethoxazole* (D)(G)
Bactrim, Septra <12 years: not recommended; ≥12 years: 2 tabs bid x 10 days
Tab: trim 80 mg/sulfa 400 mg*
Bactrim DS, Septra DS <12 years: not recommended; ≥12 years: 1 tab bid x 10 days
Tab: trim 160 mg/sulfa 800 mg*
Bactrim Pediatric Suspension, Septra Pediatric Suspension <2 months: not recommended; ≥2 months-12 years: 40 mg/kg/day of *sulfamethoxazole* in 2 doses bid; >12 years: use tabs
Oral susp: trim 40 mg/sulfa 200 mg per 5 ml (100 ml) (cherry) (alcohol 0.3%)

BLEPHARITIS

OPHTHALMIC AGENTS

➤ *erythromycin* ophthalmic ointment (B) apply 1/2 inch bid-qid x 14 days; then q HS x 10 days
Ilotycin *Oint:* 5 mg/g (1/2 oz)

➤ *polymyxin/bacitracin* ophthalmic ointment (C) apply 1/2 inch bid-qid x 14 days; then q HS
Polysporin *Oint:* poly B 10,000 U/baci 500 U (3.75 gm)

➤ *polymyxin B/bacitracin/neomycin* ophthalmic ointment (C) apply 1/2 inch bid-qid x 14 days; then q HS
Neosporin *Oint:* poly B 10,000 U/baci 400 U/neo 3.5 mg/g (3.75 gm)

➤ *sodium sulfacetamide* (C)
Bleph-10 Ophthalmic Solution <2 years: not recommended; 2-12 years: years: 1-2 drops q 2-3 hours during the day x 7-14 days; >12 years: 2 drops q 4 hours x 7-14 days
Ophth soln: 10% (2.5, 5, 15 ml) (benzalkonium chloride)

Bleph-10 Ophthalmic Ointment <2 years: not recommended; ≥2 years: apply 1/2 inch qid and HS x 7-14 days
Ophth oint: 10% (3.5 gm) (phenylmercuric acetate)

SYSTEMIC AGENTS

 tetracycline (D)(G) <8 years: not recommended; ≥8 years, ≤100 lb: 25-50 mg/kg/day in 4 divided doses x 7-10 days; *see page 574 for dose by weight table;* >8 years, >100 lb: 250 mg qid x 7-10 days
Achromycin V *Cap:* 250, 500 mg
Sumycin *Tab:* 250, 500 mg; *Cap:* 250, 500 mg; *Oral susp:* 125 mg/5 ml (100, 200 ml) (fruit) (sulfites)
Comment: *tetracycline* is contraindicated <8 years-of-age, in pregnancy, and lactation (discolors developing tooth enamel). A side effect may be photo-sensitivity (photophobia). Do not give with antacids, calcium supplements, milk or other dairy, or within two hours of taking another drug.

BRONCHIOLITIS

Inhaled Beta₂-Agonists (Bronchodilators) *see Asthma page* 29
Oral Beta₂-Agonists (Bronchodilators) *see Asthma page* 33
Inhaled Corticosteroids *see Asthma page* 29
Parenteral Corticosteroids *see page* 499
Oral Corticosteroids *see page* 498

BRONCHITIS: ACUTE/ACUTE EXACERBATION OF CHRONIC BRONCHITIS (AECB)

Comment: Antibiotics are seldom needed for treatment of acute bronchitis because the etiology is usually viral.
Inhaled Beta₂-Agonists (Bronchodilators) *see Asthma page* 29
Oral Beta₂-Agonists (Bronchodilators) *see Asthma page* 33

ANTI-INFECTIVES FOR SECONDARY BACTERIAL INFECTION

 amoxicillin (B)(G) <40 kg (88 lb): 20-40 mg/kg/day in 3 divided doses x 10 days or 25-45 mg/kg/day in 2 divided doses x 10 days; *see page 543 for dose by weight table;* ≥40 kg: 500-875 mg bid or 250-500 mg tid x 10 days
Amoxil *Cap:* 250, 500 mg; *Tab:* 875*mg; *Chew tab:* 125, 200, 250, 400 mg (cherry-banana-peppermint) (phenylalanine); *Oral susp:* 125, 250 mg/5 ml (80, 100, 150 ml) (strawberry); 200, 400 mg/5 ml (50, 75, 100 ml) (bubble gum); *Oral drops:* 50 mg/ml (30 ml) (bubble gum)
Moxatag *Tab:* 775 mg ext-rel
Trimox *Tab:* 125, 250 mg; *Cap:* 250, 500 mg; *Oral susp:* 125, 250 mg/5 ml (80, 100, 150 ml) (raspberry-strawberry)

➤ *amoxicillin/clavulanate* (B)(G)
  Augmentin <40 kg: 40-45 mg/kg/day divided tid x 10 days or 90 mg/kg/day divided bid x 10 days; *see page 545 for dose by weight table;* ≥40 kg: 500 mg tid or 875 mg bid x 10 days
    Tab: 250, 500, 875 mg; *Chew tab:* 125, 250 mg (lemon-lime); 200, 400 mg (cherry-banana) (phenylalanine); *Oral susp:* 125 mg/5 ml (banana), 250 mg/5 ml (75, 100, 150 ml) (orange); 200, 400 mg/5 ml (50, 75, 100 ml) (orange) (phenylalanine)
  Augmentin ES-600 <3 months: not recommended; ≥3 months, <40 kg: 90 mg/kg/day divided q 12 hours x 10 days; *see page 546 for dose by weight table;* ≥40 kg: not recommended
    Oral susp: 600 mg/5 ml (50, 75, 100, 125, 150, 200 ml) (strawberry cream) (phenylalanine)
  Augmentin XR <16 years: use other forms; ≥16 years: 2 tabs q 12 hours x 7-10 days
    Tab: 1000*mg ext-rel
➤ *ampicillin* (B) <12 years: not recommended for bronchitis in children; ≥12 years: 250-500 mg qid x 10 days
  Omnipen, Principen *Cap:* 250, 500 mg; *Oral susp:* 125, 250 mg/5 ml (100, 150, 200 ml) (fruit)
➤ *azithromycin* (B)(G) <12 years: not recommended for bronchitis in children; ≥12 years: 500 mg x 1 dose on day 1, then 250 mg daily on days 2-5 or 500 mg once daily x 3 days or 2 gm in a single dose
  Zithromax *Tab:* 250, 500, 600 mg; *Oral susp:* 100 mg/5 ml (15 ml); 200 mg/5 ml(15, 22.5, 30 ml) (cherry); *Pkt:* 1 gm for reconstitution (cherry-banana)
  Zithromax Tri-pak *Tab:* 3 x 500 mg tabs/pck
  Zithromax Z-pak *Tab:* 6 x 250 mg tabs/pck
  Zmax *Oral susp:* 2 gm ext-rel for reconstitution (cherry-banana) (148 mg Na⁺)
➤ *cefaclor* (B)(G) <16 years: not recommended; ≥16 years: 250-500 mg q 8 hours x 10 days; max 2 gm/day
    Tab: 500 mg; *Cap:* 250, 500 mg; *Susp:* 125 mg/5 ml (75, 150 ml) (strawberry); 187 mg/5 ml (50, 100 ml) (strawberry); 250 mg/5 ml (75, 150 ml) (strawberry); 375 mg/5 ml (50, 100 ml) (strawberry)
  Cefaclor Extended Release <16 years: not recommended; ≥16 years: 500 mg bid (clinically equivalent to 250 mg immed-rel caps tid); swallow whole; take with meals
    Tab: 375, 500 mg ext-rel
➤ *cefadroxil* (B) <12 years: 30 mg/kg/day in 2 divided doses x 10 days; *see page 550 for dose by weight table;* ≥12 years: 1-2 gm in 1-2 divided doses x 10 days
  Duricef *Tab:* 1 g; *Cap:* 500 mg; *Oral susp:* 250 mg/5 ml (100 ml); 500 mg/5 ml (75, 100 ml) (orange-pineapple)
➤ *cefdinir* (B) <6 months: not recommended; 6 months-12 years: 14 mg/kg/day in 1-2 divided doses x 10 days; *see page 551 for dose by weight table;* >12 years: 300 mg bid x 10 days or 600 mg daily x 10 days
  Omnicef *Cap:* 300 mg; *Oral susp:* 125 mg/5 ml (60, 100 ml) (strawberry)
➤ *cefditoren pivoxil* (B) <12 years: not recommended; ≥12 years: 400 mg bid x 10 days
  Spectracef *Tab:* 200 mg
  Comment: **Spectracef** is contraindicated with milk protein allergy or carnitine deficiency.

▷ *cefixime* (B)(G) <6 months: not recommended; 6 months-12 years, <50 kg: 8 mg/kg/day in 1-2 divided doses x 10 days; *see page 552 for dose by weight table;* >12 years, >50 kg: 400 mg once daily x 10 days
  Suprax *Tab:* 400 mg; *Cap:* 400 mg; *Oral susp:* 100, 200, 500 mg/5 ml (50, 75, 100 ml)(strawberry)

▷ *cefpodoxime proxetil* (B) <2 months: not recommended; ≥2 months-12 years: 10 mg/kg/day (max 400 mg/dose) or 5 mg/kg/day bid (max 200 mg/dose) x 10 days; *see page 553 for dose by weight table;* >12 years: 200 mg bid x 10 days

▷ *cefprozil* (B) <2 years: not recommended; 2-12 years: 15 mg/kg bid x 10 days; *see page 554 for dose by weight table;* >12 years: 250-500 mg bid or 500 mg daily x 10 days
  Cefzil *Tab:* 250, 500 mg; *Oral susp:* 125, 250 mg/5 ml (50, 75, 100 ml) (bubble gum) (phenylalanine)

▷ *ceftibuten* (B) <12 years: 9 mg/kg daily x 10 days; max 400 mg/day; *see page 555 for dose by weight table;* ≥12 years: 400 mg daily x 10 days
  Cedax *Cap:* 400 mg; *Oral susp:* 90 mg/5 ml (30, 60, 90, 120 ml); 180 mg/5 ml (30, 60, 120 ml) (cherry)

▷ *ceftriaxone* (B)(G) <12 years: 50 mg/kg IM daily; continue 2 days after clinical stability; ≥12 years: 1-2 gm IM daily; continue 2 days after signs of infection have disappeared; max 4 gm/day
  Rocephin *Vial:* 250, 500 mg; 1, 2 g

▷ *cefuroxime axetil* (B)(G) <12 years: 15 mg/kg bid x 10 days; *see page 556 for dose by weight table;* ≥12 years: 250-500 mg bid x 10 days
  Ceftin *Tab:* 250, 500 mg; *Oral susp:* 125, 250 mg/5 ml (50, 100 ml) (tutti-frutti)

▷ *cephalexin* (B)(G) <12 years: 25-50 mg/kg/day in 4 divided doses x 10 days; *see page 557 for dose by weight table;* ≥12 years: 250-500 mg qid x 10 days
  Keflex *Cap:* 250, 333, 500, 750 mg; *Oral susp:* 125, 250 mg/5 ml (100, 200 ml) (strawberry)

▷ *clarithromycin* (C)(G) <6 months: not recommended; ≥6 months-12 years: 7.5 mg/kg bid x 7 days; *see page 558 for dose by weight table;* >12 years: 500 mg or 500 mg ext-rel once daily x 7 days
  Biaxin *Tab:* 250, 500 mg
  Biaxin Oral Suspension *Oral susp:* 125, 250 mg/5 ml (50, 100 ml) (fruit punch)
  Biaxin XL *Tab:* 500 mg ext-rel

▷ *dirithromycin* (C)(G) <12 years: not recommended; ≥12 years: 500 mg daily x 7 days
  Dynabac *Tab:* 250 mg

▷ *doxycycline* (D)(G) <8 years: not recommended; ≥8 years, ≤100 lb: 2 mg/lb on first day in 2 divided doses, followed by 1 mg/lb/day in 1-2 divided doses; ≥8 years, >100 lb: 40-100 mg bid; *see page 561 for dose by weight table*
  Acticlate *Tab:* 75, 150** mg
  Adoxa *Tab:* 50, 75, 100, 150 mg ent-coat
  Doryx *Tab:* 50, 75, 100, 150, 200 mg del-rel
  Monodox *Cap:* 50, 75, 100 mg
  Oracea *Cap:* 40 mg del-rel
  Vibramycin *Tab:* 100 mg; *Cap:* 50, 100 mg; *Syr:* 50 mg/5 ml (raspberry-apple) (sulfites); *Oral susp:* 25 mg/5 ml (raspberry)
  Vibra-Tab *Tab:* 100 mg film-coat

  Comment: *doxycycline* is contraindicated <8 years-of-age, in pregnancy, and lactation (discolors developing tooth enamel). A side effect may be photo-sensitivity (photophobia). Do not give with antacids, calcium supplements, milk or other dairy, or within 2 hours of taking another drug.

➤ *erythromycin ethylsuccinate* (B)(G) 30-50 mg/kg/day in 4 divided doses x 7 days; may double dose with severe infection; max 100 mg/kg/day or 400 mg qid; *see page 563 for dose by weight table*

    EryPed *Oral susp:* 200 mg/5 ml (100, 200 ml) (fruit); 400 mg/5 ml (60, 100, 200 ml) (banana); *Oral drops:* 200, 400 mg/5 ml (50 ml) (fruit); *Chew tab:* 200 mg wafer (fruit)

    E.E.S. *Oral susp:* 200, 400 mg/5 ml (100 ml) (fruit)

    E.E.S. Granules *Oral susp:* 200 mg/5 ml (100, 200 ml) (cherry)

    E.E.S. 400 Tablets *Tab:* 400 mg

➤ *gemifloxacin* (C) <18 years: not recommended; ≥18 years: 320 mg once daily x 5-7 days

    Factive *Tab:* 320*mg

Comment: *gemifloxacin* is contraindicated <18 years-of-age, and during pregnancy and lactation. Risk of tendonitis or tendon rupture.

➤ *levofloxacin* (C) <18 years: not recommended; ≥18 years: *Uncomplicated:* 500 mg daily x 7 days; *Complicated:* 750 mg daily x 7 days

    Levaquin *Tab:* 250, 500, 750 mg

Comment: *levofloxacin* is contraindicated <18 years-of-age, and during pregnancy and lactation. Risk of tendonitis or tendon rupture.

➤ *loracarbef* (B) <12 years: 15 mg/kg/day in 2 divided doses x 7 days; *see page 570 for dose by weight table;* ≥12 years: 200-400 mg bid x 7 days

    Lorabid *Pulvule:* 200, 400 mg; *Oral susp:* 100 mg/5 ml (50, 100 ml); 200 mg/5 ml (50, 75, 100 ml) (strawberry bubble gum)

➤ *moxifloxacin* (C)(G) <18 years: not recommended; ≥18 years: 400 mg daily x 5 days

    Avelox *Tab:* 400 mg; *IV soln:* 400 mg/250 mg (latex-free, preservative-free)

Comment: *moxifloxacin* is contraindicated <18 years-of-age and during pregnancy and lactation. Risk of tendonitis or tendon rupture.

➤ *ofloxacin* (C)(G) <18 years: not recommended; ≥18 years: 400 mg bid x 10 days

    Floxin *Tab:* 200, 300, 400 mg

Comment: *ofloxacin* is contraindicated <18 years-of-age and during pregnancy and lactation. Risk of tendonitis or tendon rupture.

➤ *telithromycin* (C) <18 years: not recommended; ≥18 years: 2 x 400 mg tabs in a single dose daily x 5 days

    Ketek *Tab:* 400 mg

➤ *tetracycline* (D)(G) <8 years: not recommended; ≥8 years, ≤100 lb: 25-50 mg/kg/day in 4 divided doses x 7 days; *see page 574 for dose by weight table;* ≥8 years, >100 lb: 250-500 mg qid x 7 days

    Achromycin V *Cap:* 250, 500 mg

    Sumycin *Tab:* 250, 500 mg; *Cap:* 250, 500 mg; *Oral susp:* 125 mg/5 ml (100, 200 ml) (fruit) (sulfites)

Comment: *tetracycline* is contraindicated <8 years-of-age, in pregnancy, and lactation (discolors developing tooth enamel). A side effect may be photo-sensitivity (photophobia). Do not give with antacids, calcium supplements, milk or other dairy, or within two hours of taking another drug.

➤ *trimethoprim/sulfamethoxazole* (D)(G)

    Bactrim, Septra <12 years: not recommended; ≥12 years: 2 tabs bid x 10 days

    Tab: trim 80 mg/sulfa 400 mg*

Bactrim DS, Septra DS <12 years: not recommended; ≥12 years: 1 tab bid x 10 days
> *Tab: trim* 160 mg/*sulfa* 800 mg*

Bactrim Pediatric Suspension, Septra Pediatric Suspension <2 months: not recommended; ≥2 months-12 years: 40 mg/kg/day of *sulfamethoxazole* in 2 doses bid; >12 years: use tabs
> *Oral susp: trim* 40 mg/*sulfa* 200 mg per 5 ml (100 ml) (cherry) (alcohol 0.3%)

BULIMIA NERVOSA

SELECTIVE SEROTONIN REUPTAKE INHIBITOR (SSRI)

▷ *fluoxetine* (C)(G)
Prozac <8 years: not recommended; 8-17 years: initially 10 mg/day; may increase after 1 week to 20 mg/day; range 20-60 mg/day; range for lower weight children, 20-30 mg/day; >17 years: initially 20 mg daily; may increase after 1 week; doses >20 mg/day should be divided into AM and noon doses; max 80 mg/day
> *Cap:* 10, 20, 40 mg; *Tab:* 30*, 60*mg; *Oral soln:* 20 mg/5 ml (4 oz) (mint)

Prozac Weekly <12 years: not recommended; ≥12 years: following daily *fluoxetine* therapy at 20 mg/day for 13 weeks, may initiate **Prozac Weekly** 7 days after the last 20 mg *fluoxetine* dose
> *Cap:* 90 mg ent-coat del-rel pellets

BURN: MINOR

▷ *silver sulfadiazine* (B)(G) <12 years: not established; ≥12 years: apply bid
Silvadene *Crm:* 1% (20 gm tube; 20, 50, 85, 400, 1,000 gm jar)
Comment: *silver sulfadiazine* is contradicted in sulfa allergy, late pregnancy, within the first 2 months after birth, premature infants.

TOPICAL/TRANSDERMAL ANESTHETICS

Comment: *lidocaine* gel, cream, lotion, or patch is not recommended <12 years-of-age and should not be applied to non-intact skin and
▷ *lidocaine* burn gel (B)(G)
▷ *lidocaine* cream (B)(G)
LidaMantle *Crm:* 3% (1, 2 oz)
Lidoderm *Crm:* 3% (85 gm)
▷ *lidocaine* lotion (B)(G)
LidaMantle *Lotn:* 3% (177 ml)
▷ *lidocaine* 5% patch (B)(G) apply up to 3 patches at one time for up to 12 hours/24 hour period (12 hours on/12 hours off); patches may be cut into smaller sizes before removal of the release liner; do not reuse
Lidoderm *Patch:* 5% (10 x 14 cm; 30/carton)
▷ *lidocaine* 2.5%/*prilocaine* 2.5%
Emla Cream (B) (5, 30 gm)

BURSITIS

Acetaminophen for IV Infusion *see **Pain** page* 296
Oral Prescription NSAIDs *see page* 490
Other Oral Analgesics *see **Pain** page* 298
Topical/Transdermal NSAIDs *see **Pain** page* 298
Parenteral Corticosteroids *see page* 499
Oral Corticosteroids *see page* 498
Topical Analgesic and Anesthetic Agents *see page* 488

CANDIDIASIS: ABDOMEN, BLADDER, ESOPHAGUS, KIDNEY

▷ *voriconazole* (D)(G) *PO*: <40 kg: 100 mg q 12 hours; may increase to150 mg q 12
hours if inadequate response; ≥40 kg: 200 mg q 12 hours; may increase to 300 mg q
12 hours if inadequate; *IV*: 6 mg/kg q 12 hours x 2 doses; then 4 mg/kg q 12 hour;
max rate 3 mg/kg/hour over 1-2 hours
Vfend *Tab*: 50, 200 mg
Vfend I.V. for Injection *Vial*: 200 mg pwdr for reconstitution (preservative-free)
Vfend *Oral susp*: 40 mg/ml pwdr for reconstitution (75 ml) (orange)

 CANDIDIASIS: ORAL (THRUSH)

ORAL ANTIFUNGALS

▷ *clotrimazole* (C) <3 years: not recommended; ≥3 years: *Prophylaxis:* 1 troche dissolved in mouth tid; *Treatment:* 1 troche dissolved in mouth 5 times/day x 10-14 days
Mycelex Troches *Troches*: 10 mg
▷ *fluconazole* (C) <2 weeks: not recommended; 2 weeks-12 years: 6 mg/kg x 1 day;
then 3 mg/kg/day for at least 3 weeks; *see page 566 for dose by weight table*; >12
years: 200 mg x 1 dose first day; then 100 mg once daily x 13 days
Diflucan *Tab*: 50, 100, 150, 200 mg; *Oral susp*: 10, 40 mg/ml (35 ml) (orange)
(sucrose)
▷ *gentian violet* (NE)(G) apply to oral mucosa with a cotton swab tid x 3 days
▷ *itraconazole* (C) <12 years: 5 mg/kg daily x 7-14 days; max 200 mg/day; *see page
569 for dose by weight table*; ≥12 years: 200 mg daily x 7-14 days
Sporanox *Oral soln*: 10 mg/ml (150 ml) (cherry-caramel)
▷ *miconazole* (C) <16 years: not recommended; ≥16 years: 1 buccal tab once daily x
14 days; apply to upper gum region; hold place 30 seconds; do not crush, chew, or
swallow
Oravig *Buccal tab*: 50 mg (14/pck)
▷ *nystatin* (C)(G)
Mycostatin 1-2 pastilles dissolved slowly in mouth 4-5 times/day x 10-14 days;
max 14 days
Pastille: 200,000 units/pastille (30 pastilles/pck)
Mycostatin Suspension *Infants*: 1 ml in each cheek qid after feedings; *Older
children*: 4-6 ml qid swish and swallow
Oral susp: 100,000 units/ml (60 ml w. dropper)

INVASIVE INFECTION

▷ *posaconazole* (D) <13 years: not recommended; ≥13 years: take with food; 100 mg bid on day one; then 100 mg once daily x 13 days; refractory, 400 mg bid

Noxafil *Oral susp:* 40 mg/ml (105 ml) (cherry)

Comment: **Noxafil** is indicated as prophylaxis for invasive aspergillus and candida infections in patients >13 years old who are at high risk due to being severely compromised.

CANDIDIASIS: SKIN

TOPICAL ANTIFUNGALS

▷ *butenafine* (B) <12 years: not recommended; ≥12 years: apply bid x 1 week <u>or</u> once daily x 4 weeks

Lotrimin Ultra (C)(OTC) *Crm:* 1% (12, 24 gm)

Mentax *Crm:* 1% (15, 30 gm)

Comment: *butenafine* is a benzylamine, not an azole. Fungicidal activity continues for at least 5 weeks after the last application.

▷ *ciclopirox* (B)

Loprox Cream <10 years: not recommended; ≥10 years: apply bid; max 4 weeks
Crm: 0.77% (15, 30, 90 gm)

Loprox Lotion <10 years: not recommended; ≥10 years: apply bid; max 4 weeks
Lotn: 0.77% (30, 60 ml)

Loprox Gel <16 years: not recommended; ≥16 years: apply bid; max 4 weeks
Gel: 0.77% (30, 45 gm)

▷ *clotrimazole* (B) apply bid x 7 days

Lotrimin *Crm:* 1% (15, 30, 45 gm)

Lotrimin AF (OTC) *Crm:* 1% (12 gm); *Lotn:* 1% (10 ml); *Soln:* 1% (10 ml)

▷ *econazole* (C) apply bid x 14 days

Spectazole *Crm:* 1% (15, 30, 85 gm)

▷ *ketoconazole* (C) apply once daily x 14 days

Nizoral Cream *Crm:* 2% (15, 30, 60 gm)

▷ *miconazole* 2% (C) apply once daily x 2 weeks

Lotrimin AF Spray Liquid (OTC) *Spray liq:* 2% (113 gm) (alcohol 17%)

Lotrimin AF Spray Powder (OTC) *Spray pwdr:* 2% (90 gm) (alcohol 10%)

Monistat-Derm *Crm:* 2% (1, 3 oz); *Spray liq:* 2% (3.5 oz); *Spray pwdr:* 2%(3 oz)

▷ *nystatin* (C)

Nystop Powder dust affected skin freely bid-tid
Pwdr: nystatin 100,000 U/g (15 gm)

ORAL ANTIFUNGALS

▷ *amphotericin b* (B) apply tid-qid x 7-14 days

Fungizone *Oral susp:* 100 mg/ml (24 ml w. dropper)

▷ *ketoconazole* (C)(G) <2 years: not recommended; ≥2 years-12 years: 3.3-6.6 mg/ kg once daily x 4 weeks; >12 years: initially 200 mg once daily; max 400 mg/day x 4 weeks

Nizoral *Tab:* 200 mg

Comment: Caution with *ketoconazole* due to potential for hepatotoxicity.

INVASIVE INFECTION

▷ *posaconazole* (D) <13 years: not recommended; ≥13 years: take with food; 100 mg bid on day one; then 100 mg once daily x 13 days; refractory, 400 mg bid x 13 days

    Noxafil *Oral susp:* 40 mg/ml (105 ml) (cherry)

    Comment: **Noxafil** is indicated as prophylaxis for invasive aspergillus and candida infections in patients >13 years old who are at high risk due to being severely compromised.

 # CANDIDIASIS: VULVOVAGINAL (MONILIASIS)

PROPHYLAXIS

▷ *acetic acid/oxyquinolone* (C) <12 years: not recommended; ≥12 years: one full applicator intravaginally bid for up to 30 days

    Relagard *Gel: acetic acid* 0.9%/*oxyquin* 0.025% (50 gm tube w. applicator)

    Comment: The following treatment regimens for vulvovaginal candidiasis (VVC) are published in the **2015 CDC Sexually Transmitted Diseases Treatment Guidelines**. Treatment regimens are presented by generic drug name first, followed by information about brands and dose forms. Complicated VVC (recurrent, severe, non-albicans, <u>or</u> females with uncontrolled diabetes, debilitation, <u>or</u> immunosuppression) may require more intensive treatment <u>and/or</u> longer duration of treatment. VVC frequently occurs during pregnancy. Only topical azole therapies, applied for 7 days, are recommended during pregnancy.

ORAL RX AGENT

▷ *fluconazole* 150 mg in a single dose; complicated VVC, 150 mg x 3 doses on days 1, 4, 7 <u>or</u> weekly x 6 months

RX INTRAVAGINAL AGENTS

Regimen 1

▷ *butoconazole* 2% cream (bioadhesive product) 5 gm intravaginally in a single dose

Regimen 2

▷ *nystatin* 100,000-unit vaginal tablet once daily x 14 days

Regimen 3

▷ *terconazole* 0.4% cream 5 gm intravaginally once daily x 7 days

Regimen 4

▷ *terconazole* 0.8% cream 5 gm intravaginally once daily x 3 days

Regimen 5

▷ *terconazole* 80 mg vaginal suppository intravaginally once daily x 3 days

OTC INTRAVAGINAL AGENTS

Regimen 1

▷ *butoconazole* 2% cream 5 gm intravaginally once daily x 3 days

Regimen 2

▷ *clotrimazole* 1% cream intravaginally once daily x 7-14 days

Regimen 3

▷ *clotrimazole* 2% cream intravaginally once daily x 3 days

Regimen 4

▷ *miconazole* 2% cream intravaginally once daily x 7 days

Regimen 5

▷ *miconazole* 4% cream intravaginally once daily x 3 days

Regimen 6

▷ *miconazole* 100 mg vaginal suppository intravaginally once daily x 7 days

Regimen 7

▷ *miconazole* 200 mg vaginal suppository intravaginally once daily x 3 days

Regimen 8

▷ *miconazole* 1,200 mg vaginal suppository intravaginally in a single application

Regimen 9

▷ *tioconazole* 6.5% ointment 5 gm intravaginally in a single application

DRUG BRANDS AND DOSE FORMS

▷ *butoconazole* cream 2% (C)
    Gynazole-12% Vaginal Cream *Prefilled vag applicator:* 5 g
    Femstat-3 Vaginal Cream (OTC) *Vag crm:* 2% (20 gm w. 3 applicators); *Prefilled vag applicator:* 5 gm (3/pck)
▷ *clotrimazole* (B)(OTC)
    Gyne-Lotrimin Vaginal Cream (OTC) *Vag crm:* 1% (45 gm w. applicator)
    Gyne-Lotrimin Vaginal Suppository (OTC) *Vag supp:* 100 mg (7/pck)
    Gyne-Lotrimin 3 Vaginal Suppository (OTC) *Vag supp:* 200 mg (3/pck)
    Gyne-Lotrimin Combination Pack (OTC) *Combination pck:* 7-100 mg supp with 7 gm 1% cream
    Gyne-Lotrimin 3 Combination Pack (OTC) *Combination pck:* 200 mg supp (7/pck) plus 1% cream (7 gm)
    Mycelex-G Vaginal Cream *Vag crm:* 1% (45, 90 gm w. applicator)
    Mycelex-G Vaginal Tab 1 *Tab:* 500 mg (1/pck)
    Mycelex Twin Pack *Twin pck:* 500 mg tab (7/pck) with 1% crm (7 gm)
    Mycelex-7 Vaginal Cream (OTC) *Vag crm:* 1% (45 gm w. applicator)

      Mycelex-7 Vaginal Inserts (OTC) *Vag insert:* 100 mg insert (7/pck)
      Mycelex-7 Combination Pack (OTC) *Combination pck:* 100 mg inserts (7/pck)
      plus 1% crm (7 gm)
▶ *fluconazole* (C)
      Diflucan *Tab:* 50, 100, 150, 200 mg; *Oral susp:* 10, 40 mg/ml (35 ml) (orange)
      (sucrose)
▶ *miconazole* (B)
      Monistat-3 Combination Pack (OTC) *Combination pck:* 200 mg supp (3/pck)
      plus 2% crm (9 gm)
      Monistat-7 Combination Pack (OTC) *Combination pck:* 100 mg supp (7/pck)
      plus 2% crm (9 gm)
      Monistat-7 Vaginal Cream (OTC) *Vag crm:* 2% (45 gm w. applicator)
      Monistat-7 Vaginal Suppositories (OTC) *Vag supp:* 100 mg supp (7/pck)
      Monistat-3 Vaginal Suppositories (OTC) *Vag supp:* 200 mg supp (3/pck)
▶ *nystatin* (C)
      Mycostatin *Vag tab:* 100,000 U (1/pck)
▶ *terconazole* (C)
      Terazol-3 Vaginal Cream *Vag crm:* 0.8% (20 gm w. applicator)
      Terazol-3 Vaginal Suppositories *Vag supp:* 80 mg supp (3/pck)
      Terazol-7 Vaginal Cream *Vag crm:* 0.4% (45 gm w. applicator)
▶ *tioconazole* (C)
      1-Day (OTC) *Vag oint:* 6.5% (prefilled applicator x 1)
      Monistat 1 Vaginal Ointment (OTC) *Vag oint:* 6.5% (prefilled applicator x 1)
      Vagistat-1 Vaginal Ointment (OTC) *Vag oint:* 6.5% (prefilled applicator x 1)

INVASIVE INFECTION

▶ *posaconazole* (D) <13 years: not recommended; ≥13 years: take with food; 100 mg
   bid on day 1; then 100 mg once daily x 13 days; refractory, 400 mg bid
      Noxafil *Oral susp:* 40 mg/ml (105 ml) (cherry)
      Comment: **Noxafil** is indicated as prophylaxis for invasive aspergillus and
      candida infections in patients ≥13 years old who are at high risk due to being
      severely compromised.

CARCINOID SYNDROME DIARRHEA

TRIPTOPHAN HYDROXYLASE

▶ *telotristat* <18 years: not established; ≥18 years: take with food; 250 mg tid
      Xermelo *Tab:* 250 mg (4 x 7 daily dose packs/carton)
  Comment: Take **Xermelo** in combination with somatostatin analog (SSA) therapy
  to treat patients inadequately controlled by SSA therapy. Breastfeeding females
  should monitor the infant for constipation.

CARPAL TUNNEL SYNDROME (CTS)

Acetaminophen for IV Infusion *see* **Pain** *page* 296
Oral Prescription NSAIDs *see page* 490

Other Oral Analgesics *see* ***Pain*** *page* 298
Topical/Transdermal NSAIDs *see* ***Pain*** *page* 298
Parenteral Corticosteroids *see page* 499
Oral Corticosteroids *see page* 498
Topical Analgesic and Anesthetic Agents *see page* 488

CAT SCRATCH FEVER (*BARTONELLA* INFECTION)

Comment: Cat scratch fever is usually self-limited. Treatment should be limited to severe <u>or</u> debilitating cases.

ANTI-INFECTIVES

▷ *azithromycin* (B)(G) <12 years: 12 mg/kg/day x 5 days; *see page* 548 *for dose by weight table*; max 500 mg/day; ≥12 years: 500 mg x 1 dose on day 1, then 250 mg daily on days 2-5 <u>or</u> 500 mg daily x 3 days <u>or</u> **Zmax** 2 gm in a single dose
 Zithromax *Tab:* 250, 500, 600 mg; *Oral susp:* 100 mg/5 ml (15 ml); 200 mg/5 ml (15, 22.5, 30 ml) (cherry); *Pkt:* 1 gm for reconstitution (cherry-banana)
 Zithromax Tri-pak *Tab:* 3 x 500 mg tabs/pck
 Zithromax Z-pak *Tab:* 6 x 250 mg tabs/pck
 Zmax *Oral susp:* 2 gm ext-rel for reconstitution (cherry-banana) (148 mg Na+)
▷ *doxycycline* (D)(G) <8 years: not recommended; ≥8 years, ≤100 lb: 2 mg/lb on first day in 2 divided doses, followed by 1 mg/lb/day in 1-2 divided doses; ≥8 years, >100 lb: 100 mg bid; *see page* 561 *for dose by weight table*
 Acticlate *Tab:* 75, 150** mg
 Adoxa *Tab:* 50, 75, 100, 150 mg ent-coat
 Doryx *Tab:* 50, 75, 100, 150, 200 mg del-rel
 Monodox *Cap:* 50, 75, 100 mg
 Oracea *Cap:* 40 mg del-rel
 Vibramycin *Tab:* 100 mg; *Cap:* 50, 100 mg; *Syr:* 50 mg/5 ml (raspberry-apple) (sulfites); *Oral susp:* 25 mg/5 ml (raspberry)
 Vibra-Tab *Tab:* 100 mg film-coat
Comment: *doxycycline* is contraindicated <8 years-of-age, in pregnancy, and lactation (discolors developing tooth enamel). A side effect may be photo-sensitivity (photophobia). Do not give with antacids, calcium supplements, milk <u>or</u> other dairy, <u>or</u> within 2 hours of taking another drug.
▷ *erythromycin base* (B)(G) 45 kg: 30-50 mg in 2-4 divided doses x 4 weeks; ≥45 kg: 500-1000 mg qid x 4 weeks
 Ery-Tab *Tab:* 250, 333, 500 mg ent-coat
 PCE *Tab:* 333, 500 mg
▷ *erythromycin ethylsuccinate* (B)(G) 30-50 mg/kg/day in 4 divided doses x 4 weeks; may double dose with severe infection; max 100 mg/kg/day <u>or</u> 400 mg qid; *see page* 563 *for dose by weight table*
 EryPed *Oral susp:* 200 mg/5 ml (100, 200 ml) (fruit); 400 mg/5 ml (60, 100, 200 ml) (banana); *Oral drops:* 200, 400 mg/5 ml (50 ml) (fruit); Chew tab: 200 mg wafer (fruit)
 E.E.S. *Oral susp:* 200, 400 mg/5 ml (100 ml) (fruit)
 E.E.S. Granules *Oral susp:* 200 mg/5 ml (100, 200 ml) (cherry)
 E.E.S. 400 Tablets *Tab:* 400 mg

➤ *trimethoprim/sulfamethoxazole* (D)(G)

> **Bactrim, Septra** <12 years: not recommended; ≥12 years: 2 tabs bid x 10 days
> *Tab:* trim 80 mg/*sulfa* 400 mg*
> **Bactrim DS, Septra DS** <12 years: not recommended; ≥12 years: 1 tab bid x 10 days
> *Tab:* trim 160 mg/*sulfa* 800 mg*
> **Bactrim Pediatric Suspension, Septra Pediatric Suspension** <2 months: not recommended; ≥2 months-12 years: 40 mg/kg/day of *sulfamethoxazole* in 2 doses bid; >12 years: use tabs
> *Oral susp:* trim 40 mg/*sulfa* 200 mg per 5 ml (100 ml) (cherry) (alcohol 0.3%)

CELLULITIS

Comment: Duration of treatment should be 10-30 days. Obtain culture from site. Consider blood cultures.

ANTI-INFECTIVES

➤ *amoxicillin* (B)(G) <40 kg (88 lb): 20-40 mg/kg/day in 3 divided doses x 10 days or 25-45 mg/kg/day in 2 divided doses x 10 days; *see page 543 for dose by weight table;* ≥40 kg: 500-875 mg bid or 250-500 mg tid x 10 days

> **Amoxil** *Cap:* 250, 500 mg; *Tab:* 875*mg; *Chew tab:* 125, 200, 250, 400 mg (cherry-banana-peppermint) (phenylalanine); *Oral susp:* 125, 250 mg/5 ml (80, 100, 150 ml) (strawberry); 200, 400 mg/5 ml (50, 75, 100 ml) (bubble gum); *Oral drops:* 50 mg/ml (30 ml) (bubble gum)
> **Moxatag** *Tab:* 775 mg ext-rel
> **Trimox** *Tab:* 125, 250 mg; *Cap:* 250, 500 mg; *Oral susp:* 125, 250 mg/5 ml (80, 100, 150 ml) (raspberry-strawberry)

➤ *amoxicillin/clavulanate* (B)(G)

> **Augmentin** <40 kg: 40-45 mg/kg/day divided tid x 10 days or 90 mg/kg/day divided bid x 10 days; *see page 545 for dose by weight table;* ≥40 kg: 500 mg tid or 875 mg bid x 10 days
> *Tab:* 250, 500, 875 mg; *Chew tab:* 125, 250 mg (lemon-lime); 200, 400 mg (cherry-banana) (phenylalanine); *Oral susp:* 125 mg/5 ml (banana), 250 mg/5 ml (75, 100, 150 ml) (orange); 200, 400 mg/5 ml (50, 75, 100 ml) (orange) (phenylalanine)
> **Augmentin ES-600** <3 months: not recommended; ≥3 months, <40 kg: 90 mg/kg/day divided q 12 hours x 10 days; *see page 546 for dose by weight table;* ≥40 kg: not recommended
> *Oral susp:* 600 mg/5 ml (50, 75, 100, 125, 150, 200 ml) (strawberry cream) (phenylalanine)
> **Augmentin XR** <16 years: use other forms; ≥16 years: 2 tabs q 12 hours x 7-10 days
> *Tab:* 1000*mg ext-rel

➤ *azithromycin* (B)(G) <12 years: 12 mg/kg/day x 5 days; *see page 548 for dose by weight table;* max 500 mg/day; ≥12 years: 500 mg x 1 dose on day 1, then 250 mg daily on days 2-5 or 500 mg daily x 3 days **oarsman** 2 gm in a single dose

> **Zithromax** *Tab:* 250, 500, 600 mg; *Oral susp:* 100 mg/5 ml (15 ml); 200 mg/5 ml (15, 22.5, 30 ml) (cherry); *Pkt:* 1 gm for reconstitution (cherry-banana)

Zithromax Tri-pak *Tab:* 3 x 500 mg tabs/pck
Zithromax Z-pak *Tab:* 6 x 250 mg tabs/pck
Zmax *Oral susp:* 2 gm ext-rel for reconstitution (cherry-banana) (148 mg Na⁺)

▷ *cefaclor* **(B)(G)** <1 month: not recommended; 1 month-12 years: 20-40 mg/kg in 2 or 3 divided doses x 10 days; *see page 549 for dose by weight table;* max 1 gm/day; >12 years: 375 mg q 12 hours x 10 days; max 2 gm/day
   Tab: 500 mg; *Cap:* 250, 500 mg; *Susp:* 125 mg/5 ml (75, 150 ml) (strawberry); 187 mg/5 ml (50, 100 ml) (strawberry); 250 mg/5 ml (75, 150 ml) (strawberry); 375 mg/5 ml (50, 100 ml) (strawberry)
   Cefaclor Extended Release <16 years: not recommended; ≥16 years: 500 mg bid x 10 days (clinically equivalent to 250 mg immed-rel caps tid); swallow whole; take with food
   Tab: 375, 500 mg ext-rel

▷ *cefpodoxime proxetil* **(B)(G)** <2 months: not recommended; ≥2 months-12 years: 10 mg/kg/day (max 400 mg/dose) or 5 mg/kg/day bid (max 200 mg/dose) x 7-14 days; *see page 553 for dose by weight table;* >12 years: 400 mg bid x 7-14 days

▷ *cefprozil* **(B)** <2 years: not recommended; 2-12 years: 15 mg/kg bid x 10 days; *see page 554 for dose by weight table;* >12 years: 250-500 mg bid or 500 mg daily x 10 days
   Cefzil *Tab:* 250, 500 mg; *Oral susp:* 125, 250 mg/5 ml (50, 75, 100 ml) (bubble gum) (phenylalanine)

▷ *ceftaroline fosamil* **(B)** <18 years: not established; ≥18 years: administer 600 mg once every 12 hours, by IV infusion over 5-60 minutes, x 5-14 days
   Teflaro *Vial:* 400, 600 mg pwdr for reconstitution, single use (10/carton)
   Comment: **Teflaro** is indicated for the treatment of acute bacterial skin and skin structures infection (ABSSSI).

▷ *ceftriaxone* **(B)(G)** <12 years: 50-75 mg/kg IM in 1-2 divided doses x 5-14 days; max 2 gm/day; ≥12 years: 1-2 gm IM daily x 5-14 days; max 4 gm daily
   Rocephin *Vial:* 250, 500 mg; 1, 2 g

▷ *cefuroxime axetil* **(B)(G)** <3 months: not recommended; ≥3 months-12 years: 30 mg/kg/day in 2 divided doses x 10 days; *see page 556 for dose by weight table;* ≥12 years: 250-500 mg bid x 10 days
   Ceftin *Tab:* 250, 500 mg; *Oral susp:* 125, 250 mg/5 ml (50, 100 ml) (tutti-frutti)

▷ *cephalexin* **(B)(G)** <12 years: 25-50 mg/kg/day in 4 divided doses x 10 days; *see page 557 for dose by weight table;* ≥12 years: 500 mg bid x 10 days
   Keflex *Cap:* 250, 333, 500, 750 mg; *Oral susp:* 125, 250 mg/5 ml (100, 200 ml) (strawberry)

▷ *clarithromycin* **(C)(G)** <6 months: not recommended; ≥6 months-12 years: 7.5 mg/kg bid x 10 days; *seepage 558 for dose by weight table;* >12 years: 500 mg q 12 hours or 500 mg ext-rel once daily x 10 days
   Biaxin *Tab:* 250, 500 mg
   Biaxin Oral Suspension *Oral susp:* 125, 250 mg/5 ml (50, 100 ml) (fruit punch)
   Biaxin XL *Tab:* 500 mg ext-rel

▷ *dalbavancin* **(C)** <18 years: not established; ≥18 years: 1,000 mg administered once as a single dose via IV infusion over 30 minutes or initially 1,000 mg once, followed by 500 mg 1 week later; infuse over 30 minutes; *CrCl <30 mL/min, not receiving dialysis:* initially 750 mg, followed by 375 mg 1 week later
   Dalvance *Vial:* 500 mg pwdr for reconstitution, single use (preservative-free)
   Comment: **Dalvance** is indicated for the treatment of acute bacterial skin and skin structures infection (ABSSSI) caused by gram positive bacteria.

▷ *dicloxacillin* **(B)(G)** <12 years: 12.5-25 mg/kg/day in 4 divided doses x 10 days; *see page* 560 *for dose by weight table;* ≥12 years: 500 mg q 6 hours x 10 days
    Dynapen *Cap:* 125, 250, 500 mg; *Oral susp:* 62.5 mg/5 ml (80, 100, 200 ml)

▷ *dirithromycin* **(C)(G)** <12 years: not recommended; ≥12 years: 500 mg once daily x 7-10 days
    Dynabac *Tab:* 250 mg

▷ *erythromycin base* **(B)(G)** <45 kg: 30-50 mg in 2-4 divided doses x 7-10 days; ≥45 kg: 250 mg qid *or* 333 mg tid *or* 500 mg bid x 7-10 days; then taper to lowest effective dose
    Ery-Tab *Tab:* 250, 333, 500 mg ent-coat
    PCE *Tab:* 333, 500 mg

▷ *erythromycin ethylsuccinate* **(B)(G)** 30-50 mg/kg/day in 4 divided doses x 7-10 days; may double dose with severe infection; max 100 mg/kg/day *or* 400 mg qid; *see page* 563 *for dose by weight table*
    EryPed *Oral susp:* 200 mg/5 ml (100, 200 ml) (fruit); 400 mg/5 ml (60, 100, 200 ml) (banana); *Oral drops:* 200, 400 mg/5 ml (50 ml) (fruit); *Chew tab:* 200 mg wafer (fruit)
    E.E.S. *Oral susp:* 200, 400 mg/5 ml (100 ml) (fruit)
    E.E.S. Granules *Oral susp:* 200 mg/5 ml (100, 200 ml) (cherry)
    E.E.S. 400 Tablets *Tab:* 400 mg

▷ *linezolid* **(C)(G)** <5 years: 10 mg/kg q 8 hours x 10-14 days; 5-11 years: 10 mg/kg q 12 hours x 10-14 days; >11 years: 400-600 mg q 12 hours x 10-14 days
    Zyvox *Tab:* 400, 600 mg; *Oral susp:* 100 mg/5 ml (150 ml) (orange) (phenylalanine)
    Comment: *linezolid* is indicated to treat susceptible vancomycin-resistant *E. faecium* infections of skin and skin structures, including diabetic foot without osteomyelitis.

▷ *loracarbef* **(B)** <12 years: 15 mg/kg/day in 2 divided doses x 10 days; *see page* 570 *for dose by weight table;* ≥12 years: 200 mg bid x 10 days
    Lorabid *Pulvule:* 200, 400 mg; *Oral susp:* 100 mg/5 ml (50, 100 ml); 200 mg/5 ml (50, 75, 100 ml) (strawberry bubble gum)

▷ *moxifloxacin* **(C)(G)** <18 years: not recommended; ≥18 years: 400 mg daily x 5 days
    Avelox *Tab:* 400 mg; IV soln: 400 mg/250 mg (latex-free, preservative-free)
    Comment: *moxifloxacin* is contraindicated <18 years-of-age and during pregnancy and lactation. Risk of tendonitis *or* tendon.

▷ *oritavancin* **(C)** <18 years: not established; ≥18 years: administer 1,200 mg as a single dose by IV infusion over 3 hours
    Orbactiv *Vial:* 400 mg pwdr for reconstitution, single use (10/carton) (mannitol; preservative-free)
    Comment: **Orbactiv** is indicated for the treatment of acute bacterial skin and skin structures infection (ABSSSI).

▷ *penicillin V potassium* **(B)** <12 years: 25-75 mg/kg day divided q 6-8 hours x 5-7 days; *see page* 572 *for dose by weight table;* ≥12 years: 250-500 mg q 6 hours x 5-7 days
    Pen-VK *Tab:* 250, 500 mg; *Oral soln:* 125 mg/5 ml (100, 200 ml); 250 mg/5 ml (100, 150, 200 ml)

▷ *tedizolid phosphate* **(C)** <18 years: not established; ≥18 years: administer 200 mg once daily x 6 days, via PO *or* IV infusion over 1 hour
    Sivextro *Tab:* 200 mg (6/blister pck)

Comment: **Sivextro** is indicated for the treatment of acute bacterial skin and skin structures infection (ABSSSI).

▷ **tigecycline** (D)(G) <18 years: not recommended; ≥18 years: 100 mg as a single dose; then 50 mg q 12 hours x 5-14 days; with severe hepatic impairment (Child Pugh C), 100 mg as a single dose; then 25 mg q 12 hours

    Tygacil *Vial:* 50 mg pwdr for reconstitution and IV infusion (preservative-free)

    Comment: **Tygacil** is contraindicated in pregnancy, and lactation (discolors developing tooth enamel). A side effect may be photo-sensitivity (photophobia). Do not give with antacids, calcium supplements, milk <u>or</u> other dairy, <u>or</u> within two hours of taking another drug.

CERUMEN IMPACTION

OTIC ANALGESIC

▷ **antipyrine/benzocaine/zinc acetate dihydrate** otic (C) fill ear canal with solution; then moisten cotton plug with solution and insert into meatus; may repeat every 1-2 hours prn

    Otozin *Otic soln:* antipyr 5.4%/benz 1%/zinc 1% per ml (10 ml w. dropper)

CERUMINOLYTICS

▷ **triethanolamine** (NE)(OTC)(G) fill ear canal and insert cotton plug for 15-30 minutes before irrigating with warm water

    Cerumenex *Soln:* 10% (6, 12 ml)

▷ **carbamide peroxide** (NE)(OTC)(G) instill 5-10 drops in ear canal; keep drops in ear several minutes; then irrigate with warm water; repeat bid for up to 4 days

    Debrox *Soln:* 15, 30 ml squeeze bottle w. applicator

CHAGAS DISEASE (AMERICAN TRYPANOSOMIASIS)

Comment: Chagas Disease is a protozoal parasite (*Trypanosoma cruzi*) infection with increasing prevalence in the US attributed to immigration from *T. cruzi*- endemic areas of South and Central Latin America. Approximately 300,000 persons in the US have chronic Chagas Disease and up to 30% of them will develop clinically evident cardiovascular and/or gastrointestinal disease. Chagas Disease is one of the five neglected parasitic infections (NPIs) targeted by CDC for public health action. Transmitted by the bite of the triatomine bug ("kissing bug") which feeds on human blood, maternal-fetus vertical transmission, blood transfusion, consumption of contaminated food, and organ donation. A clinical marker is Romaña sign (periorbital swelling), chagoma (skin nodule), Schizotrypanides (nonpruritic morbilliform rash). Only two antiparasitic drugs, **benznidazole** and **nifurtimox**, have demonstrated effectiveness altering the progression of this chronic disease. These drugs are not FDA approved and are available only from CDC under investigational protocols. Treatment is indicated for all cases of acute <u>or</u> reactivated Chagas Disease and for chronic *Trypanosoma cruzi* infection in children ≤18. Congenital infections are considered acute disease. Treatment is strongly recommended up to 50 years old with chronic infection who do not already have advanced Chagas cardiomyopathy. For adults older than 50 years with chronic *T. cruzi* infection, the decision to treat with antiparasitic drugs should be individualized, weighing the potential benefits and risks for the patient. Patients taking either of these drugs should have a CBC and CMP at the start of treatment and then bi-monthly for the duration of treatment to monitor for rare bone marrow suppression. Contraindications for treatment include severe hepatic and/or renal disease. As safety for infants exposed through breastfeeding has not been documented, withholding treatment while breastfeeding is also recommended. For emergencies (for example, acute Chagas Disease with severe manifestations, Chagas Disease in a newborn, or Chagas Disease in an immunocompromised person) outside of regular business hours, call the CDC Emergency Operations Center (770-488-7100) and ask for the person on call for Parasitic Diseases. For more detailed information about screening, assessment, and treatment of this public health threat, see McDonald, J, & Mattingly, J. (November, 2016). Chagas disease: Creeping into family practice in the United States, *Clinician Reviews*, pp. 38-45, or call 404-718-4745 or e-mail questions to chagas@cdc.gov.

ANTI-PARASITIC AGENTS

➤ *benznidazole* **(NR)(G)** take with a meal to avoid GI upset; <12 years: 5-7.5 mg/kg/day divided bid x 60 days; ≥12 years: 5-7 mg/kg/day divided bid x 60 days
Comment: Common side effects of *benznidazole* are allergic dermatitis, peripheral neuropathy, insomnia, anorexia with weight loss.

➤ *nifurtimox* **(NR)(G)** take with a meal to avoid GI upset; ≤10 years: 15-20 mg/kg/day divided tid-qid x 90 days; 11-16 years: 12.5-15 mg/kg/day divided tid-qid x 90 days; ≥17 years: 8-10 mg/kg/day divided tid-qid x 90 days
Comment: Common side effects of *nifurtimox* are anorexia and weight loss, nausea, vomiting, polyneuropathy, headache, dizziness or vertigo.

CHANCROID

ANTI-INFECTIVES

➤ *azithromycin* **(B)(G)** <12 years: 12 mg/kg/day x 5 days; *see page* 548 *for dose by weight table*; max 500 mg/day; ≥12 years: 500 mg x 1 dose on day 1, then 250 mg daily on days 2-5 or 500 mg daily x 3 days **oarsman** 2 gm in a single dose
Zithromax *Tab:* 250, 500, 600 mg; *Oral susp:* 100 mg/5 ml (15 ml); 200 mg/5 ml (15, 22.5, 30 ml) (cherry); *Pkt:* 1 gm for reconstitution (cherry-banana)
Zithromax Tri-pak *Tab:* 3 x 500 mg tabs/pck
Zithromax Z-pak *Tab:* 6 x 250 mg tabs/pck
Zmax *Oral susp:* 2 gm ext-rel for reconstitution (cherry-banana) (148 mg reconstitution (cherry-banana))

➤ *ceftriaxone* **(B)(G)** <45 kg: 125 mg IM in a single dose; ≥45 kg: 250 mg IM in a single dose
Rocephin *Vial:* 250, 500 mg; 1, 2 g

➤ *ciprofloxacin* **(C)** <18 years: not recommended; ≥18 years: 500 mg bid x 10 days; max 1.5 gm/day
Cipro (G) *Tab:* 250, 500, 750 mg; *Oral susp:* 250, 500 mg/5 ml (100 ml) (strawberry)
Cipro XR *Tab:* 500, 1,000 mg ext-rel
ProQuin XR *Tab:* 500 mg ext-rel
Comment: *ciprofloxacin* is contraindicated <18 years-of-age, and during pregnancy and lactation. Risk of tendonitis or tendon rupture.

▷ *erythromycin base* **(B)(G)** <45 kg: 30-50 mg/kg/day divided bid-qid; max 100 mg/kg/day; >45 kg: 500 mg qid x 7 days
Ery-Tab *Tab:* 250, 333, 500 mg ent-coat
PCE *Tab:* 333, 500 mg
▷ *erythromycin ethylsuccinate* **(B)(G)** 30-50 mg/kg/day in 4 divided doses x 7 days; may double dose with severe infection; max 100 mg/kg/day <u>or</u> 400 mg qid; *see page 563 for dose by weight table*
EryPed *Oral susp:* 200 mg/5 ml (100, 200 ml) (fruit); 400 mg/5 ml (60, 100, 200 ml) (banana); *Oral drops:* 200, 400 mg/5 ml (50 ml) (fruit); *Chew tab:* 200 mg wafer (fruit)
E.E.S. *Oral susp:* 200, 400 mg/5 ml (100 ml) (fruit)
E.E.S. Granules *Oral susp:* 200 mg/5 ml (100, 200 ml) (cherry)
E.E.S. 400 Tablets *Tab:* 400 mg

CHICKENPOX (VARICELLA)

PROPHYLAXIS

▷ *Varicella virus* vaccine, live, attenuated **(C)**
Varivax <12 months: not recommended; 12 months-12 years: 1 dose of 0.5 ml SC; repeat 4-6 weeks later; >12 years: 0.5 ml SC; repeat 4-8 weeks later
Vial: 1350 PFU/0.5 ml single dose w. diluent (preservative-free)
Comment: Administer **Varivax** SC in the deltoid for all ages.

TREATMENT

Antipyretics *see Fever page* 136

ORAL ANTIPRURITICS

▷ *diphenhydramine* **(B)(G)**
Benadryl (OTC) <2 years: not recommended; 2-6 years: 6.25 mg q 4-6 hours; max 37.5 mg/day; >6-12 years: 12.5-25 mg q 4-6 hours; max 150 mg/day; >12 years: 25-50 mg q 6-8 hours; max 100 mg/day
Chew tab: 12.5 mg (grape) (phenylalanine); *Liq:* 12.5 mg/5 ml (4, 8 oz); *Cap:* 25 mg; *Tab:* 25 mg; *Dye-free soft gel:* 25 mg;
Dye-free liq: 12.5 mg/5 ml (4, 8 oz)
▷ *diphenhydramine* injectable **(B)(G)**
Benadryl Injectable <12 years: *See mfr pkg insert:* 1.25 mg/kg up to 25 mg IM x 1 dose; then q 6 hours prn; ≥12 years: 25-50 mg IM immediately; then q 6 hours prn
Vial: 50 mg/ml (1 ml single use); 50 mg/ml (10 ml multi-dose); *Amp:* 10 mg/ml (1 ml); *Prefilled syringe:* 50 mg/ml (1 ml)
▷ *hydroxyzine* **(C)(G)** <6 years: 50 mg/day divided qid; 6-12 years: 50-100 mg/day divided qid; >12 years: 50-100 mg qid; max 600 mg/day
Atarax *Tab:* 10, 25, 50, 100 mg; *Syr:* 10 mg/5 ml (alcohol 0.5%)
Vistaril *Cap:* 25, 50, 100 mg; *Oral susp:* 25 mg/5 ml (4 oz) (lemon)
Comment: *hydroxyzine* is contraindicated in early pregnancy and in patients with a prolonged QT interval. It is not known whether this drug is excreted in human milk; therefore, *hydroxyzine* should not be given to nursing mothers.

ANTIVIRALS

▷ *acyclovir* (B)(G) <2 years: not recommended; ≥2 years, <40 kg: 20 mg/kg qid x 5 days;≥2 years, >40 kg: 800 mg qid x 5 days; *see page 541 for dose by weight table*
  Zovirax *Cap:* 200 mg; *Tab:* 400, 800 mg
  Zovirax Oral Suspension *Oral susp:* 200 mg/5 ml (banana)

CHLAMYDIA TRACHOMATIS

Comment: The following treatment regimens for *C. trachomatis* are published in the **2015 CDC Sexually Transmitted Diseases Treatment Guidelines**. Treatment regimens are presented by generic drug name first, followed by information about brands and dose forms. Treat all sexual contacts. Patients who are HIV-positive should receive the same treatment as those who are HIV-negative. Sexual abuse must be considered a cause of chlamydial infection in preadolescent children, although perinatally transmitted *C. trachomatis* infections of the nasopharynx, urogenital tract, and rectum may persist for >1 year.

RECOMMENDED REGIMENS: ADOLESCENT AND ≥18 YEARS, NON-PREGNANT

Regimen 1

▷ *azithromycin* 1 gm in a single dose

Regimen 2

▷ *doxycycline* 100 mg bid x 7 days

ALTERNATIVE REGIMENS: ADOLESCENT AND ≥18 YEARS, NON-PREGNANT

Regimen 1

▷ *erythromycin base* 500 mg qid x 7 days

Regimen 2

▷ *erythromycin ethylsuccinate* 800 mg qid x 7 days

Regimen 3

▷ *levofloxacin* 500 mg once daily x 7 days

Regimen 4

▷ *ofloxacin* 300 mg bid x 7 days

RECOMMENDED REGIMENS: PREGNANCY

Regimen 1

▷ *azithromycin* 1 gm in a single dose

Regimen 2

▷ *amoxicillin* (B)(G) <40 kg (88 lb): 20-40 mg/kg/day in 3 divided doses x 10 days <u>or</u> 25-45 mg/kg/day in 2 divided doses x 10 days; *see page* 543 *for dose by weight table*; ≥40 kg: 500 mg tid x 7 days

ALTERNATE REGIMENS: PREGNANCY

Regimen 1

▷ *erythromycin base* 500 mg qid x 7 days

Regimen 2

▷ *erythromycin base* 250 mg qid x 14 days

Regimen 3

▷ *erythromycin ethylsuccinate* 800 mg qid x 7 days

Regimen 4

▷ *erythromycin ethylsuccinate* 400 mg qid x 14 days

ALTERNATE REGIMENS: CHILDREN ≤8 YEARS

Regimen 1

▷ *azithromycin* 1 gm in a single dose

Regimen 2

▷ *doxycycline* 100 mg bid x 7 days

ALTERNATE REGIMEN: CHILDREN >45 KG; <8 YEARS

Regimen 1

▷ *azithromycin* 1 gm in a single dose

ALTERNATE REGIMENS: INFANTS

Regimen 1

▷ *erythromycin base* 50 mg/kg/day in divided doses qid x 14 days

Regimen 2

▷ *erythromycin ethylsuccinate* 50 mg/kg/day divided qid x 14 days

DRUG BRANDS AND DOSE FORMS

▷ *azithromycin* (B)(G) <12 years: 12 mg/kg/day x 5 days; *see page* 548 *for dose by weight table*; max 500 mg/day; ≥12 years: 500 mg x 1 dose on day 1, then 250 mg daily on days 2-5 <u>or</u> 500 mg daily x 3 days <u>or</u> **Zmax** 2 gm in a single dose
    Zithromax *Tab:* 250, 500, 600 mg; *Oral susp:* 100 mg/5 ml (15 ml); 200 mg/5 ml (15, 22.5, 30 ml) (cherry); *Pkt:* 1 gm for reconstitution (cherry-banana)
    Zithromax Tri-pak *Tab:* 3 x 500 mg tabs/pck
    Zithromax Z-pak *Tab:* 6 x 250 mg tabs/pck

Zmax *Oral susp:* 2 gm ext-rel for reconstitution (cherry-banana) (148 mg Na⁺)
➤ **doxycycline** (D)(G) <8 years: not recommended; ≥8 years, ≤100 lb: 2 mg/lb on first day in 2 divided doses, followed by 1 mg/lb/day in 1-2 divided doses; ≥8 years, >100 lb: 100 mg bid; *see page 561 for dose by weight table*
  Acticlate *Tab:* 75, 150** mg
  Adoxa *Tab:* 50, 75, 100, 150 mg ent-coat
  Doryx *Tab:* 50, 75, 100, 150, 200 mg del-rel
  Monodox *Cap:* 50, 75, 100 mg
  Oracea *Cap:* 40 mg del-rel
  Vibramycin *Tab:* 100 mg; *Cap:* 50, 100 mg; *Syr:* 50 mg/5 ml (raspberry-apple) (sulfites); *Oral susp:* 25 mg/5 ml (raspberry)
  Vibra-Tab *Tab:* 100 mg film-coat
Comment: **doxycycline** is contraindicated <8 years-of-age, in pregnancy, and lactation (discolors developing tooth enamel). A side effect may be photo-sensitivity (photophobia). Do not take with antacids, calcium supplements, milk <u>or</u> other dairy, <u>or</u> within 2 hours of taking another drug.
➤ **erythromycin base** (B)(G)
  Ery-Tab *Tab:* 250, 333, 500 mg ent-coat
  PCE *Tab:* 333, 500 mg
➤ **erythromycin ethylsuccinate** (B)(G)
  EryPed *Oral susp:* 200 mg/5 ml (100, 200 ml) (fruit); 400 mg/5 ml (60, 100, 200 ml) (banana); *Oral drops:* 200, 400 mg/5 ml (50 ml) (fruit); *Chew tab:* 200 gaffer (fruit)
  E.E.S. *Oral susp:* 200, 400 mg/5 ml (100 ml) (fruit)
  E.E.S. Granules *Oral susp:* 200 mg/5 ml (100, 200 ml) (cherry)
  E.E.S. 400 Tablets *Tab:* 400 mg
➤ **levofloxacin** (C)
  Levaquin *Tab:* 250, 500, 750 mg
Comment: **levofloxacin** is contraindicated; <18 years-of-age, and during pregnancy and lactation. Risk of tendonitis <u>or</u> tendon rupture.
➤ **ofloxacin** (C)(G)
  Floxin *Tab:* 200, 300, 400 mg
Comment: **ofloxacin** is contraindicated <18 years-of-age, and during pregnancy and lactation. Risk of tendonitis <u>or</u> tendon rupture.

CHOLELITHIASIS

➤ **ursodiol** (B) <12 years: not recommended; ≥12 years: 8-10 mg/kg/day in 2-3 divided doses
  Actigall *Cap:* 300 mg
  Comment: **Actigall** is indicated for the dissolution of radiolucent, non-calciferous, gallstones <20 mm in diameter and for prevention of gallstones during rapid weight loss.

CHOLERA (*VIBRIO CHOLERAE*)

Comment: June 10, 2016, the FDA approved the first vaccine for the prevention of cholera caused by serogroup O1 (the most predominant cause of cholera globally

[WHO]) in patients aged 18-64 years traveling to cholera-affected areas (https://www.drugs.com/newdrugs/fda-approves-vaxchora-cholera-vaccine-live-oral-prevent-cholera-travelers-4396.html). **Vaxchora** (R) is the only FDA-approved vaccine for the prevention of cholera. The bacterium *Vibrio cholerae* is acquired by ingesting contaminated water or food and causes nausea, vomiting, and watery diarrhea that may be mild to severe. Profuse fluid loss may cause life-threatening dehydration if antibiotics and fluid replacement are not initiated promptly.

VACCINE PROPHYLAXIS

▷ *Vibrio cholerae* vaccine

Vaxchora reconstitute the buffer component in 100 ml purified bottled water; then add the active component (lyophilized *V. cholerae* CVD 103-HgR); total dose after reconstitution is 100 ml; instruct the patient to avoid eating or drinking fluids for 60 minutes before and after ingestion of the dose

Comment: **Vaxchora** is a live, attenuated vaccine that is taken as a single oral dose at least 10 days before travel to a cholera-affected area and at least 10 days before starting antimalarial prophylaxis. Diminished immune response occurs when taken concomitantly with *chloroquine*. Avoid concomitant administration with systemic antibiotics since these agents may be active against the vaccine strain. Do not administer to patients who have received an oral or parental antibiotic within 14 days prior to vaccination. **Vaxchora** may be shed in the stool of recipients for at least 7 days. There is potential for transmission of the vaccine strain to non-vaccinated and immunocompromised close contacts. The Centers for Disease Control and Prevention and several health professional organizations state that vaccines given to a nursing mother do not affect the safety of breastfeeding for mothers or infants and that breastfeeding is not a contraindication to cholera vaccine. **Vaxchora** is not absorbed systemically, and maternal use is not expected to result in fetal exposure to the drug. The **Vaxchora** pregnancy exposure registry for reporting adverse events is 800-533-5899. There are 0 disease interactions, but at least 165 drug-drug interactions with **Vaxchora** (see mfr pkg insert).

TREATMENT

Comment: The first-line treatment for *V. cholerae* is oral rehydration therapy (ORT) and intravenous fluid replacement as indicated. Antibiotic therapy may shorten the duration and severity of symptoms, but is optional in other than severe cases. Although *doxycycline* is contraindicated in pregnancy and in children <8 years-of-age, the benefits may outweigh the risks (WHO, CDC, UNICEF). Although *ciprofloxacin* is contraindicated in children <18 years-of-age, the benefits may outweigh the risks (WHO, CDC, UNICEF). Cholera is not transmitted from person to person, but rather the fecal-oral route. Therefore, chemoprophylaxis is not usually required with strict hand hygiene and sanitation measures, and avoidance of contaminated food and water. Drugs and dosages for chemoprophylaxis are the same as for treatment.

NON-PREGNANT FEMALES ≤15 YEARS-OF-AGE

Regimen 1

▷ *doxycycline* (D)(G) 300 mg in a single dose

Acticlate *Tab:* 75, 150** mg

Adoxa *Tab:* 50, 75, 100, 150 mg ent-coat
Doryx *Tab:* 50, 75, 100, 150, 200 mg del-rel
Monodox *Cap:* 50, 75, 100 mg
Oracea *Cap:* 40 mg del-rel
Vibramycin *Tab:* 100 mg; *Cap:* 50, 100 mg; *Syr:* 50 mg/5 ml (raspberry-apple) (sulfites); *Oral susp:* 25 mg/5 ml (raspberry)
Vibra-Tab *Tab:* 100 mg film-coat

Comment: *doxycycline* is contraindicated <8 years-of-age, in pregnancy, and lactation (discolors developing tooth enamel). A side effect may be photosensitivity (photophobia). Do not take with antacids, calcium supplements, milk or other dairy, or within 2 hours of taking another drug.

Regimen 2

▷ *azithromycin* (B) 1000 mg in a single dose
    Zithromax *Tab:* 250, 500, 600 mg
    Zmax *Oral susp:* 2 gm ext-rel for reconstitution (cherry-banana) (148 mg Na$^+$)
    or
▷ *ciprofloxacin* (C) <18 years: not recommended; ≥18 years: 1000 mg in a single dose
    Cipro (G) *Tab:* 250, 500, 750 mg; *Oral susp:* 250, 500 mg/5 ml (100 ml) (strawberry)
    Cipro XR *Tab:* 500, 1000 mg ext-rel
    ProQuin XR *Tab:* 500 mg ext-rel

PREGNANT FEMALES ≤15 YEARS-OF-AGE

▷ *azithromycin* (B) 1,000 mg in a single dose
    Zithromax *Tab:* 250, 500, 600 mg
    Zmax *Oral susp:* 2 gm ext-rel for reconstitution (cherry-banana) (148 mg Na$^+$)
    or
▷ *erythromycin* (B)(G) 500 mg q 6 hours x 3 days
    E.E.S. 400 Tablets *Tab:* 400 mg
    Ery-Tab *Tab:* 250, 333, 500 mg ent-coat
    PCE *Tab:* 333, 500 mg

CHILDREN 3-15 YEARS-OF-AGE WHO CAN SWALLOW TABLETS

Regimen 1

▷ *erythromycin* (B)(G) 12.5 mg/kg q 6 hours x 3 days
    E.E.S. 400 Tablets *Tab:* 400 mg
    Ery-Tab *Tab:* 250, 333, 500 mg ent-coat
    PCE *Tab:* 333, 500 mg
    or
▷ *azithromycin* (B) 20 mg/kg in a single dose; max 1 gm
    Zithromax *Tab:* 250, 500, 600 mg; *Oral susp:* 100 mg/5 ml (15 ml); 200 mg/5 ml (15, 22.5, 30 ml) (cherry)
    Zmax *Oral susp:* 2 gm ext-rel for reconstitution (cherry-banana) (148 mg Na$^+$)

Regimen 2

▷ *ciprofloxacin* (D) <18 years: not recommended; ≥18 years: 20 mg/kg in a single dose

    Cipro (G) *Tab:* 250, 500, 750 mg; *Oral susp:* 250, 500 mg/5 ml (100 ml)
    (strawberry)
    Cipro XR *Tab:* 500, 1000 mg ext-rel
    ProQuin XR *Tab:* 500 mg ext-rel
       or
▷ *doxycycline* (D)(G) 2-4 mg/kg in a single dose
    Acticlate *Tab:* 75, 150**mg
    Adoxa *Tab:* 50, 75, 100, 150 mg ent-coat
    Doryx *Tab:* 50, 75, 100, 150, 200 mg del-rel
    Monodox *Cap:* 50, 75, 100 mg
    Oracea *Cap:* 40 mg del-rel
    Vibramycin *Tab:* 100 mg; *Cap:* 50, 100 mg; *Syr:* 50 mg/5 ml (raspberry-apple)
    (sulfites); *Oral susp:* 25 mg/5 ml (raspberry)
    Vibra-Tab *Tab:* 100 mg film-coat

CHILDREN <3 YEARS-OF-AGE

Regimen 1

▷ *erythromycin ethylsuccinate* (B)(G) 12.5 mg/kg q 6 hours x 3 days; use suspension
    E.E.S. *Oral susp:* 200, 400 mg/5 ml (100 ml) (fruit)
    E.E.S. Granules *Oral susp:* 200 mg/5 ml (100, 200 ml) (cherry, fruit); *Chew tab*
    200 mg wafer (fruit)
    EryPed *Oral susp:* 200 mg/5 ml (100, 200 ml) (fruit); 400 mg/5 ml (60, 100, 200
    ml) (banana); *Oral drops:* 200, 400 mg/5 ml (50 ml) (fruit); *Chew tab:* 200 mg wafer
    (fruit)
       or
▷ *azithromycin* (B) 20 mg/kg in a single dose; max 1 g; use suspension
    Zithromax *Tab:* 250, 500, 600 mg; *Oral susp:* 100 mg/5 ml (15 ml); 200 mg/5
    ml(15, 22.5, 30 ml) (cherry)
    Zmax *Oral susp:* 2 gm ext-rel for reconstitution (cherry-banana) (148 mg Na⁺)

Regimen 2

▷ *ciprofloxacin* (C) <18 years: not recommended; ≥18 years: 20 mg/kg in a single
    dose; use suspension
    Cipro (G) *Oral susp:* 250, 500 mg/5 ml (100 ml) (strawberry)
       or
▷ *doxycycline* (D)(G) <8 years: not recommended; ≥8 years: 2-4 mg/kg in a single
    dose; use suspension or syrup
    Vibramycin *Tab:* 100 mg; *Cap:* 50, 100 mg; *Syr:* 50 mg/5 ml (raspberry-apple)
    (sulfites); *Oral susp:* 25 mg/5 ml (raspberry)

COLIC: INFANTILE

▷ *hyoscyamine* (C)(G) 3-4 kg: 4 drops q 4 hours prn; max 24 drops/day; 5 kg: 5 drops
    q 4 hours prn; max 30 drops/day; 7 kg: 6 drops q 4 hours prn; max 36 drops/day; 10
    kg: 8 drops q 4 hours prn; max 40 drops/day
    Levsin Drops *Oral drops:* 0.125 mg/ml (15 ml) (orange) (alcohol 5%)
▷ *simethicone* (C) 0.3 ml qid pc and HS
    Mylicon Drops (OTC) *Oral drops:* 40 mg/0.6 ml (30 ml)

COMMON COLD (VIRAL UPPER RESPIRATORY INFECTION [URI])

Oral Prescription Drugs for the Management of Allergy, Cough, and Cold *see page* 523
Oral Antipyretic-Analgesics *see Fever page* 136

NASAL SALINE DROPS/SPRAYS

▷ *saline* nasal spray (NE)(G)
　　Afrin Saline Mist w. Eucalyptol and Menthol (OTC) 1 month-2 years: 1-2 sprays in each nostril prn; >2-12 years: 1-4 sprays in each nostril prn; >12 years: 2-6 sprays in each nostril
　　　　Squeeze bottle: 45 ml
　　Afrin Moisturizing Saline Mist (OTC) 1 month-2 years: 1-2 sprays in each nostril prn; >2-12 years: 1-4 sprays in each nostril prn; >12 years: 2-6 sprays in each nostril prn
　　　　Squeeze bottle: 45 ml
　　Ocean Mist (OTC) 1 month-2 years: 1-2 sprays in each nostril prn; >2-12 years: 1-4 sprays in each nostril prn; >12 years: 2-6 sprays in each nostril prn
　　　　Squeeze bottle: saline 0.65% (45 ml) (alcohol-free)
　　Pediamist (OTC) 1 month-2 years: 1-2 sprays in each nostril prn; >2-12 years: 1-4 sprays in each nostril prn; >12 years: 2-6 sprays in each nostril prn
　　　　Squeeze bottle: saline 0.5% (15 ml) (alcohol-free)

NASAL SYMPATHOMIMETICS

▷ *oxymetazoline* (C)(OTC) <6 years: not recommended; 6-12 years: use 4-hour formulation; 2-3 drops <u>or</u> sprays q 4 hours prn; max duration 5 days; >12 years: may use 12-hour formulation; 2-3 drops <u>or</u> sprays in each nostril q 10-12 hours prn; max 2 doses/day; max duration 5 days
　　Afrin 12-Hour Extra Moisturizing Nasal Spray
　　Afrin 12-Hour Nasal spray Pump Mist
　　Afrin 12-Hour Original Nasal spray
　　Afrin 12-Hour Original Nose Drops
　　Afrin 12-Hour Severe Congestion Nasal Spray
　　Afrin 12-Hour Sinus Nasal Spray
　　　　Nasal spray: 0.05% (45 ml); *Nasal drops:* 0.05% (45 ml)
　　Afrin 4-Hour Nasal Spray
　　Neo-Synephrine 12 Hour Nasal Spray
　　Neo-Synephrine 12 Hour Extra Moisturizing Nasal Spray
　　　　Nasal spray: 0.05% (15 ml)
▷ *phenylephrine* (C)
　　Afrin Allergy Nasal Spray (OTC) <12 years: not recommended; ≥12 years: 2-3 sprays in each nostril q 4 hours prn; max duration 5 days
　　　　Nasal spray: 0.5% (15 ml)
　　Afrin Nasal Decongestant Children's Pump Mist (OTC) <6 years: not recommended; ≥6 years: 2-3 sprays in each nostril q 4 hours prn; max duration 5 days

Nasal spray: 0.25% (15 ml)
Neo-Synephrine Extra Strength (OTC) <12 years: not recommended; ≥12 years: 2-3 sprays <u>or</u> drops in each nostril q 4 hours prn; max duration 5 days
Nasal spray: 0.1% (15 ml); *Nasal drops:* 0.1% (15 ml)
Neo-Synephrine Mild Formula (OTC) <6 years: not recommended; ≥6 years: 2-3 sprays <u>or</u> drops in each nostril q 4 hours prn; max duration 5 days
Nasal spray: 0.25% (15 ml)
Neo-Synephrine Regular Strength (OTC) <12 years: not recommended; ≥12 years: 2-3 sprays <u>or</u> drops in each nostril q 4 hours prn; max duration 5 days
Nasal spray: 0.5% (15 ml); *Nasal drops:* 0.5% (15 ml)
➤ *tetrahydrozoline* (C)
Tyzine <6 years: not recommended; ≥6 years: 2-4 drops <u>or</u> 3-4 sprays in each nostril q 3-8 hours prn; max duration 5 days
Nasal spray: 0.1% (15 ml); *Nasal drops:* 0.1% (30 ml)
Tyzine Pediatric Nasal Drops 2-3 sprays <u>or</u> drops in each nostril q 3-6 hours prn
Nasal drops: 0.05% (15 ml)

CONJUNCTIVITIS: ALLERGIC

Oral Prescription Drugs for the Management of Allergy, Cough, and Cold Symptoms
page 523

OPHTHALMIC CORTICOSTEROIDS

Comment: Concomitant contact lens wear is contraindicated during therapy. Ophthalmic steroids are contraindicated with ocular, fungal, mycobacterial, viral (except herpes zoster), and untreated bacterial infection. Ophthalmic steroids may mask <u>or</u> exacerbate infection, and may increase intraocular pressure, optic nerve damage, cataract formation, <u>or</u> corneal perforation. Limit ophthalmic steroid use to 2-3 days if possible; usual max 2 weeks. With prolonged or frequent use, there is risk of corneal and scleral thinning and cataract formation.
➤ *dexamethasone* (C) <12 years: not recommended; ≥12 years: initially 1-2 drops hourly during the day and q 2 hours at night; then prolong dosing interval to 4-6 hours as condition improves
Maxidex *Ophth susp:* 0.1% (5, 15 ml) (benzalkonium chloride)
➤ *dexamethasone phosphate* (C) <12 years: not recommended; ≥12 years: initially 1-2 drops hourly during the day and q 2 hours at night; then 1 drop q 4-8 hours <u>or</u> more as condition improves
Decadron *Ophth soln:* 0.1% (5 ml) (sulfites)
➤ *fluorometholone* (C) <12 years: not recommended; ≥12 years: 1 drop bid-qid <u>or</u> 1/2 inch of ointment once daily-tid; may increase dose frequency during initial 24-48 hours
FML *Ophth susp:* 0.1% (5, 10, 15 ml) (benzalkonium chloride)
FML Forte *Ophth susp:* 0.25% (5, 10, 15 ml) (benzalkonium chloride)
FML S.O.P. Ointment *Ophth oint:* 0.1% (3.5 gm)
➤ *fluorometholone acetate* (C) <12 years: not recommended; ≥12 years: initially 2 drops q 2 hours during the first 24-48 hours; then 1-2 drops qid as condition improves

       Flarex *Ophth susp:* 0.1% (2.5, 5 10 ml) (benzalkonium chloride)
▷ *loteprednol etabonate* (**C**)
       Alrex <12 years: not recommended; ≥12 years: 1 drop qid
         Ophth susp: 0.2% (5, 10 ml) (benzalkonium chloride)
       Lotemax <12 years: not recommended; ≥12 years: 1-2 drops qid
         Ophth susp: 0.5% (5, 10, 15 ml) (benzalkonium chloride)
▷ *medrysone* (**C**) <12 years: not recommended; ≥12 years: 1 drop up to q 4 hours
       HMS *Ophth susp:* 1% (5, 10 ml) (benzalkonium chloride)
▷ *rimexolone* (**C**) <12 years: not recommended; ≥12 years: initially 1-2 drops hourly while awake x 1 week; then 1 drop q 2 hours while awake x 1 week; then taper as condition improves
       Vexol *Ophth susp:* 0.1% (5, 10 ml) (benzalkonium chloride)
▷ *prednisolone acetate* (**C**)(**G**)
       Econopred <12 years: not recommended; ≥12 years: 2 drops qid
         Ophth susp: 0.125% (5, 10 ml)
       Econopred Plus <12 years: not recommended; ≥12 years: 2 drops qid
         Ophth susp: 1% (5, 10 ml)
       Pred Forte <12 years: not recommended; ≥12 years: initially 2 drops hourly x 24-48 hours; then 1-2 drops bid-qid
         Ophth susp: 1% (1, 5, 10, 15 ml) (benzalkonium chloride, sulfites)
       Pred Mild <12 years: not recommended; ≥12 years: initially 2 drops hourly x 24-48 hours; then 1-2 drops bid-qid
         Ophth susp: 0.12% (5, 10 ml) (benzalkonium chloride)
▷ *prednisolone sodium phosphate* (**C**) <12 years: not recommended; ≥12 years: initially 1-2 drops hourly during the day and q 2 hours at night; then 1 drop q 4 hours; then 1 drop tid-qid as condition improves
       Inflamase Forte *Ophth soln:* 1% (5, 10, 15 ml) (benzalkonium chloride)
       Inflamase Mild *Ophth soln:* 1/8% (5, 10 ml) (benzalkonium chloride)

OPHTHALMIC H₁ ANTAGONISTS (ANTIHISTAMINES)

Comment: May insert contact lens 10 minutes after administration of ophthalmic antihistamine.
▷ *emedastine* (**C**) <3 years: not recommended; ≥3 years: 1 drop qid prn
       Emadine *Ophth soln:* 0.05% (5 ml) (benzalkonium chloride)
▷ *levocabastine* (**C**) <12 years: not recommended; ≥12 years: 1 drop qid prn
       Livostin *Ophth susp:* 0.05% (2.5, 5, 10 ml) (benzalkonium chloride)

OPHTHALMIC MAST CELL STABILIZERS

Comment: Concomitant contact lens wear is contraindicated during treatment.
▷ *cromolyn sodium* (**B**) <4 years: not recommended; ≥4 years: 1-2 drops 4-6 x/day at regular intervals
       Crolom *Ophth soln:* 4% (10 ml) (benzalkonium chloride)
▷ *lodoxamide tromethamine* (**B**) <2 years: not recommended; ≥2 years: 1-2 drops qid up to 3 months
       Alomide *Ophth soln:* 1% (10 ml) (benzalkonium chloride)
▷ *nedocromil* (**B**) <3 years: not recommended; ≥3 years: 1-2 drops bid
       Alocril *Ophth soln:* 2% (5 ml) (benzalkonium chloride)

▷ *pemirolast potassium* (C) 3 years: not recommended; ≥3 years: 1-2 drops qid
   Alamast *Ophth soln:* 0.1% (10 ml) (lauralkonium chloride)

OPHTHALMIC ANTIHISTAMINE/MAST CELL STABILIZER COMBINATIONS

▷ *alcaftadine* (B) <2 years: not recommended; ≥2 years: 1 drop each eye daily
   Lastacaft *Ophth soln:* 0.25% (6 ml) (benzalkonium chloride)
   Comment: May insert contact lens 10 minutes after ophthalmic administration.
▷ *azelastine* (C) <3 years: not recommended; ≥3 years: 1 drop each eye bid
   Optivar *Ophth soln:* 0.05% (6 ml) (benzalkonium chloride)
   Comment: May insert contact lens 10 minutes after ophthalmic administration.
▷ *bepotastine besilate* (C) <2 years: not recommended; ≥2 years: 1 drop each eye bid
   Bepreve *Ophth soln:* 1.5% (10 ml) (benzalkonium chloride)
   Comment: May insert contact lens 10 minutes after ophthalmic administration.
▷ *epinastine* (C)(G) <3 years: not recommended; ≥3 years: 1 drop each eye bid
   Elestat *Ophth soln:* 0.05% (5 ml) (benzalkonium chloride)
▷ *ketotifen fumarate* (C) <3 years: not recommended; ≥3 years: 1 drop each eye q
   8-12 hours
   Alaway (OTC) *Ophth soln:* 0.025% (10 ml) (benzalkonium chloride)
   Claritin Eye (OTC) *Ophth soln:* 0.025% (5 ml) (benzalkonium chloride)
   Refresh Eye Itch Relief (OTC) *Ophth soln:* 0.025% (5 ml) (benzalkonium chloride)
   Zaditor (OTC) *Ophth soln:* 0.025% (5 ml)(benzalkonium chloride)
   Zyrtec Itchy Eye (OTC) *Ophth soln:* 0.025% (5 ml) (benzalkonium chloride)
▷ *olopatadine* (C) <3 years: not recommended; ≥3 years: 1 drop each eye bid
   Pataday (G) *Ophth soln:* 0.2% (2.5 ml) (benzalkonium chloride)
   Patanol *Ophth soln:* 0.1% (5 ml) (benzalkonium chloride)
   Pazeo *Ophth soln:* 0.7% (2.5 ml) (benzalkonium chloride)
   Comment: May insert contact lens 10 minutes after administration.

OPHTHALMIC VASOCONSTRICTORS

Comment: Concomitant contact lens wear is contraindicated during treatment.
▷ *naphazoline* (C) <12 years: not recommended; ≥12 years: 1-2 drops each eye qid
   prn
   Vasocon-A *Ophth soln:* 0.1% (15 ml) (benzalkonium chloride)
▷ *oxymetazoline* (NE)(OTC) <6 years: not recommended; ≥6 years: 1-2 drops each
   eye qid prn
   Visine L-R *Ophth soln:* 0.025% (15, 30 ml)
▷ *tetrahydrozoline* (NE)(OTC)(G) <6 years: not recommended; ≥6 years: 1-2 drops
   each eye qid prn
   Visine *Ophth soln:* 0.05% (15, 22.5, 30 ml)

OPHTHALMIC VASOCONSTRICTOR/MOISTURIZER COMBINATION

Comment: Concomitant contact lens wear is contraindicated during treatment.
▷ *tetrahydrozoline/polyethylene glycol 400/povidone/dextran 70* (NE)(OTC) <6 years:
   not recommended; ≥6 years: 1-2 drops each eye qid prn
   Advanced Relief Visine *Ophth soln:* tetra 0.025%/poly 1%/pov 1%/dex 0.1% (15,
   30 ml)

OPHTHALMIC VASOCONSTRICTOR/ASTRINGENT COMBINATION

Comment: Concomitant contact lens wear is contraindicated during treatment.
➤ *tetrahydrozoline/zinc sulfate* (NE)(OTC) <6 years: not recommended; ≥6 years: 1-2 drops each eye qid prn
    Visine AC *Ophth soln: tetra* 0.025%/*zinc* 0.05% (15, 30 ml)

OPHTHALMIC VASOCONSTRICTOR/ANTIHISTAMINE COMBINATIONS

Comment: Concomitant contact lens wear is contraindicated during treatment.
➤ *naphazoline/pheniramine* (C) <6 years: not recommended; ≥6 years: 1-2 drops each eye qid
    Naphcon-A (OTC) *Ophth soln: naph* 0.025%/*phen* 0.3% (15 ml) (benzalkonium chloride)

OPHTHALMIC NSAIDs

Comment: Concomitant contact lens wear is contraindicated during treatment.
➤ *diclofenac* (B) <12 years: not recommended; ≥12 years: 1 drop affected eye(s) qid
    Voltaren Ophthalmic Solution *Ophth soln:* 0.1% (2.5, 5 ml)
➤ *ketorolac tromethamine* (C) <3 years: not recommended; ≥3 years: 1 drop affected eye(s) qid; max x 4 days
    Acular *Ophth soln:* 0.5% (3, 5, 10 ml) (benzalkonium chloride)
    Acular LS *Ophth soln:* 0.4% (5 ml) (benzalkonium chloride)
    Acular PF *Ophth soln:* 0.5% (0.4 ml; 12 single-use vials/carton) (preservative-free)
➤ *nepafenac* (C) <10 years: not recommended; ≥10 years: 1 drop affected eye(s) tid
    Nevanac Ophthalmic Suspension *Ophth susp:* 0.1% (3 ml) (benzalkonium chloride)

CONJUNCTIVITIS/BLEPHAROCONJUNCTIVITIS: BACTERIAL

OPHTHALMIC ANTI-INFECTIVES

➤ *azithromycin* ophthalmic solution (B)(G) <1 year: not recommended; ≥1 year: 1 drop to affected eye(s) bid x 2 days; then 1 drop once daily for the next 5 days
    AzaSite Ophthalmic Solution *Ophth susp:* 1% (2.5 ml) (benzalkonium chloride)
➤ *bacitracin* ophthalmic ointment (C)(G) apply 1/2 inch ribbon to the lower conjunctival sac of affected eye(s) 1-3 x daily x 7 days
    Bacitracin Ophthalmic Ointment *Ophth oint:* 500 units/g (3.5 gm)
➤ *besifloxacin* ophthalmic solution (C) <1 year: not recommended; ≥1 year: 1 drop to affected eye(s) tid x 7 days
    Besivance Ophthalmic Solution *Ophth susp:* 0.6% (5 ml) (benzalkonium chloride)
➤ *ciprofloxacin* ophthalmic ointment (C) <2 years: not recommended; ≥2 years: apply 1/2 inch ribbon to the lower conjunctival sac of affected eye(s) tid x 2 days; then bid x 5 days

   Ciloxan Ophthalmic Ointment *Ophth oint:* 0.3% (3.5 gm)
▷ *ciprofloxacin* ophthalmic solution **(C)** <1 years: not recommended; ≥1 year: 1-2
   drops to affected eye(s) q 2 hours while awake x 2 days; then, q 4 hours while awake
   x 5 days
   Ciloxan Ophthalmic Solution *Ophth soln:* 0.3% (2.5, 5, 10 ml) (benzalkonium
   chloride)
▷ *erythromycin* ophthalmic ointment **(B)** apply 1/2 inch ribbon to the lower conjunctival sac of affected eye(s) up to 6 x/day
   Ilotycin Ophthalmic Ointment *Ophth oint:* 5 mg/g (1/8 oz)
▷ *gatifloxacin* ophthalmic solution **(C)**
   Zymar Ophthalmic Solution <1 year: not recommended; ≥1 year: initially 1
   drop to affected eye(s) q 2 hours while awake up to 8 times/day for 2 days; then
   1 drop qid while awake x 5 more days
      Ophth soln: 0.3% (5 ml) (benzalkonium chloride)
   Zymaxid Ophthalmic Solution(G) <1 year: not recommended; ≥1 year: initially
   1 drop to affected eye(s) q 2 hours while awake up to 8 times/day on day 1; then
   1 drop bid-qid while awake on days 2-7
      Ophth soln: 0.5% (2.5 ml) (benzalkonium chloride)
▷ *gentamicin sulfate* ophthalmic ointment **(C)(G)** apply 1/2 inch ribbon to the lower
   conjunctival sac of affected eye(s) bid-tid
   Garamycin Ophthalmic Ointment *Ophth oint:* 3 mg/g (3.5 gm) (preservative-free formulation available)
   Genoptic Ophthalmic Ointment *Ophth oint:* 3 mg/g (3.5 gm)
   Gentacidin Ophthalmic Ointment *Ophth oint:* 3 mg/g (3.5 gm)
▷ *gentamicin sulfate* ophthalmic solution **(C)(G)** 1-2 drops to affected eye(s) q 4
   hours x 7-14 days; max 2 drops q 1 h
   Garamycin Ophthalmic Solution *Ophth soln:* 0.3% (5 ml) (benzalkonium
   chloride)
   Genoptic Ophthalmic Solution *Ophth soln:* 0.3% (3, 5 ml)
▷ *levofloxacin* ophthalmic solution **(C)** <1 year: not recommended; ≥1 years: 1-2
   drops to affected eye(s) q 2 hours while awake on days 1 and 2 (max 8 times/day);
   then 1-2 drops q 4 hours while awake on days 3-7; max 4 x/day
   Quixin Ophthalmic Solution *Ophth soln:* 0.5% (2.5, 5 ml) (benzalkonium
   chloride)
▷ *moxifloxacin* ophthalmic solution **(C)** <1 year: not recommended; ≥1 year: 1 drop
   to affected eye(s) tid x 7 days
   Moxeza Ophthalmic Solution (G) *Ophth soln:* 0.5% (3 ml)
   Vigamox Ophthalmic Solution *Ophth soln:* 0.5% (3 ml)
▷ *ofloxacin* ophthalmic solution **(C)** <1 year: not recommended; ≥1 year: 1-2 drops to
   affected eye(s) q 2-4 hours x 2 days; then qid x 5 days
   Ocuflox Ophthalmic Solution *Ophth soln:* 0.3% (5, 10 ml) (benzalkonium
   chloride)
▷ *sulfacetamide* ophthalmic solution and ointment **(C)**
   Bleph-10 Ophthalmic Solution 1-2 drops to affected eye(s) q 2-3 hours during
   the day x 7-10 days
      Ophth soln: 10% (2.5, 5, 15 ml) (benzalkonium chloride)
   Bleph-10 Ophthalmic Ointment <2 years: not recommended; ≥2 years: apply
   1/2 inch ribbon to the lower conjunctival sac of affected eye(s) q 3-4 hours and
   HS x 7-10 days

Ophth oint: 10% (3.5 gm) (phenylmercuric acetate)

Cetamide Ophthalmic Solution <2 years: not recommended; ≥2 years: initially 1-2 drops to affected eye(s) q 2-3 hours; then increase dosing interval as condition improves

Ophth soln: 15% (5, 15 ml)

Isopto Cetamide Ophthalmic Ointment <2 years: not recommended; ≥2 years: initially 1/2 inch ribbon in lower conjunctival sac of affected eye(s) q 3-4 hours; then increase dosing interval as condition improves

Ophth oint: 10% (3.5 gm)

Isopto Cetamide Ophthalmic Solution <2 years: not recommended; ≥2 years: initially 1-2 drops to affected eye(s)q 2-3 hours; then increase dosing interval as condition improves

Ophth soln: 15% (5, 15 ml)

▷ *tobramycin* (B)

Tobrex Ophthalmic Solution 1-2 drops to affected eye(s) q 4 hours

Ophth soln: 0.3% (5 ml) (benzalkonium chloride)

Tobrex Ophthalmic Ointment apply 1/2 inch ribbon to the lower conjunctiva sac of affected eye(s) bid-tid

Ophth oint: 0.3% (3.5 gm) (chlorobutanol)

OPHTHALMIC ANTI-INFECTIVE COMBINATIONS

▷ *polymyxin b sulfate/bacitracin* ophthalmic ointment (C) apply 1/2 inch ribbon to the lower conjunctival sac of affected eye(s) q 3-4 hours x 7-10 days

Polysporin Ophthalmic Ointment *Ophth oint: poly b* 10,000 U/*bac* 500 U (3.75 gm)

▷ *polymyxin b sulfate/bacitracin zinc/neomycin sulfate* ophthalmic ointment (C) apply 1/2 inch ribbon to the lower conjunctival sac of affected eye(s) q 3-4 hours x 7-10 days

Neosporin Ophthalmic Ointment *Ophth oint: poly b* 10,000 U/*bac* 400 U/*neo* 3.5 mg/g (3.75 gm)

▷ *polymyxin b sulfate/gramicidin/neomycin* ophthalmic solution (C) <12 years: not recommended; ≥12 years: 1-2 drops to affected eye(s) q 1 hour x 2-3 doses; then 1-2 drops bid-qid x 7-10 days

Neosporin Ophthalmic Solution *Ophth soln: poly b* 10,000 U/*gram* 0.025 mg/*neo* 1.7 mg/g (10 ml)

▷ *trimethoprim/polymyxin b sulfate* <2 years: not recommended; ≥2 years: ophthalmic solution (C) 1 drop to affected eye(s)q 3 hours x 7-10 days; max 6 doses/day

Polytrim *Ophth soln: trim* 1 mg/*poly b* 10,000 U/ml (10 ml) (benzalkonium chloride)

OPHTHALMIC ANTI-INFECTIVE/STEROID COMBINATIONS

Comment: Ophthalmic corticosteroids are contraindicated after removal of a corneal foreign body, epithelial herpes simplex keratitis, *varicella*, other viral infections of the cornea or conjunctiva, fungal ocular infections, and mycobacterial ocular infections. Limit ophthalmic steroid use to 2-3 days if possible; usual max 2 weeks. With prolonged or frequent use, there is risk of corneal and scleral thinning and cataract formation.

▷ *gentamicin sulfate/prednisolone acetate* ophthalmic suspension **(C)**
    Pred-G Ophthalmic Suspension <12 years: not recommended; ≥12 years: 1 drop to affected eye(s) bid-qid; max 20 ml/therapeutic course
        Ophth susp: gent 0.3%/pred 1%/ml (2, 5, 10 ml) (benzalkonium chloride)
    Pred-G Ophthalmic Ointment <12 years: not recommended; ≥12 years: apply 1/2 inch ribbon to the lower conjunctiva sac of affected eye(s) once daily-tid; max 8 gm/therapeutic course
        Ophth oint: gent 0.3%/pred 0.6%/g (3.5 gm)

▷ *neomycin sulfate/polymyxin B sulfate/dexamethasone* ophthalmic suspension **(C)**
    Maxitrol Ophthalmic Suspension <12 years: not recommended; ≥12 years: 1-2 drops to affected eye(s) q 1 hour (severe infection) or qid (mild to moderate infection)
        Ophth susp: neo 0.35%/poly b 10,000 U/dexa 1%/ml (5 ml) (benzalkonium chloride)
    Maxitrol Ophthalmic Ointment <12 years: not recommended; ≥12 years: apply 1/2 inch ribbon to the lower conjunctiva sac of affected eye(s) q 1 hour (severe infection) or qid (mild to moderate infection)
        Ophth oint: neo 0.35%/poly b 10,000 U/dexa 0.1%/g (3.5 gm)

▷ *neomycin sulfate/polymyxin B sulfate/prednisolone acetate ophthalmic suspension* **(C)** <12 years: not recommended; ≥12 years: 1-2 drops to affected eye(s) q 3-4 hours; more often as necessary; max 20 ml/therapeutic course
    Poly-Pred Ophthalmic Suspension *Ophth susp: neo 0.35%/poly b 10,000 U/pred 0.5%/ml (10 ml)*

▷ *polymyxin B sulfate/neomycin sulfate/hydrocortisone* ophthalmic suspension **(C)** <12 years: not recommended; ≥12 years: 1-2 drops to affected eye(s) tid-qid; more often if necessary; max 20 ml/therapeutic course
    Cortisporin Ophthalmic Suspension *Ophth susp: poly b 10,000 U/neo 0.35%/hydro 1%/ml (7.5 ml) (thimerosal)*

▷ *polymyxin B sulfate/neomycin sulfate/bacitracin zinc/hydrocortisone* ophthalmic ointment **(C)** <12 years: not recommended; ≥12 years: apply 1/2 inch ribbon to the lower conjunctival sac of affected eye(s) tid-qid; more often if necessary; max 8 gm/therapeutic course
    Cortisporin Ophthalmic Ointment *Ophth oint: poly b 10,000 U/neo 0.35%/bac 400 U/hydro 1%/g (3.5 gm)*

▷ *sulfacetamide sodium/fluorometholone* suspension **(C)** <12 years: not recommended; ≥12 years: 1 drop to affected eye(s) qid; max 20 ml/therapeutic course
    FML-S *Ophth susp: sulfa 10%/fluoro 0.1%/ml (5, 10, 15 ml) (benzalkonium chloride)*

▷ *sulfacetamide sodium/prednisolone acetate* ophthalmic suspension and ointment **(C)**
    Blephamide Liquifilm <6 years: not recommended; ≥6 years: 2 drops to affected eye(s) qid and HS
        Ophth susp: sulfa 10%/pred 0.2%/ml (5, 10 ml) (benzalkonium chloride)
    Blephamide S.O.P. Ophthalmic Ointment <6 years: not recommended; ≥6 years: apply 1/2 inch ribbon to the lower conjunctival sac of affected eye(s) tid-qid
        Ophth oint: sulfa 10%/pred 0.2%/g (3.5 gm) (benzalkonium chloride)

▷ *sulfacetamide sodium/prednisolone sodium phosphate* ophthalmic solution **(C)** <6 years: not recommended; ≥6 years: 2 drops to affected eye(s) q 4 hours
    Vasocidin Ophthalmic Solution *Ophth soln: sulfa 10%/pred 0.25%/ml (5, 10 ml)*

➤ *tobramycin/dexamethasone* ophthalmic solution and ointment (C)
TobraDex Ophthalmic Solution <2 years: not recommended; ≥2 years: 1-2 drops q 4-6 hours; may start with 1-2 drops q 2 hours first 1-2 days; then 1-2 drops to affected eye(s) q 2-6 hours x 24-48 hours; then 4-6 hours; reduce frequency of dose as condition improves; max 20 ml per therapeutic course
Ophth susp: tobra 0.3%/*dexa* 0.1%/ml (2.5, 5 ml) (benzalkonium chloride)
TobraDex Ophthalmic Ointment <2 years: not recommended; ≥2 years: apply 1/2 inch ribbon to the lower conjunctival sac of affected eye(s) tid-qid; may use at HS in conjunction with daytime drops; max 8 gm/therapeutic course
Ophth oint: tobra 0.3%/*dexa* 0.1%/g (3.5 gm) (chlorobutanol chloride)
TobraDex ST <12 years: not recommended; ≥12 years: 1-2 drops to affected eye(s) q 2-6 hours x 24-48 hours; then 4-6 hours; reduce frequency of dose as condition improves; max 20 ml per therapeutic course
Ophth susp: tobra 0.3%/*dexa* 0.05%/ml (2.5, 5, 10 ml) (benzalkonium chloride)
➤ *tobramycin/loteprednol etabonate* ophthalmic suspension (C) <12 years: not recommended; ≥12 years: 1-2 drops to affected eye(s) q 1-2 hours first 24-48 hours; reduce frequency of dose to q 4-6 hours as condition improves; max 20 ml per therapeutic course
Zylet
Ophth susp: tobra 0.3%/*lote etab* 0.5%/ml (2.5, 5, 10 ml) (benzalkonium chloride)

CONJUNCTIVITIS: CHLAMYDIAL

Comment: A chlamydial etiology should be considered for all infants aged ≤30 days that have conjunctivitis, especially if the mother has a history of chlamydia infection. Topical antibiotic therapy alone is inadequate for treatment for ophthalmia neonatorum caused by chlamydia and is unnecessary when systemic treatment is administered.

ANTI-INFECTIVES

➤ *amoxicillin* (B)(G) <40 kg (88 lb): 20-40 mg/kg/day in 3 divided doses x 7 days or 25-45 mg/kg/day in 2 divided doses x 7 days; *see page 543 for dose by weight table;* ≥40 kg: 500-875 mg bid or 250-500 mg tid x 7 days
Amoxil *Cap:* 250, 500 mg; *Tab:* 875*mg; *Chew tab:* 125, 200, 250, 400 mg (cherry-banana-peppermint) (phenylalanine); Oral susp: 125, 250 mg/5 ml (80, 100, 150 ml) (strawberry); 200, 400 mg/5 ml (50, 75, 100 ml) (bubble gum); Oral drops: 50 mg/ml (30 ml) (bubble gum)

RECOMMENDED 1ST LINE REGIMEN

➤ *erythromycin base* (B)(G) <45 kg: 50 mg/kg/day in 4 divided doses x 14 days; ≥45 kg: 250 mg qid x 14 days or 500 mg qid x 7 days
Ery-Tab *Tab:* 250, 333, 500 mg ent-coat
PCE *Tab:* 333, 500 mg
➤ *erythromycin ethylsuccinate* (B)(G) 50 mg/kg/day in 4 divided doses x 14 days; max 100 mg/kg/day or 400 mg qid; *see page 563 for dose by weight table*

EryPed *Oral susp:* 200 mg/5 ml (100, 200 ml) (fruit); 400 mg/5 ml (60, 100, 200 ml) (banana); Oral drops: 200, 400 mg/5 ml (50 ml) (fruit); *Chew tab:* 200 mg wafer (fruit)
E.E.S. *Oral susp:* 200, 400 mg/5 ml (100 ml) (fruit)
E.E.S. Granules *Oral susp:* 200 mg/5 ml (100, 200 ml) (cherry)
E.E.S. 400 Tablets *Tab:* 400 mg

ALTERNATE REGIMEN

▷ *azithromycin* (B)(G) <12 years: 12 mg/kg/day x 5 days; *see page 548 for dose by weight table;* max 500 mg/day; ≥12 years: 500 mg x 1 dose on day 1, then 250 mg daily on days 2-5 or 500 mg daily x 3 days or Zmax 2 gm in a single dose
Zithromax *Tab:* 250, 500, 600 mg; *Oral susp:* 100 mg/5 ml (15 ml); 200 mg/5 ml (15, 22.5, 30 ml) (cherry); *Pkt:* 1 gm for reconstitution (cherry-banana)
Zithromax Tri-pak *Tab:* 3 x 500 mg tabs/pck
Zithromax Z-pak *Tab:* 6 x 250 mg tabs/pck
Zmax *Oral susp:* 2 gm ext-rel for reconstitution (cherry-banana) (148 mg Na$^+$)

CONJUNCTIVITIS: FUNGAL

▷ *natamycin* ophthalmic suspension (C) <1 year: not recommended; ≥1 year: 1 drop q 1-2 hours x 3-4 days; then 1 drop every 6 hours; treat for 14-21 days; withdraw dose gradually at 4- to 7-day intervals
Natacyn Ophthalmic Suspension *Ophth susp:* 0.5% (15 ml) (benzalkonium chloride)

CONJUNCTIVITIS: GONOCOCCAL

RECOMMENDED REGIMENS

Regimen 1

▷ *ceftriaxone* (B)(G) <45 kg: 50 mg/kg IM x 1 dose; max 125 mg IM; ≥45 kg: 250 mg IM x 1 dose
Rocephin *Vial:* 250, 500 mg; 1, 2 g

Regimen 2

▷ *erythromycin base* (B)(G) <45 kg: 50 mg/kg/day in 4 divided doses x 10-14 days; ≥45 kg: 250 mg qid x 10-14 days
Ery-Tab *Tab:* 250, 333, 500 mg ent-coat
PCE *Tab:* 333, 500 mg
▷ *erythromycin ethylsuccinate* (B)(G) 50 mg/kg/day in 4 divided doses x 7 days; max 100 mg/kg/day or 400 mg qid; *see page 563 for dose by weight table*
EryPed *Oral susp:* 200 mg/5 ml (100, 200 ml) (fruit); 400 mg/5 ml (60, 100, 200 ml) (banana); *Oral drops:* 200, 400 mg/5 ml (50 ml) (fruit); *Chew tab:* 200 mg wafer (fruit)
E.E.S. *Oral susp:* 200, 400 mg/5 ml (100 ml) (fruit)
E.E.S. Granules *Oral susp:* 200 mg/5 ml (100, 200 ml) (cherry)
E.E.S. 400 Tablets *Tab:* 400 mg

ALTERNATE REGIMEN

➤ *azithromycin* (B) <12 years: not recommended for bronchitis in children; ≥12 years: 500 mg x 1 dose on day 1; then 250 mg once daily on days; 2-5 or 500 mg daily x 3 days or 2 gm in a single dose

Zithromax *Tab:* 250, 500, 600 mg; *Oral susp:* 100 mg/5 ml (15 ml); 200 mg/5 ml (15, 22.5, 30 ml) (cherry); Pkt: 1 gm for reconstitution (cherry-banana)

Zithromax Tri-pak *Tab:* 3 x 500 mg tabs/pck

Zithromax Z-pak *Tab:* 6 x 250 mg tabs/pck

Zmax *Oral susp:* 2 gm ext-rel for reconstitution (cherry-banana) (148 mg Na$^+$)

CONJUNCTIVITIS: VIRAL

Comment: For prevention of secondary bacterial infection, see agents listed under bacterial conjunctivitis. Ophthalmic corticosteroids are contraindicated with herpes simplex, keratitis, *Varicella*, and other viral infections of the cornea.

➤ *trifluridine* ophthalmic suspension (C) <6 years: not recommended; ≥6 years: 1 drop q 2 hours while awake; max 9 drops/day; after re-epithelialization, 1 drop q 4 h x 7 days (at least 5 drops/day); max 21 days of therapy

Viroptic Ophthalmic Solution *Ophth soln:* 1% (7.5 ml) (thimerosal)

CONSTIPATION

CHRONIC IDIOPATHIC CONSTIPATION (CIC)

➤ *lubiprostone (chloride channel activator [GI motility enhancer])* (C) <12 years: not recommended; ≥12 years: 1 cap bid with food

Amitiza *Cap:* 24 mcg

➤ *linaclotide (guanylate cyclase-c agonist)* (C) <6 years: not recommended; 6-17 years: avoid; >17 years: 290 mcg once daily; take on an empty stomach at least 30 minutes before the first meal of the day; swallow whole

Linzess *Cap:* 145, 290 mcg

BULK-FORMING AGENTS

➤ *calcium polycarbophil* (C)

FiberCon (OTC) <6 years: not recommended; 6-12 years: 1 tab daily to qid; >12 years: 2 tabs once daily-qid

Cplt: 625 mg

Konsyl Fiber Tablets (OTC) *Tab:* 625 mg

➤ *methylcellulose*

Citrucel <6 years: not recommended; 6-12 years: 1/2 heaping tbsp in 4 oz cold water; >12 years: 1 heaping tbsp in 8 oz cold water tid

Oral pwdr: 16, 24, 30 oz and single-dose pkts (orange)

Citrucel Sugar-Free <6 years: not recommended; 6-12 years: 1 level tbsp in 4 oz cold water; >12 years: 1 heaping tbsp in 8 oz cold water tid

Oral pwdr: 16, 24, 30 oz and single-dose pkts (orange) (sugar-free, phenylalanine)

▷ *psyllium husk* (B) <6 years: not recommended; 6-12 years: 1/2 wafer, cap, or pkt in 8 oz liquid tid; >12 years: wafer or cap or 1 pkt or 1 rounded tsp (1 rounded tbsp for sugar-containing form) in 8 oz liquid tid

    Metamucil (OTC)
        Cap: psyllium husk 5.2 gm (100, 150/carton); *Wafer:* psyllium husk 3.4 gm/ rounded tsp (24/carton) (apple crisp, cinnamon spice); *Plain and flavored pwdr:* 3.4 g/rounded tsp (15, 20, 24, 29, 30, 36, 44, 48 oz); *Efferv sugar-free flav pkts:* 3.4 g/pkt (30/pkt) (phenylalanine)

▷ *psyllium* hydrophilic mucilloid (B) <6 years: not recommended; 6-12 years: 1 rounded tsp in 8 oz liquid tid; >12 years: 2 rounded tsp in 8 oz water qid

    Konsyl (OTC) *Pwdr:* 6 gm/rounded tsp (10.6, 15.9 oz); *Pwdr pkt:* 6 gm/rounded tsp (30/carton)
    Konsyl-D (OTC) *Pwdr:* 3.4 gm/rounded tsp (11.5, 17.59 oz); *Pwdr pkt:* 3.4 gm/ rounded tsp (30/carton)
    Konsyl Easy Mix Formula (OTC) *Pwdr:* 3.4 gm/rounded tsp (8 oz) (sugar-free, low sodium)
    Konsyl Orange (OTC) *Pwdr:* 3.4 gm/rounded tsp (19 oz); *Pwdr pkt:* 3.4 gm/ rounded tsp (30/carton)
    Konsyl Orange SF (OTC) *Pwdr:* 3.5 gm/rounded tsp (15 oz) (phenylalanine); *Pwdr pkt:* 3.5 gm/rounded tsp (30/carton) (phenylalanine)

STOOL SOFTENERS

▷ *docusate sodium* (OTC) <3 years: 10-40 mg/day; 3-6 years: 20-60 mg/day; >6-12 years: 40-120 mg/day; >12 years: 50-200 mg/day

    Cap: 50, 100 mg; *Liq:* 10 mg/ml (30 ml w. dropper); *Syr:* 20 mg/5 ml (8 oz) (alcohol ≤1%)
    Dialose 6 years: not recommended; ≥6 years: 1 tab q HS
    Tab: 100 mg
    Surfak (OTC) 12 years: not recommended; ≥12 years: 240 mg/day
    Cap: 240 mg

OSMOTIC LAXATIVES

▷ *lactulose* (B)(G) 6 years: not recommended; ≥6 years: take 10-20 gm dissolved in 4 oz water once daily prn; max 40 gm/day

    Kristalose *Crystals for oral soln:* 10, 20 gm single-dose pkts (30/carton)

▷ *magnesium citrate* (B)(G) <2 years: not recommended; 2-6 years: 4-12 ml once daily prn; ≥6-12 years: 50-100 ml once daily prn; >12 years: 1 full bottle (120-300 ml) once daily prn

    Citrate of Magnesia (OTC) *Oral soln:* 300 ml

▷ *magnesium hydroxide* (B) <2 years: not recommended; 2-5 years: 5-15 ml/day in a single or divided doses; 6-11 years: 15-30 ml/day in a single or divided doses; >11 years: 30-60 ml/day in a single or divided doses prn

    Milk of Magnesia *Liq:* 390 mg/5 ml (10, 15, 20, 30, 100, 120, 180, 360, 720 ml)

▷ *polyethylene glycol (PEG)* (C)(OTC)(G) ≤17: not recommended; >17 years: 1 tbsp (17 gm) dissolved in 4-8 oz water per day for up to max 7 days; may need 2-4 days for results

    GlycoLax Powder for Oral Solution *Oral pwdr:* 7, 14, 30, and 45 dose bottles w. 17 gm dosing cup (gluten-free, sugar-free); 17 gm single-dose pkts (20/ carton)

MiraLAX Powder for Oral Solution *Oral pwdr:* 7, 14, 30, and 45 dose bottles w. 17 gm dosing cup (gluten-free, sugar-free)
Polyethylene Glycol 3350 Powder for Oral Solution (G) *Oral pwdr:* 3350 gm w. dosing cup; 17 gm/scoop

Comment: *PEG* is an osmotic indicated for occasional constipation without affecting glucose and electrolyte levels. Contraindicated with suspected or known bowel obstruction.

STIMULANTS

▷ *bisacodyl* (B)(OTC) 2-3 tabs or 1 suppository bid prn
Dulcolax, Gentlax <12 years: 1/2 suppository once daily prn; 6-12 years: 1 tablet or 1/2 suppository once daily prn; >12 years: 1 tab or 1 rectal suppository
Tab: 5 mg; *Rectal supp:* 10 mg
Senokot <2 years: not recommended; 2-6 years: 1/4 tab or 1/2 tsp once daily prn; max 1 tab or 1/2 tsp bid; 6-12 years: 1 tab or 1/2 tsp once daily prn; max 2 tabs or 1 tsp once daily; >12 years: initially 2-4 tabs or 1 level tsp at HS prn; max 4 tabs or 2 tsp bid
Tab: 8.6*mg; *Granules:* 15 mg/tsp (2, 6, 12 oz) (cocoa)
Senokot Syrup <12 years: use Children's Syrup; ≥12 years: initially 10-15 ml at HS prn; max 15 ml bid
Syr: 8.8 mg/5 ml (2, 8 oz) (chocolate) (alcohol-free)
Senokot Children's Syrup (OTC) <2 years: not recommended; 2-6 years: 2.5-3.75 ml once daily prn; max 3.75 ml bid prn; ≥6-12 years: 5-7.5 ml once daily prn; max 7.5 ml bid
Syr: 8.8 mg/5 ml (2.5 oz) (chocolate) (alcohol-free)
Senokot Xtra (OTC) <2 years: not recommended; 2-6 years: use Children's Syrup; 6-12 years: 1/2 tab once daily at HS; max 1 tab bid; >12 years: 1 tab at HS prn; max 2 tabs bid
Tab: 17*mg

BULK-FORMING AGENT/STIMULANT COMBINATIONS

▷ *psyllium/senna* (B)
Perdiem (OTC) <7 years: not recommended; 7-11 years: 1 rounded tsp swallowed with 8 oz cool liquid qd-bid; >11 years: 1-2 rounded tsp swallowed with 8 oz cool liquid daily bid
Canister: 8.8, 14 oz; *Individual pkt:* 6 gm (6/pck)
SennaPrompt (OTC) <12 years: not recommended; ≥12 years: initially 2-5 caps bid
Cap: psyl 500 mg/*senna* 9 mg

STOOL SOFTENER/STIMULANT COMBINATIONS

▷ *docusate/casanthranol* (C)
Doxidan (OTC) <2 years: not recommended; ≥2 years-12 years: 1 cap/day; >12 years: 1-3 caps/day; max 1 week
Cap: doc 60 mg/*cas* 30 mg
Peri-Colace (OTC) <12 years: 5-15 ml q HS; ≥12 years: 1-2 caps or 15-30 ml q HS; max 2 caps or 30 ml bid or 3 caps q HS
Cap: doc 100 mg/*cas* 30 mg; *Syr: doc* 60 mg/*cas* 30 mg per 15 ml (8, 16 oz)

▷ *docusate/senna* concentrate (C)
    Senokot S (OTC) <2 years: not recommended; 2-6 years: 1/2 tab daily; max 1 tab bid; >6-12 years: 1 tab daily; max 2 tabs bid; >12 years: 2 tabs q HS; max 4 tabs bid
      Tab: doc 50 mg/*senna* 8.6 mg

ENEMAS AND OTHER AGENTS

▷ *sodium biphosphate/sodium phosphate* enema (C)(OTC)
    Fleets Adult <2 years: not recommended; 2-12 years: 59 ml rectally; >12 years: 59-118 ml rectally
      Enema: Na biphos 19 gm/*Na phos* 7 gm (59, 118 ml w. applicator)
    Fleets Pediatric <12 years: 59 ml rectally; ≥12 years: use **Fleets Adult**
      Enema: sod biphos 19 gm/*sod phos* 7 gm (59 ml w. applicator)
▷ *glycerin* suppositories (C)(OTC) <6 years: 1 pediatric suppository; ≥6 years: 1 adult suppository

CORNEAL EDEMA

▷ *sodium chloride* (NE)(G)
    Various (OTC) 1-2 drops <u>or</u> 1 inch ribbon q 3-4 hours prn; reduce frequency as edema subsides
      Ophth soln: 2, 5% (15, 30 ml); *Ophth oint:* 5% (3.5 gm)

CORNEAL ULCERATION

ANTIBACTERIAL OPHTHALMIC SOLUTION/OINTMENT

see Conjunctivitis/Blepharoconjunctivitis: Bacterial page 81

COSTOCHONDRITIS (CHEST WALL SYNDROME)

Acetaminophen for IV Infusion *see **Pain** page* 296
Oral Prescription NSAIDs *see page* 490
Other Oral Analgesics *see **Pain** page* 298
Topical/Transdermal NSAIDs *see **Pain** page* 298
Parenteral Corticosteroids *see page* 499
Oral Corticosteroids *see page* 498
Topical Analgesic and Anesthetic Agents *see page* 488

CRAMPS: ABDOMINAL, INTESTINAL

ANTISPASMODIC/ANTICHOLINERGIC COMBINATIONS

▷ *dicyclomine* (B)(G) <12 years: not recommended; ≥12 years: initially 20 mg bid-qid; may increase to 40 mg qid PO; usual IM dose 80 mg/day divided qid; do not use IM route for more than 1-2 days

Bentyl *Tab:* 20 mg; *Cap:* 10 mg; *Syr:* 10 mg/5 ml (16 oz); *Vial:* 10 mg/ml (10 ml); *Amp:* 10 mg/ml (2 ml)

➢ *methscopolamine bromide* (B) <12 years: not recommended; ≥12 years: 1 tab q 6 hours prn

Pamine *Tab:* 2.5 mg
Pamine Forte *Tab:* 5 mg

ANTICHOLINERGICS

➢ *hyoscyamine* (C)(G)

Anaspaz <2 years: not recommended; 2-12 years: 0.0625-0.125 mg q 4 hours prn; max 0.75 mg/day; >12 years: 1-2 tabs q 4 hours prn; max 12 tabs/day
Tab: 0.125*mg

Levbid <12 years: not recommended; ≥12 years: 1-2 tabs q 12 hours prn; max 4 tabs/day
Tab: 0.375*mg ext-rel

Levsin <6 years: not recommended; ≥6-12 years: 1 tab q 4 hours prn; >12 years: 1-2 tabs q 4 hours prn; max 12 tabs/day
Tab: 0.125*mg

Levsinex SL <2 years: not recommended; 2-12 years: 1 tab SL or PO q 4 hours; max 6 tabs/day; >12 years: 1-2 tabs q 4 hours SL or PO; max 12 tabs/day
Tab: 0.125 mg sublingual

Levsinex Timecaps <2 years: not recommended; 2-12 years: 1 cap q 12 hours; max 2 caps/day; >12 years: 1-2 caps q 12 hours; may adjust to 1 cap q 8 hours
Cap: 0.375 mg time-rel

NuLev <2 years: not recommended; 2-12 years: dissolve 1 tab on tongue, with or without water, q 4 hours prn; max 6 tabs/day; >12 years: dissolve 1-2 tabs on tongue, with or without water, q 4 hours prn; max 12 tabs/day
ODT: 0.125 mg (mint) (phenylalanine)

➢ *simethicone* (C)(G) 0.3 ml qid pc and HS

Mylicon Drops (OTC) *Oral drops:* 40 mg/0.6 ml (30 ml)

➢ *phenobarbital/hyoscyamine/atropine/scopolamine* (C)(IV)(G)

Donnatal <12 years: not recommended; ≥12 years: 1-2 tabs ac and HS
Tab: pheno 16.2 mg/*hyo* 0.1037 mg/*atro* 0.0194 mg/*scop* 0.0065 mg

Donnatal Elixir 20 lb: 1 ml q 4 hours or 1.5 ml q 6 hours; 30 lb: 1.5 ml q 4 hours or 2 ml q 6 hours; 50 lb: 1/2 tsp q 4 hours or 3/4 tsp q 6 hours; 75 lb: 3/4 tsp q 4 hours or 1 tsp q 6 hours; 100 lb: 1 tsp q 4 hours or 1 tsp q 6 hours; ≥12 years: 1-2 tsp ac and HS
Elix: pheno 16.2 mg/*hyo* 0.1037 mg/*atro* 0.0194 mg/*scop* 0.0065 mg per 5 ml (4, 16 oz)

Donnatal Extentabs <12 years: not recommended; ≥12 years: 1 tab q 12 hours
Tab: pheno 48.6 mg/*hyo* 0.3111 mg/*atro* 0.0582 mg/*scop* 0.0195 mg ext-rel

ANTICHOLINERGIC/SEDATIVE COMBINATION

➢ *chlordiazepoxide/clidinium* (D)(IV) <12 years: not recommended; ≥12 years: 1-2 caps ac and HS; max 8 caps/day
Librax *Cap: chlor* 5 mg/*clid* 2.5 mg

CROHN'S DISEASE

Comment: Standard treatment regimen for active disease (flare) is: antibiotic, antispasmodic, and bowel rest; progress to clear liquids; then progress to high-fiber diet.

Parenteral Corticosteroids *see page* 499
Oral Corticosteroids *see page* 498

▷ *azathioprine* (D)(G)

Imuran *Tab:* 50*mg; *Injectable:* 100 mg
Comment: **Imuran** is usually administered on a daily basis. The initial dose should be approximately 1.0 mg/kg (50 to 100 mg) as a single dose or divided bid. Dose may be increased beginning at 6-8 weeks, and thereafter at 4-week intervals, if there are no serious toxicities and if initial response is unsatisfactory. Dose increments should be 0.5 mg/kg/day, up to max 2.5 mg/kg per day. Therapeutic response usually occurs after 6-8 weeks of treatment. An adequate trial should be a minimum of 12 weeks. Patients not improved after 12 weeks can be considered refractory. **Imuran** may be continued long-term in patients with clinical response, but patients should be monitored carefully, and gradual dosage reduction should be attempted to reduce risk of toxicities. Maintenance therapy should be at the lowest effective dose, and the dose given can be lowered decrementally with changes of 0.5 mg/kg or approximately 25 mg daily every 4 weeks while other therapy is kept constant. The optimum duration of maintenance **Imuran** has not been determined. **Imuran** can be discontinued abruptly, but delayed effects are possible.

▷ *infliximab (tumor necrosis factor-alpha blocker)* (B) <12 years: not recommended; ≥12 years: administer 5 mg/kg/dose by IV infusion over at least 2 h; *Fistulizing disease:* initial dose; repeat dose at 2 weeks and 6 weeks (total 3 doses); then repeat dose every 8 weeks; *Maintenance:* usually 5 mg/kg every 8 weeks; may increase to 10 mg/kg/dose

Remicade *Vial:* 100 mg pwdr for IV infusion single use (preservative-free)

▷ *mesalamine* (B)

Asacol <12 years: not recommended; ≥12 years: 800 mg tid x 6 weeks; maintenance 1.6 gm/day in divided doses; swallow whole, do not crush or chew
Tab: 400 mg del-rel

Comment: 2 **Asacol** 400 mg tabs are not bioequivalent to 1 **Asacol HD** 800 mg tab.

Asacol HD <12 years: not recommended; ≥12 years: 1,600 mg tid x 6 weeks; swallow whole, do not crush or chew
Tab: 800 mg del-rel

Comment: 1 **Asacol HD** 800 mg tab is not bioequivalent to 2 **Asacol** 400 mg tabs

Canasa <12 years: not established; ≥12 years: 1 gm qid for up to 8 weeks
Rectal supp: 1 gm del-rel (30, 42/pck)

Delzicol <5 years: not established; >5 years: *Treatment:* 800 mg tid x 6 weeks; maintenance 1.6 gm/day in 2-4 divided doses daily; swallow whole; do not crush or chew
Cap: 400 mg del-rel

Comment: 2 **Delzicol** 400 mg caps are not bioequivalent to 1 *mesalamine* 800 mg del-rel tab

Lialda <18 years: not established; ≥18 years: 2.4-4.8 gm daily in a single dose for up to 8 weeks; swallow whole, do not crush or chew

Tab: 1.2 gm del-rel

Pentasa <12 years: not established; ≥12 years: 1 gm qid for up to 8 weeks; swallow whole, do not crush or chew

Cap: 250 mg cont-rel

Rowasa Enema <12 years: not established; ≥12 years: 4 gm rectally by enema q HS; retain for 8 hours x 3-6 weeks

Enema: 4 gm/60 ml (7, 14, 28/pck; kit, 7, 14, 28/pck w. wipes)

Rowasa Suppository <12 years: not established; ≥12 years: 1 suppository rectally bid x 3-6 weeks; retain for 1-3 hours or longer

Rectal supp: 500 mg

Sulfite-Free Rowasa Rectal Suspension <12 years: not established; ≥12 years: 4 gm rectally by enema q HS; retain for 8 hours x 3-6 weeks

Enema: 4 gm/60 ml (7, 14, 28/pck; kit, 7, 14, 28/pck w. wipes)

▷ *olsalazine* (C)

Dipentum <12 years: not established; ≥12 years: 1 gm/day in 2 divided doses; max 2 gm/day

Cap: 250 mg

Comment: Indicated in persons who cannot tolerate *sulfasalazine*.

▷ *sulfasalazine* (B)(G)

Azulfidine <2 years: not recommended; 2-16 years: initially 40-60 mg/kg/day in 3-6 divided doses; max 2 gm/day; >16 years: initially 1-2 gm/day; increase to 3-4 gm/day in divided doses pc until clinical symptoms controlled; maintenance 2 gm/day; max 4 gm/day

Tab: 500*mg

Azulfidine EN <2 years: not recommended; 2-16 years: initially 40-60 mg/kg/day in 3-6 divided doses; max 2 gm/day; >16 years: initially 500 mg in the PM x 7 days; then 500 mg bid x 7 days; then 500 mg in the AM and 1 gm in the PM x 7 days; then 1 gm bid; max 4 gm/day

Tab: 500 mg ent-coat

▷ *vedolizumab* (B) <2 years: not recommended; 2-16 years: initially 40-60 mg/kg/day in 3-6 divided doses; max 2 gm/day; >16 years: administer by IV infusion over 30 minutes; 300 mg at weeks 0, 2, 6; then once every 8 weeks

Entyvio *Vial:* 300 mg (20 ml) single dose, pwdr for IV infusion after reconstitution (preservative-free)

▷ *budesonide micronized* (C)(G) <12 years: not established; ≥12 years: *Treatment* 9 mg once daily in the AM for up to 8 weeks; may repeat an 8-week course; *Maintenance of remission*: 6 mg once daily for up to 3 months

Entcort EC *Cap:* 3 mg ent-coat ext-rel granules

Comment: Taper other systemic steroids when transferring to **Entocort EC.** When corticosteroids are used chronically, systemic effects such as hypercorticism and adrenal suppression may occur. Corticosteroids can reduce the response of the hypothalamus-pituitary-adrenal (HPA) axis to stress. In situations where patients are subject to surgery or other stress situations, supplementation with a systemic corticosteroid is recommended. General precautions concerning corticosteroids should be followed.

ORAL ANTI-INFECTIVES

▷ *metronidazole* (not for use in 1st; B in 2nd, 3rd)(G) <12 years: 35-50 mg/kg/day in 3 divided doses x 10 days; ≥12 years: 500 mg tid or 750 mg bid; max 8 weeks

Flagyl *Tab:* 250*, 500*mg

Flagyl 375 *Cap:* 375 mg

Flagyl ER *Tab:* 750 mg ext-rel

Comment: Alcohol is contraindicated during treatment with oral *metronidazole* and for 72 hours after therapy due to a possible *disulfiram*-like reaction (nausea, vomiting, flushing, headache).

TUMOR NECROSIS FACTOR (TNF) BLOCKER

▷ *adalimumab* (B) <2 years, <10 kg: not recommended; 10-<15 kg: 10 mg every other week; 15-<30 kg: 20 mg every other week; ≥30 kg: 40 mg every other week; 2-17 years, supervise first dose; ≥12 years: 40 mg SC once every other week; may increase to once weekly without MTX; administer in abdomen or thigh; rotate sites

Humira *Prefilled syringe:* 20 mg/0.4 ml; 40 mg/0.8 ml single dose (2/pck; 2, 6/ starter pck) (preservative-free)

Comment: May use with methotrexate (MTX), DMARDs, corticosteroids, salicylates, NSAIDs, or analgesics.

▷ *certolizumab* (B) <12 years: not established; ≥12 years: 400 mg SC (2 x 200 mg inj at two different sites on day 1); then, 400 mg SC at weeks 2 and 4; maintenance 400 mg SC every 4 weeks; administer in abdomen or thigh; rotate sites

Cimzia *Vial:* 200 mg (2/pck); *Prefilled syringe:* 200 mg/ml single dose (2/pck; 2, 6/starter pck) (preservative-free)

▷ *infliximab* (B) <6 years: not recommended; ≥6 years: administer by IV infusion over 2 hours; 5 mg/kg weeks 0, 2, 6; then once every 8 weeks

Remicade

Vial: 100 mg pwdr for reconstitution for IV infusion (preservative-free)

▷ *vedolizumab* (B) <6 years: not recommended; ≥6 years: administer by IV infusion over 30 minutes; 300 mg at weeks 0, 2, 6; then 300 mg once every 8 weeks

Entyvio

Vial: 300 mg (20 ml) single dose, pwdr for IV infusion after reconstitution (preservative-free)

INTEGRIN RECEPTOR ANTAGONIST (IMMUNOMODULATOR)

▷ *natalizumab* (C) <6 years: not established; ≥6 years: administer by IV infusion over 1 hour; monitor during and for 1 hour post infusion; 300 mg every 4 weeks; discontinue after 12 weeks if no therapeutic response, or if unable to taper off chronic concomitant steroids within 6 months; may continue aminosalicylates

Tysabri *Vial:* 300 mg single-dose, soln after dilution for IV infusion (preservative-free)

CRYPTOSPORIDIUM PARVUM

▷ *nitazoxanide* (B) <12 months: not recommended; 12-47 months: 5 ml q 12 hours x 3 days; 4-11 years: 10 ml q 12 hours x 3 days; ≥12 years: 500 mg by mouth q 12 hours x 3 days

Alinia *Oral susp:* 100 mg/5 ml (60 ml)
Comment: **Alinia** is an antiprotozoal for the treatment of diarrhea due to
G. lamblia or *C. parvum.*

CYSTIC FIBROSIS

▶ *acetylcysteine* (B)(G) administer via face mask, mouth piece, tracheostomy T-piece,
mist tent, or croupette; routine tracheostomy care, 1 to 2 ml of a 10% to 20%
solution may be administered by direct instillation into the tracheostomy every 1 to
4 hours
   Mucomyst *Vial:* 10, 20% (4, 10, 30 ml) soln for inhalation
   Comment: **Mucomyst** is a mucolytic. For inhalation, the 10% concentration
   may be used undiluted; the 20% concentration should be diluted with sterile
   water or normal saline (either for injection or inhalation).
▶ *lumacaftor/ivacaftor* (B) <12 years: not established; ≥12 years: 2 tabs q 12 hours;
reduce dose with moderate to severe hepatic impairment
   Orkambi *Tab: luma* 200 mg/*iva* 125 mg film-coat

CYSTIC FIBROSIS TRANSMEMBRANE CONDUCTANCE REGULATOR (CFTR) POTENTIATOR

▶ *ivacaftor* (B) <6 years: not established; ≥6 years: 150 mg every 12 hours; administer
with fat-containing food (e.g., eggs, butter, peanut butter, cheese pizza); avoid food
containing grapefruit or Seville oranges.
   Kalydeco *Tab:* 150 mg film-coat
   Comment: **Kalydeco** is indicated for the treatment of CF in patients who have a
   G551D comutation in the *CFTR* gene. If the patient's genotype is unknown, an
   FDA-cleared CF mutation test should be used to detect the presence of the *G551D*
   mutation. **Kalydeco** is not effective in patients with CF who are homozygous for
   the *F508del* mutation in the *CFTR* gene. Transaminases (ALT and AST) should
   be assessed prior to initiating **Kalydeco**, every 3 months during the first year of
   treatment, and annually thereafter. Patients who develop increased transaminase
   levels should be closely monitored until the abnormalities resolve. Dosing should
   be interrupted in patients with ALT or AST greater than 5 times the upper limit
   of normal (ULN). Following resolution of transaminase elevations, consider the
   benefits and risks of resuming **Kalydeco** dosing. Concomitant use with strong
   CYP3A inducers (e.g., *rifampin*, St. John's Wort) substantially decreases exposure
   of **Kalydeco** (which may diminish effectiveness); therefore, co-administration is
   not recommended. Reduce dose to 150 mg twice weekly when co-administered
   with strong CYP3A inhibitors (e.g., *ketoconazole*). Reduce dose to 150 mg
   once daily when co-administered with moderate CYP3A inhibitors. Caution is
   recommended in patients with severe renal impairment (CrCl <30 mL/min) or
   ESRD. No dose adjustment is necessary for patients with mild hepatic impairment
   (Child-Pugh Class A). A reduced dose of 150 mg once daily is recommended in
   patients with moderate hepatic impairment (Child-Pugh Class B). No studies
   have been conducted in patients with severe hepatic impairment (Child-Pugh
   Class C). The most commonly reported adverse reactions are headache, sore
   throat, nasopharyngitis, URI, nasal congestion, abdominal pain, nausea, diarrhea,
   dizziness, and rash. Excretion of **Kalydeco** into human milk is probable. To report

suspected adverse reactions, contact Vertex Pharmaceuticals Incorporated at 1-877-752-5933 or FDA at 1-800-FDA-1088 or www.fda.gov/medwatch.

ANTI-INFECTIVE

▷ *ciprofloxacin* (C) <18 years: 20-40 mg/kg/day divided q 12 hours; ≥18 years: 500 mg bid x 7-10 days; max 1.5 gm/day

Cipro (G) *Tab:* 250, 500, 750 mg; *Oral susp:* 250, 500 mg/5 ml (100 ml) (strawberry)
Cipro XR *Tab:* 500, 1000 mg ext-rel
ProQuin XR *Tab:* 500 mg ext-rel

DEEP VEIN THROMBOSIS (DVT)

Anticoagulation Therapy *see page* 515

DEHYDRATION

ORAL REHYDRATION AND ELECTROLYTE REPLACEMENT THERAPY

▷ *oral electrolyte replacement* (NE)(OTC)(G)

KaoLectrolyte <12 years: not indicated; ≥12 years: 1 pkt dissolved in 8 oz water q 3-4 hours

Pkt: sod 12 mEq/*pot* 5 mEq/*chlor* 10 mEq/*citrate* 7 mEq/*dextrose* 5 gm/ calories 22 per 6.2 g
Pedialyte <2 years: as desired and as tolerated; ≥2 years: 1-2 liters/day

Oral soln: dextrose 20 gm/*fructose* 5 gm/*sodium* 25 mEq/*potassium* 20 mEq/ *chloride* 35 mEq/*citrate* 30 mEq/*calories* 100 per liter (8 oz, 1 L)
Pedialyte Freezer Pops as desired and as tolerated

Pops: dextrose 1.6 gm/*sodium* 2.8 mEq/*potassium* 1.25 mEq/*chloride* 2.2 mEq/*citrate* 1.88 mEq/*calories* 6.25 per 62.5 ml (2.1 fl oz) pop

DENTAL ABSCESS

▷ *amoxicillin/clavulanate* (B)(G)

Augmentin <40 kg: 40-45 mg/kg/day divided tid x 10 days or 90 mg/kg/day divided bid x 10 days; *see page* 545 *for dose by weight table;* ≥40 kg: 500 mg tid or 875 mg bid x 10 days

Tab: 250, 500, 875 mg; *Chew tab:* 125, 250 mg (lemon-lime); 200, 400 mg (cherry-banana) (phenylalanine); *Oral susp:* 125 mg/5 ml (banana), 250 mg/5 ml (75, 100, 150 ml) (orange); 200, 400 mg/5 ml (50, 75, 100 ml) (orange) (phenylalanine)
Augmentin ES-600 <3 months: not recommended; ≥3 months, <40 kg: 90 mg/ kg/day divided q 12 hours x 10 days; *see page* 546 *for dose by weight table;* ≥40 kg: not recommended

Oral susp: 600 mg/5 ml (50, 75, 100, 125, 150, 200 ml) (strawberry cream) (phenylalanine)
Augmentin XR <16 years: use other forms; ≥16 years: 2 tabs q 12 hours x 7-10 days

Tab: 1000*mg ext-rel

➤ *clindamycin*(B)(G) <12 years: 8-16 mg/kg/day in 3-4 divided doses x 10 days; *see page 559 for dose by weight table;* administer with TMP-SMX; ≥12 years: 300 mg qid x 10 days; administer with fluoroquinolone

 Cleocin *Cap:* 75 (tartrazine), 150 (tartrazine), 300 mg
 Cleocin Pediatric Granules *Oral susp:* 75 mg/5 ml (100 ml) (cherry)

➤ *erythromycin base* (B)(G) <45 kg: 50 mg/kg/day in 4 divided doses x 10-14 days; ≥45 kg: 500 mg q 6 hours x 10 days

 Ery-Tab *Tab:* 250, 333, 500 mg ent-coat
 PCE *Tab:* 333, 500 mg

➤ *erythromycin ethylsuccinate* (B)(G) 30-50 mg/kg/day in 4 divided doses x 7 days; may double dose with severe infection; max 100 mg/kg/day <u>or</u> 400 mg qid; *see page 563 for dose by weight table*

 EryPed *Oral susp:* 200 mg/5 ml (100, 200 ml) (fruit); 400 mg/5 ml (60, 100, 200 ml) (banana); *Oral drops:* 200, 400 mg/5 ml (50 ml) (fruit); *Chew tab:* 200 mg wafer (fruit)
 E.E.S. *Oral susp:* 200, 400 mg/5 ml (100 ml) (fruit)
 E.E.S. Granules *Oral susp:* 200 mg/5 ml (100, 200 ml) (cherry)
 E.E.S. 400 Tablets *Tab:* 400 mg

➤ *penicillin V potassium* (B) <12 years: 25-75 mg/kg day divided q 6-8 hours x 5-7 days; *see page 572 for dose by weight table;* ≥12 years: 250-500 mg q 6 hours x 5-7 days

 Pen-VK *Tab:* 250, 500 mg; *Oral soln:* 125 mg/5 ml (100, 200 ml); 250 mg/5 ml(100, 150, 200 ml)

DEPRESSION, MAJOR DEPRESSIVE DISORDER (MDD)

Comment: Abrupt withdrawal or interruption of treatment with an antidepressant medication is sometimes associated with an *antidepressant discontinuation syndrome* which may be mediated by gradually tapering the drug over a period of two weeks or longer, depending on the dose strength and length of treatment. Common symptoms of antidepressant withdrawal include flu-like symptoms, insomnia, nausea, imbalance, sensory disturbances, and hyperarousal. These medications include SSRIs, TCAs, MAOIs, and atypical agents such as *venlafaxine* (**Effexor**), *mirtazapine* (**Remeron**), *trazodone* (**Desyrel**), and *duloxetine* (**Cymbalta**). Common symptoms of the *serotonin discontinuation syndrome* include flu-like symptoms (nausea, vomiting, diarrhea, headaches, sweating), sleep disturbances (insomnia, nightmares, constant sleepiness), mood disturbances (dysphoria, anxiety, agitation), cognitive disturbances (mental confusion, hyperarousal), sensory and movement disturbances (imbalance, tremors, vertigo, dizziness, electric-shock-like sensations in the brain, often described by sufferers as "brain zaps").

SELECTIVE SEROTONIN REUPTAKE INHIBITORS (SSRIs)

Comment: Co-administration of SSRIs with TCAs requires extreme caution. Concomitant use of MAOIs and SSRIs is absolutely contraindicated. Avoid St. John's wort and other serotonergic agents. A potentially fatal adverse event is *serotonin syndrome*, caused by serotonin excess. Milder symptoms require HCP intervention to avert severe symptoms that can be rapidly fatal without urgent/emergent medical care.

Symptoms include restlessness, agitation, confusion, tachycardia, hypertension, dilated pupils, muscle twitching, muscle rigidity, loss of muscle coordination, diaphoresis, diarrhea, headache, shivering, piloerection, hyperpyrexia, cardiac arrhythmias, seizures, loss of consciousness, coma, death. Common symptoms of the *serotonin discontinuation syndrome* include flu-like symptoms (nausea, vomiting, diarrhea, headaches, sweating), sleep disturbances (insomnia, nightmares, constant sleepiness), mood disturbances (dysphoria, anxiety, agitation), cognitive disturbances (mental confusion, hyperarousal, hallucinations), sensory and movement disturbances (imbalance, tremors, vertigo, dizziness, electric-shock-like sensations in the brain, often described by sufferers as "brain zaps").

▷ *citalopram* (C)(G) <12 years: not recommended; ≥12 years: initially 20 mg once daily; may increase after one week to 40 mg once daily; max 40 mg

    Celexa *Tab:* 10, 20, 40 mg; *Oral soln:* 10 mg/5 ml (120 ml) (pepper mint) (sugar-free, alcohol-free, parabens)

▷ *escitalopram* (C)(G) <12 years: not recommended; 12-17 years: initially 10 mg daily; may increase to 20 mg daily after 3 weeks; >17 years: initially 10 mg daily; may increase to 20 mg daily after 1 week; *Hepatic impairment:* 10 mg once daily

    Lexapro *Tab:* 5, 10*, 20*mg

    Lexapro Oral Solution *Oral soln:* 1 mg/ml (240 ml) (peppermint) (parabens)

▷ *fluoxetine* (C)(G)

    Prozac <8 years: not recommended; 8-17 years: initially 10 mg/day; may increase after 1 week to 20 mg/day; range 20-60 mg/day; range for lower weight children, 20-30 mg/day; >17 years: initially 20 mg daily; may increase after 1 week; doses >20 mg/day should be divided into AM and noon doses; max 80 mg/day

        Cap: 10, 20, 40 mg; *Tab:* 30*, 60*mg; *Oral soln:* 20 mg/5 ml (4 oz) (mint)

    Prozac Weekly <12 years: not recommended; ≥12 years: following daily *fluoxetine* therapy at 20 mg/day for 13 weeks, may initiate **Prozac Weekly** 7 days after the last 20 mg *fluoxetine* dose

        Cap: 90 mg ent-coat del-rel pellets

▷ *levomilnacipran* (C) <12 years: not recommended; ≥12 years: swallow whole; initially 20 mg once daily for 2 days; then increase to 40 mg once daily; may increase dose in 40 mg increments at intervals of ≥2 days; max 120 mg once daily; *CrCl 30-59 mL/min:* max 80 mg once daily; *CrCl 15-29 mL/min:* max 40 mg once daily

    Fetzima *Cap:* 20, 40, 80, 120 mg ext-rel

▷ *paroxetine maleate* (D)(G)

    Paxil <12 years: not recommended; ≥12 years: initially 20 mg daily in AM; may increase by 10 mg/day at weekly intervals as needed; max 60 mg/day

        Tab: 10*, 20*, 30, 40 mg

    Paxil CR <12 years: not recommended; ≥12 years: initially 25 mg daily in AM; may increase by 12.5 mg at weekly intervals as needed; max 62.5 mg/day

        Tab: 12.5, 25, 37.5 mg cont-rel ent-coat

    Paxil Suspension <12 years: not recommended; ≥12 years: initially 20 mg daily in AM; may increase by 10 mg/day at weekly intervals as needed; max 60 mg/day

        Oral susp: 10 mg/5 ml (250 ml) (orange)

▷ *sertraline* (C)(G) <6 years: not recommended; 6-<12 years: initially 25 mg daily; max 200 mg/day; 12-17 years: initially 50 mg daily; max 200 mg/day >17 years: initially 50 mg daily; increase at 1 week intervals if needed; max 200 mg daily; dilute oral concentrate immediately prior to administration in 4 oz water, ginger ale, lemon/lime soda, lemonade, *or* orange juice

    Zoloft *Tab:* 25*, 50*, 100*mg; *Oral conc:* 20 mg per ml (60 ml) (alcohol 12%)

SEROTONIN AND NOREPINEPHRINE REUPTAKE INHIBITORS (SNRIs)

▷ *desvenlafaxine* (C)(G) <18 years: not recommended; ≥18 years: swallow whole; initially 50 mg once daily; max 120 mg/day
   Pristiq *Tab:* 50, 100 mg ext-rel
▷ *duloxetine* (C)(G) <12 years: not recommended; ≥12 years: swallow whole; initially 30 mg once daily x 1 week; then, increase to 60 mg once daily; max 120 mg/day
   Cymbalta *Cap:* 20, 30, 40, 60 mg del-rel
▷ *venlafaxine* (C)(G)
   Effexor initially <12 years: not recommended; ≥12 years: 75 mg/day in 2-3 divided doses; may increase at 4 day intervals in 75 mg increments to 150 mg/day; max 225 mg/day
      Tab: 37.5, 75, 150, 225 mg
   Effexor XR <18 years: not recommended; ≥18 years: initially 75 mg q AM; may start at 37.5 mg daily x 4-7 days, then increase by increments of up to 75 mg/day at intervals of at least 4 days; usual max 375 mg/day
      Tab/Cap: 37.5, 75, 150 mg ext-rel
▷ *vortioxetine* (C) <18 years: not established; ≥18 years: initially 10 mg once daily; max 30 mg/day
   Brintellix *Tab:* 5, 10, 15, 20 mg

SELECTIVE SEROTONIN REUPTAKE INHIBITOR (SSRI)/5-HT-14 RECEPTOR PARTIAL AGONIST COMBINATION

▷ *vilazodone* (C) <18 years: not established; ≥18 years: take with food; initially 10 mg once daily x 7 days; then, 20 mg once daily x 7 days; then, 40 mg once daily
   Viibryd *Tab:* 10, 20, 40 mg

THIENOBENZODIAZEPINE/SSRI COMBINATION

▷ *olanzapine/fluoxetine* (C) <10 years: not established; ≥10 years: initially one 6/25 cap in the PM; titrate; max one 18/75 cap once daily in the PM
   Symbyax
      Cap: **Symbyax 3/25:** *olan* 3 mg/*fluo* 25 mg
         Symbyax 6/25: *olan* 6 mg/*fluo* 25 mg
         Symbyax 6/50: *olan* 6 mg/*fluo* 50 mg
         Symbyax 12/25: *olan* 12 mg/*fluo* 25 mg
         Symbyax 12/50: *olan* 12 mg/*fluo* 50 mg
   Comment: **Symbyax** is a thienobenzodiazepine-SSRI indicated for the treatment of depressive episodes associated with bipolar depression disorder and treatment resistant depression (TRD).

TRICYCLIC ANTIDEPRESSANTS (TCAs)

Comment: Co-administration of SSRIs and TCAs requires extreme caution.
▷ *amitriptyline* (C)(G) <12 years: not recommended; ≥12 years: 10-20 mg q HS
   Tab: 10, 25, 50, 75, 100, 150 mg

▷ *amoxapine* (C) <12 years: not recommended; ≥12 years: initially 50 mg bid-tid; after 1 week may increase to 100 mg bid-tid; usual effective dose 200-300 mg/day; if total dose exceeds 300 mg/day, give in divided doses (max 400 mg/day); may give as a single bedtime dose (max 300 mg q HS)
    Tab: 25, 50, 100, 150 mg
▷ *clomipramine* (C)(G) <10 years: not recommended; 10-<16 years: initially 25 mg daily in divided doses; gradually increase; max 3 mg/kg or 100 mg, whichever is smaller; >16 years: initially 25 mg daily in divided doses; gradually increase to 100 mg during first 2 weeks; max 250 mg/day; total maintenance dose may be given at HS
    Anafranil *Cap:* 25, 50, 75 mg
▷ *desipramine* (C)(G) <12 years: not recommended; ≥12 years: 100-200 mg/day in single or divided doses; max 300 mg/day
    Norpramin *Tab:* 10, 25, 50, 75, 100, 150 mg
▷ *doxepin* (C)(G) <12 years: not recommended; ≥12 years: 75 mg/day; max 150 mg/day
    Cap: 10, 25, 50, 75, 100, 150 mg; *Oral conc:* 10 mg/ml (4 oz w. dropper)
▷ *imipramine* (C)(G) <12 years: not recommended; ≥12 years:
    Tofranil initially 75 mg daily (max 200 mg); adolescents initially 30-40 mg daily (max 100 mg/day); if maintenance dose exceeds 75 mg daily, may switch to
    Tofranil PM for divided or bedtime dose
        Tab: 10, 25, 50 mg
    Tofranil PM initially 75 mg daily 1 hour before HS; max 200 mg
        Cap: 75, 100, 125, 150 mg
▷ *nortriptyline* (D)(G) <12 years: not recommended; ≥12 years: initially 25 mg tid-qid; max 150 mg/day
    Pamelor *Cap:* 10, 25, 50, 75 mg; *Oral soln:* 10 mg/5 ml (16 oz)
▷ *protriptyline* (C) <12 years: not recommended; ≥12 years: initially 5 mg tid; usual dose 15-40 mg/day in 3-4 divided doses; max 60 mg/day
    Vivactil *Tab:* 5, 10 mg
▷ *trimipramine* (C) <12 years: not recommended; ≥12 years: initially 75 mg/day in divided doses; max 200 mg/day
    Surmontil *Cap:* 25, 50, 100 mg

AMINOKETONES

▷ *bupropion HBr* (C)(G)
    Aplenzin <18 years: not recommended; ≥18 years: initially 100 mg bid for at least 3 days; may increase to 375 or 400 mg/day after several weeks; then after at least 3 more days, 450 mg in 4 divided doses; max 450 mg/day, 174 mg/single dose
        Tab: 174, 348, 522 mg
    Forfivo XL <18 years: not recommended; ≥18 years: do not use for initial treatment; use immediate-release bupropion forms for initial titration; switch to **Forfivo XL** 450 mg once daily when total dose/day reaches 450 mg; may switch to **Forfivo XL** when total dose/day reaches 300 mg for 2 weeks and patient needs 450 mg/day to reach therapeutic target; swallow whole, do not crush or chew
        Tab: 450 mg ext-rel
▷ *bupropion HCl* (C)(G)
    Wellbutrin <18 years: not recommended; ≥18 years: initially 100 mg bid for at least 3 days; may increase to 375 or 400 mg/day after several weeks; then after at least 3 more days, 450 mg in 4 divided doses; max 450 mg/day, 150 mg/single dose

Tab: 75, 100 mg

Wellbutrin SR <18 years: not recommended; ≥18 years: initially 150 mg in AM for at least 3 days; increase to 150 mg bid if well tolerated; usual dose 300 mg/day; max 400 mg/day

Tab: 100, 150 mg sust-rel

Wellbutrin XL <18 years: not recommended; ≥18 years: initially 150 mg in AM for at least 3 days; increase to 150 mg bid if well tolerated; usual dose 300 mg/day; max 450 mg/day

Tab: 150, 300 mg sust-rel

MONOAMINE OXIDASE INHIBITORS (MAOIs)

Comment: Many drug and food interactions with this class of drugs; use cautiously. Should be reserved for refractory depression that has not responded to other classes of antidepressants. Concomitant use of MAOIs and SSRIs is an absolute contraindication. See mfr pkg insert for drug and food interactions.

▷ *isocarboxazid* (C)(G) <16 years: not recommended; ≥16 years: initially 10 mg bid; increase by 10 mg every 2-4 days up to 40 mg/day; may increase by 20 mg/week to max 60 mg/day divided bid-qid

Marplan *Tab:* 10 mg

▷ *phenelzine* (C)(G) <16 years: not recommended; ≥16 years: initially 15 mg tid; max 90 mg/day

Nardil *Tab:* 15 mg

▷ *selegiline* (C) initially 10 mg tid; max 60 mg/day

Emsam *Transdermal patch:* 6 mg/24 h, 9 mg/24 h, 12 mg/24 h

Comment: With the **Emsam** transdermal patch 6 mg/24 h dose, the dietary restrictions commonly required when using non-selective MAOIs are not necessary.

▷ *tranylcypromine* (C) initially 10 mg tid; may increase in 10 mg/day every 1-3 weeks; max 60 mg/day

Parnate *Tab:* 10 mg

TETRACYCLICS

▷ *maprotiline* (B)(G) <18 years: not recommended; ≥18 years: initially 75 mg/day for 2 weeks then change gradually as needed in 25 mg increments; max 225 mg/day

Ludiomil *Tab:* 25, 50, 75 mg

▷ *mirtazapine* (C) <12 years: not recommended; ≥12 years: initially 15 mg q HS; increase at intervals of 1-2 weeks; usual range 15-45 mg/day; max 45 mg/day

Remeron *Tab:* 15*, 30*, 45*mg

Remeron SolTab *ODT:* 15, 30, 45 mg (orange) (phenylalanine)

▷ *chlordiazepoxide/amitriptyline* (C)(IV)

Limbitrol <12 years: not recommended; ≥12 years: 3-4 tabs in divided doses

Tab: chlor 5 mg/*amit* 12.5 mg

Limbitrol DS <18 years: not recommended; ≥18 years: 3-4 tabs in divided doses; max 6 tabs/day

Tab: chlor 10 mg/*amit* 25 mg

▷ *trazodone* (C)(G) <18 years: not recommended; ≥18 years: initially 150 mg/day in divided doses with food; increase by 50 mg/day q 3-4 days; max 400 mg/day in divided doses or 50-400 mg at HS

ATYPICAL ANTIPSYCHOTICS

➤ *aripiprazole* (C)(G) <10 years: not recommended; 10-17 years: initially 2 mg/day for 2 days; then, increase to 5 mg/day for 2 days; then, increase to target dose of 10 mg/day; may increase by 5 mg/day at 1 week intervals as needed to max 30 mg/day; >17 years: initially 15 mg daily; may increase to max 30 mg/day

Abilify *Tab:* 2, 5, 10, 15, 20, 30 mg

Abilify Discmelt *Tab:* 15 mg orally disintegrating (vanilla) (phenylalanine)

Abilify Maintena *Vial:* 300, 400 mg ext-rel pwdr for IM injection after reconstitution; 300, 400 mg single-dose prefilled dual-chamber syringes w. supplies

Comment: Abilify is indicated for acute and maintenance treatment of manic or mixed episodes in bipolar I disorder, as monotherapy or as an adjunct to *lithium* or *valproate*, as adjunct to antidepressants for major depressive disorder (MDD), and for irritability associated with autistic disorder.

➤ *brexpiprazole* (C) <12 years: not recommended; ≥12 years: initially 0.5 or 1 mg once daily; titrate weekly up to target 2 mg/day; max 3 mg/day; *Moderate-severe hepatic impairment, renal impairment, or ESRD:* max 2 mg/day

Rexulti *Tab:* 0.25, 0.5, 1, 2, 3, 4 mg

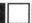

DERMATITIS: ATOPIC (ECZEMA)

Oral Drugs for the Management of Allergy, Cough, and Cold Symptoms *see page* 523
Parenteral Corticosteroids *see page 499*
Oral Corticosteroids *see page 498*

SECOND GENERATION ANTIHISTAMINES

Comment: Second generation antihistamines are sedating, but much less so than the first generation antihistamines. All antihistamines are excreted into breast milk.

➤ *cetirizine* (C)(OTC)(G) <6 years: not recommended; ≥6-<65 years: initially 5-10 mg once daily; ≥65 years: 5 mg once daily

Children's Zyrtec Chewable *Chew tab:* 5, 10 mg (grape)

Children's Zyrtec Allergy Syrup *Syr:* 1 mg/ml (4 oz) (grape, bubble gum) (sugar-free, dye-free)

Zyrtec *Tab:* 10 mg

Zyrtec Hives Relief *Tab:* 10 mg

Zyrtec Liquid Gels *Liq gel:* 10 mg

➤ *desloratadine* (C)

Clarinex <6 years: not recommended; ≥6 years: 1/2-1 tab once daily

Tab: 5 mg

Clarinex RediTabs <6 years: not recommended; 6-12 years: 2.5 mg once daily; ≥12 years: 5 mg once daily

ODT: 2.5, 5 mg (tutti-frutti) (phenylalanine)

Clarinex Syrup <6 months: not recommended; 6-11 months: 1 mg (2 ml) once daily; 1-5 years: 1.25 mg (2.5 ml) once daily; 6-11 years: 2.5 mg (5 ml) once aily; ≥12 years: 5 mg (10 ml) once daily

Tab: 0.5 mg per ml (4 oz) (tutti-frutti) (phenylalanine)

Desloratadine ODT

▷ *fexofenadine* (C)(OTC)(G) 6 months-2 years: 15 mg bid; *CrCl ≤90 mL/min:* 15 mg once daily; 2-11 years: 30 mg bid; *CrCl ≤90 mL/min:* 30 mg once daily ≥12 years and older: ≥12 years: 60 mg once daily-bid <u>or</u> 180 mg once daily; *CrCl <90 mL/min:* 60 mg once daily **Allegra** *Tab:* 30, 60, 180 mg film-coat
    Allegra Allergy *Tab:* 60, 180 mg film-coat
    Allegra ODT *ODT:* 30 mg (phenylalanine)
    Allegra Oral Suspension *Oral susp:* 30 mg/5 ml (6 mg/ml) (4 oz)
▷ *loratadine* (C)(OTC)(G) <2 years: not recommended; 2-5 years: 5 mg once daily; ≥6 years: 5 mg bid or 10 mg once daily; *Hepatic <u>or</u> Renal Insufficiency:* (see mfr pkg insert)
    Children's Claritin Chewables *Chew tab:* 5 mg (grape) (phenylalanine)
    Children's Claritin Syrup 1 mg/ml (4 oz) (fruit) (sugar-free, alcohol-free, dye-free; sodium 6 mg/5 ml)
    Claritin *Tab:* 10 mg
    Claritin Hives Relief *Tab:* 10 mg
    Claritin Liqui-Gels *Liq gel:* 10 mg
    Claritin RediTabs 12 Hours *ODT:* 5 mg (mint)
    Claritin RediTabs 24 Hours *ODT:* 10 mg (mint)
▷ *levocetirizine* (B)(OTC) administer dose in the PM; *Seasonal Allergic Rhinitis:* <2 years: not recommended; may start at ≥2 years; *Chronic Idiopathic Urticaria (CIU), Perennial Allergic Rhinitis:* <6 months: not recommended; may start at ≥6 months; *Dosing by Age:* 6 months-5 years: max 1.25 mg once daily; 6-11 years: max 2.5 mg once daily; ≥12 years: 2.5-5 mg once daily; *Renal Dysfunction <12 years:* contraindicated; *Renal Dysfunction ≥12 years:* CrCl 50-80 ml/min: 2.5 mg once daily; CrCl 30-50 mL/min: 2.5 mg every other day; CrCl: 10-30 mL/min: 2.5 mg twice weekly (every 3-4 days); CrCl <10 mL/min, ESRD <u>or</u> hemodialysis: contraindicated;
    Children's Xyzal Allergy 24HR *Oral Soln:* 0.5 mg/ml (150 ml)
    Xyzal Allergy 24HR *Tab:* 5*mg

FIRST GENERATION ANTIHISTAMINES

▷ *hydroxyzine* (C)(G) <6 years: 50 mg/day divided qid prn; ≥6 years: 50-100 mg/day divided qid prn; max 600 mg/day; 25 mg tid prn; max 600 mg/day
    AtaraxR *Tab:* 10, 25, 50, 100 mg; *Syr:* 10 mg/5 ml (alcohol 0.5%)
    VistarilR *Cap:* 25, 50, 100 mg; *Oral susp:* 25 mg/5 ml (4 oz) (lemon)

TOPICAL STEROIDS

(For other topical steroids, *see* **Topical Corticosteroids** page 494)
Comment: Topical steroids should be applied sparingly and for the shortest time necessary. Do not use in the diaper area. Do not use an occlusive dressing. Systemic absorption of topical corticosteroids can induce reversible hypothalamic-pituitary-adrenal (HPA) axis suppression with the potential for clinical glucocorticoid insufficiency.
▷ *desonide* 0.05% topical gel (C) <3 months: not recommended; ≥3 months: apply sparingly bid-tid; max 4 weeks
    Desonate *Gel:* 0.05% (60 gm) (89% purified water; fragrance-free, surfactant-free, alcohol-free)

PHOSPHODIESTERASE 4 INHIBITOR

▷ *crisaborole 2%* (C) <2 years: not recommended; ≥2 years: apply sparingly bid; max 4 weeks
    Eucrisa *Oint: 2%* (60 g)

INTERLEUKIN-4 RECEPTOR ALPHA ANTAGONIST

▷ *dupilumab* <18 years: not recommended; ≥18 years: administer SC into the upper arm, abdomen, or thigh; rotate sites; initially 600 mg (2 x 300 mg injections at different sites) followed by 300 mg SC once every other week; may use with or without topical corticosteroids; may use with calcineurin inhibitors, but reserve only for problem areas (e.g., face, neck, intertriginous, and genital areas); avoid live vaccines.
    Dupixent *Prefill syr:* 300 mg/2 ml (2/pck without needle) (preservative-free)
    Comment: *dupilumab* is a human monoclonal IgG4 antibody that inhibits interleukin-4 (IL-4) and interleukin-13 (IL-13) signaling by specifically binding to the IL4Rα subunit shared by the IL-4 and IL-13 receptor complexes, thereby inhibiting the release of pro-inflammatory cytokines, chemokines, and IgE. *dupilumab* is indicated for moderate-to-severe atopic dermatitis in patients who are not adequately controlled with topical prescription therapies or when they are not advisable.

MOISTURIZING AGENTS

Aquaphor Healing Ointment (OTC) *Oint:* 1.75, 3.5, 14 oz (alcohol)
Eucerin Daily Sun Defense (OTC) *Lotn:* 6 oz (fragrance-free)
Comment: **Eucerin Daily Sun Defense** is a moisturizer with SPF-15 sunscreen.
Eucerin Facial Lotion (OTC) *Lotn:* 4 oz
Eucerin Light Lotion (OTC) *Lotn:* 8 oz
Eucerin Lotion (OTC) *Lotn:* 8, 16 oz
Eucerin Original Creme (OTC) *Crm:* 2, 4, 16 oz (alcohol)
Eucerin Plus Creme (OTC) *Crm:* 4 oz
Eucerin Plus Lotion (OTC) *Lotn:* 6, 12 oz
Eucerin Protective Lotion (OTC) *Lotn:* 4 oz (alcohol)
Comment: **Eucerin Protective Lotion** is a moisturizer with SPF-25 sunscreen.
Lac-Hydrin Cream (OTC) *Crm:* 280, 385 g
Lac-Hydrin Lotion (OTC) *Lotn:* 25, 400 g
Lubriderm Dry Skin Scented (OTC) *Lotn:* 6, 10, 16, 32 oz
Lubriderm Dry Skin Unscented (OTC) *Lotn:* 3.3, 6, 10, 16 oz (fragrance-free)
Lubriderm Sensitive Skin Lotion (OTC) *Lotn:* 3.3, 6, 10, 16 oz (lanolin-free)
Lubriderm Dry Skin (OTC) *Lotn (scented):* 2.5, 6, 10, 16 oz;
    Lotn (fragrance-free): 1, 2.5, 6, 10, 16 oz
Lubriderm Bath 1-2 capfuls in bath or rub onto wet skin as needed, then rinse
    Oil: 8 oz
Moisturel apply as needed
    Crm: 4, 16 oz; *Lotn:* 8, 12 oz; *Clnsr:* 8.75 oz

OATMEAL COLLOIDS

Aveeno (OTC) add to bath as needed

Regular: 1.5 oz (8/pck); *Moisturizing:* 0.75 oz (8/pck)
Aveeno Oil (OTC) add to bath as needed
    Oil: 8 oz
Aveeno Moisturizing (OTC) apply as needed
    Lotn: 2.5, 8, 12 oz; *Crm:* 4 oz
Aveeno Cleansing Bar (OTC) *Bar:* 3 oz
Aveeno Gentle Skin Cleanser (OTC) *Liq clnsr:* 6 oz

TOPICAL OIL

▷ *fluocinolone acetamide* 0.01% topical oil (C)
    Derma-Smoothe/FS Topical Oil <6 years: not recommended; 6-12 years: apply
    sparingly bid for up to 4 weeks; >12 years: apply sparingly tid
        Topical oil: 0.01% (4 oz) (peanut oil)

TOPICAL ANALGESICS

▷ *capsaicin* cream (B)(G) <2 years: not recommended; 2-12 years: apply sparingly to
intact skin bid prn; >12 years: apply tid-qid prn
    Axsain *Crm:* 0.075% (1, 2 oz)
    Capsin (OTC) *Lotn:* 0.025, 0,075% (59 ml)
    Capzasin-P (OTC) *Crm:* 0.025% (1.5 oz); *Lotn:* 0.025% (2 oz)
    Capzasin-HP (OTC) *Crm:* 0.075% (1.5 oz); *Lotn:* 0.075% (2 oz)
    Dolorac *Crm:* 0.025% (28 gm)
    Double Cap (OTC) *Crm:* 0.05% (2 oz)
    R-Gel *Gel:* 0.025% (15, 30 gm)
    Zostrix (OTC) *Crm:* 0.025% (0.7, 1.5, 3 oz)
    Zostrix HP (OTC) *Emol crm:* 0.075% (1, 2 oz)
    Comment: Provides some relief by 1-2 weeks; optimal benefit may take 4-6 weeks.
Avoid contact with mucous membranes.
▷ *doxepin* cream (B) <12 years: not recommended; ≥12 years: apply to affected area
qid at intervals of at least 3-4 hours; max 8 days
    Prudoxin *Crm:* 5% (45 gm)
    Zonalon *Crm:* 5% (30, 45 gm)
▷ *pimecrolimus* 1% cream (C) <2 years: not recommended; ≥2 years: apply to affected
area bid; do not occlude
    Elidel *Crm:* 1% (30, 60, 100 gm)
    Comment: *pimecrolimus* is indicated for short-term and intermittent long-term
use. Discontinue use when resolution occurs. Contraindicated if the patient is
immunosuppressed. Change to the 0.1% preparation or if secondary bacterial
infection is present.
▷ *tacrolimus* (C) <2 years: not recommended; 2-15 years: use 0.03% strength; apply to
affected area bid; continue for 1 week after clearing; >15 years: apply to affected area
bid; do not occlude or apply to wet skin; continue for 1 week after clearing
    Protopic *Oint:* 0.03, 0.1% (30, 60, 100 gm)
▷ *trolamine salicylate* (NE) <2 years: not recommended; ≥2 years: apply tid-qid prn
to intact skin
    Mobisyl *Crm:* 10%
    Comment: Provides some relief by 1-2 weeks; optimal benefit may take 4-6 weeks.

TOPICAL ANESTHETIC

➤ *lidocaine* (B) reduce dosage commensurate with age, body weight, and physical condition (see pkg insert); apply to affected area bid-tid prn
   Lidoderm *Crm:* 3% (85 gm)

DERMATITIS: CONTACT

PROPHYLAXIS

➤ *bentoquatam* (NE) <6 years: not recommended; ≥6 years: apply as a wet film to exposed skin at least 15 minutes prior to possible contact; reapply at least q 4 hours; remove with soap and water
   IvyBlock (OTC) *Soln:* 120 ml
   Comment: Provides protection against genus rhus (poison ivy, oak, and sumac).

TREATMENT

Oatmeal Colloids

   Aveeno (OTC) add to bath as needed
      Regular: 1.5 oz (8/pck); *Moisturizing:* 0.75 oz (8/pck)
   Aveeno Oil (OTC) add to bath as needed
      Oil: 8 oz
   Aveeno Moisturizing (OTC) apply as needed
      Lotn: 2.5, 8, 12 oz; *Crm:* 4 oz
   Aveeno Cleansing Bar (OTC) *Bar:* 3 oz
   Aveeno Gentle Skin Cleanser (OTC) *Liq clnsr:* 6 oz
Oral Prescription Drugs for the Management of Allergy, Cough, and Cold Symptoms *see page* 523
Topical Corticosteroids *see page* 494
Parenteral Corticosteroids *see page* 499
Oral Corticosteroids *see page* 498

SECOND GENERATION ANTIHISTAMINES

Comment: The following drugs are second generation antihistamines. As such they minimally sedating, much less so than the first generation antihistamines. All antihistamines are excreted into breast milk.
➤ *cetirizine* (C)(OTC)(G) <6 years: not recommended; ≥6-<65 years: initially 5-10 mg once daily; ≥65 years: 5 mg once daily
   Children's Zyrtec Chewable *Chew tab:* 5, 10 mg (grape)
   Children's Zyrtec Allergy Syrup *Syr:* 1 mg/ml (4 oz) (grape, bubble gum) (sugar-free, dye-free)
   Zyrtec *Tab:* 10 mg
   Zyrtec Hives Relief *Tab:* 10 mg
   Zyrtec Liquid Gels *Liq gel:* 10 mg
➤ *desloratadine* (C)
   Clarinex <6 years: not recommended; ≥6 years: 1/2-1 tab once daily
      Tab: 5 mg

Clarinex RediTabs <6 years: not recommended; 6-12 years: 2.5 mg once daily; ≥12 years: 5 mg once daily
   ODT: 2.5, 5 mg (tutti-frutti) (phenylalanine)
Clarinex Syrup <6 months: not recommended; 6-11 months: 1 mg (2 ml) once daily; 1-5 years: 1.25 mg (2.5 ml) once daily; 6-11 years: 2.5 mg (5 ml) once daily; ≥12 years: 5 mg (10 ml) once daily
   Tab: 0.5 mg per ml (4 oz) (tutti-frutti) (phenylalanine)
Desloratadine ODT <6 years: not recommended; 6-11 years: ½ tab once daily; ≥12 years: 1 tab once daily
   ODT: 5 mg

▷ *fexofenadine* (C)(OTC)(G) <6 months: not recommended; 6 months-<2 years: 15 mg bid; *CrCl ≤90 mL/min:* 15 mg once daily; 2-11 years: 30 mg bid; *CrCl ≤90 mL/min:* 30 mg once daily; ≥12 years: 60 mg once daily-bid or 180 mg once daily; *CrCl <90 mL/min:* 60 mg once daily **Allegra** *Tab:* 30, 60, 180 mg film-coat
   Allegra Allergy *Tab:* 60, 180 mg film-coat
   Allegra ODT *ODT:* 30 mg (phenylalanine)
   Allegra Oral Suspension *Oral susp:* 30 mg/5 ml (6 mg/ml) (4 oz)

▷ *loratadine* (C)(OTC)(G) <2 years: not recommended; 2-5 years: 5 mg once daily; ≥6 years: 5 mg bid or 10 mg once daily; *Hepatic or Renal Insufficiency:* (see mfr pkg insert)
   Children's Claritin Chewables *Chew tab:* 5 mg (grape) (phenylalanine)
   Children's Claritin Syrup 1 mg/ml (4 oz) (fruit) (sugar-free, alcohol-free, dye-free; sodium 6 mg/5 ml)
   Claritin *Tab:* 10 mg
   Claritin Hives Relief *Tab:* 10 mg
   Claritin Liqui-Gels *Liq gel:* 10 mg
   Claritin RediTabs 12 Hours *ODT:* 5 mg (mint)
   Claritin RediTabs 24 Hours *ODT:* 10 mg (mint)

▷ *levocetirizine* (B)(OTC) administer dose in the PM; *Seasonal Allergic Rhinitis:* <2 years: not recommended; may start at ≥2 years; *Chronic Idiopathic Urticaria (CIU), Perennial Allergic Rhinitis:* <6 months: not recommended; may start at ≥ 6 months; *Dosing by Age:* 6 months-5 years: max 1.25 mg once daily; 6-11 years: max 2.5 mg once daily; ≥12 years: 2.5-5 mg once daily; *Renal Dysfunction <12 years:* contraindicated; *Renal Dysfunction ≥12 years:* CrCl 50-80 ml/min: 2.5 mg once daily; CrCl 30-50 mL/min: 2.5 mg every other day; CrCl: 10-30 mL/min: 2.5 mg twice weekly (every 3-4 days); CrCl <10 mL/min, ESRD or hemodialysis: contraindicated;
   Children's Xyzal Allergy 24HR *Oral Soln:* 0.5 mg/ml (150 ml)
   Xyzal Allergy 24HR *Tab:* 5*mg

FIRST GENERATION ANTIHISTAMINES

▷ *diphenhydramine* (B)(G)
   Benadryl (OTC) <2 years: not recommended; 2-6 years: 6.25 mg q 4-6 hours; max 37.5 mg/day; >6-12 years: 12.5-25 mg q 4-6 hours; max 150 mg/day; >12 years: 25-50 mg q 6-8 hours; max 100 mg/day
   Chew tab: 12.5 mg (grape) (phenylalanine); *Liq:* 12.5 mg/5 ml (4, 8 oz); *Cap:* 25 mg; *Tab:* 25 mg; *Dye-free soft gel:* 25 mg;
   Dye-free liq: 12.5 mg/5 ml (4, 8 oz)

▷ *diphenhydramine* injectable **(B)(G)**
    Benadryl Injectable <12 years: *See mfr pkg insert:* 1.25 mg/kg up to 25 mg IM x
    1 dose; then q 6 hours prn; ≥12 years: 25-50 mg IM immediately; then q 6 hours
    prn
    Vial: 50 mg/ml (1 ml single use); 50 mg/ml (10 ml multi-dose); *Amp:* 10 mg/ml
    (1 ml); *Prefilled syringe:* 50 mg/ml (1 ml)
▷ *hydroxyzine* **(C)(G)** <6 years: 50 mg/day divided qid prn; ≥6 years: 50-100 mg/day
divided qid prn
    Atarax *Tab:* 10, 25, 50, 100 mg; *Syr:* 10 mg/5 ml (alcohol 0.5%)
    Vistaril *Cap:* 25, 50, 100 mg; *Oral susp:* 25 mg/5 ml (4 oz) (lemon)
    Comment: *hydroxyzine* is contraindicated in early pregnancy and in patients with
a prolonged QT interval. It is not known whether this drug is excreted in human
milk; therefore, *hydroxyzine* should not be given to nursing mothers.

DERMATITIS: GENUS RHUS (POISON OAK, POISON IVY, POISON SUMAC)

PROPHYLAXIS

▷ *bentoquatam* **(NE)** <6 years: not recommended; ≥6 years: apply as a wet film to
exposed skin at least 15 minutes prior to possible contact; reapply at least q 4 hours;
remove with soap and water
    IvyBlock (OTC) *Soln:* 120 ml
    Comment: Provides protection against genus rhus (poison oak, poison ivy, and
poison sumac).

TREATMENT

Oatmeal Colloids

Aveeno (OTC) add to bath as needed
    Regular: 1.5 oz (8/pck); *Moisturizing:* 0.75 oz (8/pck)
Aveeno Oil (OTC) add to bath as needed
    Oil: 8 oz
Aveeno Moisturizing (OTC) apply as needed
    Lotn: 2.5, 8, 12 oz; *Crm:* 4 oz
Aveeno Cleansing Bar (OTC) *Bar:* 3 oz
Aveeno Gentle Skin Cleanser (OTC) *Liq clnsr:* 6 oz
Oral Drugs for Allergy, Cough, and Cold *see page 523*
Topical Corticosteroids *see page 494*
Parenteral Corticosteroids *see page 499*
Oral Corticosteroids *see page 498*

SECOND GENERATION ANTIHISTAMINES

Comment: The following drugs are second generation antihistamines. As such
they minimally sedating, much less so than the first generation antihistamines. All
antihistamines are excreted into breast milk.
▷ *cetirizine* **(C)(OTC)(G)** <6 years: not recommended; ≥6-<65 years: initially 5-10
mg once daily; ≥65 years: 5 mg once daily

Children's Zyrtec Chewable *Chew tab:* 5, 10 mg (grape)
Children's Zyrtec Allergy Syrup *Syr:* 1 mg/ml (4 oz) (grape, bubble gum) (sugar-free, dye-free)
Zyrtec *Tab:* 10 mg
Zyrtec Hives Relief *Tab:* 10 mg
Zyrtec Liquid Gels *Liq gel:* 10 mg

▷ *desloratadine* (C)
Clarinex <6 years: not recommended; ≥6 years: 1/2-1 tab once daily
  Tab: 5 mg
Clarinex RediTabs <6 years: not recommended; 6-12 years: 2.5 mg once daily; ≥12 years: 5 mg once daily
  ODT: 2.5, 5 mg (tutti-frutti) (phenylalanine)
Clarinex Syrup <6 months: not recommended; 6-11 months: 1 mg (2 ml) once daily; 1-5 years: 1.25 mg (2.5 ml) once daily; 6-11 years: 2.5 mg (5 ml) once daily; ≥12 years: 5 mg (10 ml) once daily
  Tab: 0.5 mg per ml (4 oz) (tutti-frutti) (phenylalanine)
Desloratadine ODT <6 years: not recommended; 6-11 years: ½ tab once daily; ≥12 years: 1 tab once daily
  ODT: 5 mg

▷ *fexofenadine* (C)(OTC)(G) <6 months: not recommended; 6 months-<2 years: 15 mg bid; *CrCl ≤90 mL/min:* 15 mg once daily; 2-11 years: 30 mg bid; *CrCl ≤90 mL/min:* 30 mg once daily; ≥12 years: 60 mg once daily-bid *or* 180 mg once daily; *CrCl <90 mL/min:* 60 mg once daily Allegra *Tab:* 30, 60, 180 mg film-coat
Allegra Allergy *Tab:* 60, 180 mg film-coat
Allegra ODT *ODT:* 30 mg (phenylalanine)
Allegra Oral Suspension *Oral susp:* 30 mg/5 ml (6 mg/ml) (4 oz)

▷ *loratadine* (C)(OTC)(G) <2 years: not recommended; 2-5 years: 5 mg once daily; ≥6 years: 5 mg bid *or* 10 mg once daily; *Hepatic or Renal Insufficiency:* (see mfr pkg insert)
Children's Claritin Chewables *Chew tab:* 5 mg (grape) (phenylalanine)
Children's Claritin Syrup 1 mg/ml (4 oz) (fruit) (sugar-free, alcohol-free, dye-free; sodium 6 mg/5 ml)
Claritin *Tab:* 10 mg
Claritin Hives Relief *Tab:* 10 mg
Claritin Liqui-Gels *Liq gel:* 10 mg
Claritin RediTabs 12 Hours *ODT:* 5 mg (mint)
Claritin RediTabs 24 Hours *ODT:* 10 mg (mint)

▷ *levocetirizine* (B)(OTC) administer dose in the PM; *Seasonal Allergic Rhinitis:* <2 years: not recommended; may start at ≥2 years; *Chronic Idiopathic Urticaria (CIU), Perennial Allergic Rhinitis:* <6 months: not recommended; may start at ≥ 6 months; *Dosing by Age:* 6 months-5 years: max 1.25 mg once daily; 6-11 years: max 2.5 mg once daily; ≥12 years: 2.5-5 mg once daily; *Renal Dysfunction <12 years:* contraindicated; *Renal Dysfunction ≥12 years:* CrCl 50-80 ml/min: 2.5 mg once daily; CrCl 30-50 mL/min: 2.5 mg every other day; CrCl: 10-30 mL/min: 2.5 mg twice weekly (every 3-4 days); CrCl <10 mL/min, ESRD *or* hemodialysis: contraindicated;
Children's Xyzal Allergy 24HR *Oral Soln:* 0.5 mg/ml (150 ml)
Xyzal Allergy 24HR *Tab:* 5*mg

FIRST GENERATION ANTIHISTAMINES

▷ *diphenhydramine* (B)(G)
  Benadryl (OTC) <2 years: not recommended; 2-6 years: 6.25 mg q 4-6 hours; max 37.5 mg/day; >6-12 years: 12.5-25 mg q 4-6 hours; max 150 mg/day; >12 years: 25-50 mg q 6-8 hours; max 100 mg/day
    Chew tab: 12.5 mg (grape) (phenylalanine); *Liq:* 12.5 mg/5 ml (4, 8 oz); *Cap:* 25 mg; *Tab:* 25 mg; *Dye-free soft gel:* 25 mg;
    Dye-free liq: 12.5 mg/5 ml (4, 8 oz)
▷ *diphenhydramine* injectable (B)(G)
  Benadryl Injectable <12 years: *See mfr pkg insert:* 1.25 mg/kg up to 25 mg IM x 1 dose; then q 6 hours prn; ≥12 years: 25-50 mg IM immediately; then q 6 hours prn
    Vial: 50 mg/ml (1 ml single use); 50 mg/ml (10 ml multi-dose); *Amp:* 10 mg/ml (1 ml); *Prefilled syringe:* 50 mg/ml (1 ml)
▷ *hydroxyzine* (C)(G) <6 years: 50 mg/day divided qid prn; ≥6 years: 50-100 mg/day divided qid prn
  Atarax *Tab:* 10, 25, 50, 100 mg; *Syr:* 10 mg/5 ml (alcohol 0.5%)
  Vistaril *Cap:* 25, 50, 100 mg; *Oral susp:* 25 mg/5 ml (4 oz) (lemon)
  Comment: *hydroxyzine* is contraindicated in early pregnancy and in patients with a prolonged QT interval. It is not known whether this drug is excreted in human milk; therefore, *hydroxyzine* should not be given to nursing mothers.

DERMATITIS: SEBORRHEIC

ANTIFUNGAL SHAMPOOS AND TOPICAL AGENTS

▷ *chloroxine* shampoo (C) <12 years: not recommended; ≥12 years: massage onto wet scalp; wait 3 minutes, rinse, repeat, and rinse thoroughly; use twice weekly
  Capitrol Shampoo *Shampoo:* 2% (4 oz)
▷ *ciclopirox* (B) apply gel once daily <u>or</u> apply cream <u>or</u> lotion twice daily, x 4 weeks <u>or</u> shampoo twice weekly; massage shampoo onto wet scalp; wait 3 minutes, rinse, repeat, and rinse thoroughly; shampoo twice weekly
  Loprox Cream <10 years: not recommended
    Crm: 0.77% (15, 30, 90 gm)
  Loprox Gel <16 years: not recommended
    Gel: 0.77% (30, 45 gm)
  Loprox Lotion <10 years: not recommended
    Lotn: 0.77% (30, 60 ml)
  Loprox Shampoo *Shampoo:* 1% (120 ml)
▷ *coal tar* (C)(G)
  Scytera (OTC) apply once daily-qid; use lowest effective dose
    Foam: 2%
  T/Gel Shampoo Extra Strength (OTC) use every other day; max 4 x/week; massage into wet scalp for 5 minutes; rinse; repeat
    Shampoo: 1%
  T/Gel Shampoo Original Formula (OTC) use every other day; max 7 x/week; massage into wet scalp for 5 minutes; rinse; repeat
    Shampoo: 0.5%

T/Gel Shampoo Stubborn Itch Control (OTC) use every other day; max 7 x/week; massage into wet scalp for 5 minutes; rinse; repeat
    Shampoo: 0.5%

▷ *fluocinolone acetamide* (C)
    Derma-Smoothe/FS Shampoo <12 years: not recommended; ≥12 years: apply up to 1 oz to scalp daily, lather, and leave on x 5 minutes, then rinse twice
        Shampoo: 0.01% (4 oz)
    Derma-Smoothe/FS Topical Oil *fluocinolone acetamide* 0.01% topical oil (C) <6 years: not recommended; ≥6-12 years: apply sparingly bid for up to 4 weeks; >12 years: apply sparingly tid; for scalp psoriasis wet or dampen hair or scalp, then apply a thin film, massage well, cover with a shower cap and leave on for at least 4 hours or overnight, then wash hair with regular shampoo and rinse
        Topical oil: 0.01% (4 oz) (peanut oil)

▷ *ketoconazole* (C) <12 years: not recommended; ≥12 years: apply cream or gel once daily x 4 week or apply up to 1 oz shampoo to scalp daily, lather, leave on x 5 minutes, then rinse twice
    Nizoral Cream *Crm:* 2% (15, 30, 60 gm)
    Nizoral Shampoo *Shampoo:* 2% (4 oz)
    Xolegel *Gel:* 2% (45 gm)
    Xolegel Duo *Kit:* **Xolegel** *Gel:* 2% (45 gm) + **Xolex** *Shampoo:* 2% (4 oz)

▷ *selenium sulfide* (C) <12 years: not recommended; ≥12 years: massage cream into scalp twice weekly x 2 weeks or massage into wet scalp, wait 2-3 minutes, rinse; repeat twice weekly x 2 weeks; may continue treatment with lotion of shampoo 1-2 x weekly as needed
    Exsel Shampoo *Shampoo:* 2.5% (4 oz)
    Selsun Rx *Lotn:* 2.5% (4 oz)
    Selsun Shampoo *Shampoo:* 1% (120, 210, 240, 330 ml); 2.5% (120 ml)

▷ *sodium sulfacetamide/sulfur* (C)
    Clenia Emollient Cream apply daily tid
        Emol crm: sod sulfa 10%/*sulfur* 5% (10 oz) (alcohol-free)
    Clenia Foaming Wash wash 1-2 x/daily
        Wash: sod sulfa 10%/*sulfur* 5% (6, 12 oz) (alcohol-free)
    Rosula Gel apply daily tid
        Gel: sod sulfa 10%/*sulfur* 4.5% (45 ml)
    Rosula Lotion apply daily tid
        Lotn: sod sulfa 10%/*sulfur* 4.5% (45 ml) (alcohol-free)
    Rosula Wash wash bid
        Clnsr: sod sulfa 10%/*sulfur* 4.5% (12 oz) (alcohol-free)

TOPICAL STEROID

▷ *betamethasone valerate* 0.12% foam (C)(G) <12 years: not recommended; ≥12 years: apply twice daily in AM and PM; invert can and dispense a small amount of foam onto a clean saucer or another cool surface (do not apply directly to hand) and massage a small amount into affected area until foam disappears
    Luxiq *Foam:* 100 g
    Other Topical Corticosteroids *see page* 494

DIABETIC PERIPHERAL NEUROPATHY

NUTRITIONAL SUPPLEMENT

▷ *L-methylfolate calcium(as metafolin)/pyridoxal 5-phosphate/methyl-cobalamin*
(NE) <12 years: not recommended; ≥12 years: 1 cap twice daily or 2 caps once daily

> Metanx *Cap: meta* 3 mg/*pyr* 35 mg/*methyl* 2 mg

> Comment: **Metanx** is indicated as adjunct treatment for patients with endothelial cell dysfunction, who have loss of protective sensation and neuropathic pain associated with diabetic peripheral neuropathy.

Acetaminophen for IV Infusion *see Pain page* 296

ORAL ANALGESICS

▷ *acetaminophen* (B)(G) *see Fever page* 137
▷ *aspirin* (D)(G) *see Fever page* 137

> Comment: *aspirin*-containing medications are contraindicated with history of allergic-type reaction to *aspirin*, children and adolescents with *Varicella* or other viral illness, and 3rd trimester pregnancy.

▷ *tramadol* (C)(IV)(G)

> Comment: *Tramadol* is known to be excreted in breast milk. The FDA and the European Medicines Agency (EMA) are investigating the safety of using *tramadol*-containing medications to treat pain in children 12-18 years because of the potential for serious side effects, including slowed or difficult breathing.

> **Rybix ODT** <12 years: contraindicated; 12-<18: use extreme caution; not recommended for children and adolescents with obesity, asthma, obstructive sleep apnea, or other chronic breathing problem, or for post-tonsillectomy/adenoidectomy pain; ≥18 years: initially 100 mg once daily; may increase by 100 mg every 5 days; max 300 mg/day; *CrCl <30 mL/min or severe hepatic impairment:* not recommended; *Cirrhosis:* max 50 mg q 12 hours

> > *ODT:* 50 mg (mint) (phenylalanine)

> **Ryzolt** <12 years: contraindicated; 12-<18: use extreme caution; not recommended for children and adolescents with obesity, asthma, obstructive sleep apnea, or other chronic breathing problem, or for post-tonsillectomy/adenoidectomy pain; ≥18 years: initially 100 mg once daily; may increase by 100 mg every 5 days; max 300 mg/day; *CrCl <30 mL/min or severe hepatic impairment:* not recommended

> > *Tab:* 100, 200, 300 mg ext-rel

> **Ultram** <12 years: contraindicated; 12-<18: use extreme caution; not recommended for children and adolescents with obesity, asthma, obstructive sleep apnea, or other chronic breathing problem, or for post-tonsillectomy/adenoidectomy pain; ≥18 years: 50-100 mg q 4-6 hours prn; max 400 mg/day; *CrCl <30 mL/min:* max 100 mg q 12 hours; *Cirrhosis:* max 50 mg q 12 hours

> > *Tab:* 50*mg

> **Ultram ER** <12 years: contraindicated; 12-<18: use extreme caution; not recommended for children and adolescents with obesity, asthma, obstructive sleep apnea, or other chronic breathing problem, or for post-tonsillectomy/adenoidectomy pain; ≥18 years: initially 100 mg once daily; may increase by 100 mg every 5 days; max 300 mg/day; *CrCl <30 mL/min: or severe hepatic impairment:* not recommended

Tab: 100, 200, 300 mg ext-rel

▷ *tramadol/acetaminophen* (C)(IV)(G) <12 years: contraindicated; 12-<18: use extreme caution; not recommended for children and adolescents with obesity, asthma, obstructive sleep apnea, or other chronic breathing problem, or for post-tonsillectomy/adenoidectomy pain; ≥18 years: 2 tabs q 4-6 hours; max 8 tabs/day; 5 days; *CrCl <30 mL/min:* max 2 tabs q 12 hours; max 4 tabs/day x 5 days

    Ultracet *Tab:* tram 37.5/acet 325 mg

    Other Oral Analgesics *see Pain page* 298

Comment: *Tramadol* is known to be excreted in breast milk. The FDA and the European Medicines Agency (EMA) are investigating the safety of using *tramadol*-containing medications to treat pain in children 12-18 years because of the potential for serious side effects, including slowed or difficult breathing.

TOPICAL ANALGESICS

▷ *capsaicin* cream (B)(G) <2 years: not recommended; 2-12 years: apply sparingly to intact skin bid prn; >12 years: apply tid-qid prn

    Axsain *Crm:* 0.075% (1, 2 oz)
    Capsin (OTC) *Lotn:* 0.025, 0,075% (59 ml)
    Capzasin-P (OTC) *Crm:* 0.025% (1.5 oz); *Lotn:* 0.025% (2 oz)
    Capzasin-HP (OTC) *Crm:* 0.075% (1.5 oz); *Lotn:* 0.075% (2 oz)
    Dolorac *Crm:* 0.025% (28 gm)
    Double Cap (OTC) *Crm:* 0.05% (2 oz)
    R-Gel *Gel:* 0.025% (15, 30 gm)
    Zostrix (OTC) *Crm:* 0.025% (0.7, 1.5, 3 oz)
    Zostrix HP (OTC) *Emol crm:* 0.075% (1, 2 oz)

Comment: Provides some relief by 1-2 weeks; optimal benefit may take 4-6 weeks. Avoid contact with mucous membranes.

▷ *capsaicin* 8% patch (B) <18 years: not recommended; ≥18 years: apply up to 4 patches for one 60-minute application to clean dry skin; may prep area with topical anesthetic; wear non-latex gloves; patches may be cut to size/shape; treatment may be repeated every 3 months

    Qutenza *Patch:* 8% 1640 mcg/cm (179 mg) (1 or 2 patches w. 1-50 gm tube cleansing gel/carton)

▷ *lidocaine* 5% patch (B)(G) <12 years: not recommended; ≥12 years: apply up to 3 patches at one time for up to 12 hours/24-hour period (12 hours on/12 hours off); patches may be cut into smaller sizes before removal of the release liner; do not reuse

    Lidoderm *Patch:* 5% 10 x 14 cm (30 patches/carton)

ANTICONVULSANTS

Gamma Aminobutyric Acid Analog

▷ *gabapentin* (C) <3 years: not recommended; 3-12 years: initially 10-15 mg/kg/day in 3 divided doses; max 12 hours between doses; titrate over 3 days; 3-4 years: titrate to 40 mg/kg/day; 5-12 years: titrate to 25-35 mg/kg/day; max 50 mg/kg/day; >12 years: initially 300 mg on Day 1; then 600 mg on Day 2; then 900 mg on Days 3-6; then 1,200 mg on Days 7-10; then 1,500 mg on Days 11-14; titrate up to 1,800 mg on Day 15; take entire dose once daily with the evening meal; do not crush, split, or chew

Gralise (C) *Tab*: 300, 600 mg
Neurontin (G) *Tab*: 600*, 800* mg; *Cap*: 100, 300, 400 mg; *Oral soln*: 250 mg/5 ml (480 ml) (strawberry-anise)

▷ *gabapentin enacarbil* (C) <18 years: not recommended; ≥18 years: 600 mg once daily at about 5:00 PM; if dose not taken at recommended time, next dose should be taken the following day; swallow whole; take with food; *CrCl 30-59 mL/min*: 600 mg on Day 1, Day 3, and every day thereafter; *CrCl <30 mL/min*: or hemodialysis: not recommended

Horizant *Tab*: 300, 600 mg ext-rel

Comment: Avoid abrupt cessation of *gabapentin enacarbil*. To discontinue, withdraw gradually over 1 week or longer.

▷ *pregabalin (GABA analog)* (C)(V) <18 years: not recommended; ≥18 years: initially 50 mg tid; may titrate to 100 mg tid within one week; max 600 mg divided tid; discontinue over 1 week

Lyrica *Cap*: 25, 50, 75, 100, 150, 200, 225, 300 mg; *Oral soln*: 20 mg/ml

TRICYCLIC ANTIDEPRESSANTS (TCAs)

Comment: Co-administration of SSRIs and TCAs requires extreme caution.

▷ *amitriptyline* (C)(G) <12 years: not recommended; ≥12 years: 10-20 mg q HS *Tab*: 10, 25, 50, 75, 100, 150 mg

▷ *amoxapine* (C) <12 years: not recommended; ≥12 years: initially 50 mg bid-tid; after 1 week may increase to 100 mg bid-tid; usual effective dose 200-300 mg/day; if total dose exceeds 300 mg/day, give in divided doses (max 400 mg/day); may give as a single bedtime dose (max 300 mg q HS)

Tab: 25, 50, 100, 150 mg

▷ *clomipramine* (C)(G) <10 years: not recommended; 10-<16 years: initially 25 mg daily in divided doses; gradually increase; max 3 mg/kg or 100 mg, whichever is smaller; >16 years: initially 25 mg daily in divided doses; gradually increase to 100 mg during first 2 weeks; max 250 mg/day; total maintenance dose may be given at HS

Anafranil *Cap*: 25, 50, 75 mg

▷ *desipramine* (C)(G) <12 years: not recommended; ≥12 years: 100-200 mg/day in single or divided doses; max 300 mg/day

Norpramin *Tab*: 10, 25, 50, 75, 100, 150 mg

▷ *doxepin* (C)(G) <12 years: not recommended; ≥12 years: 75 mg/day; max 150 mg/day

Cap: 10, 25, 50, 75, 100, 150 mg; Oral conc: 10 mg/ml (4 oz w. dropper)

▷ *imipramine* (C)(G) <12 years: not recommended; ≥12 years:

Tofranil initially 75 mg daily (max 200 mg); adolescents initially 30-40 mg daily (max 100 mg/day); if maintenance dose exceeds 75 mg daily, may switch to **Tofranil PM** for divided or bedtime dose

Tab: 10, 25, 50 mg

Tofranil PM initially 75 mg daily 1 hour before HS; max 200 mg

Cap: 75, 100, 125, 150 mg

▷ *nortriptyline* (D)(G) <12 years: not recommended; ≥12 years: initially 25 mg tid-qid; max 150 mg/day

Pamelor *Cap*: 10, 25, 50, 75 mg; *Oral soln*: 10 mg/5 ml (16 oz)

▷ *protriptyline* (C) <12 years: not recommended; ≥12 years: initially 5 mg tid; usual dose 15-40 mg/day in 3-4 divided doses; max 60 mg/day

Vivactil *Tab*: 5, 10 mg

▷ *trimipramine* (C) <12 years: not recommended; ≥12 years: initially 75 mg/day in divided doses; max 200 mg/day
  Surmontil *Cap:* 25, 50, 100 mg

DIABETIC RETINOPATHY

Comment: Diabetic retinopathy is the leading cause of blindness among working-age adults in the US.

▷ *ranibizumab* (D) <18 years: not established; ≥18 years:
  Neovascular (wet) Age-related Macular Degeneration (AMD): Intravitreal: 0.5 mg once a month (approximately every 28 days). Frequency may be reduced (e.g., 4 to 5 injections over 9 months) after the first 3 injections or may be reduced after the first 4 injections to once every 3 months if monthly injections are not feasible. *Note:* A regimen averaging 4 to 5 doses over 9 months is expected to maintain visual acuity and an every 3-month dosing regimen has reportedly resulted in a ~5 letter (1 line) loss of visual acuity over 9 months, as compared to monthly dosing which may result in an additional ~1 to 2 letter gain
  Diabetic macular edema (DME): Intravitreal: 0.3 mg once a month (approximately every 28 days); in clinical trials, monthly doses of 0.5 mg were also studied
  Diabetic retinopathy (DR): Intravitreal: 0.3 mg once a month (approximately every 28 days)
  Macular edema following retinal vein occlusion (RVO): Intravitreal: 0.5 mg once a month (approximately every 28 days)
  Myopic choroidal neovascularization (mCNV): Intravitreal: 0.5 mg once a month (approximately every 28 days) for up to 3 months; may re-treat if necessary
    Lucentis *Prefilled Syringe:* 0.3 mg/0.05 mL (0.05 ml); 0.5 mg/0.05 ml (0.05 ml); for intravitreal injection (preservative free);
    Vial: 10 mg/ml (**Lucentis** 0.5 mg); 6 mg/ml solution (**Lucentis** 0.3 mg); single use; a 5-micron sterile filter needle (19 gauge x 1-1/2 inch) is required for preparation, but not included; Keep refrigerated. Do not freeze. Protect vial from light; see mfr pkg insert.

Comment: Lucentis is a recombinant humanized monoclonal antibody fragment which binds to and inhibits human vascular endothelial growth factor A (VEGF-A). **Lucentis** inhibits VEGF from binding to its receptors and thereby suppressing neovascularization and slowing vision loss. Contraindications include ocular <u>or</u> periocular infection, and active intraocular inflammation. For ophthalmic intravitreal injection only. Each vial or prefilled syringe should only be used for the treatment of a single eye. If the contralateral eye requires treatment, a new vial or prefilled syringe should be used and the sterile field, syringe, gloves, drapes, eyelid speculum, filter, and injection needles should be changed before **Lucentis** is administered to the other eye. Adequate anesthesia and a topical broad-spectrum antimicrobial agent should be administered prior to the procedure. Refer to manufacturer labeling for additional detailed information. Based on its mechanism of action, adverse effects on pregnancy would be expected. Information related to use in pregnancy is limited. The intravitreal injection procedure should be carried out under controlled aseptic conditions, which include the use of sterile gloves, a sterile drape, and a sterile eyelid speculum (or equivalent). Adequate anesthesia and a broad-spectrum microbicide should be given prior to the injection. Prior to and 30 minutes following the intravitreal injection, patients should be monitored for elevation in intraocular pressure using tonometry. Each prefilled syringe or vial should only be used for the treatment of a single eye. If the contralateral eye requires treatment, a new prefilled syringe or vial should be used and the sterile field, syringe, gloves, drapes, eyelid speculum, filter needle (vial only), and injection needles should be changed. Solomon, SD, Chew, E, Duh, EJ, *et al.* Diabetic retinopathy: A position statement by the American Diabetes Association [published online February 21, 2017]. *ADA.*

DIAPER RASH

Topical Corticosteroids *see page* 494
Comment: Low to intermediate potency topical corticosteroids are indicated if inflammation is present.

PROTECTIVE BARRIERS

▷ *aloe/vitamin E/zinc oxide* (NE) ointment apply at each diaper change after thoroughly cleansing skin
  Balmex *Oint:* 2, 4 oz tube; 16 oz jar
▷ *vitamin A&D* (NE) (G) ointment apply at each diaper change after thoroughly cleansing skin
  A&D Ointment *Oint:* 1.5, 4 oz
▷ *zinc oxide* (NE)(G) cream and ointment apply at each diaper change after thoroughly cleansing the skin
  A&D Ointment with Zinc Oxide *Oint:* 10% (1.5, 4 oz)
  Desitin *Oint:* 40% (1, 2, 4, 9 oz)
  Desitin Cream *Crm:* 10% (2, 4 oz)

TOPICAL ANTIFUNGALS

Comment: Use if caused by *Candida albicans.*
▷ *butenafine* (B)(G) <12 years: not recommended; ≥12 years: apply bid x 1 week or once daily x 4 weeks
  Lotrimin Ultra (C)(OTC) *Crm:* 1% (12, 24 gm)
  Mentax *Crm:* 1% (15, 30 gm)
  Comment: *butenafine* is a benzylamine, not an azole. Fungicidal activity continues for at least 5 weeks after last application.
▷ *clotrimazole* (B) apply to affected area bid x 7 days
  Lotrimin (OTC) *Crm:* 1% (15, 30, 45 gm)
  Lotrimin AF (OTC) *Crm:* 1% (12 gm); *Lotn:* 1% (10 ml); *Soln:* 1% (10 ml)
▷ *econazole* (C) apply bid x 7 days
  Spectazole *Crm:* 1% (15, 30, 85 gm)
▷ *ketoconazole* (C) apply to affected area bid x 7 days
  Nizoral Cream *Crm:* 2% (15, 30, 60 gm)
▷ *nystatin* (C)(G) apply bid x 7 days
  Mycostatin *Crm:* 100,000 U/g (15, 30 gm)

COMBINATION AGENT

▷ *clotrimazole/betamethasone* cream (C)(G) apply bid x 7 days
  Lotrisone *Crm:* 15, 45 g

DIARRHEA: ACUTE

▷ *attapulgite* (C)
  Donnagel (OTC) <3 years: not recommended; 3-6 years: 7.5 ml; >6-12 years: 15 ml; >12 years: 30 ml after each loose stool; max 7 doses/day x 2 days
    Liq: 600 mg/15 ml (120, 240 ml)
  Donnagel Chewable Tab (OTC) <3 years: not recommended; 3-6 years: 1/2 tab after each loose stool; max 7 doses/day; >6-12 years: 1 tab after each loose stool; max tabs/day; >12 years: 2 tabs after each loose stool; max 14 tabs/day
    Chew tab: 600 mg
  Kaopectate (OTC) <3 years: not recommended; 3-6 years: 7.5 ml after each loose stool; >6-12 years: 15 ml after each loose stool; >12 years: 30 ml after each loose stool; max 7 doses/day x 2 days
    Liq: 600 mg/15 ml (120, 240 ml)
▷ *bismuth subsalicylate* (C; D in 3rd)(G)
  Pepto-Bismol (OTC) <3 years (14-18 lb): 2.5 ml q 4 hours; max 6 doses/day; <3 years(18-28 lb): 5 ml q 4 hours; max 6 doses/day; 3-6 years: 1/3 tab or 5 ml q 30-60 minutes; max 8 doses/day; >6-9 years: 2/3 tab or 10 ml q 30-60 minutes; max 8 doses/day; >9-12 years: 1 tab or 15 ml q 30-60 minutes; max 8 doses/day; >12 years: 2 tabs or 30 ml q 30-60 minutes as needed; max 8 doses/day
    Chew tab: 262 mg; *Liq:* 262 mg/15 ml (4, 8, 12, 16 oz)
  Pepto-Bismol Maximum Strength (OTC) <3 years: not recommended; 3-6 years: 5 ml q 60 minutes; max 4 doses/day; >6-9 years: 10 ml q 60 minutes; max 4 doses/day; >9-12 years: 15 ml q 60 minutes; max 4 doses/day; >12 years: 30 ml q 60 minutes; max 4 doses/day
    Liq: 525 mg/15 ml (4, 8, 12, 16 oz)
Comment: *aspirin*-containing medications are contraindicated with history of allergic type reaction to *aspirin*, children and adolescents with *Varicella* or other viral illness, and 3rd trimester pregnancy.
▷ *calcium polycarbophil* (C)
  Fibercon (OTC) <6 years: not recommended; 6-12 years: 1 tab daily qid; >12 years: 2 tabs daily qid
    Cplt: 625 mg
▷ *crofelemer* (C) <12 years: not recommended; ≥12 years: 2 tabs once daily; swallow whole with or without food; do not crush or chew
  Mytesi *Tab:* 125 mg del-rel
  Comment: *crofelemer* is indicated for the symptomatic relief of non-infectious diarrhea in patients ≥18 years with HIV/AIDS on antiretroviral therapy.
▷ *difenoxin/atropine* (C)
  Motofen <2 years: not recommended; ≥2 years: 2 tabs, then 1 tab after each loose stool or 1 tab q 3-4 hours as needed; max 8 tab/day x 2 days
    Tab: dif 1 mg/atro 0.025 mg
▷ *diphenoxylate/atropine* (C)(V)(G) <2 years: not recommended; 2-12 years: initially 0.3-0.4 mg/kg/day in 4 divided doses; >12 years: 2 tabs or 10 ml qid until diarrhea is controlled

Lomotil *Tab:* diphen 2.5 mg/*atrop* 0.025 mg; *Liq:* diphen 2.5 mg/*atrop* 0.025 mg per 5 ml (2 oz)

▷ *loperamide* (B)(OTC)(G)
Imodium <5 years: not recommended; ≥5 years: 4 mg initially, then 2 mg after each loose stool; max 16 mg/day x 2 days
Cap: 2 mg
Imodium A-D <2 years: not recommended; 2-5 years (24-47 lb): 1 mg up to tid x 2 days; 6-8 years (48-59 lb): 2 mg initially, then 1 mg after each loose stool; max 4 mg/day x 2 days; 9-11 years (60-95 lb): 2 mg initially, then 1 after each loose stool; max 6 mg/day x 2 days; >11 years: 4 mg initially, then 2 mg after each loose stool; usual max 8 mg/day x 2 days
Cplt: 2 mg; *Liq:* 1 mg/5 ml (2, 4 oz) (cherry-mint) (alcohol 0.5%)

▷ *loperamide/simethicone* (B)(OTC)(G)
Imodium Advanced <6 years: not recommended; 6-8 years: chew 1 tab after loose stool, then chew 1/2 tab after next loose stool; ≥8-11 years: chew 1 tab after loose stool, then chew 1/2 tab after next loose stool; max 3 tabs/day; >11 years: 2 tabs chewed after loose stool, then 1 after the next loose stool; max 4 tabs/day
Chew tab: loper 2 mg/*simeth* 125 mg (vanilla-mint)

ORAL REHYDRATION AND ELECTROLYTE REPLACEMENT THERAPY

▷ *oral electrolyte replacement* (NE)(OTC)
CeraLyte 50 <4 years: not indicated; ≥4 years: dissolve in 8 oz water
Pkt: sodium 50 mEq/*potassium* 20 mEq/*chloride* 40 mEq/*citrate* 30 mEq/*rice syrup solids* 40 gm/*calories* 190 per liter (mixed berry) (gluten-free)
CeraLyte 70 <4 years: not indicated; ≥4 years: dissolve in 8 oz water
Pkt: sodium 70 mEq/*potassium* 20 mEq/*chloride* 60 mEq/*citrate* 30 mEq/*rice syrup solids* 40 gm/*calories* 165 per liter (natural or lemon) (gluten-free)
KaoLectrolyte <2 years: not indicated; ≥2 years: 1 pkt dissolved in 8 oz water q 3-4 hours
Pkt: sod 12 mEq/*pot* 5 mEq/*chlor* 10 mEq/*citrate* 7 mEq/*dextrose* 5 gm/calories 22 per 6.2 g
Pedialyte <2 years: as desired and as tolerated; ≥2 years: 1-2 L/day
Oral soln: dextrose 20 gm/*fructose* 5 gm/*sodium* 25 mEq/*potassium* 20 mEq/*chloride* 35 mEq/*citrate* 30 mEq/*calories* 100 per liter (8 oz, 1 L)
Pedialyte Freezer Pops as desired and as tolerated
Pops: dextrose 1.6 gm/*sodium* 2.8 mEq/*potassium* 1.25 mEq/*chloride* 2.2 mEq/*citrate* 1.88 mEq/*calories* 6.25 per 6.25 ml pop (8 oz, 1 L)

DIARRHEA: CARCINOID SYNDROME

TRIPTOPHAN HYDROXYLASE

▷ *telotristat* <18 years: not established; ≥18 years: take with food; 250 mg tid
Xermelo *Tab:* 250 mg (4 x 7 daily dose packs/carton
Comment: Take **Xermelo** in combination with somatostatin analog (SSA) therapy to treat patients inadequately controlled by SSA therapy. Breastfeeding females should monitor the infant for constipation.

DIARRHEA: CHRONIC

▷ *cholestyramine* (C)

Questran Powder for Oral Suspension initially 1 pkt or scoop daily; usual maintenance 2-4 pkts or scoops daily in 2 doses; max 6 pkts or scoops daily

Oral pwdr: 9 gm pkts; 9 gm equals 4 gm *anhydrous cholestyramine resin* (60/pck); *Bulk can:* 378 gm w. scoop

Questran Light initially 1 pkt or scoop daily; usual maintenance 2-4 pkts or scoops daily in 2 doses

Light: 5 gm pkts; 5 gm equals 4 gm *anhydrous cholestyramine resin* (60/pck); *Bulk can:* 210 gm w. scoop

Comment: Use *cholestyramine* only if diarrhea is due to bile salt malabsorption.

▷ *crofelemer* (C) not established; <12 years: not recommended; ≥12 years: 2 tabs daily; swallow whole with or without food; do not crush or chew

Mytesi *Tab:* 125 mg del-rel

Comment: *crofelemer* is indicated for the symptomatic relief of non-infectious diarrhea in patients ≥18 years with HIV/AIDS on antiretroviral therapy.

▷ *difenoxin/atropine* (C)

Motofen <2 years: not recommended; ≥2 years: 2 tabs, then 1 tab after each loose stool or 1 tab q 3-4 hours prn; max 8 tab/day x 2 days

Tab: dif 1 mg/*atrop* 0.025 mg

▷ *diphenoxylate/atropine* (B)(V)(G)

Lomotil <2 years: not recommended; 2-12 years: initially 0.3-0.4 mg/kg/day in 4 divided doses; >12 years: 5-20 mg/day in divided doses

Tab: diphen 2.5 mg/*atrop* 0.025 mg; *Liq:* diphen 2.5 mg/*atrop* 0.025 mg per 5 ml (2 oz w. dropper)

▷ *attapulgite* (C)(G)

Donnagel (OTC) <2 years: not recommended; 2-6 years: 7.5 ml after each loose stool; >6 years: 30 ml after each loose stool; max 7 doses/day

Liq: 600 mg/15 ml (120, 240 ml)

Donnagel Chewable Tab <3 years: not recommended; 3-6 years: 1/2 tab after each stool; max 7 doses/day; >6-12 years: 1 tab after each loose stool; max 7 tabs/day; >12 years: 2 tabs after loose stool; max 14 tabs/day

▷ *loperamide* (B)(OTC)(G)

Imodium (OTC) <5 years: not recommended; ≥5 years: 4-16 mg/day in divided doses

Cap: 2 mg

Imodium A-D (OTC) <2 years: not recommended; 2-5 years (24-47 lb): 1 mg up to tid x 2 days; >5-8 years (48-59 lb): 2 mg initially, then 1 mg after each loose stool; max 4 mg/day x 2 days; >8-11 years (60-95 lb): 2 mg initially, then 1 mg after each loose stool; max 6 mg/day x 2 days; >11 years: 4-16 mg/day in divided doses

Cplt: 2 mg; *Liq:* 1 mg/5 ml (2, 4 oz)

▷ *loperamide/simethicone* (B)(OTC)(G)

Imodium Advanced <6 years: not recommended; 6-8 years: chew 1 tab after loose stool, then chew 1/2 tab after next loose stool; 9-11 years: chew 1 tab after loose stool, then chew 1/2 tab after next loose stool; max 3 tabs/day; >11 years: 2 tabs chewed after loose stool, then 1 after the next loose stool; max 4 tabs/day

Chew tab: loper 2 mg/*simeth* 125 mg

DIARRHEA: TRAVELERS

▶ *ciprofloxacin* (C) <18 years: not recommended; ≥18 years: 500 mg bid x 3 days; max 1.5 gm/day

Cipro (G) *Tab:* 250, 500, 750 mg; *Oral susp:* 250, 500 mg/5 ml (100 ml) (strawberry)

Cipro XR *Tab:* 500, 1000 mg ext-rel

ProQuin XR *Tab:* 500 mg ext-rel

Comment: *ciprofloxacin* is contraindicated <18 years-of-age, and during pregnancy, and lactation. Risk of tendonitis or tendon rupture.

▶ *rifaximin* (C) <12 years: not recommended; ≥12 years: 200 mg tid x 3 days; discontinue if diarrhea worsens or persists more than 24 hours; not for use if diarrhea is accompanied by fever or blood in the stool or if causative organism other than *E. coli* is suspected.

Xifaxan *Tab:* 200 mg

▶ *trimethoprim/sulfamethoxazole* (C)(G)

Bactrim, Septra <12 years: not recommended; ≥12 years: 2 tabs bid x 10 days
Tab: trim 80 mg/*sulfa* 400 mg*

Bactrim DS, Septra DS <12 years: not recommended; ≥12 years: 1 tab bid x 10 days
Tab: trim 160 mg/*sulfa* 800 mg*

Bactrim Pediatric Suspension, Septra Pediatric Suspension <2 months: not recommended; ≥2 months-12 years: 40 mg/kg/day of *sulfamethoxazole* in 2 doses bid; >12 years: use tabs
Oral susp: trim 40 mg/*sulfa* 200 mg per 5 ml (100 ml) (cherry) (alcohol 0.3%)

DIGITALIS TOXICITY

Comment: The digitalis therapeutic index is narrow, 0.8-1.2 ng/mL. Whether acute or chronic toxicity, the patient should be treated in the emergency department and/or admitted to in-patient service for continued monitoring and care. Signs and symptoms of digitalis toxicity include: loss of appetite, nausea, vomiting, abdominal pain, diarrhea, visual disturbances (diplopia, blurred, or yellow vision, yellow-green halos around lights and other visual images, spots, blind spots), decreased urine output, generalized edema, orthopnea, confusion, dilirium, decreased consciousness, potentially lethal cardiac arrhythmias (ranging from ventricular tachycardia (VT) and ventricular fibrillation (VF) to sino-atrial heart block AVB). Treatment measures include repeated doses of charcoal via NG tube administered after gastric lavage for acute ingestion (methods to induce vomiting are usually discouraged because vomiting can worsen bradyarrhythmias), digitalis binders. Monitoring includes: serial ECGs, serum digitalis level, chemistries, potassium (hyperkalemia), magnesium (hypomagnesemia), BUN and creatinine.

DIGOXIN BINDER

▶ *digoxin (immune fab [ovine])*(B)contents of one vial of **Digibind** or **Digifab** neutralizes 0.5 mg *digoxin*; dose based on amount of *digoxin* or *digitoxin* to be neutralized; see mfr pkg insert

Digibind *Vial:* 38 mg

Digifab *Vial:* 40 mg for IV injection after reconstitution (preservative-free)

DIPHTHERIA

Prophylaxis *see Childhood Immunizations page* 473

POSTEXPOSURE PROPHYLAXIS FOR NON-IMMUNIZED PERSONS

▷ *erythromycin base* (B)(G) 45 kg: 50 mg/kg/day in 4 divided doses x 14 days; ≥45 kg: 500 mg qid x 14 days

　　Ery-Tab *Tab:* 250, 333, 500 mg ent-coat
　　PCE *Tab:* 333, 500 mg

▷ *erythromycin ethylsuccinate* (B)(G) 30-50 mg/kg/day in 4 divided doses x 14 days; may double dose with severe infection; max 100 mg/kg/day or 400 mg qid; *see page 563 for dose by weight table*

　　EryPed *Oral susp:* 200 mg/5 ml (100, 200 ml) (fruit); 400 mg/5 ml (60, 100, 200 ml) (banana); *Oral drops:* 200, 400 mg/5 ml (50 ml) (fruit); *Chew tab:* 200 mg wafer (fruit)
　　E.E.S. *Oral susp:* 200, 400 mg/5 ml (100 ml) (fruit)
　　E.E.S. Granules *Oral susp:* 200 mg/5 ml (100, 200 ml) (cherry)
　　E.E.S. 400 Tablets *Tab:* 400 mg

▷ *Immunization Series*
　　see *Childhood Immunizations page* 473

POSTEXPOSURE PROPHYLAXIS FOR IMMUNIZED PERSONS

▷ *Diphtheria* immunization booster

DIVERTICULITIS

▷ *amoxicillin* (B)(G) <40 kg (88 lb): 20-40 mg/kg/day in 3 divided doses x 10 days or 25-45 mg/kg/day in 2 divided doses x 10 days; *see page 543 for dose by weight table;* ≥40 kg: 500-875 mg bid x 10 days

　　Amoxil *Cap:* 250, 500 mg; *Tab:* 875*mg; *Chew tab:* 125, 200, 250, 400 mg(cherry-banana-peppermint) (phenylalanine); *Oral susp:* 125, 250 mg/5 ml(80, 100, 150 ml) (strawberry); 200, 400 mg/5 ml (50, 75, 100 ml) (bubble gum); *Oral drops:* 50 mg/ml (30 ml) (bubble gum)
　　Moxatag *Tab:* 775 mg ext-rel
　　Trimox *Tab:* 125, 250 mg; *Cap:* 250, 500 mg; *Oral susp:* 125, 250 mg/5 ml (80, 100, 150 ml) (raspberry-strawberry)

▷ *amoxicillin/clavulanate* (B)(G)

　　Augmentin <40 kg: 40-45 mg/kg/day divided tid x 10 days or 90 mg/kg/day divided bid x 10 days; *see page 545 for dose by weight table;* ≥40 kg: 500 mg tid or 875 mg bid x 10 days

　　Tab: 250, 500, 875 mg; *Chew tab:* 125, 250 mg (lemon-lime); 200, 400 mg (cherry-banana) (phenylalanine); *Oral susp:* 125 mg/5 ml (banana), 250 mg/5 ml (75, 100, 150 ml) (orange); 200, 400 mg/5 ml (50, 75, 100 ml) (orange) (phenylalanine)

　　Augmentin ES-600 <3 months: not recommended; ≥3 months, <40 kg: 90 mg/kg/day divided q 12 hours x 10 days; *see page 546 for dose by weight table;* ≥40 kg: not recommended

Oral susp: 600 mg/5 ml (50, 75, 100, 125, 150, 200 ml) (strawberry cream) (phenylalanine)

Augmentin XR <16 years: use other forms; ≥16 years: 2 tabs q 12 hours x 7-10 days

Tab: 1000*mg ext-rel

▶ *ciprofloxacin* (C) <18 years: not recommended; ≥18 years: 500 mg bid x 7 days; max 1.5 gm/day

Cipro (G) *Tab:* 250, 500, 750 mg; *Oral susp:* 250, 500 mg/5 ml (100 ml) (strawberry)

Cipro XR *Tab:* 500, 1000 mg ext-rel

ProQuin XR *Tab:* 500 mg ext-rel

Comment: *ciprofloxacin* is contraindicated <18 years-of-age, and during pregnancy, and lactation. Risk of tendonitis or tendon rupture.

▶ *metronidazole* **(not for use in 1st; B in 2nd, 3rd)(G)** 250-500 mg q 8 hours or 750 mg q 12 hours x 7 days

Flagyl *Tab:* 250*, 500*mg

Flagyl 375 *Cap:* 375 mg

Flagyl ER *Tab:* 750 mg ext-rel

Comment: Alcohol is contraindicated during treatment with oral *metronidazole* and for 72 hours after therapy due to a possible *disulfiram*-like reaction (nausea, vomiting, flushing, headache).

▶ *trimethoprim/sulfamethoxazole* **(D)(G)**

Bactrim, Septra <12 years: not recommended; ≥12 years: 2 tabs bid x 10 days

Tab: trim 80 mg/*sulfa* 400 mg*

Bactrim DS, Septra DS <12 years: not recommended; ≥12 years: 1 tab bid x 10 days

Tab: trim 160 mg/*sulfa* 800 mg*

Bactrim Pediatric Suspension, Septra Pediatric Suspension <2 months: not recommended; ≥2 months-12 years: 40 mg/kg/day of *sulfamethoxazole* in 2 doses bid; >12 years: use tabs

Oral susp: trim 40 mg/*sulfa* 200 mg per 5 ml (100 ml) (cherry) (alcohol 0.3%)

DIVERTICULOSIS

BULK-PRODUCING AGENTS

see **Constipation** *page 87*

DRY EYE SYNDROME

OPHTHALMIC IMMUNOMODULATOR/ANTI-INFLAMMATORY

▶ *cyclosporine* (C) <16 years: not recommended; ≥16 years: 1 drop q 12 hours

Restasis *Ophth emul:* 0.05% (0.4 ml) (preservative-free)

Comment: Ophthalmic Immunomodulators are contraindicated with active ocular infection. Allow at least 15 minutes between doses of artificial tears. May reinsert contact lenses 15 minutes after treatment.

OCULAR LUBRICANTS

Comment: Remove contact lens prior to using an ocular lubricant.

➤ *dextran 70/hypromellose* (NE) 1-2 drops prn
> **Bion Tears** (OTC) *Ophth soln:* single-use containers (28/pck) (preservative-free)

➤ *hydroxypropyl cellulose* (NE) apply 1/2 inch ribbon <u>or</u> 1 insert in each inferior cul-de-sac 1-2 times/day prn
> **Lacrisert** *Ophth inserts:* 5 mg (60/pck) (preservative-free)
> **Hypotears Ophthalmic Ointment** (OTC) *Ophth oint:* 1% (3.5 gm) (preservative-free)

Comment: Place insert in the inferior cul-de-sac of the eye, beneath the base of the tarsus, not in opposition to the cornea nor beneath the eyelid at the level of the tarsal plate.

➤ *hydroxypropyl methylcellulose* (NE) 1-2 drops prn
> **GenTeal Mild, GenTeal Moderate** (OTC) *Ophth soln:* (15 ml) (perborate)
> **GenTeal Severe** (OTC) *Ophth soln:* (15 ml) (carbopol 980, perborate)

➤ *petrolatum/mineral oil* (NE) apply 1/2 inch ribbon prn
> **Hypotears Ophthalmic Ointment** (OTC) *Ophth oint:* 1% (3.5 gm) (benzalkonium chloride, alcohol 1%)
> **Hypotears PF Ophthalmic Ointment** (OTC) *Ophth oint:* 1% (3.5 gm) (preservative-free, alcohol 1%)
> **Lacri-Lube** (OTC) *Ophth oint:* 1% (3.5, 7 gm)
> **Lacri-Lube NP** (OTC) *Ophth oint:* 1% (0.7 g, 24/pck) (preservative-free)

➤ *petrolatum/lanolin/mineral oil* (NE) apply 1/4 inch ribbon prn
> **Duratears Naturale** (OTC) *Ophth oint:* 3.5 gm (preservative-free)

➤ *polyethylene glycol/glycerin/hydroxypropyl methylcellulose* (NE) 1-2 drops prn
> **Visine Tears** (OTC) *Ophth soln:* 1% (15, 30 ml)

➤ *polyethylene glycol 400* 0.4%/*propylene glycol* 0.3% (NE) 1-2 drops prn
> **Systane** (OTC) *Ophth soln:* (15, 30, 40 ml) (polyquaternium-1, zinc chloride); *Vial:* 0.01 oz (28) (preservative-free)
> **Systane Ultra** (OTC) *Ophth soln:* (10, 20 ml) (aminomethylpropanol, polyquaternium-1, sorbitol (zinc chloride); *Vial:* 0.01 oz (24) (preservative-free)

➤ *polyvinyl alcohol* (NE) 1-2 drops prn
> **Hypotears** (OTC) *Ophth soln:* 1% (15, 30 ml)
> **Hypotears PF** (OTC) 1-2 drops q 3-4 hours prn
> *Ophth soln:* 1% (0.02 oz single-use containers, 30/pck) (preservative-free)

➤ *propylene glycol* 0.6% (NE) 1-2 drops prn
> **Systane Balance** (OTC) *Ophth soln:* (10 ml) (polyquaternium-1)

DUCHENNE MUSCULAR DYSTROPHY

➤ *deflazacort* (B) <5 years: not established; ≥ 5 years: 0.9 mg/kg/day administered once daily; take with <u>or</u> without food; may crush and mix with applesauce (then take immediately)
> **Emflaza** *Tab:* 6, 18, 30, 36 mg; *Oral susp:* 22.75 mg/ml (13 ml)

Comment: **Emflaza** is the first FDA-approved HYPERLINK\t "corticosteroid indicated for this condition to decrease inflammation and reduce the activity of the immune system. The side effects caused by **Emflaza** are similar to those experienced with other corticosteroids. The most common side effects include facial puffiness

(Cushingoid appearance), weight gain, increased appetite, upper respiratory tract infection, cough, extraordinary daytime urinary frequency (pollakiuria), hirsutism, and central obesity. Other side effects that are less common include problems with endocrine function, increased susceptibility to infection, elevation in blood pressure, risk of gastrointestinal perforation, serious skin rashes, behavioral and mood changes, decrease in the density of the bones and vision problems such as cataracts. Patients receiving immunosuppressive doses of corticosteroids should not be given live or live attenuated vaccines (LAVs). Moderate or strong CYP3A4 inhibitors, give one third of the recommended dosage of **Emflaza**. Avoid use of moderate or strong CYP3A4 inducers with **Emflaza**, as they may reduce efficacy. Dosage must be decreased gradually if the drug has been administered for more than a few days. Use only the oral dispenser provided with the product. After withdrawing the appropriate dose into the oral dispenser, slowly add the oral suspension into 3 to 4 ounces of juice or milk and mix well. The dose should then be administered immediately. Do not administer with grapefruit. Discard any unused EMFLAZA Oral Suspension remaining after 1 month of first opening the bottle.

DYSHIDROSIS

Topical Corticosteroids *see page* 494
Comment: Intermediate to high potency ophthalmic steroid treatment is indicated for dyshidrosis.

DYSFUNCTIONAL UTERINE BLEEDING (DUB)

▷ *medroxyprogesterone acetate* (X) 10 mg daily x 10-13 days
  Provera *Tab:* 2.5, 5, 10 mg
▷ *Oral contraceptives* (X) with 35 mcg estrogen equivalent
  see **Combined Oral Contraceptives** *page* 476
  Oral Prescription NSAIDs *see page* 490
  Other Oral Analgesics *see Pain page* 298

DYSLIPIDEMIA (HYPERCHOLESTEROLEMIA, HYPERLIPIDEMIA, MIXED DYSLIPIDEMIA)

OMEGA 3-ACID ETHYL ESTERS

▷ *omega 3-acid ethyl esters* (C)(G) <18 years: not recommended; ≥18 years: 2 gm bid or 4 gm once daily
  Lovaza *Soft gel cap:* 1 gm (α-tocopherol 4 mg/cap)

MICROSOMAL TRIGLYCERIDE-TRANSFER PROTEIN (MTP) INHIBITOR

▷ *lomitapide mesylate* (X) <12 years: not recommended; ≥12 years: 10 mg daily
  Juxtapid *Cap:* 5, 10, 20 mg
  Comment: **Juxtapid** is an adjunct to low-fat diet and other lipid-lowering treatments, including LDL apheresis where available, to reduce LDL-C, total

cholesterol, apo-B, and non-HDL-C in patients with homozygous familial hypercholesterolemia (HoFH); not for patients with hypercholesterolemia who do not have HoFH.

OLIGONUCLEOTIDE INHIBITOR OF APO B-100 SYNTHESIS

▷ *mipomersen* (B) <12 years: not established; ≥12 years: administer 200 mg SC once weekly, on the same day, in the upper arm, abdomen, or thigh; administer 1st injection under appropriate professional supervision

Kynamro *Vial/Prefilled syringe:* 200 mg mg/ml soln for SC inj single-use vial (preservative-free)

Comment: **Kynamro** is an adjunct to low-fat diet and other lipid-lowering treatments, to reduce LDL-C, apo-B, total cholesterol (TC), non-HDL-C in patients with homozygous familial hypercholesterolemia (HoFH).

CHOLESTEROL ABSORPTION INHIBITOR

▷ *ezetimibe* (C)(G) <10 years: not recommended; ≥10 years: 10 mg daily

Zetia *Tab:* 10 mg

Comment: *ezetimibe* is contraindicated with concomitant statins in liver disease, persistent elevations in serum transaminase, pregnancy, and nursing mothers. Concomitant fibrates are not recommended. Potentiated by *fenofibrate*, *gemfibrozil*, and possibly *cyclosporine*. Separate dosing of bile acid sequestrants is required; take *ezetimibe* at least 2 hours before or 4 hours after.

PROPROTEIN CONVERTASE SUBTILISIN KEXIN TYPE 9 (PCSK9) INHIBITOR

Comment: PCSK9 inhibitors are an adjunct to maximally tolerated statin therapy in persons who require additional lowering of LDL-C.

▷ *alirocumab* (NE)

Praluent <12 years: not established; ≥12 years: administer SC in the upper outer arm, abdomen, or thigh; initially 75 mg SC once every 2 weeks; measure LDL 4-8 weeks after initiation or titration; if inadequate response, may increase to 150 mg SC every 2 weeks

Soln for SC inj: 75, 150 mg/ml single-use prefilled syringe (preservative-free)

Comment: Although **Praluent** does not have an assigned pregnancy category, it is contraindicated in the 2nd and 3rd trimester of pregnancy.

▷ *evolocumab* (NE)

Repatha <12 years: HeFH, primary hyperlipidemia: not established; HoFH: <13 years: not established; >13 years: administer SC in the upper outer arm, elbow, or thigh; measure LDL 4-8 weeks after initiation; *HeFH or primary hyperlipidemia:* 140 mg SC once every 2 weeks or 420 mg once monthly; *HoFH:* 420 mg once monthly

Soln for SC inj: single-use prefilled syringe; 140 mg/syringe; single-use prefilled SureClick Autoinjector (140 mg/syringe preservative-free)

Comment: To administer 420 mg of **Repatha**, administer 150 mg SC x 3 within 30 minutes. Although **Repatha** does not have an assigned pregnancy category, it is contraindicated in pregnancy.

HMG-COA REDUCTASE INHIBITORS (STATINS)

Comment: The statins decrease total cholesterol, LDL-C, TG, and apo-B, and increase HDL-C. Before initiating and at 4-6 weeks, 3 months, and 6 months of therapy, check fasting lipid profile and LFTs. Side effects include myopathy and increased liver enzymes. Relative contraindications include concomitant use of cyclosporine, a macrolide antibiotic, various oral antifungal agents, and CYP-450 inhibitors. An absolute contraindication is active or chronic liver disease.

▷ *atorvastatin* (X)(G) <10 years: not recommended; ≥10 years (female post-men-arche): initially 10 mg daily; usual range 10-80 mg/day
   Lipitor *Tab:* 10, 20, 40, 80 mg

▷ *fluvastatin* (X)(G) <18 years: not recommended; ≥18 years; initially 20-40 mg q HS; usual range 20-80 mg/day
   Lescol *Cap:* 20, 40 mg
   Lescol XL *Tab:* 80 mg ext-rel

▷ *lovastatin* (X)
   Mevacor <10 years: not recommended; 10-17 years: initially 10-20 mg daily at evening meal; may increase at 4-week intervals; max 40 mg daily; >17 years: initially 20 mg daily at evening meal; may increase at 4-week intervals; max 80 mg/day in single or divided doses; if concomitant fibrates, niacin, or *CrCl <30 mL/min*, usual max 20 mg/day
      Tab: 10, 20, 40 mg
   Altoprev <20 years: not recommended; ≥20 years: initially 20 mg daily at evening meal; may increase at 4-week intervals; max 60 mg/day; if concomitant fibrates, or *niacin*; >1 gm/day, usual max 40 mg/day; if concomitant cyclospo-rine, *amiodarone*, or *verapamil*, or *CrCl <30 mL/min*, usual max 20 mg/day
      Tab: 10, 20, 40, 60 mg ext-rel

▷ *pitavastatin* (X)(G) <12 years: not established; initially 2 mg q HS; may increase to 4 mg after 4 weeks; max 4 mg/day; if concomitant *erythromycin* or *CrCl <60 ml/min;* 1 mg/day with usual max 2 mg/day; if concomitant *rifampin*, max 2 mg once daily
   Livalo *Tab:* 1, 2, 4 mg

▷ *pravastatin* (X) <8 years: not recommended; 8-13 years: 20 mg daily; >13-18 years: 40 mg daily; >18 years: initially 10-20 mg q HS; usual range 10-40 mg/day; may start at 40 mg/day
   Pravachol *Tab:* 10, 20, 40, 80 mg

▷ *rosuvastatin* (X)(G) <10 years: not recommended; 10-17 years: 5-20 mg/day; max 20 mg/day; >17 years: initially 10-20 mg q HS; usual range 5-40 mg/day; adjust at 4-week intervals
   Crestor *Tab:* 5, 10, 20, 40 mg

▷ *simvastatin* (X) <10 years: not recommended; ≥10 years (female post menarche): initially 20 mg q PM; usual range 5-80 mg/day; adjust at 4-week intervals
   Zocor *Tab:* 5, 10, 20, 40, 80 mg

CHOLESTEROL ABSORPTION INHIBITOR/HMG-COA REDUCTASE INHIBITOR COMBINATION

▷ *ezetimibe/simvastatin* (X)(G) <17 years: not recommended; ≥17 years: take once daily in the PM; may start at 10/40; swallow whole
   Vytorin
      Tab: **Vytorin 10/10** *ezet* 10 mg/*simva* 10 mg
         Vytorin 10/20 *ezet* 10 mg/*simva* 20 mg

Vytorin 10/40 *ezet* 10 mg/*simva* 40 mg
Vytorin 10/80 *ezet* 10 mg/*simva* 80 mg

ISOBUTYRIC ACID DERIVATIVES AND FIBRATE

Comment: These agents decrease total cholesterol, LDL-C, and TG; increase HDL-C. They are indicated when the primary problem is very high TG level. Side effects include epigastric discomfort, dyspepsia, abdominal pain, cholelithiasis, myopathy, and neutropenia. Before initiating, and at 4-6 weeks, 3 months, and 6 months of therapy, check fasting CBC, lipid profile, LFT, and serum creatinine. Absolute contraindications include severe renal disease and severe hepatic disease.

ISOBUTYRIC ACID DERIVATIVES

▷ *gemfibrozil* (C)(G) <12 years: not recommended; ≥12 years: 600 mg bid 30 minutes before AM and PM meal
Lopid *Tab:* 600*mg

FIBRATES (FIBRIC ACID DERIVATIVES)

▷ *fenofibrate* (C)(G) <12 years: not recommended; ≥12 years: take with meals; adjust at 4- to 8-week intervals; discontinue if inadequate response after 2 months; lowest dose or contraindicated with renal impairment
Antara 43-130 mg daily; max 130 mg/day
Cap: 43, 87, 130 mg
Fenoglide 40-120 mg daily; max 120 mg/day
Tab: 40, 120 mg
FibriCor 30-105 mg daily; max 105 mg/day
Tab: 30, 105 mg
TriCor 48-145 mg daily; max 145 mg/day
Tab: 48, 145 mg
TriLipix 45-135 mg daily; max 135 mg/day
Cap: 45, 135 mg del-rel
Lipofen 50-150 mg daily; max 150 mg/day
Cap: 50, 150 mg
Lofibra 67-200 mg daily; max 200 mg/day
Tab: 67, 134, 200 mg

NICOTINIC ACID DERIVATIVES

Comment: Nicotinic acid derivatives decrease total cholesterol, LDL-C, and TG; increase HDL-C. Before initiating and at 4-6 weeks, 3 months, and 6 months of therapy, check fasting lipid profile, LFT, glucose, and uric acid. Side effects include hyperglycemia, upper GI distress, hyperuricemia, hepatotoxicity, and significant transient skin flushing. Take with food and take *aspirin* 325 mg 30 minutes before dose to decrease flushing. Relative contraindications include diabetes, hyperuricemia (gout), and PUD and absolute contraindications include severe gout and chronic liver disease.
▷ *niacin* (C)
Niaspan (G) <21 years: not recommended; 375 mg daily for 1st week, then 500 mg daily for 2nd week, then 750 mg daily for 3rd week, then 1 gm daily for weeks 4-7; may increase by 500 mg q 4 weeks; usual range 1-2 gm/day; max 2 gm/day

Tab: 500, 750, 1000 mg ext-rel

Slo-Niacin <12 years: not recommended; ≥12 years: one 250 <u>or</u> 500 mg tab q AM <u>or</u> HS <u>or</u> one-half 750 mg tab q AM <u>or</u> HS

Tab: 250, 500, 750 mg cont-rel

BILE ACID SEQUESTRANTS

Comment: Bile acid sequestrants decrease total cholesterol, LDL-C, and increase HDL-C, but have no effect on triglycerides. A relative contraindication is TG ≥200 mg/dL and an absolute contraindication is TG ≥400 mg/dL. Before initiating and at 4-6 weeks, 3 months, and 6 months of therapy, check fasting lipid profile. Side effects include sandy taste in mouth, abdominal gas, abdominal cramping, and constipation. These agents decrease the absorption of many other drugs.

▷ *cholestyramine* (C)

Questran Powder for Oral Suspension <12 years: see mfr pkg insert; ≥12 years: initially 1 pkt <u>or</u> scoop daily; usual maintenance 2-4 pkts <u>or</u> scoops daily in 2 divided doses; max 6 pkts <u>or</u> scoops daily

Pwdr: 9 gm pkts; 9 gm equals 4 gm anhydrous *cholestyramine* resin for reconstitution (60/pck); Bulk can: 378 gm w. scoop

Questran Light <12 years: see mfr pkg insert; ≥12 years: initially 1 pkt <u>or</u> scoop daily; usual maintenance 2-4 pkts <u>or</u> scoops daily in 2 doses

Light: 5 gm pkts; 5 gm equals 4 gm anhydrous *cholestyramine* resin (60/pck): Bulk can: 210 gm w. scoop

▷ *colesevelam* (B)

Monotherapy: <12 years: not recommended; ≥12 years: 3 tabs bid <u>or</u> 6 tabs once daily <u>or</u> one 1.875 gm pkt bid <u>or</u> one 3.75 gm pkt once daily

WelChol *Tab:* 625 mg; *Pwdr for oral susp:* 1.875 gm pwdr pkts (60/carton); 3.75 g pwdr pkts (30/carton) (citrus) (phenylalanine)

Comment: WelChol is indicated as adjunctive therapy to improve glycemic control in patients >18 years with type 2 diabetes. It can be added to *metformin*, sulfonylureas, <u>or</u> insulin alone <u>or</u> in combination with other antidiabetic agents

▷ *colestipol* (C)

Colestid <12 years: not recommended; ≥12 years: 2-16 gm daily in a single <u>or</u> divided doses; granules: 5-30 gm daily in a single <u>or</u> divided dose

Tab: 1 gm (120); *Granules:* unflavored: 5 gm pkt (30, 90/carton); unflavored bulk: 300, 500 gm w. scoop; orange-flavored: 7.5 gm pkt (60/carton) (aspartame, phenylalanine); orange-flavored bulk: 450 gm w. scoop (aspartame); flavored: 7.5 gm pkt

Colestid Tab initially 2 gm bid; increase by 2 gm bid at 1-2-month intervals; usual maintenance 2-16 gm/day

Tab: 1 g

Comment: *colestipol* lowers LDL and total cholesterol.

ANTILIPID COMBINATIONS

Nicotinic Acid Derivative/HMG-CoA Reductase Inhibitors

▷ *niacin/lovastatin* (X)

Advicor <18 years: not recommended; ≥18 years: swallow whole at bedtime with a low-fat snack; may pretreat with aspirin; start at lowest niacin dose; may titrate niacin by no more than 500 mg/day every 4 weeks; max 2000/40 daily

Tab: **Advicor 500/20** *nia* 500 mg ext-rel/*lova* 20 mg
Advicor 750/20 *nia* 750 mg ext-rel/*lova* 20 mg
Advicor 1000/20 *nia* 1000 mg ext-rel/*lova* 20 mg
Advicor 1000/40 *nia* 1000 mg ext-rel/*lova* 40 mg

▷ *niacin/simvastatin* (X)
Simcor <18 years: not recommended; ≥18 years: swallow whole at bedtime with a low-fat snack; may pretreat with *aspirin*; start at lowest *niacin* dose; may titrate *niacin* by no more than 500 mg/day every 4 weeks; max 2000/40 daily
Tab: **Simcor 500/20** *nia* 500 mg ext-rel/*simva* 20 mg
Simcor 750/20 *nia* 750 mg ext-rel/*simva* 20 mg
Simcor 1000/20 *nia* 1000 mg ext-rel/*simva* 20 mg
Simcor 500/40 *nia* 500 mg ext-rel/*simva* 40 mg
Simcor 1000/40 *nia* 1000 mg ext-rel/*simva* 40 mg

ANTIHYPERTENSIVE/ANTILIPID COMBINATIONS

Calcium Channel Blocker/HMG-CoA Reductase Inhibitor (Statin) Combinations

▷ *amlodipine/atorvastatin* (X)(G)
Caduet <10 years: not recommended; ≥10 years (female, post-menarche):select according to blood pressure and lipid values; titrate amlodipine over 7-14 days; titrate atorvastatin according to monitored lipid values; max amlodipine 10 mg/day and max atorvastatin 80 mg/day; for contraindications and precautions for CCB and statin therapy, see to mfr pkg insert
Tab: **Caduet 5/10** *amlo* 5 mg/*ator* 10 mg
Caduet 5/20 *amlo* 5 mg/*ator* 20 mg
Caduet 5/40 *amlo* 5 mg/*ator* 40 mg
Caduet 5/80 *amlo* 5 mg/*ator* 80 mg
Caduet 10/10 *amlo* 10 mg/*ator* 10 mg
Caduet 10/20 *amlo* 10 mg/*ator* 20 mg
Caduet 10/40 *amlo* 10 mg/*ator* 40 mg
Caduet 10/80 *amlo* 10 mg/*ator* 80 mg

DYSMENORRHEA: PRIMARY

Oral Prescription NSAIDs *see page* 490
Other Oral Analgesics *see Pain page* 298

BENZENEACETIC ACID DERIVATIVE

▷ *diclofenac* (C) <14 years: not recommended; ≥14 years: 50-100 mg once; then 50 tid
Cataflam *Tab:* 50 mg
Voltaren *Tab:* 25, 50, 75 mg ent-coat
Voltaren-XR *Tab:* 100 mg ext-rel
Comment: *diclofenac* is contraindicated with *aspirin* allergy and late (≥30 weeks) pregnancy.

FENAMATE

▷ *mefenamic acid* (C) <14 years: not recommended; >14 years: 500 mg once; then 250 mg q 6 hours for up to 2-3 days; take with food
Ponstel *Cap:* 250 mg

Comment: Avoid *aspirin* with a fenamate.

COX-2 INHIBITORS

Comment: Cox-2 inhibitors are contraindicated with history of asthma, urticaria, and allergic-type reactions to *aspirin*, other NSAIDs, and sulfonamides, 3rd trimester of pregnancy, and coronary artery bypass graft (CABG) surgery.

▷ *celecoxib* (C)(G) <18 years: not recommended; ≥18 years: 100-400 mg bid; max 800 mg/day
Celebrex *Cap:* 50, 100, 200, 400 mg

▷ *meloxicam*(C)(G)
Mobic <2 years, <60 kg: not recommended; ≥2, ≥60 kg: 0.125 mg/kg; max 7.5 mg once daily; ≥18 years: initially 7.5 mg once daily; max 15 mg once daily; *Hemodialysis:* max 7.5 mg/day
Tab: 7.5, 15 mg; *Oral susp:* 7.5 mg/5 ml (100 ml) (raspberry)
Vivlodex <18 years: not established; ≥18 years: initially 5 mg qd; may increase to max 10 mg/day; *Hemodialysis:* max 5 mg/day
Cap: 5, 10 mg

EDEMA

THIAZIDE DIURETICS

▷ *chlorthalidone* (B)(G) initially 30-60 mg daily or 60 mg on alternate days; max 90-120 mg/day
Thalitone *Tab:* 15 mg

▷ *chlorothiazide* (B)(G) <6 months: up to 15 mg/lb/day in 2 divided doses; ≥6 months-12 years: 10 mg/lb/day in 2 divided doses; max 375 mg/day; >12 years: 0.5-1 gm/day in a single or divided doses; max 2 gm/day
Diuril *Tab:* 250*, 500*mg; *Oral susp:* 250 mg/5 ml (237 ml)

▷ *hydrochlorothiazide* (B)(G) <12 years: not recommended; ≥12 years:
Esidrix 25-200 mg daily
Tab: 25, 50, 100 mg
Microzide 12.5 mg daily; usual max 50 mg/day
Cap: 12.5 mg

▷ *hydroflumethiazide* (B) <2 years: not recommended; ≥2 years: 50-200 mg/day in a single or 2 divided doses
Saluron *Tab:* 50 mg

▷ *polythiazide* (C) <2 years: not recommended; ≥2 years: 1-4 mg daily
Renese *Tab:* 1, 2, 4 mg

POTASSIUM-SPARING DIURETICS

▷ *amiloride* (B)(G) <12 years: not recommended; ≥12 years: initially 5 mg; may increase to 10 mg; max 20 mg
Tab: 5 mg

▷ *spironolactone* (D)(G) <12 years: not recommended; ≥12 years: initially 25-200 mg in a single <u>or</u> divided doses; titrate at 2-week intervals
    Aldactone *Tab:* 25, 50*, 100*mg
▷ *triamterene* (B) <12 years: not recommended; ≥12 years: 100 mg bid; max 300 mg
    Dyrenium *Cap:* 50, 100 mg

LOOP DIURETICS

▷ *bumetanide* (C)(G) <18 years: not recommended; ≥18 years: 0.5-2 mg daily; may repeat at 4-5 hour intervals; max 10 mg/day
    Tab: 1* mg
  Comment: *bumetanide* is contraindicated with sulfa drug allergy.
▷ *ethacrynic acid* (B)(G) ≤1 month: not recommended; >1 month-12 years: initially 25 mg/day; then adjust dose in 25 mg increments; >12 years: max 50-200 mg once daily
    Edecrin *Tab:* 25, 50 mg
▷ *ethacrynate sodium* (B)(G) <1 month: not recommended; ≥1 month-12 years: use the smallest effective dose; initially 25 mg; then careful stepwise increments in dosage of 25 mg to achieve effective maintenance; ≥12 years: administer smallest dose required to produce gradual weight loss (about 1-2 pounds per day); onset of diuresis usually occurs at 50-100 mg in children ≥12 years; after diuresis has been achieved, the minimally effective dose (usually 50-200 mg/day) may be administered on a continuous <u>or</u> intermittent dosage schedule; dose titrations are usually in 25-50 mg increments to avoid derangement electrolyte and water excretion; the patient should be weighed under standard conditions before and during administration of *ethacrynate sodium;* the following schedule may be helpful in determining the lowest effective dose: *Day 1:* 50 mg once daily after a meal; *Day 2:* 50 mg bid after meals, if necessary; *Day 3:* 100 mg in the morning and 50-100 mg following the afternoon <u>or</u> evening meal, depending upon response to the morning dose; a few patients may require initial and maintenance doses as high as 200 mg bid; these higher doses, which should be achieved gradually, are most often required in patients with severe, refractory edema
    Sodium Edecrin *Vial:* 50 mg single dose
  Comment: **Sodium Edecrin** is more potent than more commonly used loop and thiazide diuretics. Treatment of the edema associated with congestive heart failure, cirrhosis of the liver, and renal disease, including the nephrotic syndrome, short-term management of ascites due to malignancy, idiopathic edema, and lymphedema, short-term management of hospitalized pediatric patients, other than infants, with congenital heart disease or the nephrotic syndrome. IV Sodium Edecrin is indicated when a rapid onset of diuresis is desired, e.g., in acute pulmonary edema <u>or</u> when gastrointestinal absorption is impaired <u>or</u> oral medication is not practical.
▷ *furosemide* (C)(G) <12 years: not recommended; ≥12 years: initially 20-80 mg as a single dose
    Lasix *Tab:* 20, 40*, 80 mg; *Oral soln:* 10 mg/ml (2, 4 oz w. dropper)
  Comment: *furosemide* is contraindicated with sulfa drug allergy.
▷ *torsemide* (B) <12 years: not recommended; ≥12 years: 5 mg daily; may increase to 10 mg daily
    Demadex *Tab:* 5*, 10*, 20*, 100*mg

OTHER DIURETICS

➤ *indapamide* (B) <12 years: not recommended; ≥12 years: initially 1.25 mg daily; may titrate every 4 weeks if needed; max 5 mg/day

Lozol *Tab:* 1.25, 2.5 mg

Comment: *indapamide* is contraindicated with sulfa drug allergy.

➤ *metolazone* (B)

Mykrox <12 years: not recommended; ≥12 years: initially 0.5 mg q AM; max 1 mg/day

Tab: 0.5 mg

Zaroxolyn <12 years: not recommended; ≥12 years: 2.5-5 mg once daily

Tab: 2.5, 5, 10 mg

Comment: *metolazone* is contraindicated with sulfa drug allergy.

DIURETIC COMBINATIONS

➤ *amiloride/hydrochlorothiazide* (B)(G) <12 years: not recommended; ≥12 years: initially 1 tab daily; may increase to 2 tabs/day in a single or divided doses

Moduretic *Tab: amil* 5 mg/*hydro* 50 mg*

➤ *spironolactone/hydrochlorothiazide* (D)(G) <12 years: not recommended; ≥12 years: usual maintenance is 100 mg each of spironolactone and hydrochlorothiazide daily, in a single dose or in divided doses; range 25-200 mg of each component daily depending on the response to the initial titration

Aldactazide 25 *Tab: spiro* 25 mg/*hydro* 25 mg

Aldactazide 50 *Tab: spiro* 50 mg/*hydro* 50 mg

➤ *triamterene/hydrochlorothiazide* (C)(G) <12 years: not recommended; ≥12 years:

Dyazide 1-2 caps once daily

Cap: triam 37.5 mg/*hydro* 25 mg

Maxzide 1 tab once daily

Tab: triam 75 mg/*hydro* 50 mg*

Maxzide-25 1-2 tabs once daily

Tab: triam 37.5 mg/*hydro* 25 mg*

 ENCOPRESIS

INITIAL BOWEL EVACUATION

➤ *mineral oil* (C) 1 oz x 1 day

➤ *bisacodyl* (B) <12 years: 1/2 suppository daily prn; ≥12 years: 1 suppository daily prn

Dulcolax *Rectal supp:* 10 mg

➤ *glycerin* suppository <6 years: 1 pediatric suppository; ≥6 years: 1 adult suppository

MAINTENANCE

➤ *mineral oil* (C) 5-15 ml once daily

➤ *multivitamin* (A) 1 daily

Comment: Mineral oil can inhibit absorption of fat-soluble vitamins.

ENURESIS: PRIMARY, NOCTURNAL

VASOPRESSIN

▷ *desmopressin acetate* (B)

DDAVP <6 years: not recommended; ≥6 years: usual dosage 0.1-1.2 mg/day in 2-3 divided doses; 0.2 mg q HS prn for nocturnal enuresis

Tab: 0.1*, 0.2*mg

DDAVP Rhinal Tube <6 years: not recommended; ≥6 years: 10 mcg or 0.1 ml of soln each nostril (20 mcg total dose) q HS prn; max 40 mcg total dose

Nasal spray: 10 mcg/actuation (5 ml, 50 sprays); *Rhinal tube:* 0.1 mg/ml (2.5 ml)

TRICYCLIC ANTIDEPRESSANT (TCA)

Comment: Co-administration of SSRIs and TCAs requires extreme caution.

▷ *amitriptyline* (C)(G) <12 years: not recommended; ≥12 years: 10-20 mg q HS

Tab: 10, 25, 50, 75, 100, 150 mg

▷ *amoxapine* (C) <12 years: not recommended; ≥12 years: initially 50 mg bid-tid; after 1 week may increase to 100 mg bid-tid; usual effective dose 200-300 mg/day; if total dose exceeds 300 mg/day, give in divided doses (max 400 mg/day); may give as a single bedtime dose; max 300 mg q HS

Tab: 25, 50, 100, 150 mg

▷ *clomipramine* (C)(G) <10 years: not recommended; 10-16 years: initially 25 mg daily in divided doses; gradually increase; max 3 mg/kg or 100 mg, whichever is smaller; >16 years: initially 25 mg daily in divided doses; gradually increase to 100 mg during first 2 weeks; max 250 mg/day; total maintenance dose may be given at HS

Anafranil *Cap:* 25, 50, 75 mg

▷ *desipramine* (C)(G) <12 years: not recommended; ≥12 years: 100-200 mg/day in single or divided doses; max 300 mg/day

Norpramin *Tab:* 10, 25, 50, 75, 100, 150 mg

▷ *doxepin* (C)(G) <12 years: not recommended; ≥12 years: 75 mg/day; max 150 mg/day

Cap: 10, 25, 50, 75, 100, 150 mg; *Oral conc:* 10 mg/ml (4 oz w. dropper)

▷ *imipramine* (C)(G) <12 years: not recommended; ≥12 years:

Tofranil initially 75 mg daily (max 200 mg); adolescents initially 30-40 mg daily (max 100 mg/day); if maintenance dose exceeds 75 mg daily, may switch to **Tofranil PM** for divided or bedtime dose

Tab: 10, 25, 50 mg

Tofranil PM initially 75 mg daily 1 hour before HS; max 200 mg

Cap: 75, 100, 125, 150 mg

▷ *nortriptyline* (D)(G) <12 years: not recommended; ≥12 years: initially 25 mg tid-qid; max 150 mg/day

Pamelor *Cap:* 10, 25, 50, 75 mg; *Oral soln:* 10 mg/5 ml (16 oz)

▷ *protriptyline* (C) <12 years: not recommended; ≥12 years: initially 5 mg tid; usual dose 15-40 mg/day in 3-4 divided doses; max 60 mg/day

Vivactil *Tab:* 5, 10 mg

▷ *trimipramine* (C) <12 years: not recommended; ≥12 years: initially 75 mg/day in divided doses; max 200 mg/day

Surmontil *Cap:* 25, 50, 100 mg

EPICONDYLITIS

Acetaminophen for IV Infusion *see Pain page* 296
Oral Prescription NSAIDs *see page* 490
Other Oral Analgesics *see Pain page* 298
Topical/Transdermal NSAIDs *see Pain page* 298
Parenteral Corticosteroids *see page* 499
Oral Corticosteroids *see page* 498
Topical Analgesic and Anesthetic Agents *see page* 488

EPIDIDYMITIS

Comment: The following treatment regimens for epididymitis are published in the **2015 CDC Transmitted Diseases Treatment Guidelines**. Treatment regimens are presented by generic drug name first, followed by information about brands and dose forms. Empiric treatment requires concomitant treatment of chlamydia. Treat all sexual contacts. Patients who are HIV-positive should receive the same treatment as those who are HIV-negative.

RECOMMENDED REGIMEN

Regimen 1

▷ *ceftriaxone* (B)(G) 250 mg IM in a single dose
       plus
▷ *doxycycline* (D)(G) 100 mg bid x 10 days

RECOMMENDED REGIMENS: LIKELY CAUSED BY ENTERIC ORGANISMS

Regimen 1

▷ *levofloxacin* (C) 500 mg daily x 10 days

Regimen 2

▷ *ofloxacin* (C)(G) 300 mg bid x 10 day

DRUG BRANDS AND DOSE FORMS

▷ *ceftriaxone* (B)(G)
       Rocephin *Vial:* 250, 500 mg; 1, 2 g
▷ *doxycycline* (D)(G)
       Acticlate *Tab:* 75, 150** mg
       Adoxa *Tab:* 50, 75, 100, 150 mg ent-coat
       Doryx *Tab:* 50, 75, 100, 150, 200 mg del-rel
       Monodox *Cap:* 50, 75, 100 mg
       Oracea *Cap:* 40 mg del-rel
       Vibramycin *Tab:* 100 mg; *Cap:* 50, 100 mg; *Syr:* 50 mg/5 ml (raspberry-apple) (sulfites); *Oral susp:* 25 mg/5 ml (raspberry)
       Vibra-Tab *Tab:* 100 mg film-coat

Comment: *doxycycline* is contraindicated <8 years-of-age, in pregnancy, and lactation (discolors developing tooth enamel). A side effect may be photo-sensitivity (photophobia). Do not take with antacids, calcium supplements, milk or other dairy, or within 2 hours of taking another drug.

▷ *levofloxacin* (C)
    Levaquin *Tab:* 250, 500, 750 mg; *Oral soln:* 25 mg/ml (480 ml) (benzyl alcohol)
    Comment: is contraindicated <18 years-of-age, and during pregnancy, and lactation. Risk of tendonitis or tendon rupture.

▷ *ofloxacin* (C)(G)
    Floxin *Tab:* 200, 300, 400 mg
    Comment: *ofloxacin* is contraindicated <18 years-of-age, and during pregnancy and lactation. Risk of tendonitis or tendon rupture.

ERYSIPELAS

Comment: Erysipelas is most commonly due to GABHS (Group A beta-hemolytic Strept).

TREATMENT OF CHOICE

▷ *penicillin V potassium* (B) <12 years: 25-75 mg/kg day divided q 6-8 hours x 10 days; *see page 572 for dose by weight table;* ≥12 years: 250-500 mg q 6 hours x 10 days
    Pen-VK *Tab:* 250, 500 mg; *Oral soln:* 125 mg/5 ml (100, 200 ml); 250 mg/5 ml (100, 150, 200 ml)

TREATMENT IF PENICILLIN ALLERGIC

▷ *erythromycin base* (B)(G) 30-40 mg/kg/day divided q 6 hours x 10 days; >40 kg: 250 mg q 6 hours x 10 days
    Ery-Tab *Tab:* 250, 333, 500 mg ent-coat
    PCE *Tab:* 333, 500 mg

▷ *erythromycin ethylsuccinate* (B)(G) 30-50 mg/kg/day in 4 divided doses x 7 days; may double dose with severe infection; max 100 mg/kg/day or 400 mg qid; *see page 563 for dose by weight table*
    EryPed *Oral susp:* 200 mg/5 ml (100, 200 ml) (fruit); 400 mg/5 ml (60, 100, 200 ml) (banana); *Oral drops:* 200, 400 mg/5 ml (50 ml) (fruit); *Chew tab:* 200 mg wafer (fruit)
    E.E.S. *Oral susp:* 200, 400 mg/5 ml (100 ml) (fruit)
    E.E.S. Granules *Oral susp:* 200 mg/5 ml (100, 200 ml) (cherry)
    E.E.S. 400 Tablets *Tab:* 400 mg

EYE PAIN

Acetaminophen for IV Infusion *see **Pain** page 296*

OPHTHALMIC NSAIDs

Comment: Concomitant contact lens wear is contraindicated during therapy. Etiology of eye pain must be known prior to use of these agents

➤ *diclofenac* (B) <12 years: not recommended; ≥12 years: 1 drop affected eye qid
Voltaren Ophthalmic Solution *Ophth soln:* 0.1% (2.5, 5 ml)
➤ *ketorolac tromethamine* (C) <3 years: not recommended; ≥3 years: 1 drop affected
eye qid for up to 4 days
Acular *Ophth soln:* 0.5% (3, 5, 10 ml; benzalkonium chloride)
Acular LS *Ophth soln:* 0.4% (5 ml; benzalkonium chloride)
Acular PF *Ophth soln:* 0.5% (0.4 ml; 12 single-use vials/carton) (preservative-free)
➤ *nepafenac* (C) <10 years: not recommended; ≥10 years: 1 drop affected eye tid
Nevanac Ophthalmic Suspension *Ophth susp:* 0.1% (3 ml) (benzalkonium
chloride)

OPHTHALMIC STEROIDS

Comment: Contraindications: ocular fungal, viral, or mycobacterial infections.
Effectiveness of treatment should be assessed after 2 days. The corticosteroid should be
tapered and treatment concluded within 14 days if possible due to risk of corneal and/
or scleral thinning with prolonged use.
➤ *difluprednate* (C) <12 years: not recommended; ≥12 years: 1 drop affected eye qid;
Post-op pain: beginning 24 hours after surgery, 1 drop affected eye qid; continue for
2 weeks post-op; then bid x 1 week; then taper until resolved
Durezol Ophthalmic Solution *Ophth emul:* 0.05% (5 ml)
➤ *etabonate* (C) <12 years: not recommended; ≥12 years: 1 drop affected eye qid
Alrex Ophthalmic Solution *Ophth emul:* 0.2% (5 ml) (benzalkonium chloride)

FACIAL HAIR, EXCESSIVE/UNWANTED

TOPICAL HAIR GROWTH RETARDANT

➤ *eflornithine* 13.9% cream (C) <12 years: not recommended; ≥12 years: apply a thin
layer to affected areas of face and under the chin bid at least 8 hours apart; rub in
thoroughly; do not wash treated area for at least 4 hours following application
Vaniqa *Crm:* 13.9% (30, 60 gm)
Comment: After **Vaniqa** dries, may apply cosmetics or sunscreen. Hair removal
techniques may be continued as needed.

FECAL ODOR

➤ *bismuth subgallate powder* (B)(OTC) 1-2 tabs tid with meals
Devrom *Chew tab:* 200 mg; *Cap:* 200 mg
Comment: **Devron** is an internal (oral) deodorant for control of odors from
ileostomy or colostomy drainage or fecal incontinence.

FEVER (PYREXIA)

ACETAMINOPHEN FOR IV INFUSION

➤ *acetaminophen* injectable (B)(G) <2 years: not recommended; 2-13 years <50 kg:
15 mg/kg q 6 hours prn or 12.5 mg/kg q 4 hours prn; max 750 mg single dose; max

75 mg/kg per day; >13 years: administer by IV infusion over 15 minutes; 1,000 mg q 6 hours prn <u>or</u> 650 mg q 4 hours prn; max 4,000 mg/day

Ofirmev *Vial:* 10 mg/ml (100 ml) (preservative-free)

Comment: The **Ofirmev** vial is intended for single use. If any portion is withdrawn from the vial, use within 6 hours. Discard the unused portion. For pediatric patients, withdraw the intended dose and administer via syringe pump. Do not admix **Ofirmev** with any other drugs. **Ofirmev** is physically incompatible with *diazepam* and *chlorpromazine hydrochloride.*

▷ *acetaminophen* (B)(G)

Children's Tylenol (OTC) 10-20 mg/kg q 4-6 hours prn

Oral susp: 80 mg/tsp

4-11 months (12-17 lb): 1/2 tsp q 4 hours prn; 12-23 months (18-23 lb): 3/4 tsp q 4 hours prn; 2-3 years (24-35 lb): 1 tsp q 4 hours prn; 4-5 years(36-47 lb): 1 tsp q 4 hours prn; 6-8 years (48-59 lb): 2 tsp q 4 hours prn; 9-10 years (60-71 lb): 2 tsp q 4 hours prn; 11 years (72-95 lb): 3 tsp q 4 hours prn; All: max 5 doses/day

Elix: 160 mg/5 ml (2, 4 oz)

Chew tab: 80 mg

2-3 years (24-35 lb): 2 tabs q 4 hours prn; 4-5 years (36-47 lb): 3 tabs q 4 hours prn; 6-8 years (48-59 lb): 4 tabs q 4 hours prn; 9-10 years (60-71 lb): 5 tabs q 4 hours prn; 11 years (72-95 lb): 6 tabs q 4 hours prn; All: max 5 doses/day

Junior Strength:

6-8 years: 2 tabs q 4 hours prn; 9-10 years: 2 tabs q 4 hours prn; 11 years: 3 tabs q 4 hours prn; 12 years: 4 tabs q 4 hours prn; All: max 5 doses/day

Chew tab: 160 mg

Junior cplt: 160 mg

Infant's Drops and Suspension: 80 mg/0.8 ml (1/2, 1 oz)

<3 months: 0.4 ml q 4 hours prn; 4-11 months: 0.8 ml q 4 hours prn; 12-23 months: 1.2 ml q 4 hours prn; 2-3 years (24-35 lb): 1.6 ml q 4 hours prn; 4-5 years (36-47 lb): 2.4 ml q 4 hours prn; All: max 5 doses/day

Extra Strength Tylenol (G)(OTC) <12 years: not recommended; ≥12 years: 500-1000 mg q 4-6 hours prn; max 4 gm/day

Tab/Cplt/Gel tab/Gel cap: 500 mg; *Liq:* 500 mg/15 ml (8 oz)

FeverAll Extra Strength Tylenol (OTC) <3 months: not recommended; 3-36 months: 80 mg q 4 hours prn; 3-6 years: 120 mg q 4 hours prn; ≥6 years: 325 mg q 4 hours prn; *Rectal supp:* 80, 120, 325 mg (6/carton)

Maximum Strength Tylenol Sore Throat (OTC) <12 years: not recommended; ≥12 years: 500-1000 mg q 4-6 hours prn

Liq: 1000 mg/30 ml (8 oz)

Tylenol (OTC) <6 years: not recommended; 6-11 years: 325 mg q 4-6 hours prn; max 1.625 gm/day; ≥12 years: 650 mg q 4-6 hours; max 4 gm/day

▷ *aspirin* (D)(G)

Bayer (OTC) <6 years: not recommended; 6-11 years: 325 mg q 4-6 hours prn; max 1.625 gm/day; >11 years: 325-650 mg q 4 hours prn; max: 5 doses/day

Tab/Cplt: 325 mg ext-rel

Extra Strength Bayer (OTC) <6 years: not recommended; 6-11 years: 325 mg q 4-6 hours prn; max 1.625 gm/day; ≥12 years: 500-1000 mg q 4-6 hours prn; max 4 gm/day

Cplt: 500 mg
Extended-Release Bayer 8 Hour (OTC) <12 years: not recommended; ≥12 years: 650-1300 mg q 8 hours prn
Cplt: 650 mg ext-rel

Comment: *aspirin*-containing medications are contraindicated with history of allergic-type reaction to *aspirin*, children and adolescents with *Varicella* or other viral illness, and 3rd trimester pregnancy.

▷ *aspirin/caffeine* (D)(G)
Anacin (OTC) <6 years: not recommended; 6-12 years: 400 mg q 4 hours prn; max 2 gm/day; ≥12 years: 800 mg q 4 hours prn; max 4 gm/day
Tab/Cplt: 400 mg
Anacin Maximum Strength (OTC) <12 years: not recommended; ≥12 years: 1 gm tid-qid
Tab: 500 mg

Comment: *aspirin*-containing medications are contraindicated with history of allergic-type reaction to aspirin, children and adolescents with *Varicella* or other viral illness, and 3rd trimester pregnancy.

▷ *aspirin/antacid* (D)(G)
Extra Strength Bayer Plus (OTC) <12 years: not recommended; ≥12 years: 500 mg-1 gm q 4-6 hours prn; usual max 4 gm/day
Cplt: 500 mg *aspirin* with *calcium carbonate*
Bufferin (OTC) <12 years: not recommended; ≥12 years: 650 mg q 4 hours; max 3.9 mg/day
Tab: 325 mg *aspirin* with *calcium carbonate*, *magnesium carbonate*, and *magnesium oxide*

Comment: *aspirin*-containing medications are contraindicated with history of allergic-type reaction to *aspirin*, children and adolescents with *Varicella* or other viral illness, and 3rd trimester pregnancy.

▷ *ibuprofen* (B; not for use in 3rd)(G)
Comment: *ibuprofen* is contraindicated in children <6 months-of-age.
Children's Advil (OTC), ElixSure IB (OTC), Motrin (OTC), PediaCare (OTC), PediaProfen (OTC)5-10 mg/kg q 6-8 hours; max 40 mg/kg/day; <24 lb (<2 years):individualize; 24-35 lb (2-3 years): 5 ml q 6-8 hours prn; 36-47 lb (4-5 years): 7.5 ml q 6-8 hours prn; 48-59 lb (6-8 years): 10 ml or 2 tabs q 6-8 hours prn; 60-71 lb (9-10 years): 12.5 ml or 2 tabs q 6-8 hours prn; 72-95 lb (11 years): 15 ml or 3 tabs q 6-8 hours prn
Oral susp: 100 mg/5 ml (2, 4 oz) (berry); *Junior tabs:* 100 mg
Children's Motrin Drops (OTC), PediaCare Drops (OTC) n <24 lb (<2 years): individualize; 24-35 lb (2-3 years): 2.5 ml q 6-8 hours prn; *Oral drops:* 50 mg/1.25 ml (15 ml; berry)
Children's Motrin Chewables and Caplets (OTC) 48-59 lb (6-8 years): 200 mg q 6-8 hours prn; 60-71 lb (9-10 years): 250 mg q 6-8 hours prn; 72-95 lb (11 years): 300 mg q 6-8 hours prn; ≥12 years: 400 mg q 4 hours prn
Chew tab: 100*mg (citrus; phenylalanine)
Cplt: 100 mg
Motrin (OTC) <6 months: not recommended; >6 months, fever <102.5: 5 mg/kg q6-8 hours prn; >6 months, fever >102.5: 10 mg/kg q 6-8 hours prn; *All:* max 40 mg/kg/day; ≥12 years: 400 mg q 6 hours prn

Tab: 400 mg; *Cplt:* 100*mg; *Chew tab:* 50*, 100*mg (citrus; phenylalanine); *Oral susp:* 100 mg/5 ml (4, 16 oz) (berry); *Oral drops:* 40 mg/ml (15 ml) (berry)

Advil (OTC), Motrin IB (OTC), Nuprin (OTC) <12 years: not recommended; ≥12 years: 200-400 mg q 4-6 hours; max 1.2 gm/day
Tab/Cplt/Gel cap: 200 mg

▷ *naproxen* (B)(G)
Aleve (OTC) <2 years: not recommended; ≥2 years-6 years: 2.5-5 mg/kg bid-tid; max: 15 mg/kg/day; 400 mg x 1 dose; then 200 mg q 8-12 hours prn; max 10 days
Tab/Cplt/Gel cap: 200 mg
Anaprox <12 years: not recommended; ≥12 years: 550 mg x 1 dose; then 550 mg q 12 hours or 275 mg q 6-8 hours prn; max 1.375 gm first day and 1.1 gm/day thereafter
Tab: 275 mg
Anaprox DS <12 years: not recommended; ≥12 years: 1 tab bid
Tab: 550 mg
EC-Naprosyn <12 years: not recommended; ≥12 years: 375 or 500 mg bid prn; may increase dose up to max 1500 mg/day as tolerated
Tab: 375, 500 mg del-rel
Naprelan <12 years: not recommended; ≥12 years: 1 gm daily or 1.5 gm daily for limited time; max 1 gm/day thereafter
Tab: 375, 500 mg
Naprosyn <12 years: not recommended; ≥12 years: initially 500 mg, then 500 mg q 12 hours or 250 mg q 6-8 hours prn; max 1.25 gm first day and 1 gm/day thereafter
Tab: 250, 375, 500 mg; *Oral susp:* 125 mg/5 ml (473 ml) (pineapple-orange)

▮ FIBROMYALGIA

Acetaminophen for IV Infusion *see Pain page 296*
Oral Prescription NSAIDs *see page 490*
Other Oral Analgesics *see Pain page 298*
Topical/Transdermal NSAIDs *see Pain page 298*
Parenteral Corticosteroids *see page 499*
Oral Corticosteroids *see page 498*
Topical Analgesic and Anesthetic Agents *see page 488*

SEROTONIN AND NOREPINEPHRINE REUPTAKE INHIBITORS (SNRIs)

▷ *duloxetine* (C)(G) <12 years: not recommended; ≥12 years: swallow whole; initially 30 mg once daily x 1 week; then increase to 60 mg once daily; max 120 mg/day
Cymbalta *Cap:* 20, 30, 60 mg ent-coat pellets
▷ *milnacipran* (C)(G) <17 years: not recommended; ≥17 years: *Day 1:* 12.5 mg once; *Days 2-3:* 12.5 mg bid; *Days 4-7:* 25 mg bid; max 100 mg bid
Savella *Tab:* 12.5, 25, 50, 100 mg

GAMMA-AMINOBUTYRIC ACID ANALOG

➤ *gabapentin* (C) <3 years: not recommended; 3-12 years: initially 10-15 mg/kg/day in 3 divided doses; max 12 hours between doses; titrate over 3 days; 3-4 years: titrate to 40 mg/kg/day; 5-12 years: titrate to 25-35 mg/kg/day; max 50 mg/kg/day; >12 years: initially 300 mg on Day 1; then 600 mg on Day 2; then 900 mg on Days 3-6; then 1200 mg on Days 7-10; then 1500 mg on Days 11-14; titrate up to 1800 mg on Day 15; take entire dose once daily with the evening meal; do not crush, split, or chew
    Gralise (C) *Tab:* 300, 600 mg
    Neurontin (G) *Tab:* 600*, 800* mg; *Cap:* 100, 300, 400 mg; *Oral soln:* 250 mg/5 ml (480 ml) (strawberry-anise)
    Comment: Avoid abrupt cessation of *gabapentin*. To discontinue, withdraw gradually over 1 week or longer.

➤ *gabapentin enacarbil* (C) <12 years: not recommended: ≥12 years: 600 mg once daily at about 5: 00 PM; if dose not taken at recommended time, next dose should be taken the following day; swallow whole; take with food; *CrCl 30-59 mL/min:* 600 mg on Day 1, Day 3, and every day thereafter; *CrCl <30 mL/min:* or on hemodialy-sis: not recommended
    Horizant *Tab:* 300, 600 mg ext-rel
    Comment: Avoid abrupt cessation of *gabapentin enacarbil*. To discontinue, withdraw gradually over 1 week or longer.

α₂-DELTA LIGAND

➤ *pregabalin (GABA analog)* (C)(V) <18 years: not recommended; ≥18 years: initially 50 mg tid; may titrate to 100 mg tid within one week; max 600 mg divided tid; discontinue over one week
    Lyrica *Cap:* 25, 50, 75, 100, 150, 200, 225, 300 mg; *Oral soln:* 20 mg/ml

OTHER AGENTS

➤ *amitriptyline* (C)(G) <12 years: not recommended; ≥12 years: 20 mg q HS; may increase gradually to max 50 mg q HS
    Tab: 10, 25, 50, 75, 100, 150 mg

➤ *cyclobenzaprine* (B)(G) <15 years: not recommended; ≥15 years: 10 mg tid; usual range 20-40 mg/day in divided doses; max 60 mg/day x 2-3 weeks or 15 mg ext-rel once daily; max 30 mg ext-rel/day x 2-3 weeks
    Amrix *Cap:* 15, 30 mg ext-rel
    Fexmid *Tab:* 7.5 mg
    Flexeril *Tab:* 5, 10 mg

➤ *eszopiclone* (pyrrolopyrazine) (C)(IV)(G) <18 years: not recommended; ≥18 years: 1-3 mg; max 3 mg/day x 1 month; do not take if unable to sleep for at least 8 hours before required to be active again; delayed effect if taken with a meal
    Lunesta *Tab:* 1, 2, 3 mg

➤ *flurazepam* (X)(IV)(G) <18 years: not recommended; ≥18 years: 15 mg q HS; may increase to 30 mg q HS
    Dalmane *Cap:* 15, 30 mg

➤ *trazodone* (C)(G) <18 years: not recommended; ≥18 years: 50 mg q HS
    Desyrel *Tab:* 50, 100, 150, 300 mg

➤ *triazolam* (X)(IV)(G) <18 years: not recommended; ≥18 years: 0.125 mg q HS, may increase gradually to 0.5 mg
    Halcion *Tab:* 0.125, 0.25*mg

➤ *zaleplon* (imidazopyridine) **(C)(IV)** <12 years: not recommended; ≥12 years: 5-10 mg at HS or after going to bed if unable to sleep; do not take if unable to sleep for at least 4 hours before required to be active again; max 20 mg/day x 1 month; delayed effect if taken with a meal

    Sonata *Cap:* 5, 10 mg (tartrazine)

    Comment: **Sonata** is indicated for the treatment of insomnia when a middle-of-the-night awakening is followed by difficulty returning to sleep.

➤ *zolpidem* oral solution spray (imidazopyridine hypnotic) **(C)(IV)** <12 years: not recommended; ≥12 years: 2 actuations (10 mg) immediately before bedtime; *Debilitated,* or *hepatic impairment:* 2 actuations (5 mg); max 2 actuations (10 mg)

    ZolpiMist *Oral soln spray:* 5 mg/actuation (60 metered actuations) (cherry)

Comment: The lowest dose of *zolpidem* in all forms is recommended for females as drug elimination is slower than in men.

➤ *zolpidem* tabs (pyrazolopyrimidine hypnotic) **(B)(IV)(G)** <18 years: not recommended; ≥18 years: 5-10 mg or 6.25-12.5 ext-rel q HS prn; max 12.5 mg/day x 1 month; do not take if unable to sleep for at least 8 hours before required to be active again; delayed effect if taken with a meal

    Ambien *Tab:* 5, 10 mg

    Ambien CR *Tab:* 6.25, 12.5 mg ext-rel

Comment: The lowest dose of *zolpidem* in all forms is recommended for females as drug elimination is slower than in males.

➤ *zolpidem* sublingual tabs (imidazopyridine hypnotic) **(C)(IV)** <18 years: not recommended; ≥18 years: dissolve 1 tab under the tongue; allow to disintegrate completely before swallowing; take only once per night and only if at least 4 hours of bedtime remain before planned time for awakening

    Edluar *SL Tab:* 5, 10 mg

    Intermezzo *SL Tab:* 1.75, 3.5 mg

Comment: **Intermezzo** is indicated for the treatment of insomnia when a middle-of-the-night awakening is followed by difficulty returning to sleep. The lowest dose of *zolpidem* in all forms is recommended for females as drug elimination is slower than in males.

▮ FIFTH DISEASE (ERYTHEMA INFECTIOSUM)

Antipyretics *see Fever page 136*

▮ FLATULENCE

➤ *simethicone* **(C)(G)**

    Gas-X (OTC) 2-4 tabs pc and HS prn

        Tab: 40, 80, 125 mg; *Cap:* 125 mg

    Mylicon (OTC) 2-4 tabs pc and HS prn

        Tab: 40, 80, 125 mg; *Cap:* 125 mg

    Phazyme-95 1-2 tabs with each meal and HS prn

        Tab: 95 mg

    Phazyme Infant Oral Drops <2 years: 0.3 ml qid pc and HS prn; 2-12 years: 0.6 ml qid pc and HS prn; >12 years: 1.2 ml qid pc and HS prn; *Oral drops:* 40 mg/0.6 ml (15, 30 ml w. calibrated dropper) (orange)(alcohol-free)

Maximum Strength Phazyme 1-2 caps with each meal and HS prn
Cap: 125 mg

FLUORIDATION, WATER, <0.6 PPM

▷ *fluoride* (NE)(G)
   Luride *Water fluoridation 0.3-0.6 ppm:* <3 years: use drops; 6 months-3 years: 0.125 mg daily; 4-6 years: 0.25 mg daily; 7-16 years: 0.5 mg daily; *Water fluoridation <0.3 ppm:* <3 years: use drops; 6 months-3 years: 0.25 mg daily; 3-6 years: 0.5 mg daily; >6-16 years: 1 mg daily
      Chew tab: 0.25, 0.5, 1 mg (sugar-free)
   Luride Drops *Water fluoridation 0.3-0.6 ppm:* 6 months-3 years: 0.25 ml once daily; 4-6 years: 0.5 ml once daily; 7-16 years: 1 ml once daily; *Water fluoridation <0.3 ppm:* 6 months-3 years: 0.5 ml once daily; 4-6 years: 1 ml once daily; 7-16 years: 2 ml daily
      Oral drops: 0.5 mg/ml (50 ml) (sugar-free)

COMBINATION AGENTS

▷ *fluoride/vitamin a/vitamin d/vitamin c* (NE)(G) *Water fluoridation 0.3-0.6 ppm:* <3 years: not recommended; 3-6 years: 0.25 mg fluoride/day; 7-16 years: 0.5 mg fluoride/day; *Water fluoridation <0.3 ppm:* <6 months: not recommended; 6 months-3 years: 0.25 mg fluoride/day; 4-6 years: 0.5 mg fluoride/day; 7-16 years: 1 mg fluoride/day
   Tri-Vi-Flor Drops
      Oral drops: fluoride 0.25 mg/*vit a* 1500 u/*vit d* 400 u/*vit c* 35 mg per ml (50 ml)
      Oral drops: fluoride 0.5 mg/*vit a* 1500 u/*vit d* 400 u/*vit c* 35 mg per ml (50 ml)
▷ *fluoride/vitamin a/vitamin d/vitamin c/iron* (NE) *Water fluoridation 0.3-0.6 ppm:* <3 years: not recommended; 3-6 years: 0.25 mg fluoride/day; 7-16 years: 0.5 mg fluoride/day; *Water fluoridation <0.3 ppm:* <6 months: not recommended; 6 months-3 years: 0.25 mg fluoride/day; 4-6 years: 0.5 mg fluoride/day; 7-16 years: 1 mg fluoride/day
   Tri-Vi-Flor w. Iron Drops
      Oral drops: fluoride 0.25 mg/*vit a* 1500 u/*vit d* 400 u/*vit c* 35 mg/*iron* 10 mg per ml (50 ml)

FOLLICULITIS BARBAE

TOPICAL AGENTS

▷ *benzoyl peroxide* (B) apply after shaving; may discolor clothing and linens.
   Benzac-W initially apply to affected area once daily; increase to bid-tid as tolerated
      Gel: 2.5, 5, 10% (60 gm)
   Benzac-W Wash wash affected area bid
      Wash: 5% (4, 8 oz); 10% (8 oz)
   Benzagel apply to affected area one or more times/day
      Gel: 5, 10% (1.5, 3 oz) (alcohol 14%)
   Benzagel Wash wash affected area bid
      Gel: 10% (6 oz)

Desquam X₅ wash affected area bid
   Wash: 5% (5 oz)
Desquam X₁₀ wash affected area bid
   Wash: 10% (5 oz)
Triaz apply to affected area daily bid
   Lotn: 3, 6, 9% (bottle), 3% (tube); *Pads:* 3, 6, 9% (jar)
ZoDerm apply once <u>or</u> twice daily
   Gel: 4.5, 6.5, 8.5% (125 ml); *Crm:* 4.5, 6.5, 8.5% (125 ml); *Clnsr:* 4.5, 6.5, 8.5% (400 ml)
➤ *clindamycin* topical **(B)** apply bid
   Cleocin T *Pad:* 1% (60/pck; alcohol 50%); *Lotn:* 1% (60 ml); *Gel:* 1% (30, 60 gm);*Soln w. applicator:* 1% (30, 60 ml) (alcohol 50%)
   Clindagel *Gel:* 1% (42, 77 gm)
   Clindets *Pad:* 1% (60/pck)
   Evoclin *Foam:* 1% (50, 100 gm) (alcohol)
➤ *clindamycin/benzoyl peroxide* topical **(C)** *benzoyl peroxide* may discolor clothing and linens; <12 years: not recommended; ≥12 years:
   Acanya (G) apply qd-bid
      Gel: clin 1.2%/*benz* 2.5% (50 gm)
   BenzaClin apply bid
      Gel: clin 1%/*benz* 5% (25, 50 gm)
   Duac apply daily in the evening
      Gel: clin 1%/*benz* 5% (45 gm)
   Onexton Gel apply once daily
      Gel: clin 1.2%/*benz* 3.75% (50 gm pump) (alcohol-free) (preservative-free)
➤ *dapsone* topical **(C)** <12 years: not recommended; ≥12 years: apply bid
   Aczone *Gel:* 5% (30 gm)
➤ *hydrocortisone* 1% **(C)(OTC)(G)** apply q HS; *see Topical Corticosteroids page 494*
➤ *tazarotene* **(X)(G)** <12 years: not recommended; ≥12 years: apply daily at HS
   Avage Cream *Crm:* 0.1% (30 gm)
   Tazorac Cream *Crm:* 0.05, 0.1% (15, 30, 60 gm)
   Tazorac Gel *Gel:* 0.05, 0.1% (30, 100 gm)
➤ *tretinoin* **(C)** <12 years: not recommended; ≥12 years: apply q HS
   Avita *Crm/Gel:* 0.025% (20, 45 gm)
   Renova *Crm:* 0.02% (40 gm); 0.05% (40, 60 gm)
   Retin-A Cream *Crm:* 0.025, 0.05, 0.1% (20, 45 gm)
   Retin-A Gel *Gel:* 0.01, 0.025% (15, 45 gm) (alcohol 90%)
   Retin-A Liquid *Liq:* 0.05% (28 ml) (alcohol 55%)
   Retin-A Micro *Microspheres:* 0.04, 0.1% (20, 45 gm)

FOREIGN BODY: ESOPHAGUS

➤ *glucagon* **(B)** 0.02 mg/kg IV <u>or</u> IM with serial x-rays; max 1 mg
   Glucagon (rDNA origin <u>or</u> beef/pork derived)
      Vial: 1 mg/ml w. diluent
   Comment: *glucagon* facilitates passage of foreign body from esophagus into stomach.

FOREIGN BODY: EYE

▷ *proparacaine* (NE) 1-2 drops to anesthetize surface of eye; then flush with normal saline

Ophthaine *Ophth soln:* 0.5% (15 ml)

Comment: *proparacaine* facilitates the search, location, and removal of foreign body and examination of the cornea.

GASTRITIS

Antacids *see GERD page 144*
H₂ Antagonists *see GERD page 146*

GASTROESOPHAGEAL REFLUX DISEASE (GERD)

Comment: Precipitators of gastric reflux include narcotics, benzodiazepines, calcium antagonists, alcohol, nicotine, chocolate, and peppermint.

ANTACIDS

Comment: Antacids with *aluminum hydroxide* may potentiate constipation. Antacids with *magnesium hydroxide* may potentiate diarrhea.

▷ *aluminum hydroxide* (C) <12 years: not recommended; ≥12 years:

ALTernaGEL (OTC) 5-10 ml between meals and HS prn; max 90 ml/day
Liq: 500 mg/5 ml (5, 12 oz)

Amphojel (OTC) 10 ml 5-6 times/day between meals and HS prn; max 60 ml/day
Oral susp: 320 mg/5 ml (12 oz)

Amphojel Tab (OTC) 600 mg 5-6 times/day between meals and HS prn; max 3.6 gm/day
Tab: 300, 600 mg

▷ *aluminum hydroxide/magnesium hydroxide* (C)(OTC)(G) <12 years: not recommended; ≥12 years:

Maalox 10-20 ml qid and HS prn
Oral susp: 200 mg per 5 ml (5, 12, 26 oz) (mint, lemon, cherry)

Maalox Therapeutic Concentrate 10-20 ml qid pc and HS prn
Oral susp: alum 600 mg/*mag* 300 mg per 5 ml (12 oz) (mint)

▷ *aluminum hydroxide/magnesium hydroxide/simethicone* (C)(OTC)(G) <12 years: not recommended; ≥12 years:

Maalox Plus 10-20 ml qid pc and HS prn
Tab: alum 200 mg/*mag* 200 mg/*sim* 25 mg

Extra Strength Maalox Plus 10-20 ml qid pc and HS prn
Tab: alum 350 mg/*mag* 350 mg/*sim* 30 mg
Oral susp: alum 500 mg/*mag* 450 mg/*sim* 40 mg per 5 ml (5, 12, 26 oz)

Extra Strength Maalox Plus Tab 1-3 tabs qid pc and HS prn
Tab: alum 350 mg/*mag* 350 mg/*sim* 30 mg

Mylanta 10-20 ml between meals and HS prn
Liq: alum 200 mg/*mag* 200 mg/*sim* 20 mg per 5 ml (5, 12, 24 oz)

Mylanta Double Strength 10-20 ml between meals and HS prn
Liq: alum 700 mg/*mag* 400 mg/*sim* 40 mg per 5 ml (5, 12, 24 oz)

▷ *aluminum hydroxide/magnesium carbonate* (C)(OTC)(G) <12 years: not recommended; ≥12 years:

    Maalox HRF 10-20 ml qid pc and HS prn
      Oral susp: alum 280 mg/*mag* 350 mg per 10 ml (10 oz)

▷ *aluminum hydroxide/magnesium trisilicate* (C)(G) <12 years: not recommended; ≥12 years:

    Gaviscon chew 2-4 tabs qid pc and HS prn
      Tab: alum 80 mg/*mag* 20 mg
    Gaviscon Liquid 15-30 ml qid pc and HS prn
      Liq: alum 95 mg/*mag* 359 mg per 15 ml (6, 12 oz)
    Gaviscon Extra Strength 2-4 tabs qid pc and HS prn
      Tab: alum 160 mg/*mag* 105 mg
    Gaviscon Extra Strength Liquid 10-20 ml qid prn
      Liq: alum 508 mg/*mag* 475 mg per 10 ml (12 oz)

▷ *aluminum hydroxide/magnesium hydroxide/simethicone* (C)(OTC)(G) <12 years: not recommended; ≥12 years:

    Maalox Maximum Strength 10-20 ml qid prn; max 60 ml/day
      Oral susp: alum 500 mg/*mag* 450 mg/*sim* 40 mg per 5 ml (5, 12, 26 oz) (mint, cherry)

▷ *calcium carbonate* (C)(OTC)(G)

    Children's Mylanta Tab <2 years: not recommended; 2-5 years (24-47 lb): 1 tab as needed up to tid; 6-11 years (48-95 lb): 2 tabs as needed up to tid
      Tab: 400 mg
    Children's Mylanta <2 years: not recommended; 2-5 years (24-47 lb): 1 tab as needed up to tid; 6-11 years (48-95 lb): 2 tabs as needed up to tid; >11 years: 2-4 tabs as needed
      Liq: 400 mg/5 ml (4 oz)
    Maalox Tab <12 years: not recommended; ≥12 years: chew 2-4 tabs prn; max 12 tabs/day
      Chew tab: 600 mg (wild berry, lemon, wintergreen) (phenylalanine)
    Maalox Maximum Strength Tab <12 years: not recommended; ≥12 years: 1-2 tabs prn; max 8 tabs/day
      Tab: 1 gm (wild berry, lemon, wintergreen; phenylalanine)
    Rolaids Extra Strength <12 years: not recommended; ≥12 years: 1-2 tabs dissolved in mouth or chewed q 1 hour prn; max 8 tabs/day
      Tab: 1000 mg
    Tums <12 years: not recommended; ≥12 years: 1-2 tabs dissolved in mouth or chewed q 1 hour prn; max 16 tabs/day
      Tab: 500 mg
    Tums E-X <12 years: not recommended; ≥12 years: 1-2 tabs dissolved in mouth or chewed q 1 hour prn; max 16 tabs/day
      Tab: 750 mg

▷ *calcium carbonate/magnesium hydroxide* (C) <12 years: not recommended; ≥12 years:

    Mylanta Tab 2-4 tabs between meals and HS prn
      Tab: calib 350 mg/*mag* 150 mg
    Mylanta DS Tab 2-4 tabs between meals and HS prn
      Tab: calib 700 mg/*mag* 300 mg
    Rolaids Sodium-Free 1-2 tabs dissolved in mouth or chewed q 1 hour as needed
      Tab: calib 317 mg/*mag* 64 mg

▷ *calcium carbonate/magnesium carbonate* (C)
    Mylanta Gel Caps (OTC) <12 years: not recommended; ≥12 years: 2-4 caps prn
        Gel cap: calib 550 mg/*mag* 125 mg
▷ *dihydroxyaluminum* (NE)
    Rolaids (OTC) 1-2 tabs dissolved in mouth <u>or</u> chewed q 1 hour prn; max 24
    tabs/day
        Tab: 334 mg

H2 ANTAGONISTS

▷ *cimetidine* (B)(OTC)(G) <16 years: not recommended; ≥16 years: 800 mg bid <u>or</u>
400 mg qid; max 12 weeks
    Tagamet 800 mg bid or 400 mg qid; max 12 weeks
        Tab: 200, 300, 400*, 800*mg
    Tagamet HB *Prophylaxis:* 1 tab ac; *Treatment:* 1 tab bid
        Tab: 200 mg
    Tagamet HB Oral Suspension *Prophylaxis:* 1-3 tsp ac; *Treatment:* 1 tsp bid
        Oral susp: 200 mg/20 ml (12 oz)
    Tagamet Liquid *Liq:* 300 mg/5 ml (mint-peach) (alcohol 2.8%)
▷ *famotidine* (B)(OTC)(G)0.5 mg/kg/day q HS prn <u>or</u> in 2 divided doses; max 40 mg/day
    Maximum Strength Pepcid AC 1 tab ac
        Tab: 20 mg
    Pepcid 20-40 mg bid; max 6 weeks
        Tab: 20 mg; *Tab:* 40 mg; *Oral susp:* 40 mg/5 ml (50 ml)
    Pepcid AC 1 tab ac; max 2 doses/day
        Tab/Rapid dissolving tab: 10 mg
    Pepcid Complete (OTC) 1 tab ac; max 2 doses/day
        Tab: fam 10 mg/*CaCO$_2$ 800 mg/mg hydroxide* 165 mg
    Pepcid RPD *Tab:* 20, 40 mg rapid dissolv
▷ *nizatidine* (B)(OTC)(G) <12 years: not recommended; ≥12 years: 150 mg bid <u>or</u>
300 mg once daily
    Axid *Cap:* 150, 300 mg; *Oral soln:* 15 mg/ml (480 ml) (bubble gum)
▷ *ranitidine* (B)(OTC)(G) <1 month: not recommended; 1 month-16 years: 2-4 mg/
kg/day in 2 divided doses; max 300 mg/day; *Duodenal/Gastric Ulcer:* 2-4 mg/kg/day
divided bid; max 300 mg/day; *Erosive Esophagitis:* 5-10 mg/kg/day divided bid; max
300 mg/day; 20 lb, 9 kg: 0.6 ml; 30 lb, 13.6 kg: 0.9 ml; 40 lb, 18.2 kg: 1.2 ml; 50 lb,
22.7 kg: 1.5 ml; 60 lb, 27.3 kg: 1.8 ml; 70 lb, 31.8 kg: 2.1 ml
    Zantac 150 mg bid <u>or</u> 300 mg q HS
        Tab: 150, 300 mg
    Zantac 75 1 tab ac
        Tab: 75 mg
    Zantac EFFERdose dissolve 25 mg tab in 5 ml water and dissolve 150 mg tab in
    6-8 oz water
        Efferdose: 25, 150 mg effervescent
    Zantac Syrup *Syr:* 15 mg/ml (peppermint) (alcohol 7.5%)
▷ *ranitidine bismuth citrate* (C) <12 years: not recommended; ≥12 years: 400 mg bid
    Tritec *Tab:* 400 mg

PROTON PUMP INHIBITORS

▷ *dexlansoprazole* (B)(G) <18 years: not recommended; ≥18 years: 30-60 mg daily for
up to 4 weeks

Dexilant *Cap:* 30, 60 mg ent-coat del-rel granules; may open and sprinkle on applesauce; do not crush <u>or</u> chew granules

Dexilant SoluTab *Tab:* 30 mg del-rel orally-disint

➤ *esomeprazole* (B)(OTC)(G) <1 month: not established; 1 month-<1 year, 3-5 kg: 2.5 mg; 5-7.5 kg: 5 mg; >7.5-12 kg: 10 mg; 1-11 years, <20 kg: 10 mg; ≥20 kg: 10-20 mg; 12-17 years: 20 mg; max 8 weeks; >17 years: 20-40 mg once daily; max 8 weeks; take 1 hour before food; swallow whole <u>or</u> mix granules with food <u>or</u> juice and take immediately; do not crush <u>or</u> chew granules

Nexium *Cap:* 20, 40 mg ent-coat del-rel pellets

Nexium for Oral Suspension *Oral susp:* 10, 20, 40 mg ent-coat del-rel granules/pkt; mix in 2 tbsp water and drink immediately; 30 pkt/carton

➤ *lansoprazole* (B)(OTC)(G) <1 year: not recommended; ≥1 year: 15-30 mg daily for up to 8 weeks; may repeat course; take before eating

Prevacid *Cap:* 15, 30 mg ent-coat del-rel granules; swallow whole <u>or</u> mix granules with food <u>or</u> juice and take immediately; do not crush <u>or</u> chew granules; follow with water

Prevacid for Oral Suspension *Oral susp:* 15, 30 mg ent-coat del-rel granules/pkt; mix in 2 tbsp water and drink immediately; 30 pkt/carton (strawberry)

Prevacid SoluTab *ODT:* 15, 30 mg (strawberry) (phenylalanine)

Prevacid 24HR 15 mg ent-coat del-rel granules; swallow whole <u>or</u> mix granules with food <u>or</u> juice and take immediately; do not crush <u>or</u> chew granules; follow with water

➤ *omeprazole* (C)(OTC)(G) <1 year: not recommended; 5-<10 kg: 5 mg daily; 10-<20 kg: 10 mg daily; ≥20 kg: 20-40 mg daily for 14 days; may repeat course in 4 months; take before eating; swallow whole or mix granules with applesauce and take immediately; do not crush or chew granules; follow with water

Prilosec *Cap:* 10, 20, 40 mg ent-coat del-rel granules

Prilosec OTC *Tab:* 20 mg del-rel (regular, wild berry)

➤ *pantoprazole* (B)(G) <12 years: not recommended; ≥12 years: 40 mg daily

Tab: 40 mg ent-coat del-rel

Protonix for Oral Suspension

Oral susp: 40 mg ent-coat del-rel granules/pkt; mix in 1 tsp apple juice for 5 seconds <u>or</u> sprinkle on 1 tsp applesauce, and swallow immediately; do not mix in water <u>or</u> any other liquid <u>or</u> food; take approximately 30 minutes prior to a meal; 30 pkt/carton

➤ *rabeprazole* (B)(OTC)(G) <1 year: not recommended; 1-11 years, <15 kg: 5 mg once daily for up to 12 weeks; >11 years, ≥15 kg: 20 mg daily after breakfast; may open cap and sprinkle contents on a small amount of soft food <u>or</u> liquid

AcipHex *Tab:* 20 mg ent-coat del-rel

AcipHex Sprinkle *Cap:* 5, 10 mg del-rel

PROTON PUMP INHIBITORS/SODIUM BICARBONATE COMBINATION

➤ *omeprazole/na bicarbonate* (B)(G) <18 years: not recommended; ≥18 years: 20 mg daily; do not crush <u>or</u> chew; max 8 weeks

Zegerid *Cap: omep* 20 mg/*na bicarb* 1100 mg; *omep* 40 mg/*na bicarb* 1100 mg

Zegerid OTC (OTC) *Cap: omep* 20 mg/*na bicarb* 1100 mg

Zegerid for Oral Suspension *Pwdr for oral susp: omep* 20 mg/*na bicarb* 1680 mg; *omep* 40 mg/*na bicarb* 1680 mg (30 pkt/carton)

PROMOTILITY AGENT

▶ *metoclopramide* (B)(G) <18 years: not recommended; ≥18 years: 10-15 mg qid 30 minutes ac and HS prn; up to 20 mg prior to provoking situation; max 12 weeks per therapeutic course

   Metozolv ODT *ODT:* 5, 10 mg (mint)
   Reglan *Tab:* 5*, 10 mg; *Syr:* 5 mg/5 ml
   Reglan ODT *ODT:* 5, 10 mg (orange)

Comment: metoclopramide is contraindicated when stimulation of GI motility may be dangerous. Observe for tardive dyskinesia and Parkinsonism. Avoid concomitant drugs that may cause an extrapyramidal reaction (e.g., phenothiazines, *haloperidol*).

GIARDIASIS (*GIARDIA LAMBLIA*)

▶ *metronidazole* (not for use in 1st; B in 2nd, 3rd)(G) <12 years: 35-50 mg/kg/day in 3 divided doses x 10 days; ≥12 years: 250 mg tid x 5-10 days

   Flagyl *Tab:* 250*, 500*mg
   Flagyl 375 *Cap:* 375 mg
   Flagyl ER *Tab:* 750 mg ext-rel

Comment: Alcohol is contraindicated during treatment with oral *metronidazole* and for 72 hours after therapy due to a possible *disulfiram*-like reaction (nausea, vomiting, flushing, headache).

▶ *tinidazole* (not for use in 1st; B in 2nd, 3rd) <3 years: not recommended; 3-12 years: 50 mg/kg once daily x 3-5 days; take with food; max 2 gm/day; >12 years: 2 gm once daily x 3-5 days; take with food

   Tindamax *Tab:* 250*, 500*mg

▶ *nitazoxanide* (B) <1 year: not recommended; 1-3 years; 100 mg q 12 hours x 3 days; >3-11 years: 200 mg q 12 hours x 3 days; ≥11 years: 500 mg q 12 hours x 3 days; take with food

   Alinia *Tab:* 500 mg; *Oral susp:* 100 mg/5 ml (60 ml)

   Comment: **Alinia** is an antiprotozoal for the treatment of diarrhea due to *G. lamblia* <u>or</u> *C. parvum*.

GINGIVITIS/PERIODONTITIS

ANTI-INFECTIVE ORAL RINSES

Comment: Oral treatments should be preceded by brushing and flossing the teeth. Avoid foods and liquids for 2-3 hours after a treatment.

▶ *chlorhexidine gluconate* (B)(G) swish 15 ml undiluted for 30 seconds bid; do not swallow; do not rinse mouth after treatment.

   Peridex, PerioGard *Oral soln:* 0.12% (480 ml)

GLAUCOMA: OPEN ANGLE

Comment: Other ophthalmic medications should not be administered within 5-10 minutes of administering an ophthalmic antiglaucoma medication. Contact lenses should be removed prior to instillation of antiglaucoma medications and may be replaced 15 minutes later. Interactions with ophthalmic antiglaucoma agents include MAOIs, CNS depressants, beta-blockers, tricyclic antidepressants, and hypoglycemics.

OPHTHALMIC ALPHA2A-AGONISTS

Comment: Ophthalmic alpha2a-agonists are contraindicated with concomitant MAOI use. Cautious use with CNS depressants, beta-blockers (ocular and systemic), antihypertensives, cardiac glycosides, and tricyclic antidepressants.
➤ *apraclonidine* ophthalmic solution (C) <12 years: not recommended; ≥12 years: 1-2 drops affected eye tid
  Iopidine *Ophth soln:* 0.5% (5 ml) (benzalkonium chloride)
➤ *brimonidine tartrate* ophthalmic solution (B) <2 years: not recommended; ≥2 years: 1 drop affected eye q 8 hours
  Alphagan P *Ophth soln:* 0.1, 0.15% (5, 10, 15 ml) (purite)

OPHTHALMIC CARBONIC ANHYDRASE INHIBITORS

Comment: Ophthalmic carbonic anhydrase inhibitors are contraindicated in patients with sulfa allergy.
➤ *brinzolamide* ophthalmic suspension (C) <12 years: not recommended; ≥12 years: 1 drop affected eye tid
  Azopt *Ophth susp:* 1% (2.5, 5, 10, 15 ml) (benzalkonium chloride)
➤ *dorzolamide* ophthalmic solution (C)(G) <12 years: not recommended; ≥12 years: 1 drop affected eye tid
  Trusopt *Ophth soln:* 2% (10 ml) (benzalkonium chloride)

OPHTHALMIC ALPHA-2 ADRENERGIC RECEPTOR AGONIST/CARBONIC ANHYDRASE INHIBITOR

➤ *brimonidine/brinzolamide* (C) <12 years: not recommended; ≥12 years: 1 drop affected eye tid
  Simbrinza *Ophth soln:* brim 1% mg/*brinz* 0.2% per ml (10 ml)

OPHTHALMIC CHOLINERGICS (MIOTICS)

➤ *carbachol/hydroxypropyl methylcellulose* ophthalmic solution (C) <12 years: not recommended; ≥12 years: 2 drops affected eye tid
  Isopto Carbachol *Ophth soln:* carb 0.75% or 2.25%/*hydroxy* 1% (15 ml); *carb* 1.5% or 3%/*hydroxy* 1% (15, 30 ml) (benzalkonium chloride)
➤ *pilocarpine* (C)(G) <12 years: not recommended; ≥12 years:
  Isopto Carpine 2 drops affected eye tid-qid
    Ophth soln: 1, 2, 4% (15 ml) (benzalkonium chloride)
  Ocusert Pilo change ophthalmic insert once weekly
    Ophth inserts: 20 mcg/hr (8/pck)
  Pilocar Ophthalmic Solution 1-2 drops affected eye 1-6 times/day
    Ophth soln: 0.5, 1, 2, 3, 4, 6, 8% (15 ml)
  Pilopine HS apply 1/2 inch ribbon in lower conjunctival sac q HS
    Ophth gel: 4% (4 gm)

OPHTHALMIC CHOLINESTERASE INHIBITORS

➤ *demecarium bromide* ophthalmic solution (X) <12 years: not recommended; ≥12 years: 1-2 drops affected eye q 12-48 hours

      Humorsol Ocumeter *Ophth soln:* 0.125, 0.25% (5 ml)
➤ *echothiophate iodide* ophthalmic solution (C) <12 years: not recommended; ≥12 years: initially 1 drop of 0.03% affected eye bid; then increase strength as needed
      Phospholine Iodide *Ophth soln:* 0.03, 0.06, 0.125, 0.25% (5 ml)

OPHTHALMIC CARDIOSELECTIVE BETA-BLOCKERS

Comment: Ophthalmic beta-blockers are generally contraindicated in severe COPD, history of <u>or</u> current bronchial asthma, sinus bradycardia, 2nd <u>or</u> 3rd degree AV block.
➤ *betaxolol* ophthalmic solution (C)(G) <12 years: not recommended; ≥12 years: 1-2 drops affected eye bid
      Betoptic *Ophth soln:* 0.5% (5, 10, 15 ml) (benzalkonium chloride)
      Betoptic S *Ophth soln:* 0.25% (2.5, 5, 10, 15 ml) (benzalkonium chloride)

OPHTHALMIC BETA-BLOCKERS (NON-CARDIOSELECTIVE)

Comment: Ophthalmic beta-blockers are generally contraindicated in severe COPD, history of <u>or</u> current bronchial asthma, sinus bradycardia, 2nd <u>or</u> 3rd degree AV block.
➤ *carteolol* ophthalmic solution (C)(G) <12 years: not recommended; ≥12 years: 1 drop affected eye bid
      Ocupress *Ophth soln:* 1% (5, 10, 15 ml) (benzalkonium chloride)
➤ *levobunolol* ophthalmic solution (C) <12 years: not recommended; ≥12 years: 1-2 drops affected eye bid
      Betagan *Ophth soln:* 0.5% (5, 10, 15 ml) (benzalkonium chloride)
➤ *metipranolol* ophthalmic solution (C)(G) <12 years: not recommended; ≥12 years: 1 drop affected eye bid
      OptiPranolol *Ophth soln:* 0.3% (5, 10 ml) (benzalkonium chloride)
➤ *timolol* ophthalmic solution and gel (C)(G) <12 years: not recommended; ≥12 years:
      Betimol 1 drop affected eye bid
        Ophth soln: 0.25, 0.5% (5, 10, 15 ml) (benzalkonium chloride)
      Istalol 1 drop affected eye daily
        Ophth soln: 0.5% (2.5, 5 ml) (preservative-free)
      Timoptic 1 drop affected eye bid
        Ophth soln: 0.25, 0.5% (5, 10, 15 ml) (benzalkonium chloride)
      Timoptic Ocudose 1 drop bid
        Ophth soln: 0.25, 0.5% (0.2 ml/dose, 60 dose) (preservative-free)
      Timoptic-XE 1 drop affected eye bid
        Ophth gel: 0.25, 0.5% (2.5, 5 ml) (preservative-free)

OPHTHALMIC ALPHA2A-AGONIST/BETA-BLOCKER (NON-CARDIOSELECTIVE) COMBINATION

Comment: Generally contraindicated in severe COPD, history of <u>or</u> current bronchial asthma, sinus bradycardia, 2nd <u>or</u> 3rd degree AV block.
➤ *brimonidine tartrate/timolol* ophthalmic solution (C): <2 years: not recommended; ≥2 years: 1 drop affected eye bid
      Combigan *Ophth soln: brimo* 0.2%/*timo* 0.5% (5, 10, 15 ml) (benzalkonium chloride)

OPHTHALMIC PROSTAMIDE ANALOGS

▷ *bimatoprost* ophthalmic solution (C)(G) <16 years: not recommended; ≥16 years: 1 drop q affected eye HS
   Lumigan *Ophth soln:* 0.01, 0.03% (2.5, 5, 7.5 ml) (benzalkonium chloride)
▷ *latanoprost* ophthalmic solution (C) <12 years: not recommended; ≥12 years: 1 drop affected eye q HS
   Xalatan *Ophth soln:* 0.005% (2.5 ml) (benzalkonium chloride)
▷ *tafluprost* ophthalmic solution (C) <12 years: not recommended; ≥12 years: 1 drop affected eye q HS
   Zioptan *Ophth soln:* 0.0015% (0.3 ml single use, 30-60/carton) (preservative-free)
▷ *travoprost* ophthalmic solution (C)(G) <16 years: not recommended; ≥16 years: 1 drop affected eye q HS
   Travatan *Ophth soln:* 0.004% (2.5, 5 ml) (benzalkonium chloride)
   Travatan Z *Ophth soln:* 0.004% (2.5, 5 ml) (boric acid, propylene glycol, sorbitol, zinc chloride)

OPHTHALMIC SYMPATHOMIMETICS

Comment: Contraindicated in narrow-angle glaucoma. Use with caution in cardiovascular disease, hypertension, hyperthyroidism, diabetes, and asthma.
▷ *dipivefrin* ophthalmic solution (B) <12 years: not recommended; ≥12 years: 1 drop affected eye q 12 hours
   Propine *Ophth soln:* 0.1% (5, 10, 15 ml) (benzalkonium chloride)

OPHTHALMIC CARBONIC ANHYDRASE INHIBITOR/NON-CARDIOSELECTIVE OPHTHALMIC CARBONIC ANHYDRASE INHIBITOR/BETA-BLOCKER

▷ *dorzolamide/timolol* ophthalmic solution (C) <12 years: not recommended; ≥12 years: 1 drop affected eye bid
   Cosopt *Ophth soln:* dorz 2%/tim 0.5% (10 ml) (benzalkonium chloride)
   Cosopt PF *Ophth soln:* dorz 2%/tim 0.5% (10 ml) (preservative-free)

OPHTHALMIC SYNTHETIC DOCOSANOID

▷ *unoprostone isopropyl* ophthalmic solution (C) <12 years: not recommended; ≥12 years: 1 drop affected eye bid
   Rescula *Ophth soln:* 0.15% (5 ml) (benzalkonium chloride)

ORAL CARBONIC ANHYDRASE INHIBITORS

▷ *acetazolamide* (C) <12 years: not recommended; ≥12 years: 250-1000 mg/day in divided doses <u>or</u> 500 mg bid sust-rel tabs; max 1 gm/day
   Diamox *Tab:* 125*, 250*mg
   Diamox Sequels *Tab:* 500 mg sust-rel
▷ *methazolamide* (C)(G) <12 years: not recommended; ≥12 years: 50-100 mg bid-tid times daily
   Neptazane *Tab:* 25, 50 mg
Comment: Administer ophthalmic osmotic and miotic agents concomitantly.

GONORRHEA (*NEISSERIA GONORRHOEAE*)

Comment: The following treatment regimens for *N. gonorrhoeae* are published in the **2015 CDC Transmitted Diseases Treatment Guidelines**. Treatment regimens are presented by generic drug name first, followed by information about brands and dose forms. Empiric treatment requires concomitant treatment of chlamydia. Treat all sexual contacts. Patients who are HIV-positive should receive the same treatment as those who are HIV-negative. Sexual abuse must be considered a cause of gonococcal infection in preadolescent children.

RECOMMENDED REGIMENS: ≥12 YEARS; UNCOMPLICATED INFECTIONS OF THE CERVIX, URETHRA, AND RECTUM

Regimen 1

▷ *ceftriaxone* 250 mg IM in a single dose
       plus
▷ *azithromycin* 1 gm in a single dose

Regimen 2

▷ *ceftriaxone* 250 mg IM in a single dose
       plus
▷ *doxycycline* 100 mg bid x 7 days

RECOMMENDED REGIMENS: ≥12 YEARS; UNCOMPLICATED INFECTIONS OF THE PHARYNX

Regimen 1

▷ *ceftriaxone* 250 mg IM in a single dose
       plus
▷ *azithromycin* 1 gm in a single dose

Regimen 2

▷ *ceftriaxone* 250 mg IM in a single dose
       plus
▷ *doxycycline* 100 mg bid x 7 days

RECOMMENDED REGIMENS: CHILDREN ≥45 KG, ≥8 YEARS; UNCOMPLICATED INFECTIONS OF THE CERVIX, URETHRA, AND RECTUM

Regimen 1

▷ *ceftriaxone* 250 mg IM in a single dose
       plus
▷ *azithromycin* 1 gm in a single dose

RECOMMENDED REGIMEN: CHILDREN ≥45 KG

Regimen 1

▷ *ceftriaxone* 250 mg IM in a single dose

RECOMMENDED REGIMEN: CHILDREN >45 KG WHO HAVE GONOCOCCAL BACTEREMIA OR GONOCOCCAL ARTHRITIS

Regimen 1

▷ *ceftriaxone* 50 mg/kg IM or IV in a single dose daily x 7 days

RECOMMENDED REGIMENS: CHILDREN <45 KG, <8 YEARS; UNCOMPLICATED GONOCOCCAL VULVOVAGINITIS, CERVICITIS, URETHRITIS, PHARYNGITIS, OR PROCTITIS

Regimen 1

▷ *ceftriaxone* 250 mg IM in a single dose

RECOMMENDED REGIMEN: CHILDREN <45 KG, <8 YEARS WHO HAVE GONOCOCCAL BACTEREMIA OR ARTHRITIS

Regimen 1

▷ *ceftriaxone* 50 mg/kg (max dose 1 gm) IM or IV in a single dose daily x 7 days

DRUG BRANDS AND DOSE FORMS

▷ *azithromycin* (B)
    Zithromax *Tab:* 250, 500, 600 mg; *Oral susp:* 100 mg/5 ml (15 ml); 200 mg/5 ml (15, 22.5, 30 ml) (cherry); *Pkt:* 1 gm for reconstitution (cherry-banana)
    Zithromax Tri-pak *Tab:* 3 x 500 mg tabs/pck
    Zithromax Z-pak *Tab:* 6 x 250 mg tabs/pck
    Zmax *Oral susp:* 2 gm ext-rel for reconstitution (cherry-banana) (148 mg Na$^+$)
▷ *ceftriaxone* (B)(G)
    Rocephin *Vial:* 250, 500 mg; 1, 2 g
▷ *doxycycline* (D)(G) <8 years: not recommended
    Acticlate *Tab:* 75, 150** mg
    Adoxa *Tab:* 50, 75, 100, 150 mg ent-coat
    Doryx *Tab:* 50, 75, 100, 150, 200 mg del-rel
    Monodox *Cap:* 50, 75, 100 mg
    Oracea *Cap:* 40 mg del-rel
    Vibramycin *Tab:* 100 mg; *Cap:* 50, 100 mg; *Syr:* 50 mg/5 ml (raspberry-apple) (sulfites); *Oral susp:* 25 mg/5 ml (raspberry)
    Vibra-Tab *Tab:* 100 mg film-coat

ALTERNATIVE THERAPY

▷ *azithromycin* (B) <12 years: not recommended; ≥12 years: 2 gm x 1 dose
    Zithromax *Tab:* 250, 500, 600 mg; *Oral susp:* 100 mg/5 ml (15 ml); 200 mg/5 ml (15, 22.5, 30 ml) (cherry); *Pkt:* 1 gm for reconstitution (cherry-banana)
    Zithromax Tri-pak *Tab:* 3 x 500 mg tabs/pck
    Zithromax Z-pak *Tab:* 6 x 250 mg tabs/pck
    Zmax *Oral susp:* 2 gm ext-rel for reconstitution (cherry-banana) (148 mg Na$^+$)
▷ *cefotaxime* 500 mg IM x 1 dose
    Claforan *Vial:* 500 mg; 1, 2 g
▷ *cefotetan* <12 years: not recommended; ≥12 years: 1 gm IM x 1 dose

Cefotan *Vial:* 1, 2 g
➤ *cefoxitin* (B) <3 months: not recommended; ≥3 months: 2 gm IM x 1 dose
Mefoxin *Vial:* 1, 2 g
plus
➤ *probenecid* (B)(G)
Benemid <2 years: not recommended; 2-14 years: 25 mg/kg 30 minutes before
cefoxitin; >14 years: 1 gm 30 minutes before *cefoxitin*
Tab: 500*mg; *Cap:* 500 mg
➤ *cefpodoxime proxetil* (B) <2 years: not recommended; 2 months-12 years: 10 mg/
kg/day (max 400 mg/dose) or 5 mg/kg/day bid (max 200 mg/dose); ≥12 years: 200
mg x 1 dose
➤ *ceftizoxime* (B) <6 months: not recommended; ≥6 months: 1 gm IM x 1 dose
Cefizox *Vial:* 500 mg; 1, 2, 10 g
➤ *cefuroxime axetil* (B)(G) <12 years: 30 mg/kg/day x 1 dose; ≥12 years: 1000 mg x 1
dose
Ceftin *Tab:* 250, 500 mg; *Oral susp:* 125, 250 mg/5 ml (50, 100 ml) (tutti-frutti)
➤ *demeclocycline* (X) <8 years: not recommended; ≥8 years: initially 600 mg, followed
by 300 mg q 12 hours x 4 days (total 3 gm)
Declomycin *Tab:* 300 mg
Comment: *demeclocycline* is contraindicated <8 years-of-age, in pregnancy,
and lactation (discolors developing tooth enamel). A side effect may be photo-
sensitivity (photophobia). Do not give with antacids, calcium supplements, or other
dairy, or within two hours of taking another drug.
➤ *enoxacin* (C) <18 years: not recommended; ≥18 years: 400 mg x 1 dose
Penetrex *Tab:* 200, 400 mg
➤ *imipramine* (C) <18 years: not recommended; ≥18 years: 400 mg x 1 dose
Maxaquin *Tab:* 400 mg
➤ *norfloxacin* (C) <18 years: not recommended; ≥18 years: 800 mg x 1 dose
Noroxin *Tab:* 400 mg
➤ *spectinomycin* (B) <12 years: 40 mg/kg IM x 1 dose; ≥12 years: 2 gm IM x 1 dose
Trobicin *Vial:* 2 g

GOUT

Pseudogout *see Pseudogout page* 352
Acetaminophen for IV Infusion *see page* 296
Oral Prescription NSAIDs *see page* 490
Other Oral Analgesics *see page* 298
Topical/Transdermal NSAIDs *see page* 298
Parenteral Corticosteroids *see page* 499
Oral Corticosteroids *see page* 498

PEGYLATED URIC ACID SPECIFIC ENZYME

➤ *pegloticase* (C) <18 years: not recommended; ≥18 years: premedicate with antihistamine and corticosteroid; 8 mg once every 2 weeks; after dilution, administer IV
infusion over at least 2 hours; observe at least 1 hour post-infusion
Krystexxa *Vial:* 8 mg/ml (1 ml) single-use pwdr for IV infusion after dilution

Comment: Slow rate, or stop and restart at lower rate, if infusion reaction occurs (e.g., **Krystexxa** is contraindicated with G6PD deficiency; screen patients of African or Mediterranean descent). **Krystexxa** is not for the treatment of asymptomatic hyperuricemia.

PROPHYLAXIS

▷ *allopurinol* (C)(G) <12 years: not recommended; ≥12 years: initially 100 mg daily; increase by 100 mg weekly; max 800 mg/day and 300 mg/dose; usual range for mild symptoms 200-300 mg/day; for severe symptoms 400-600 mg/day; take with food

    Zyloprim *Tab:* 100*, 300*mg

Comment: Do not take concurrent with *colchicine*.

▷ *colchicine* (C)(G) <12 years: not recommended; ≥12 years: 0.6-1.2 mg at first sign of attack; then 0.6 mg every hour or 1.2 mg every 2 hours until pain relief; then consider 0.6 mg/day or every other day for maintenance

    Colcrys *Tab:* 0.6 mg
    Mitigare *Cap:* 0.6 mg

Comment: Do not take concurrently with *allopurinol*.

▷ *febuxostat* (C) <18 years: not recommended; ≥18 years: initially 40 mg daily; after 2 weeks, may increase to 80 mg daily.

    Uloric *Tab:* 40, 80 mg

Comment: Gout flare prophylaxis with *colchicine* or NSAID is recommended on initiation of *febuxostat* and up to 6 months.

URICOSURIC AGENT

▷ *probenecid* (C)(G) <12 years: not recommended; ≥12 years: 250 mg bid x 1 week; maintenance 500 mg bid

    Tab: 500*mg; *Cap:* 500 mg

Comment: Avoid concomitant use of *probenecid* and salicylates.

URICOSURIC/ANTI-INFLAMMATORY COMBINATIONS

▷ *probenecid/colchicine* (NE)(G) <12 years: not recommended; ≥12 years: 1 tab once daily x 1 week; then, 1 tab bid thereafter

    Tab: prob 500 mg/*colch* 0.5 mg

Comment: *probenecid/colchicine* is contraindicated in the treatment of acute gout attack, patients with blood dyscrasias, and patients with uric acid kidney stones. Concomitant salicylates antagonize the uricosuric effects.

▷ *sulfinpyrazone* (C) <12 years: not recommended; ≥12 years: initially 200-400 mg bid; may gradually increase to 800 mg bid

    Anturane *Cap:* 100, 200 mg

Comment: Goal is serum uric acid <6.5 mg/dL.

XANTHINE OXIDASE INHIBITOR

▷ *febuxostat* (C) <18 years: not established; ≥18 years: 40 mg once daily x 2 weeks; if serum uric acid is not <6 mg/dL, may increase to 80 mg once daily

    Uloric *Tab:* 40, 80 mg

SELECTIVE URIC ACID REABSORPTION INHIBITOR (SURI)

▶ *lesinurad* (C) <18 years: not established; ≥18 years: 200 mg once daily in combination with a xanthine oxidase inhibitor (XOI)

Zurampic *Tab:* 200 mg

Comment: **Zurampic** inhibits URATI, a urate transporter, which is responsible for the majority of renal absorption of uric acid and (OAT)4, organic anion transporter, a uric acid transporter involved in diuretic-induced hyperuricemia. Do not use as monotherapy. Use in combination with an XOI, such as *allopurinol* or *febuxostat*, (to reduce the production of uric acid). Do not initiate if *CrCl <45 mL/min*, ESRD, dialysis, or kidney transplant.

GOUTY ARTHRITIS

Acetaminophen for IV Infusion *see Pain page* 296
Oral Prescription NSAIDs *see page* 490
Other Oral Analgesics *see Pain page* 298
Topical/Transdermal NSAIDs *see Pain page* 298
Parenteral Corticosteroids *see page* 499
Oral Corticosteroids *see page* 498
Topical Analgesic and Anesthetic Agents *see page* 488

TOPICAL ANALGESICS

▶ *capsaicin* cream (B)(G) <2 years: not recommended; 2-12 years: apply sparingly to intact skin bid prn; >12 years: apply tid-qid prn

Axsain *Crm:* 0.075% (1, 2 oz)
Capsin (OTC) *Lotn:* 0.025, 0,075% (59 ml)
Capzasin-P (OTC) *Crm:* 0.025% (1.5 oz); *Lotn:* 0.025% (2 oz)
Capzasin-HP (OTC) *Crm:* 0.075% (1.5 oz); *Lotn:* 0.075% (2 oz)
Dolorac *Crm:* 0.025% (28 gm)
Double Cap (OTC) *Crm:* 0.05% (2 oz)
R-Gel *Gel:* 0.025% (15, 30 gm)
Zostrix (OTC) *Crm:* 0.025% (0.7, 1.5, 3 oz)
Zostrix HP (OTC) *Emol crm:* 0.075% (1, 2 oz)

Comment: Provides some relief by 1-2 weeks; optimal benefit may take 4-6 weeks. Avoid contact with mucous membranes.
capsaicin provides some relief by 1-2 weeks; optimal benefit may take 4-6 weeks.

ORAL SALICYLATE

▶ *indomethacin* (C) <14 years: usually not recommended; ≥2 years, if risk warranted: 1-2 mg/kg/day in divided doses; max 3-4 mg/kg/day (or 150-200 mg/day, whichever is less); <14 years: ER cap not recommended; >14 years: initially 25 mg bid-tid; increase as needed at weekly intervals by 25-50 mg/day; max 200 mg/day

Cap: 25, 50 mg; *Susp:* 25 mg/5 ml (pineapple-coconut, mint) (alcohol 1%); *Supp:* 50 mg; *ER Cap:* 75 mg ext-rel

Comment: *indomethacin* is indicated only for acute painful flares. Administer with food and/or antacids. Use lowest effective dose for shortest duration.

NSAID PLUS PPI

▷ *esomeprazole/naproxen* (C; not for use in 3rd)(G) <18 years: not recommended; ≥18 years: 1 tab bid; use lowest effective dose for the shortest duration; swallow whole; take at least 30 minutes before a meal

Vimovo *Tab:* nap 375 mg/eso 20 mg ext-rel; nap 500 mg/eso 20 mg ext-rel

Comment: **Vimovo** is indicated to improve signs/symptoms, and risk of gastric ulcer in patients at risk of developing NSAID-associated gastric ulcer.

COX-2 INHIBITORS

Comment: Cox-2 inhibitors are contraindicated with history of asthma, urticaria, and allergic-type reactions to *aspirin*, other NSAIDs, and sulfonamides, 3rd trimester of pregnancy, and coronary artery bypass graft (CABG) surgery.

▷ *celecoxib* (C)(G) <18 years: not recommended; ≥18 years: 100-400 mg bid; max 800 mg/day

Celebrex *Cap:* 50, 100, 200, 400 mg

▷ *meloxicam* (C)(G)

Mobic <2 years, <60 kg: not recommended; ≥2, >60 kg: 0.125 mg/kg; max 7.5 mg once daily; ≥18 years: initially 7.5 mg once daily; max 15 mg once daily; *Hemodialysis:* max 7.5 mg/day

Tab: 7.5, 15 mg; *Oral susp:* 7.5 mg/5 ml (100 ml) (raspberry)

Vivlodex <18 years: not established; ≥18 years: initially 5 mg qd; may increase to max 10 mg/day; *Hemodialysis:* max 5 mg/day

Cap: 5, 10 mg

GRANULOMA INGUINALE (DONOVANOSIS)

Comment: The following treatment regimens are published in the **2015 CDC Sexually Transmitted Diseases Treatment Guidelines**. Treatment regimens are for patients ≥18 years only; consult a specialist for treatment of patients less than 18 years-of-age. Treatment regimens are presented by generic drug name first, followed by information about brands and dose forms. Persons who have sexual contact with a patient who has had granuloma inguinale within the past 60 days before onset of the patient's symptoms should be examined and offered therapy. Patients who are HIV-positive should receive the same treatment as those who are HIV-negative; however, the addition of a parenteral aminoglycoside (e.g., *gentamicin*) can also be considered.

RECOMMENDED REGIMEN

▷ *doxycycline* 100 mg bid x at least 3 weeks and until all lesions have completely healed

ALTERNATE REGIMENS

▷ *azithromycin* (B)(G) 1 gm once weekly for at least 3 weeks and until all lesions have completely healed

▷ *ciprofloxacin* (C) 750 mg bid x at least 3 weeks and until all lesions have completely healed; max 1.5 gm/day

▷ *erythromycin base* 500 mg qid x 14 days or *erythromycin ethylsuccinate* 400 mg qid x 14 days
▷ *trimethoprim/sulfamethoxazole* 1 double-strength (160/800) dose bid x at least 3 weeks and until all lesions have completely healed

DRUG BRANDS AND DOSE FORMS

▷ *azithromycin* (B)(G)
   Zithromax *Tab:* 250, 500, 600 mg; *Oral susp:* 100 mg/5 ml (15 ml); 200 mg/5 ml (15, 22.5, 30 ml) (cherry); *Pkt:* 1 gm for reconstitution (cherry-banana)
   Zithromax Tri-pak *Tab:* 3 x 500 mg tabs/pck
   Zithromax Z-pak *Tab:* 6 x 250 mg tabs/pck
   Zmax *Oral susp:* 2 gm ext-rel for reconstitution (cherry-banana) (148 mg Na$^+$)
▷ *ciprofloxacin* (C)
   Cipro (G) *Tab:* 250, 500, 750 mg; *Oral susp:* 250, 500 mg/5 ml (100 ml) (strawberry)
   Cipro XR *Tab:* 500, 1000 mg ext-rel
   ProQuin XR *Tab:* 500 mg ext-rel
   Comment: *ciprofloxacin* is contraindicated <18 years-of-age, and during pregnancy, and lactation. Risk of tendonitis or tendon rupture.
▷ *doxycycline* (D)(G) <8 years: not recommended; ≥8 years, <100 lb: 2 mg/lb on first day in 2 divided doses, followed by 1 mg/lb/day in 1-2 divided doses; ≥8 years, ≥100 lb: 40-100 mg bid; *see page 561 for dose by weight table*
   Acticlate *Tab:* 75, 150** mg
   Adoxa *Tab:* 50, 75, 100, 150 mg ent-coat
   Doryx *Tab:* 50, 75, 100, 150, 200 mg del-rel
   Monodox *Cap:* 50, 75, 100 mg
   Oracea *Cap:* 40 mg del-rel
   Vibramycin *Tab:* 100 mg; *Cap:* 50, 100 mg; *Syr:* 50 mg/5 ml (raspberry-apple) (sulfites); *Oral susp:* 25 mg/5 ml (raspberry)
   Vibra-Tab *Tab:* 100 mg film-coat
   Comment: *doxycycline* is contraindicated <8 years-of-age, in pregnancy, and lactation (discolors developing tooth enamel). A side effect may be photo-sensitivity (photophobia). Do not give with antacids, calcium supplements, milk or other dairy, or within 2 hours of taking another drug.
▷ *erythromycin base* (B)(G)
   Ery-Tab *Tab:* 250, 333, 500 mg ent-coat
   PCE *Tab:* 333, 500 mg
▷ *erythromycin ethylsuccinate* (B)(G)
   EryPed *Oral susp:* 200 mg/5 ml (100, 200 ml) (fruit); 400 mg/5 ml (60, 100, 200 ml) (banana); *Oral drops:* 200, 400 mg/5 ml (50 ml) (fruit); *Chew tab:* 200 mg wafer (fruit)
   E.E.S. *Oral susp:* 200, 400 mg/5 ml (100 ml) (fruit)
   E.E.S. Granules *Oral susp:* 200 mg/5 ml (100, 200 ml) (cherry)
   E.E.S. 400 Tablets *Tab:* 400 mg
▷ *trimethoprim/sulfamethoxazole* (C)(G)
   Bactrim, Septra <12 years: not recommended; ≥12 years: 2 tabs bid x 10 days
      Tab: trim 80 mg/sulfa 400 mg*
   Bactrim DS, Septra DS <12 years: not recommended; ≥12 years: 1 tab bid x 10 days

Tab: trim 160 mg/*sulfa* 800 mg*

Bactrim Pediatric Suspension, Septra Pediatric Suspension <2 months: not recommended; ≥2 months-12 years: 40 mg/kg/day of ***sulfamethoxazole*** in 2 doses bid; >12 years: use tabs

Oral susp: trim 40 mg/*sulfa* 200 mg per 5 ml (100 ml) (cherry) (alcohol 0.3%)

GROWTH FAILURE

Comment: Administer growth hormones by SC injection into thigh, buttocks, or abdomen. Rotate sites with each dose. Contraindicated in children with fused epiphyses or evidence of neoplasia.

▷ ***mecasermin*** (recombinant human insulin-like growth factor-1 [rhIGF-1])

Increlex (B) see mfr pkg insert

Vial: 10 mg/ml (benzyl alcohol)

Comment: Increlex is indicated for growth failure in children with severe primary IGF-1 deficiency (primary IGFD) or in those with growth hormone (GH) gene deletion who have developed neutralizing antibodies to GH.

▷ ***somatropin*** (rDNA origin)

Genotropin (B) <12 years: usually 0.16-0.024 mg/kg/week divided into 6-7 doses; ≥12 years: initially not more than 0.04 mg/kg/week divided into 6-7 doses; may increase at 4-8 week intervals; max 0.08 mg/kg/week divided into 6-7 doses

Intra-Mix Device: 1.5 mg (1.3 mg/ml after reconstitution), 5.8 mg (5 mg/ml after reconstitution) (two-chamber cartridge w. diluent); *Pen or Intra-Mix Device:* 5.8 mg (5 mg/ml after reconstitution), 13.8 mg (512 mg/ml after reconstitution) (two-chamber cartridge w. diluent)

Genotropin Miniquick (B) <12 years: usually 0.16-0.024 mg/kg/week divided into 6-7 doses; ≥12 years: initially not more than 0.04 mg/kg/week divided into 6-7 doses; may increase at 4-8-week intervals; max 0.08 mg/kg/week divided into 6-7 doses

MiniQuick: 0.2, 0.4, 0.6, 0.8, 1, 1.2, 1.4, 1.6, 1.8, 2 mg/0.25 ml (pwdr for SC injection after reconstitution) (two-chamber cartridge w. diluent)

Humatrope (C) <12 years: initially 0.18 mg/kg/week IM or SC divided into equal doses give neither on 3 alternate days or 6 x/week; max 0.3 mg/kg/week

Vial: 5 mg w. 5 ml diluent

Norditropin (C) <12 years: 0.024-0.034 mg/kg 6-7 x/week SC

Vial: 4 mg (12 IU), 8 mg (24 IU); *Cartridge for inj:* 5, 10, 15 mg/1.5 ml; *Flex-Pro prefilled pen:* 5, 10, 15 mg/1.5 ml; *NordiFlex prefilled pen:* 5, 10, 15 mg/1.5 ml; 30 mg/3 ml

Nutropin (C) <12 years: 0.7 mg/kg/week SC in divided daily doses

Vial: 5, 10 mg/vial w. diluent

Nutropin AQ (C) <12 years: *Prepubertal:* up to 0.043 mg/kg SC daily; *Pubertal:* up to 0.1 mg/kg SC daily; *Turner Syndrome:* up to 0.0375 mg/kg/week divided into equal doses 3-7 x/week; ≥12 years: initially not more than 0.006 mg/kg SC daily; may increase to max 0.025 mg/kg SC daily

Vial: 5 mg/ml (2 ml)

Nutropin Depot (C) 1.5 mg/kg SC monthly on same day each month; max 22.5 mg/inj; divide injection if >22.5 mg

Vial: 13.5, 18, 22.5 mg/vial (pwdr for injection after reconstitution; single use w. diluent and needle)

Omnitrope (B) 0.16-0.24 mg/kg/week SC divided 3-7 x/week
Vial: 5.8 mg
Omnitrope Pen 5 (B) 0.16-0.24 mg/kg/week SC divided 3-7 x/week
Cartridge for inj: 5 mg/1.5 ml
Omnitrope Pen 10 (B) 0.16-0.24 mg/kg/week SC divided 3-7 x/week
Cartridge for inj: 10 mg/1.5 ml
Saizen (B)(G) 0.18 mg/kg/week IM <u>or</u> SC divided 3-7 times/week
Vial: 5 mg (pwdr for SC injection w. diluent)
Serostim (B) 0.1 mg/kg SC once daily at HS; max 6 mg
Vial: 5, 4, 6, 8.8 mg (pwdr for SC injection w. diluent) (benzyl alcohol)

HEADACHE: MIGRAINE/CLUSTER

ERGOTAMINE AGENTS

Comment: Do not use an ergotamine-type drug within 24 hours of any triptan <u>or</u> other 5-HT agonist.

▷ *dihydroergotamine mesylate* **(X)** <12 years: not recommended; ≥12 years: **DHE 45** 1 mg SC, IM, <u>or</u> IV; may repeat at 1 hour intervals; max 3 mg/day SC <u>or</u> IM/day; max 2 mg IV/day; max 6 mg/week
Amp: 1 mg/ml (1 ml)
Migranal 1 spray in each nostril; may repeat 15 minutes later; max 6 sprays/day and 8 sprays/week
Nasal spray: 4 mg/ml; 0.5 mg/spray (caffeine)

▷ *ergotamine* **(X)(G)** <12 years: not recommended; ≥12 years: 1 tab SL at onset of attack; then q 30 minutes as needed; max 3 tabs/day and 5 tabs/week
Tab: 2 mg

▷ *ergotamine/caffeine* **(X)(G)** <12 years: not recommended; ≥12 years:
Cafergot 2 tabs at onset of attack; then 1 tab every 1/2 hour if needed; max 6 tabs/attack and 10 tabs/week
Tab: ergot 1 mg/*caf* 100 mg
Cafergot Suppository 1 suppository rectally at onset of headache; may repeat x 1 after 1 hour; max 2/attack, 5/week
Rectal supp: ergot 2 mg/*caf* 100 mg

5-HT RECEPTOR AGONISTS

Comment: Contraindications to 5-HT receptor agonists include cardiovascular disease, ischemic heart disease, cerebral vascular syndromes, peripheral vascular disease, uncontrolled hypertension, hemiplegic <u>or</u> basilar migraine. Do not use any triptan within 24 hours of ergot-type drugs <u>or</u> other 5-HT1A agonists, <u>or</u> within 2 weeks of taking an MAOI.

▷ *almotriptan* **(C)(G)** <12 years: not recommended; ≥12 years: 6.25 <u>or</u> 12.5 mg; may repeat once after 2 hours; max 2 doses/day
Axert *Tab:* 6.25 mg (6/card), 12.5 mg (12/card)
Comment: *almotriptan* is indicated for patients 12-17 years-of-age with PMHx migraine headache lasting ≥4 hours untreated.

▷ *eletriptan* **(C)** <18 years: not recommended; ≥18 years: 20 <u>or</u> 40 mg; may repeat once after 2 hours; max 80 mg/day
Relpax *Tab:* 20, 40 mg

➤ *frovatriptan* (C)(G) <18 years: not recommended; ≥18 years: 2.5 mg with fluids; may repeat once after 2 hours; max 7.5 mg/day
    Frova *Tab:* 2.5 mg
➤ *naratriptan* (C) <18 years: not recommended; ≥18 years: 1 or 2.5 mg with fluids; may repeat once after 4 hours; max 5 mg/day
    Amerge *Tab:* 1, 2.5 mg
➤ *rizatriptan* (C) <18 years: not recommended; ≥18 years: initially 5 or 10 mg; may repeat in 2 hours if needed; max 30 mg/day
    Maxalt *Tab:* 5, 10 mg
    Maxalt-MLT *ODT:* 5, 10 mg (peppermint) (phenylalanine)
➤ *sumatriptan* (C)(G) <18 years: not recommended; ≥18 years:
    Alsuma 6 mg SC to the upper arm or lateral thigh only; may repeat after 1 hour if needed; max 2 doses/day
        Prefilled syringe: 6 mg/0.5 ml (2/pck with autoinjector)
    Imitrex Injectable 4-6 mg SC; may repeat after 1 hour if needed; max 2 doses/day
        Prefilled syringe: 4, 6 mg/0.5 ml (2/pck with or without autoinjector)
    Imitrex Nasal Spray (G) 5-20 mg intranasally; may repeat once after 2 hours if needed; max 40 mg/day
        Nasal spray: 5, 20 mg/spray (single dose)
    Imitrex Tab 25-200 mg x 1 dose; may be repeated at intervals of at least 2 hours if needed; max 200 mg/day
        Tab: 25, 50, 100 mg rapid-rel
    Imitrex STATdose Pen 6 mg/0.5 mg SC; may repeat once after 2 hours if needed; max 2 doses/day
        Prefilled needle-free autoinjector delivery system: 6 mg/0.5 ml (6/pck)
    Onzetra Xsail each disposable white nosepiece contains half a dose of medication (11 mg of sumatriptan); a full dose is 22 mg; do not use more than 2 nosepieces per dose; attach the mouthpiece and one nasal piece; then press the white button on the delivery device to pierce the capsule in the nasal piece, then insert the nasal piece into one nostril and blow into the mouth piece to deliver the nasal powder in the contents of one capsule (11 mg); repeat in the opposite nostril for a total single 22 mg dose
        Cap: 11 mg nasal pwdr; *Kit:* nosepieces (2), capsules (2), reusable breath powered delivery device (1)
    Sumavel DosePro 6 mg SC to the upper arm or lateral thigh only; may repeat after 1 hour if needed; max 2 doses/day
        Prefilled needle-free delivery system: 6 mg/0.5 ml (6/pck)
    Zembrace SymTouch administer 3 mg SC at onset of headache; may repeat hourly; max 12 mg/24 hours
        Autoinjector: 3 mg/0.5 ml (prefilled single-dose disposable autoinjector)
➤ *zolmitriptan* (C)(G) <18 years: not recommended; ≥18 years: initially 2.5 mg; may repeat after 2 hours if needed; max 10 mg/day
    Zomig *Tab:* 2.5*, 5 mg
    Zomig Nasal Spray *Nasal spray:* 5 mg/spray (6 single dose/carton)
    Zomig-ZMT *ODT:* 2.5 mg (6 tabs), 5*mg (3 tabs) (orange) (phenylalanine)

5-HT IB/ID RECEPTOR AGONIST/NSAID COMBINATION

➤ *sumatriptan/naproxen* (C; D in 3rd) <18 years: not recommended; ≥18 years:
    Treximet initially 1 tab; may repeat after 2 hours; max 2 doses/day
        Tab: suma 85 mg/*naprox* 500 mg (9/blister card)

Comment: Do not use *sumatriptan* within 24 hours of ergot-type drugs or other 5-HT agonists, or within 2 weeks of taking an MAOI.

OTHER ANALGESICS

➢ *acetaminophen/aspirin/caffeine* (D)(G)

Comment: *aspirin*-containing medications are contraindicated with history of allergic-type reaction to *aspirin*, children and adolescents with *Varicella* or other viral illness, and 3rd trimester pregnancy.

Excedrin Migraine (OTC) <12 years: not recommended; ≥12 years: 2 tabs q 6 hours prn; max 8 tabs/day x 2 days

Tab: acet 250 mg/*asp* 250 mg/*caf* 65 mg

➢ *diclofenac potassium powder for oral solution* (C; D ≥30 weeks)(G) <18 years: not established; ≥18 years: empty the contents of one pkt into a cup containing 1-2 oz or 2-4 tbsp (30-60 ml) of water, mix well, and drink immediately; water only, no other liquids; take on an empty stomach; use the lowest effective dose for the shortest duration of time; safety and effectiveness of a 2nd dose has not been established

Cambia *Pwdr for oral soln:* 50 mg/pkt (3 pkts/set, conjoined with a perforated border

Comment: **Cambia** is not indicated for migraine prophylaxis. May not be bioequivalent with other *diclofenac* forms (e.g., *diclofenac sodium* ent-coat tabs, *diclofenac sodium* ext-rel tabs, *diclofenac potassium* immed-rel tabs) even of the mg strength is the same, therefore, it s not possible to convert dosing from any other diclofenac formulation to **Cambia**. **Cambia** is contraindicated in the setting of coronary artery bypass graft. Use of **Cambia** should not be considered with hepatic impairment, gastric/duodenal ulcer, starting at 30 weeks gestation (risk of premature closure of the ductus arteriosus in the fetus), concomitant NSAIDs, SSRIs, anticoagulants/antiplatelets, any risk factor for potential bleeding.

➢ *isometheptene mucate/dichloralphenazone/acetaminophen* (C)(IV)

Midrin <12 years: not recommended; ≥12 years: 2 caps initially; then 1 cap q 1 hour until relieved; max 5 caps/12 hours

Cap: iso 65 mg/*dichlor* 100 mg/*acet* 325 mg

PROPHYLAXIS

➢ *topiramate* (D)(G) <12 years: not recommended; ≥12 years: initially 25 mg daily in the PM and titrate up daily as tolerated; then 25 mg bid; then, 25 mg in the AM and 50 mg in the PM; then, 50 mg bid

Topamax *Tab:* 25, 50, 100, 200 mg

Topamax Sprinkle Caps *Cap:* 15, 25 mg

Trokendi XR *Cap:* 25, 50, 100, 200 mg ext-rel

Quedexy XR *Cap:* 25, 50, 100, 150, 200 mg ext-rel

BETA-BLOCKERS

➢ *atenolol* (D)(G) <12 years: not recommended; ≥12 years: initially 25 mg bid; max 150 mg/day in divided doses

Tenormin *Tab:* 25, 50, 100 mg

➢ *metoprolol succinate* (C)(G) <12 years: not recommended; ≥12 years: initially 12.5-25 mg in a single dose daily; increase weekly if needed; reduce if symptomatic bradycardia occurs; max 400 mg/day

> **Toprol-XL** *Tab:* 25*, 50*, 100*, 200*mg ext-rel

➤ *metoprolol tartrate* (C)(G) <12 years: not recommended; ≥12 years: initially 25-50 mg bid; increase weekly if needed; max 400 mg/day
> **Lopressor** *Tab:* 25, 37.5, 50, 75, 100 mg

➤ *nadolol* (C)(G) <12 years: not recommended; ≥12 years: initially 20 mg daily; max 240 mg/day in divided doses
> **Corgard** *Tab:* 20*, 40*, 80*, 120*, 160*mg

➤ *propranolol* (C)(G)
> **Inderal** <12 years: not recommended; ≥12 years: initially 10 mg bid; usual range 160-320 mg/day in divided doses
> > *Tab:* 10*, 20*, 40*, 60*, 80*mg
> **Inderal LA** <12 years: not recommended; ≥12 years: initially 80 mg daily in a single dose; increase q 3-7 days; usual range 120-160 mg/day; max 320 mg/day in a single dose
> > *Cap:* 60, 80, 120, 160 mg sust-rel
> **InnoPran XL** <12 years: not recommended; ≥12 years: initially 80 mg q HS; max 120 mg/day
> > *Cap:* 80, 120 mg ext-rel

➤ *timolol* (C)(G) <12 years: not recommended; ≥12 years: initially 10 mg bid; increase weekly if needed; usual maintenance 20-40 mg/day; max 60 mg/day in 2 divided doses
> **Blocadren** *Tab:* 5, 10*, 20*mg

CALCIUM ANTAGONISTS

➤ *diltiazem* (C)(G) <12 years: not recommended; ≥12 years:
> **Cardizem** initially 30 mg qid; may increase gradually every 1-2 days; max 360 mg/day in divided doses
> > *Tab:* 30, 60, 90, 120 mg
> **Cardizem CD** initially 120-180 mg once daily; adjust at 1- to 2-week intervals; max 480 mg/day
> > *Cap:* 120, 180, 240, 300, 360 mg ext-rel
> **Cardizem LA** initially 180-240 mg once daily; titrate at 2-week intervals; max 540 mg/day
> > *Tab:* 120, 180, 240, 300, 360, 420 mg ext-rel
> **Cardizem SR** initially 60-120 mg bid; adjust at 2-week intervals; max 360 mg/day
> > *Cap:* 60, 90, 120 mg sust-rel

➤ *nifedipine* (C)(G) <12 years: not recommended; ≥12 years:
> **Adalat** initially 10 mg tid; usual range 10-20 mg tid; max 180 mg/day
> > *Cap:* 10, 20 mg
> **Procardia** initially 10 mg tid; titrate over 7-14 days: max 30 mg/dose and 180 mg/day in divided doses
> > *Cap:* 10, 20 mg
> **Procardia XL** initially 30-60 mg daily; titrate over 7-14 days; max 90 mg/day in divided doses

➤ *verapamil* (C)(G) <12 years: not recommended; ≥12 years:
> **Calan** 80-120 mg tid; increase daily <u>or</u> weekly if needed
> > *Tab:* 40, 80*, 120*mg
> **Covera HS** initially 180 mg q HS; titrate in steps to 240 mg; then to 360 mg; then to 480 mg if needed

Tab: 180, 240 mg ext-rel
Isoptin initially 80-120 mg tid
    Tab: 40, 80, 120 mg
Isoptin SR initially 120-180 mg in the AM; may increase to 240 mg in the AM;
then, 180 mg q 12 hours <u>or</u> 240 mg in the AM and 120 mg in the PM; then, 240
mg q 12 hours
    Tab: 120, 180*, 240*mg sust-rel

TRICYCLIC ANTIDEPRESSANTS (TCAs)

Comment: Co-administration of SSRIs and TCAs requires extreme caution.
➤ *amitriptyline* (C)(G) <12 years: not recommended; ≥12 years: 10-20 mg q HS *Tab:*
    10, 25, 50, 75, 100, 150 mg
➤ *amoxapine* (C) <12 years: not recommended; ≥12 years: initially 50 mg bid-tid;
after 1 week may increase to 100 mg bid-tid; usual effective dose 200-300 mg/day; if
total dose exceeds 300 mg/day, give in divided doses (max 400 mg/day); may give as
a single bedtime dose (max 300 mg q HS)
    Tab: 25, 50, 100, 150 mg
➤ *clomipramine* (C)(G) <10 years: not recommended; 10-<16 years: initially 25 mg daily
in divided doses; gradually increase; max 3 mg/kg <u>or</u> 100 mg, whichever is smaller;
>16 years: initially 25 mg daily in divided doses; gradually increase to 100 mg during
first 2 weeks; max 250 mg/day; total maintenance dose may be given at HS
    Anafranil *Cap:* 25, 50, 75 mg
➤ *desipramine* (C)(G) <12 years: not recommended; ≥12 years: 100-200 mg/day in
single <u>or</u> divided doses; max 300 mg/day
    Norpramin *Tab:* 10, 25, 50, 75, 100, 150 mg
➤ *doxepin* (C)(G) <12 years: not recommended; ≥12 years: 75 mg/day; max 150 mg/
day
    Cap: 10, 25, 50, 75, 100, 150 mg; Oral conc: 10 mg/ml (4 oz w. dropper)
➤ *imipramine* (C)(G) <12 years: not recommended; ≥12 years:
    Tofranil initially 75 mg daily (max 200 mg); adolescents initially 30-40 mg daily
    (max 100 mg/day); if maintenance dose exceeds 75 mg daily, may switch to
    Tofranil PM for divided <u>or</u> bedtime dose
    Tab: 10, 25, 50 mg
    Tofranil PM initially 75 mg daily 1 hour before HS; max 200 mg
    Cap: 75, 100, 125, 150 mg
➤ *nortriptyline* (D)(G) <12 years: not recommended; ≥12 years: initially 25 mg tid-
qid; max 150 mg/day
    Pamelor *Cap:* 10, 25, 50, 75 mg; *Oral soln:* 10 mg/5 ml (16 oz)
➤ *protriptyline* (C) <12 years: not recommended; ≥12 years: initially 5 mg tid; usual
dose 15-40 mg/day in 3-4 divided doses; max 60 mg/day
    Vivactil *Tab:* 5, 10 mg
➤ *trimipramine* (C) <12 years: not recommended; ≥12 years: initially 75 mg/day in
divided doses; max 200 mg/day
    Surmontil *Cap:* 25, 50, 100 mg

SSRI ANTIDEPRESSANTS

Comment: Co-administration of SSRIs with TCAs requires extreme caution.
Concomitant use of MAOIs and SSRIs is absolutely contraindicated. Avoid other

serotonergic drugs. A potentially fatal adverse event is *serotonin syndrome*, caused by serotonin excess. Milder symptoms require HCP intervention to avert severe symptoms that can be rapidly fatal without urgent/emergent medical care. Symptoms include restlessness, agitation, confusion, hallucinations, tachycardia, hypertension, dilated pupils, muscle twitching, muscle rigidity, loss of muscle coordination, diaphoresis, diarrhea, headache, shivering, piloerection, hyperpyrexia, cardiac arrhythmias, seizures, loss of consciousness, coma, death. Abrupt withdrawal or interruption of treatment with an antidepressant medication is sometimes associated with an *antidepressant discontinuation syndrome*, which may be mediated by gradually tapering the drug over a period of two weeks or longer, depending on the dose strength and length of treatment. Common symptoms of the *serotonin discontinuation syndrome* include flu-like symptoms (nausea, vomiting, diarrhea, headaches, sweating), sleep disturbances (insomnia, nightmares, constant sleepiness), mood disturbances (dysphoria, anxiety, agitation), cognitive disturbances (mental confusion, hyperarousal), sensory and movement disturbances (imbalance, tremors, vertigo, dizziness, electric-shock-like sensations in the brain, often described by sufferers as "brain zaps").

➤ *fluoxetine* (C)(G)

> **Prozac** <8 years: not recommended; 8-17 years: initially 10-20 mg/day; start lower weight children at 10 mg/day; if starting at 10 mg daily, may increase after 1 week to 20 mg once daily; ≥17 years: initially 20 mg daily; may increase after 1 week; doses >20 mg/day may be divided into AM and noon doses; max 80 mg/day
> *Cap:* 10, 20, 40 mg; *Tab:* 30*, 60*mg; *Oral soln:* 20 mg/5 ml (4 oz) (mint)
> **Prozac Weekly** <12 years: not recommended; ≥12 years: following daily *fluoxetine* therapy at 20 mg/day for 13 weeks, may initiate **Prozac Weekly** 7 days after the last 20 mg *fluoxetine* dose; 1 90 mg cap once weekly on the same day
> *Cap:* 90 mg ent-coat del-rel pellets

OTHER AGENTS

➤ *divalproex sodium* (D) <10 years: not recommended; ≥10 years: *Delayed-release*: initially 250 mg bid; titrate weekly to usual max 500 mg bid; *Extended-release*: initially 500 mg once daily; may increase after one week to 1 gm once daily

> **Depakene** *Cap:* 250 mg del-rel; *syr:* 250 mg/5 ml (16 oz)
> **Depakote** *Tab:* 125, 250, 500 mg del-rel
> **Depakote ER** *Tab:* 250, 500 mg ext-rel
> **Depakote Sprinkle** *Cap:* 125 mg del-rel

➤ *methysergide* (C) <12 years: not recommended; ≥12 years: 4-8 mg daily in divided doses with food; max 8 mg/day; max 6 month treatment course; wean off over last 2-3 weeks of treatment course; separate treatment courses by 3-4 week drug-free intervals

> **Sansert** *Tab:* 2 mg

MAGNESIUM SUPPLEMENTS

➤ *magnesium* (B) monitor serum magnesium level

> **Slow-Mag** <12 years: not recommended; ≥12 years: 2 tabs daily
> *Tab:* 64 mg (as chloride)/110 mg (as carbonate)

➤ *magnesium oxide* (B) monitor serum magnesium level

> **Mag-Ox 400** <12 years: not recommended; ≥12 years: 1-2 tabs daily
> *Tab:* 400 mg

HEADACHE: TENSION (MUSCLE CONTRACTION HEADACHE)

Acetaminophen for IV Infusion *see Pain page* 296
Oral Prescription NSAIDs *see page* 490
Other Oral Analgesics *see Pain page* 298
Topical/Transdermal NSAIDs *see Pain page* 298
Parenteral Corticosteroids *see page* 499
Oral Corticosteroids *see page* 498
Topical Analgesic and Anesthetic Agents *see page* 488

TRICYCLIC ANTIDEPRESSANTS (TCAs)

Comment: Co-administration of SSRIs and TCAs requires extreme caution.
➤ *amitriptyline* (C)(G) <12 years: not recommended; ≥12 years: 10-20 mg q HS *Tab:* 10, 25, 50, 75, 100, 150 mg
➤ *amoxapine* (C) <12 years: not recommended; ≥12 years: initially 50 mg bid-tid; after 1 week may increase to 100 mg bid-tid; usual effective dose 200-300 mg/day; if total dose exceeds 300 mg/day, give in divided doses (max 400 mg/day); may give as a single bedtime dose (max 300 mg q HS)
    Tab: 25, 50, 100, 150 mg
➤ *clomipramine* (C)(G) <10 years: not recommended; 10-<16 years: initially 25 mg daily in divided doses; gradually increase; max 3 mg/kg or 100 mg, whichever is smaller; >16 years: initially 25 mg daily in divided doses; gradually increase to 100 mg during first 2 weeks; max 250 mg/day; total maintenance dose may be given at HS
    Anafranil *Cap:* 25, 50, 75 mg
➤ *desipramine* (C)(G) <12 years: not recommended; ≥12 years: 100-200 mg/day in single or divided doses; max 300 mg/day
    Norpramin *Tab:* 10, 25, 50, 75, 100, 150 mg
➤ *doxepin* (C)(G) <12 years: not recommended; ≥12 years: 75 mg/day; max 150 mg/day
    Cap: 10, 25, 50, 75, 100, 150 mg; Oral conc: 10 mg/ml (4 oz w. dropper)
➤ *imipramine* (C)(G) <12 years: not recommended; ≥12 years:
    Tofranil initially 75 mg daily (max 200 mg); adolescents initially 30-40 mg daily (max 100 mg/day); if maintenance dose exceeds 75 mg daily, may switch to **Tofranil PM** for divided or bedtime dose
        Tab: 10, 25, 50 mg
    Tofranil PM initially 75 mg daily 1 hour before HS; max 200 mg
        Cap: 75, 100, 125, 150 mg
➤ *nortriptyline* (D)(G) <12 years: not recommended; ≥12 years: initially 25 mg tid-qid; max 150 mg/day
    Pamelor *Cap:* 10, 25, 50, 75 mg; *Oral soln:* 10 mg/5 ml (16 oz)
➤ *protriptyline* (C) <12 years: not recommended; ≥12 years: initially 5 mg tid; usual dose 15-40 mg/day in 3-4 divided doses; max 60 mg/day
    Vivactil *Tab:* 5, 10 mg
➤ *trimipramine* (C) <12 years: not recommended; ≥12 years: initially 75 mg/day in divided doses; max 200 mg/day
    Surmontil *Cap:* 25, 50, 100 mg

ANALGESICS

▷ *butalbital/acetaminophen* (C)(G) <12 years: not recommended; ≥12 years:
    Phrenilin 1-2 tabs q 4 hours prn; max 6 tabs/day
      Tab: but 50 mg/*acet* 325 mg
    Phrenilin Forte 1 tab <u>or</u> cap q 4 hours prn; max 6 caps/day
      Cap/Tab: but 50 mg/*acet* 650 mg
▷ *butalbital/acetaminophen/caffeine* (C)(G) <12 years: not recommended; ≥12 years:
    Fioricet 1-2 tabs q 4 hours prn; max 6/day
      Tab: but 50 mg/*acet* 325 mg/*caf* 40 mg
    Zebutal 1 cap q 4 hours prn; max 5/day
      Cap: but 50 mg/*acet* 500 mg/*caf* 40 mg
▷ *butalbital/acetaminophen/codeine/caffeine* (C)(III)(G) <18 years: not recommended; ≥18 years:
    Fioricet with Codeine 1-2 tabs at onset q 4 hours prn; max 6 tabs/day
      Tab: but 50 mg/*acet* 325 mg/*cod* 30 mg/*caf* 40 mg

Comment: *Codeine* is known to be excreted in breast milk. <12 years: not recommended; 12-<18: use extreme caution; not recommended for children and adolescents with asthma or other chronic breathing problem. The FDA and the European Medicines Agency (EMA) are investigating the safety of using *codeine* containing medications to treat pain, cough and colds, in children 12-<18 years because of the potential for serious side effects, including slowed or difficult breathing.

▷ *butalbital/aspirin/caffeine* (C)(III)(G) <18 years: not recommended; ≥18 years:
    Fiorinal 1-2 tabs <u>or</u> caps q 4 hours prn; max 6 caps/tabs/day
      Tab/Cap: but 50 mg/*asp* 325 mg/*caf* 40 mg
▷ *butalbital/aspirin/codeine/caffeine* (C)(III)(G) <18 years: not recommended; ≥18 years:
    Fiorinal with Codeine 1-2 caps q 4 hours prn; max 6 caps/day
      Cap: but 50 mg/*asp* 325 mg/*cod* 30 mg/*caf* 40 mg

Comment: *Codeine* is known to be excreted in breast milk. <12 years: not recommended; 12-<18: use extreme caution; not recommended for children and adolescents with asthma or other chronic breathing problem. The FDA and the European Medicines Agency (EMA) are investigating the safety of using *codeine* containing medications to treat pain, cough and colds, in children 12-<18 years because of the potential for serious side effects, including slowed or difficult breathing.

▷ *butorphanol tartrate*(C)(IV)(G) <18 years: not recommended; ≥18 years: initially 1 spray (1 mg) in one nostril and may repeat after 60-90 minutes (*Elderly* 90-120 minutes) in opposite nostril if needed <u>or</u> 1 spray in each nostril and may repeat q 3-4 hours prn
    Butorphanol Nasal Spray *Nasal spray:* 1 mg/actuation (10 mg/ml, 2.5 ml)
    Stadol Nasal Spray *Nasal spray:* 1 mg/actuation (10 mg/ml, 2.5 ml)
▷ *tramadol* (C)(IV)(G)

Comment: *Tramadol* is known to be excreted in breast milk. The FDA and the European Medicines Agency (EMA) are investigating the safety of using *tramadol*-containing medications to treat pain in children 12-18 years because of the potential for serious side effects, including slowed or difficult breathing.

    Rybix ODT <18 years: not recommended; ≥18 years: initially 100 mg once daily; may increase by 100 mg every 5 days; max 300 mg/day; *CrCl <30 mL/min* <u>or</u> *severe hepatic impairment:* not recommended; *Cirrhosis:* max 50 mg q 12 hours

      ODT: 50 mg (mint) (phenylalanine)

Ryzolt <18 years: not recommended; ≥18 years: initially 100 mg once daily; may increase by 100 mg every 5 days; max 300 mg/day; *CrCl <30 mL/min* <u>or</u> *severe hepatic impairment:* not recommended

      Tab: 100, 200, 300 mg ext-rel

Ultram <18 years: not recommended; ≥18 years: 50-100 mg q 4-6 hours prn; max 400 mg/day; *CrCl <30 mL/min:* max 100 mg q 12 hours; *Cirrhosis:* max 50 mg q 12 hours

      Tab: 50*mg

Ultram ER <18 years: not recommended; ≥18 years: initially 100 mg once daily; may increase by 100 mg every 5 days; max 300 mg/day; *CrCl <30 mL/min:* <u>or</u> *severe hepatic impairment:* not recommended

      Tab: 100, 200, 300 mg ext-rel

➤ *tramadol/acetaminophen* (C)(IV)(G) <18 years: not recommended; ≥18 years: 2 tabs q 4-6 hours; max 8 tabs/day; 5 days; *CrCl <30 mL/min:* max 2 tabs q 12 hours; max 4 tabs/day x 5 days

      Ultracet *Tab:* tram 37.5/acet 325 mg

Comment: *Tramadol* is known to be excreted in breast milk. The FDA and the European Medicines Agency (EMA) are investigating the safety of using *tramadol*-containing medications to treat pain in children 12-18 years because of the potential for serious side effects, including slowed or difficult breathing.

MAGNESIUM SUPPLEMENTS

➤ *magnesium* (B)

      Slow-Mag 2 tabs daily

        Tab: 64 mg (as chloride)/110 mg (as carbonate)

➤ *magnesium oxide* (B)

      Mag-Ox 400 1-2 tabs daily

        Tab: 400 mg

HEART FAILURE (HF)

ACE INHIBITORS (ACEIs)

➤ *captopril* (C; D in 2nd, 3rd)(G) <12 years: not recommended; ≥12 years: initially 25 mg tid; after 1-2 weeks may increase to 50 mg tid; max 450 mg/day

      Capoten *Tab:* 12.5*, 25*, 50*, 100*mg

➤ *enalapril* (D) <12 years: not recommended; ≥12 years: initially 5 mg daily; usual dosage range 10-40 mg/day; max 40 mg/day

      Epaned Oral Solution *Oral soln:* 1 mg/ml (150 ml) (mixed berry)

      Vasotec (G) *Tab:* 2.5*, 5*, 10, 20 mg

➤ *fosinopril* (C; D in 2nd, 3rd) <6 years, <50 kg: not recommended; 6-12 years, ≥50 kg: 5-10 mg daily; ≥12 years: initially 10 mg daily, usual maintenance 20-40 mg/day in a single <u>or</u> divided doses

      Monopril *Tab:* 10*, 20, 40 mg

➤ *lisinopril* (D)

      Prinivil <12 years: not recommended; ≥12 years: initially 10 mg daily; usual range 20-40 mg/day

        Tab: 5*, 10*, 20*, 40 mg

Qbrelis Oral Solution administer as a single dose once daily; <6 years, GFR <30 mL/min: not recommended; ≥6 years, GFR >30 mL/min: initially 0.07 mg/kg, max 5 mg; adjust according to BP up to a max 0.61 mg/kg (40 mg) once daily
Oral soln: 1 mg/ml (150 ml)

Zestril <12 years: not recommended; ≥12 years: initially 10 mg daily; usual range 20-40 mg/day
Tab: 2.5, 5*, 10, 20, 30, 40 mg

▷ *quinapril* (C; D in 2nd, 3rd) <12 years: not recommended; ≥12 years: initially 5 mg bid; increase weekly to 10-20 mg bid
Accupril *Tab:* 5*, 10, 20, 40 mg

▷ *ramipril* (C; D in 2nd, 3rd) <12 years: not recommended; ≥12 years: initially 2.5 mg bid; usual maintenance 5 mg bid
Altace *Tab/Cap:* 1.25, 2.5, 5, 10 mg

▷ *trandolapril* (C; D in 2nd, 3rd) <12 years: not recommended; ≥12 years: initially 1 mg daily; titrate to dose of 4 mg daily as tolerated
Mavik *Tab:* 1*, 2, 4 mg

BETA-BLOCKERS (CARDIOSELECTIVE)

▷ *carvedilol* (C)
Coreg <18 years: not recommended; ≥18 years: initially 3.125 mg bid; may increase at 1-2 week intervals to 12.5 mg bid; usual max 50 mg bid
Tab: 3.125, 6.25, 12.5, 25 mg

Coreg CR <18 years: not recommended; ≥18 years: initially 10 mg once daily x 2 weeks; may double dose at 2 week intervals; max 80 mg once daily; may open caps and sprinkle on food
Cap: 10, 20, 40, 80 mg cont-rel

▷ *metoprolol succinate* (C)(G) <12 years: not recommended; ≥12 years: initially 12.5-25 mg in a single dose daily; increase weekly if needed; reduce if symptomatic bradycardia occurs; max 400 mg/day
Toprol-XL *Tab:* 25*, 50*, 100*, 200*mg ext-rel

▷ *metoprolol tartrate* (C)(G) <12 years: not recommended; ≥12 years: initially 25-50 mg bid; increase weekly if needed; max 400 mg/day
Lopressor *Tab:* 25, 37.5, 50, 75, 100 mg

ANGIOTENSIN II RECEPTOR BLOCKERS (ARBs)

▷ *valsartan* (C; D in 2nd, 3rd) <12 years: not recommended; ≥12 years: initially 40 mg bid; increase to 160 mg bid as tolerated or 320 mg daily after 2-4 weeks; usual range 80-320 mg/day
Diovan *Tab:* 40*, 80, 160, 320 mg

NEPRILYSIN INHIBITOR/ARB COMBINATION

▷ *sacubitril/valsartan* (D) <12 years: not established; ≥12 years: initially 49/51 bid; double dose after 2-4 weeks; maintenance 97/103 bid; *GFR <30 mL/min or moderate hepatic impairment:* initially 24/26 bid; double dose every 2-4 weeks to target maintenance 97/103 bid
Entresto
Tab: **Entresto 24/26:** *sacu* 24 mg/*val* 26 mg
Entresto 49/51: *sacu* 49 mg/*val* 51 mg
Entresto 97/103: *sacu* 97 mg/*val* 103 mg

ALDOSTERONE RECEPTOR BLOCKER

▶ *eplerenone* (B) <12 years: not recommended; ≥12 years: initially 25 mg once daily; titrate within 4 weeks to 50 mg once daily; adjust dose based on serum K+
   Inspra *Tab:* 25, 50 mg
   Comment: **Inspra** is contraindicated with concomitant potent CYP3A4 inhibitors. Risk of hyperkalemia with concomitant ACEI or ARB. Monitor serum potassium at baseline, 1 week, and 1 month. Caution with serum *Cr >2 mg/dL* (male) or >1.8 mg/dL (female) and/or *CrCl <50 mL/min*, and DM with proteinuria.

THIAZIDE DIURETICS

Comment: Monitor hydration status, blood pressure, urine output, serum K+.
▶ *chlorothiazide* (C)(G) <6 months: up to 15 mg/lb/day in 2 divided doses; ≥6 months-12 years: 10 mg/lb/day in 2 divided doses; >12 years: 0.5-1 gm/day in single or divided doses; max 2 g/day
   Diuril *Tab:* 250*, 500*mg; *Oral susp:* 250 mg/5 ml (237 ml)
▶ *hydrochlorothiazide* (B)(G)
   Esidrix <12 years: not recommended; ≥12 years: 25-100 mg once daily
   Tab: 25, 50, 100 mg
   Microzide <12 years: not recommended; ≥12 years: 12.5 mg daily; usual max 50 mg/day
   Cap: 12.5 mg
▶ *polythiazide* (C) <12 years: not recommended; ≥12 years: 2-4 mg once daily
   Renese *Tab:* 1, 2, 4 mg

POTASSIUM-SPARING DIURETICS

Comment: Monitor hydration status, blood pressure, urine output, serum K+.
▶ *amiloride* (B) <12 years: not recommended; ≥12 years: initially 5 mg once daily; may increase to 10 mg; max 20 mg
   Midamor *Tab:* 5 mg
▶ *spironolactone* (D)(G) <12 years: not established; ≥12 years: initially 50-100 mg in a single or divided doses; titrate at 2 week intervals
   Aldactone *Tab:* 25, 50*, 100*mg

LOOP DIURETICS

Comment: Monitor hydration status, blood pressure, urine output, serum K+
▶ *bumetanide* (C)(G) <18 years: not recommended; ≥18 years: 0.5-2 mg as a single dose; may repeat at 4-5 hour intervals; max 10 mg/day
   Bumex *Tab:* 0.5*, 1*, 2*mg
   Comment: *bumetanide* is contraindicated with sulfa drug allergy.
▶ *ethacrynic acid* (B)(G) ≤1 month: not recommended; >1 month-12 years: initially 25 mg/day; then adjust dose in 25 mg increments; >12 years: max 50-200 mg once daily
   Edecrin *Tab:* 25, 50 mg
▶ *ethacrynate sodium* (B)(G) <1 month: not recommended; ≥1 month-12 years: **use the smallest effective dose;** initially 25 mg; then careful stepwise increments in dosage of 25 mg to achieve effective maintenance; ≥12 years: administer smallest dose required to produce gradual weight loss (about 1-2 pounds per day); onset of diuresis usually occurs at 50-100 mg in children ≥12 years; after diuresis has been achieved, the minimally effective dose (usually 50-200 mg/day) may be

administered on a continuous or intermittent dosage schedule; dose titrations are usually in 25-50 mg increments to avoid derangement electrolyte and water excretion; the patient should be weighed under standard conditions before and during administration of *ethacrynate sodium;* the following schedule may be helpful in determining the lowest effective dose: *Day 1:* 50 mg once daily after a meal; *Day 2:* 50 mg bid after meals, if necessary; *Day 3:* 100 mg in the morning and 50-100 mg following the afternoon or evening meal, depending upon response to the morning dose; a few patients may require initial and maintenance doses as high as 200 mg bid; these higher doses, which should be achieved gradually, are most often required in patients with severe, refractory edema

Sodium Edecrin *Vial:* 50 mg single dose

Comment: **Sodium Edecrin** is more potent than more commonly used loop and thiazide diuretics. Treatment of the edema associated with congestive heart failure, cirrhosis of the liver, and renal disease, including the nephrotic syndrome, short-term management of ascites due to malignancy, idiopathic edema, and lymphedema, short-term management of hospitalized pediatric patients, other than infants, with congenital heart disease or the nephrotic syndrome. IV Sodium Edecrin is indicated when a rapid onset of diuresis is desired, e.g., in acute pulmonary edema or when gastrointestinal absorption is impaired or oral medication is not practical.

➤ *furosemide* (C)(G) <12 years: not established; ≥12 years: initially 40 mg bid
Lasix *Tab:* 20, 40*, 80 mg; *Oral soln:* 10 mg/ml (2, 4 oz w. dropper)

Comment: *furosemide* is contraindicated with sulfa drug allergy.

➤ *torsemide* (B) <12 years: not established; ≥12 years: 5 mg once daily; may increase to 10 mg daily
Demadex *Tab:* 5*, 10*, 20*, 100*mg

OTHER DIURETICS

Comment: Monitor hydration status, blood pressure, urine output, serum K+.

➤ *indapamide* (B) <12 years: not established; ≥12 years: initially 1.25 mg once daily; may titrate dosage upward every 4 weeks if needed; max 5 mg/day
Lozol *Tab:* 1.25, 2.5 mg

Comment: *indapamide* is contraindicated with sulfa drug allergy.

➤ *metolazone* (B) <12 years: not established; ≥12 years: 2.5-5 mg once daily

Comment: *metolazone* is contraindicated with sulfa drug allergy.

DIURETIC COMBINATIONS

Comment: Monitor hydration status, blood pressure, urine output, serum K+.

➤ *amiloride/hydrochlorothiazide* (B)(G) <12 years: not established; ≥12 years: initially 1 tab once daily; may increase to 2 tabs/day in a single or divided doses
Moduretic *Tab: amil* 5 mg/*hydro* 50 mg*

➤ *spironolactone/hydrochlorothiazide* (D)(G)
Aldactazide <12 years: not established; ≥12 years: 25 usual maintenance 50-100 mg in a single or divided doses
Tab: spiro 25 mg/*hydro* 25 mg
Aldactazide 50 <12 years: not established; ≥12 years: usual maintenance 50-100 mg in a single or divided doses
Tab: spiro 50 mg/*hydro* 50 mg

➤ *triamterene/hydrochlorothiazide* (C)(G)
    Dyazide <12 years: not established; ≥12 years: 1-2 caps daily
      Cap: triam 37.5 mg/*hydro* 25 mg
    Maxzide <12 years: not established; ≥12 years: 1 tab once daily
      Tab: triam 75 mg/*hydro* 50 mg*
    Maxzide-25 <12 years: not established; ≥12 years: 1-2 tabs once daily
      Tab: triam 37.5 mg/*hydro* 25 mg*

NITRATE/PERIPHERAL VASODILATOR COMBINATION

➤ *isosorbide dinitrate/hydralazine* (C) <12 years: not established; ≥12 years: initially
1 tab tid; may reduce to 1/2 tab tid if not tolerated; titrate as tolerated after 3-5 days;
max 2 tabs tid
    BiDil *Tab: isosor* 20 mg/*hydral* 37.5 mg
    Comment: BiDil is an adjunct to standard therapy in self-identified Black
    persons to improve survival, to prolong time to hospitalization for heart failure,
    and to improve patient-reported functional status.

CARDIAC GLYCOSIDES

Comment: Therapeutic serum level of is 0.8-2 mcg/ml.
➤ *digoxin* (C)(G) *Total oral pediatric digitalizing dose (in 24 hours):* <2 years: 40-50
mcg/kg; 2-10 years: 30-40 mcg/kg; >10 years: 0.75-1.5 mg; *Daily oral pediatric
maintenance dose (single dose):* <2 years: 10-12 mcg/kg; 2-10 years: 8-10 mcg/kg;
>10 years: 0.125–0.5 mg; 1-1.5 mg IM, IV, or PO in divided doses over 1-3 days as a
loading dose; usual maintenance 0.125-0.5 mg/day
    Comment: For more information on the use of *digoxin* in heart failure, see Jain, S.,
    & Vaidyanathan, B. (2009). Digoxin in management of heart failure in children:
    Should it be continued or relegated to the history books? *Annals of Pediatric
    Cardiology, 2*(2), 149–152.
    Lanoxicaps <10 years: use elixir or parenteral form
      Cap: 0.05, 0.1, 0.2 mg soln-filled (alcohol)
    Lanoxin <10 years: use elixir or parenteral form
      Tab: 0.0625, 0.125*, 0.1875, 0.25*mg; *Elix:* 0.05 mg/ml (2 oz w. dropper)
      (lime) (alcohol 10%)
    Lanoxin Injection *Amp:* 0.25 mg/ml (2 ml)
    Lanoxin Injection Pediatric *Amp:* 0.1 mg/ml (1 ml)

OTHER

➤ *ivabradine* (D) <18 years: not established; ≥18 years: initially 5 mg bid with food;
assess after 2 weeks and adjust dose to achieve a resting heart rate 50-60 bpm; thereafter, adjust dose as needed based on resting heart rate and tolerability; max 7.5 mg
bid; in patients with a history of conduction defects, or for whom bradycardia could
lead to hemodynamic compromise, initiate at 2.5 mg bid before increasing the dose
based on heart rate
    Corlanor *Tab:* 5, 7.5 mg
    Comment: **Corlanor** is indicated to reduce the risk of hospitalization for
    worsening heart failure in patients with stable, symptomatic, chronic heart
    failure with left ventricular ejection fraction (LVEF) ≤35%, who are in sinus
    rhythm with resting heart rate ≤70 bpm and either are on maximally tolerated
    doses of beta-blockers or have a contraindication to beta-blocker use. **Corlanor**

is contraindicated with acute decompensated heart failure, BP <90/50, sick sinus syndrome (SSS), sino-atrial block, and 3rd degree AV block (unless patient has a functioning demand pacemaker). **Corlanor** may cause fetal toxicity when administered to pregnant females based on embryo-fetal toxicity and cardiac teratogenic effects observed in animal studies. Therefore, females should to use effective contraception when taking this drug.

☐ HELICOBACTER PYLORI (H. PYLORI) INFECTION

ERADICATION REGIMENS

Comment: There are many H₂ receptor blocker-based and PPI-based treatment regimens suggested in the professional literature for the eradication of the *H. pylori* organism and subsequent ulcer healing. Generally, regimens range from 10-14 days for eradication and 2-6 more weeks of continued gastric acid suppression. A three- or four-antibiotic combination may increase treatment effectiveness and decrease the likelihood of resistant strain emergence. Empirical treatment is not recommended. Diagnosis should be confirmed before treatment is started. Antibiotic choices include *doxycycline*, *tetracycline*, *amoxicillin*, *amoxicillin/clavulanate*, *clarithromycin*, *clindamycin*, and *metronidazole*. Follow-up visits are recommended at 2 and 6 weeks to evaluate treatment outcomes.

➤ **Regimen 1: Helidac Therapy (D)** *bismuth subsalicylate* <12 years: not recommended; ≥12 years: 525 mg qid + *tetracycline* 500 mg qid + *metronidazole* 250 mg qid x 14 days; *Pack: bismuth subsalicylate chew tab:* 262.4 mg (112/pck); *tetracycline cap:* 500 mg(56/pck); *metronidazole Tab:* 250 mg (56/pck)

➤ **Regimen 2: PrevPac (D)(G)** <12 years: not recommended; ≥12 years: *amoxicillin* 500 mg 2 caps bid + *lansoprazole* 30 mg bid+ *clarithromycin* 500 mg bid x 14 days (one card per day); *Kit: lansoprazole cap:* 30 mg (2/card); *amoxicillin cap:* 500 mg (4/card); *clarithromycin tab:* 500 mg (2/card) (14 daily cards/carton)

➤ **Regimen 3: Pylera (D)** <12 years: not recommended; ≥12 years: take 3 caps qid after meals and at bedtime x 10 days; take with 8 oz water plus *omeprazole* 20 mg bid, with breakfast and dinner, for 10 days
Cap: bismuth subsalicylate 140 mg/*tetracycline* 125 mg/*metronidazole* 125 mg (120 caps)
Comment: *omeprazole* not included with **Pylera**.

➤ **Regimen 4: Omeclamox-Pak (C)** <12 years: not recommended; ≥12 years: *omeprazole* 20 mg bid + *amoxicillin* 1000 bid +*clarithromycin* 500 mg bid x 10 days
Kit: omeprazole cap: 20 mg (2/pck); *amoxicillin cap:* 500 mg (4/pck); *clarithromycin tab:* 500 mg (2/pck) (10 pcks/carton)

➤ **Regimen 5: (C)** <12 years: not recommended; ≥12 years: *omeprazole* 40 mg daily + *clarithromycin* 500 mg tid x 2 weeks; then continue *omeprazole* 10-40 mg daily x 6 more weeks

➤ **Regimen 6: (B)** <12 years: not recommended; ≥12 years: *lansoprazole* 30 mg tid + *amoxicillin* 1 gm tid x 10 days; then continue *lansoprazole* 15-30 mg daily x 6 more weeks

➤ **Regimen 7: (C)** <12 years: not recommended; ≥12 years: *omeprazole* 40 mg daily + *amoxicillin* 1 gm bid + *clarithromycin* 500 mg bid x 10 days; then continue *omeprazole* 10-40 mg daily x 6 more weeks

➤ **Regimen 8: (D)** <12 years: not recommended; ≥12 years: *bismuth subsalicylate* 525 mg qid + *metronidazole* 250 mg qid +*tetracycline* 500 mg qid + H₂ receptor agonist x 2 weeks; then continue H₂ receptor agonist x 6 more weeks

▷ **Regimen 9: (not for use in 1st; B in 2nd, 3rd)** <12 years: not recommended; ≥12 years: *bismuth subsalicylate* 525 mg qid + *metronidazole* 250 mg qid + *amoxicillin 500 mg qid + H₂ receptor agonist x 2 weeks; then continue H₂ receptor agonist x 6 more weeks* receptor agonist x 2 weeks; then continue H₂ receptor agonist x 6 more weeks

▷ **Regimen 10: (C)** <12 years: not recommended; ≥12 years: *ranitidine bismuth citrate* 400 mg bid + *clarithromycin* 500 mg bid x 2 weeks; then continue *ranitidine bismuth citrate* 400 mg bid x 2 more weeks

▷ **Regimen 11: (D)** <12 years: not recommended; ≥12 years: *omeprazole* 20 mg <u>or</u> *lansoprazole* 30 mg q AM + *bismuth subsalicylate* 524 mg qid + *metronidazole* 500 mg tid + *tetracycline* 500 mg qid x 2 weeks; then continue *omeprazole* 20 mg <u>or</u> *lansoprazole* 30 mg q AM for 6 more weeks

HEMORRHOIDS

▷ *dibucaine* (C)(OTC)(G) <12 years: not recommended; ≥12 years: 1 applicatorful <u>or</u> suppository bid and after each stool; max 6/day

    Nupercainal (OTC) *Rectal oint:* 1% (30, 60 gm); *Rectal supp:* 1% (12, 14/pck)

▷ *hydrocortisone* (C)(OTC)(G)

    Anusol-HC 1 <12 years: not recommended; ≥12 years: suppository rectally bid-tid <u>or</u> 2 suppositories bid x 2 weeks

        Rectal supp: 25 mg (12, 24/pck)

    Anusol-HC Cream <12 years: not recommended; ≥12 years: 2.5% apply bid-qid prn

        Rectal crm: 2.5% (30 gm)

    Anusol HC-1 <12 years: not recommended; ≥12 years: apply tid-qid prn; max 7 days

        Rectal crm: 1% (0.7 oz)

    Hydrocortisone Rectal Cream <12 years: not recommended; ≥12 years: apply tid-qid prn; max 7 days

        Rectal crm: 1, 2.5% (30 gm)

    Nupercainal <12 years: not recommended; ≥12 years: apply tid-qid prn

        Rectal crm: 1% (30 gm)

    Proctocort <12 years: not recommended; ≥12 years: 1 suppository rectally bid-tid prn <u>or</u> 2 suppositories bid x 2 weeks

        Rectal supp: 30 mg (12/pck)

    Proctocream HC 2.5% <12 years: not recommended; ≥12 years: apply rectally bid-qid prn

        Rectal crm: 2.5% (30 gm)

    Proctofoam HC 1% <12 years: not recommended; ≥12 years: apply rectally tid-qid prn

        Rectal foam: 1% (14 applications/10 gm)

▷ *hydrocortisone/pramoxine* (C) <12 years: not recommended; ≥12 years: 1 applicatorful tid-qid and after each stool; max 2 weeks

    Procort *Rectal crm:* hydro 1.85%/pramox 1.15% (30 gm)

▷ *hydrocortisone/lidocaine* (B) <12 years: not recommended; ≥12 years: apply bid-tid prn

    AnaMantle HC, LidaMantle HC *Crm/Lotn:* hydrocort 5%/lido 3% (1 oz)

▷ *petrolatum/mineral oil/shark liver oil/phenylephrine* (C)(OTC)(G)

Preparation H Ointment <12 years: not recommended; ≥12 years: apply up to qid prn
> *Rectal oint:* 1, 2 oz

➤ *petrolatum/glycerin/shark liver oil/phenylephrine* (C)(OTC)(G)
Preparation H Cream <12 years: not recommended; ≥12 years: apply up to qid prn
> *Rectal crm:* 0.9, 1.8 oz

➤ *phenylephrine/cocoa butter/shark liver oil* (C)(OTC)(G)
Preparation H Suppositories <12 years: not recommended; ≥12 years: 1 suppository <u>or</u> 1 application of rectal ointment <u>or</u> cream, up to qid
> *Rectal supp: phenyle* 0.25%/*cocoa* 85.5%/*shark* 3% (12, 24, 45/pck); *Rectal oint: phenyle* 0.25%/*petro* 1.9%/*mineral oil* 14%/*shark liv* 3% (1, 2 oz); *Rectal crm: phenyle* 0.25%/*petro* 18%/*gly* 12%/*shark liv* 3% (0.9, 1.8 oz)

➤ *witch hazel* topical solution/gel (NE)(OTC)
Tucks <12 years: not recommended; ≥12 years: apply up to 6 x/day; leave on x 5-15 minutes
> *Pad:* 12, 40, 100/pck; *Gel:* 19.8 g

➤ *lidocaine* 3% cream (B) <12 years: reduce dosage commensurate with age, body weight, and physical condition; ≥12 years: apply bid-tid prn
LidaMantle *Crm:* 3% (1 oz)

Bulk-forming Agents, Stool Softeners, and Stimulant Laxatives *see Constipation page 87*

HEPATITIS A (HAV)

Comment: Administer a 2-dose series. Schedule first immunization at least 2 weeks before expected exposure. Booster dose recommended 6-12 months later. Under 1 year-of-age administer in the vastus lateralis; over 1 year-of-age administer in deltoid.

PROPHYLAXIS (HEPATITIS A)

➤ *hepatitis A vaccine, inactivated* (C)
Havrix 1,440 El.U IM <2 years: not recommended; 2-18 years: 0.5 ml IM; repeat in 6-18 months; >18 years: repeat in 6-12 months
> *Vial:* 25 U/ml single dose (preservative-free); *Prefilled syringe:* 25 U/ml, (0.5, 1 ml single dose)

Vaqta 25 U (1 ml) IM; <2 years: not recommended; 2-18 years: 0.5 ml IM; repeat in 6-18 months; >18 years: repeat in 6 months
> *Vial:* 25 U/ml single dose (preservative-free); *Prefilled syringe:* 25 U/ml, (0.5, 1 ml single dose)

PROPHYLAXIS (HEPATITIS A AND B COMBINATION)

➤ *hepatitis A inactivated/hepatitis B surface antigen (recombinant vaccine)* (C)
Twinrix <18 years: not recommended; ≥18 years: 1 ml IM in deltoid; repeat in 1 month and 6 months
> *Vial (soln): hepatitis A* inactivated 720 IU/*hepatitis B* surface antigen (recombinant) 20 mcg/ml (1, 10 ml); *Prefilled syringe: hepatitis A* inactivated 720 IU/*hepatitis B* surface antigen (recombinant) 20 mcg/ml

HEPATITIS B (HBV)

PROPHYLAXIS (HEPATITIS B)

Comment: Administer IM; under 1 year-of-age, administer in vastus lateralis. Over 1 year-of-age, administer in the deltoid. Administer a 3-dose series; *First dose:* newborn (or now); *Second dose:* 1-2 months after first dose; *Third dose:* 6 months after first dose.

▷ *hepatitis B recombinant vaccine* (C)

> **Engerix-B Adult** infant-19 years: 10 mcg (1/2 ml) IM; repeat in 1 and 6 month; >19 years: 20 mcg (1 ml) IM; repeat in 1 and 6 months
> *Vial:* 20 mcg/ml single dose (preservative-free, thimerosal); *Prefilled syringe:* 20 mcg/ml
> **Engerix-B Pediatric/Adolescent** infant-19 years: 10 mcg IM; repeat in 1 and 6 months
> *Vial:* 10 mcg/0.5 ml single dose (preservative-free, thimerosal)
> *Prefilled syringe:* 10 mcg/0.5 ml
> **Recombivax HB Adult** >19 years: 10 mcg (1 ml) IM in deltoid; repeat in 1 and 6 months
> *Vial:* 10 mcg/ml single dose; *Vial:* 10 mcg/3 ml multidose
> **Recombivax HB Pediatric/Adolescent** birth-19 years: 5 mcg (0.5 ml) IM; repeat in 1 and 6 months; ≥19 years: use adult formulation or 10 mcg (1 ml) pediatric/adolescent formulation; <19 years: 5 mcg (0.5 ml) IM; repeat in 1 and 6 months
> *Vial:* 5 mcg/0.5 ml single dose

PROPHYLAXIS (HEPATITIS A AND B COMBINATION)

Comment: Administer IM; under 1 year-of-age, administer in vastus lateralis. Over 1 year-of-age, administer in the deltoid. Administer a 3-dose series; *First dose:* newborn (or now); *Second dose:* 1-2 months after first dose; *Third dose:* 6 months after first dose.

▷ *hepatitis A inactivated/hepatitis B surface antigen (recombinant) vaccine* (C)

> **Twinrix** 1 ml IM in deltoid; repeat in 1 and 6 months
> *Vial (soln):* hepatitis A inactivated 720 IU/*hepatitis B* surface antigen (recombinant) 20 mcg/ml (1, 10 ml); *Prefilled syringe: hepatitis A* inactivated 720 IU/*hepatitis B* surface antigen (recombinant) 20 mcg/ml

CHRONIC HBV INFECTION TREATMENT

Nucleoside Analogs (Reverse Transcriptase Inhibitors and HBV Polymerase Inhibitors)

Comment: Nucleoside analogs are indicated for chronic hepatitis infection with viral replication and either elevated ALT/AST or histologically active disease.

▷ *adefovir dipivoxil* (C)(G) <12 years: not recommended; ≥12 years: 10 mg daily; *CrCl 20-49 mL/min:* 10 mg q 48 hours; *CrCl 10-19 mL/min:* 10 mg q 72 hours
> **Hepsera** *Tab:* 10 mg

▷ *entecavir* (C)(G) take on an empty stomach; <16 years: not recommended; ≥16 years: *Nucleoside naïve:* 0.5 mg daily; *Nucleoside naïve, CrCl 30-49 mL/min:* 0.25 mg daily; *Nucleoside naïve, CrCl 10-29 mL/min:* 0.15 mg daily; *Nucleoside naïve, CrCl <10 mL/min:* 0.05 mg daily; *lamivudine-refractory:* 1 mg daily; *lamivudine-refractory, renal impairment:* see mfr pkg insert
> **Baraclude** *Tab:* 0.5, 1 mg; *Oral Soln:* 0.05 mg/ml (orange; parabens)

▷ *lamivudine* (C)(G) <2 years: not recommended; 2-17 years: 3 mg/kg (max 100 mg) once daily; >17 years: 100 mg daily; *CrCl <5 mL/min:* 35 mg for 1st dose, then 10 mg once daily; *CrCl 5-14 mL/min:* 35 mg for 1st dose, then 15 mg once daily; *CrCl 15-29 mL/min:* 100 mg for 1st dose, then 25 mg once daily; *CrCl 30-49 mL/min:* 100 mg for 1st dose, then 50 mg once daily

    Epivir-HBV *Tab:* 100 mg

    Epivir-HBV Oral Solution *Oral Soln:* 5 mg/ml (240 ml) (strawberry-banana)

▷ *telbivudine* (C) <2 years: not recommended; 2-17 years: 3 mg/kg (max 100 mg) once daily; >17 years: 600 mg daily; *CrCl <40 mL/min:* 600 mg q 72 hours; *CrCl 30-49 mL/min:* 600 mg q 48 hours

    Tyzeka *Tab:* 600 mg

▷ *tenofovir alafenamide (TAF)* (C) <18 years: not established; take with food; ≥18 years: take 1 tab once daily with concomitant carbamazepine 2 tablets

    Vemlidy *Tab:* 25 mg

    Comment: No dosage adjustment of **Vemlidy** is required in patients with mild hepatic impairment (Child-Pugh A). The safety and efficacy of **Vemlidy** in patients with decompensated cirrhosis (Child-Pugh B or C) have not been established; therefore **Vemlidy** is not recommended in patients with decompensated (Child-Pugh B or C) hepatic impairment, Healthcare providers are encouraged to register patients by calling the Antiretroviral Pregnancy Registry (APR) at 1-800-258-4263.

Interferon Alpha

▷ *interferon alfa-2b* (C) <1 year: not recommended; >1 year-12 years: 3 million IU/m 23 times/week x 1 week; then increase to 6 million IU/m² 3 times/week to 16-24 weeks; max 10 million IU/dose; reduce dose by half <u>or</u> interrupt dose if WBCs, granulocyte count, <u>or</u> platelet count decreases; >12 years: 5 million IU SC <u>or</u> IM daily <u>or</u> 10 million IU SC <u>or</u> IM 3 times/week x 16 weeks; reduce dose by half <u>or</u> interrupt dose if WBCs, granulocyte count, <u>or</u> platelet count decreases

    Intron A *Vial (pwdr):* 5, 10, 18, 25, 50 million IU/vial (pwdr + diluent; single dose) (benzoyl alcohol); *Vial (soln):* 3, 5, 10 million IU/vial (single dose); *Multidose vials (soln):* 18, 25 million IU/vial soln; *Multidose pens (soln):* 3, 5, 10 million IU/0.2 ml (6 doses/pen)

HEPATITIS C (HCV)

CHRONIC HCV INFECTION TREATMENT

Nucleoside Analogs (Reverse Transcriptase Inhibitors)

Comment: Nucleoside analogs are indicated for patients with compensated liver disease previously untreated with *alpha interferon* <u>or</u> who have relapsed after *alpha interferon* therapy. Primary toxicity is hemolytic anemia. Contraindicated in male partners of pregnant females; use 2 forms of contraception during therapy and for 6 months after discontinuation.

▷ *ribavirin* (X)(G) <5 years: not established; >5-<18 years: 23-33 kg: 400 mg/day; 34-46 kg: 600 mg/day; 47-59 kg: 800 mg/day; 60-75 kg: 1 gm/day; 1.2 gm/day; >75 kg: *Genotype 2, 3:* treat for 24 weeks; *Genotype 1, 4:* treat for 48 weeks; reduce dose or discontinue if hematologic abnormalities occur; >18 years: take with food in 2 divided doses; *Genotype 2, 3:* 800 mg/day x 24 weeks; *Genotype 1, 4, <75 kg:* 1 gm/day x 48 weeks; >75 km 1.2 gm/day x 48 weeks; *HIV co-infection:* 800 mg/day x 48 weeks; *CrCl 30-50 mL/min:* alternate 200 mg and 400 mg every other day; *CrCl <30 mL/min or hemodialysis:* reduce dose or discontinue if hematologic abnormalities occur

    Copegus *Tab:* 200 mg

    Rebetol *Cap:* 200 mg

    Rebetol Oral Solution *Oral soln:* 40 mg/ml (120 ml) (bubble gum)

    Ribasphere RibaPak 600 mg *Tab:* 600 mg (14/pck)

Interferon Alpha

▷ *interferon alfacon-1* (C)

    Infergen <18 years: not recommended; ≥18 years: 9 mcg SC 3 times/week x 24 weeks, then 15 mcg SC 3 times/week x 6 months; allow at least 48 hours between doses

    Vial (soln): 9, 15 mcg/vial soln (6-single dose/pck; preservative-free)

▷ *interferon alfa-2b* (C)

    Intron A <18 years: not recommended; ≥18 years:

    Vial (pwdr): 5, 10, 18, 25, 50 million IU/vial (pwdr w. diluent; single dose) (benzoyl alcohol); *Vial (soln):* 3, 5, 10 million IU/vial (single dose); *Multidose vials (soln):* 18, 25 million IU/vial; *Multidose pens (soln):* 3, 5, 10 million IU/0.2 ml (6 doses/pen)

▷ *peginterferon alfa-2a* (C) administer 180 mcg SC once weekly (on the same day of the week); treat for 48 weeks; consider discontinuing if adequate response after 12-24 weeks

    PEGasys *Vial:* 180 mcg/ml (single dose); *Monthly pck (vials):* 180 mcg/ml (1 ml, 4/pck)

▷ *peginterferon alfa-2b* (C) <18 years: not recommended; ≥18 years: administer SC once weekly (on the same day of the week); treat for 1 year; consider discontinuing if inadequate response after 24 weeks; 37-45 kg: 40 mcg (100 mg/ml, 0.4 ml); 46-56 kg: 50 mcg (100 mg/ml, 0.5 ml); 57-72 kg: 64 mcg (160 mg/ml, 0.4 ml); 73-88 kg: 80 mcg (160 mg/ml, 0.5 ml); 89-106 kg: 96 mcg (240 mg/ml, 0.4 ml); 107-136 kg: 120 mcg (240 mg/ml, 0.5 ml); 137-160 kg: 150 mcg (300 mg/ml, 0.5 ml)

    PEG-Intron *Vial:* 50, 80, 120, 150 mcg/ml (single dose)

    PEG-Intron Redipen *Pen:* 50, 80, 120, 150 mcg/ml (disposable pens)

HCV NS5A Inhibitor

▷ *daclatasvir* (X) <18 years: not recommended; ≥18 years: 60 mg once daily for 12 weeks (with *sofosbuvir*); if *sofosbuvir* is discontinued, *daclatasvir* should also be discontinued; with concomitant CY3P inhibitors, reduce dose to 30 mg once daily; with concomitant CY3P inducers, increase dose to 90 mg once daily

    Daklinza *Tab:* 30, 60 mg

    Comment: **Daklinza** is indicated in combination with *sofosbuvir* with or without *ribavirin*, for the treatment of HCV genotypes 1 and 3, and in patients with comorbid HIV-1 infection, advanced cirrhosis, or post-liver transplant recurrence of HCV.

HCV NS5B POLYMERASE INHIBITOR

▷ *sofosbuvir* (B) <12 years: not established; ≥12-17 years, ≥35 kg (77 lb): take with or without food; taken only as a component on a combination antiviral treatment regimen; *Genotype 2:* 400 mg once daily plus *ribavirin* x 12 weeks without cirrhosis or with compensated cirrhosis; *Genotype 3:* 400 mg once daily plus *ribavirin* x 24 weeks without cirrhosis or with compensated cirrhosis; ≥18 years: *Genotype 1:* 400 mg once daily plus *simeprevir* x12 weeks or x 24 weeks; *Alternate:* 400 mg once daily with *daclatasvir* x12 weeks; *Genotype 2:* 400 mg once daily plus *daclatasvir* x12 weeks or x 16-24 weeks (duration depends on cirrhosis status--refer to AASLD/IDSA hepatitis C guidelines; *Genotype 3:* 400 mg once daily plus *daclatasvir* x12 weeks; *Genotype 4:* 400 mg once daily plus *daclatasvir* x 12 weeks; *Hepatocellular Cancer Awaiting Transplant:* 400 mg once daily plus *ribavirin*

    Sovaldi *Tab:* 400 mg film-coat

Comment: *CrCl ≥30:* no adjustment; *CrCl <30:* not defined; *Hemodialysis:* not defined; *Hepatic Impairment:* no adjustment; *Decompensated Hepatic Disease:* not defined. Refer to AASLD/IDSA hepatitis C guidelines for more information. Because **Sovaldi** is used in combination with other antiviral drugs for treatment of HCV infection, consult the prescribing information for these drugs used in combination with **Sovaldi**. Warnings and precautions related to these drugs also apply to their use in **Sovaldi** combination treatment. Hepatitis B virus (HBV) reactivation has been reported in HCV/HBV co-infected patients who were undergoing or had completed treatment with HCV direct acting antivirals, and who were not receiving HBV antiviral therapy. Some cases have resulted in fulminant hepatitis, hepatic failure, and death. Cases have been reported in patients who are HBsAg positive and also in patients with serologic evidence of resolved HBV infection (i.e., HBsAg negative and anti-HBc positive). HBV reactivation has also been reported in patients receiving certain immunosuppressant or chemotherapeutic agents; the risk of HBV reactivation associated with treatment with HCV direct-acting antivirals may be increased in these patients. HBV reactivation is characterized as an abrupt increase in HBV replication manifesting as a rapid increase in serum HBV DNA level. In patients with resolved HBV infection, reappearance of HBsAg can occur. Reactivation of HBV replication may be accompanied by hepatitis, i.e., increases in aminotransferase levels and, in severe cases, increases in bilirubin levels, liver failure, and death can occur. P-gp inducers (e.g., *rifampin*, St. John's wort) in the intestine may significantly decrease *sofosbuvir* plasma concentrations and may lead to a reduced therapeutic effect of **Sovaldi**: therefore, the use of *rifampin* and St. John's wort with **Sovaldi** is not recommended. Serious risk of symptomatic bradycardia when co-administered with *amiodarone* and another HCV direct-acting antiviral (DAA).

HCV NS5A Inhibitor/HCV NS3/4A Protease Inhibitor Combinations

▷ *elbasvir/grazoprevir* (NE) <18 years: not recommended; ≥18 years: 1 tab as a single dose once daily; see mfr pkg insert for length of treatment

    Zepatier *Tab:* *elba* 50 mg/*grazo* 100/mg

    Comment: **Zepatier** is contraindicated with moderate or severe hepatic impairment, concomitant *atazanavir*, *carbamazepine*, *cyclosporine*, *darunavir*, *efavirenz*, *lopinavir*, *phenytoin*, *rifampin*, *saquinavir*, St. John's wort, *tipranavir*. When co-administered with *ribavirin*, pregnancy category (X).

HCV NS5A Inhibitor/HCV NS3/4A Protease Inhibitor/CYP3A Inhibitor Combinations

▷ *ombitasvir/paritaprevir/ritonavir* (B) <18 years: not recommended; ≥18 years: 2 tabs once daily in the AM x 12 weeks

Technivie *Tab: omvi* 25 mg/*pari* 75 mg/*rito* 50 mg (4 x 7 daily dose pcks/carton)
Comment: **Technivie** is indicated for use in chronic HCV genotype 4 without cirrhosis. **Technivie** is not for use with moderate hepatic impairment.

HCV NS3/4A Protease Inhibitor Combinations

▷ *boceprevir* (C) <18 years: not recommended; ≥18 years: 800 mg 3 times/day; take with food (not low-fat); not for monotherapy; start after 4 weeks therapy with *peginterferon* and discontinue if HCV-RNA levels indicate futility *ribavirin*; *Without cirrhosis:* continue as indicated by HCV-RNA levels at weeks 8, 12, and 24; *With cirrhosis:* continue for 44 weeks; do not reduce dose
Victrelis *Cap:* 200 mg

▷ *simeprevir* (C) <18 years: not recommended; ≥18 years: 150 mg once daily; swallow whole; take with food, not for monotherapy; do not reduce dose or interrupt therapy; if discontinued, do not reinitiate; discontinue if HCV-RNA levels indicate futility; discontinue if *peginterferon*, *ribavirin*, or *sofosbuvir* is permanently discontinued; *Treatment-naïve, treatment relapses, with or without cirrhosis:* treat x 12 weeks (*simeprevir* + *peginterferon* + *ribavirin*) followed by additional 12 weeks *peginterferon* + *ribavirin* (total = 24 weeks). *Partial and non-responders, with or without cirrhosis:* treat x 12 weeks (*simeprevir* + *peginterferon* + *ribavirin*) followed by additional 36 weeks *peginterferon* + *ribavirin* (total = 48 weeks); *Treatment-naïve or treatment-experienced without cirrhosis:* treat x 12 weeks (*simeprevir* + *sofosbuvir*); *Treatment-naïve or treatment-experienced with cirrhosis:* treat x 24 weeks (*simeprevir* + *sofosbuvir*)
Olysio *Cap:* 150 mg

HCV NS5A Inhibitor/HCV NS5B Polymerase Inhibitor Combinations

▷ *ledipasvir/sofosbuvir* (NE) <12 years: not recommended; ≥12 years: *Treatment-naïve, without cirrhosis, with pretreatment HCV RNA <6 million IU/ml:* 1 tab daily x 8 weeks; *Treatment-naïve with or without cirrhosis or treatment-experienced without cirrhosis:* 1 tab daily x 12 weeks; *Treatment-experienced with cirrhosis:* 1 tab daily x 24 weeks; *In combination with ribavirin:* 1 tab daily x 12 weeks
Harvoni *Tab: ledi* 90 mg/*sofo* 400 mg
Comment: **Harvoni** is indicated for patients with advanced liver disease, genotype 1, 4, 5, or 6 infection: chronic HCV genotype 1- or 4-infected liver transplant recipients with or without cirrhosis or with compensated cirrhosis (Child-Pugh A), and for HCV genotype 1-infected patients with decompensated cirrhosis (Child-Pugh B/C), including those who have undergone liver transplantation. No adequate human data are available to establish whether or not **Harvoni** poses a risk to pregnancy outcomes; the background risk of major birth defects and miscarriage for the indicated population is unknown. If **Harvoni** is administered with *ribavirin*, the combination regimen is contraindicated (**X**) in pregnant females and in males whose female partners are pregnant. It is not known whether **Harvoni** and its metabolites are present in human breast milk, affect human milk production, or have effects on the breastfed infant. If **Harvoni** is administered with *ribavirin*, the nursing mother's information for *ribavirin* also applies to this combination regimen.

▷ *sofosbuvir/velpatasvir* (NE) <18 years: not established; ≥18 years: *Without cirrhosis or compensated cirrhosis (Child-Pugh A):* 1 tablet daily x 12 weeks; *Decompensated cirrhosis (Child Pugh B or C):* 1 tablet daily plus *ribavirin* (RBV)
Epclusa *Tab: sofo* 400 mg/*velpa* 100 mg

Comment: **Epclusa** is indicated for patients with chronic HCV with genotype 12, 3, 4, 5, or 6 infection.

HCV NS5A Inhibitor/HCV NS3/4A Protease Inhibitor/CYP3A Inhibitor Combination

➤ *sofosbuvir/velpatasvir* (B) <12 years: not established; ≥12 years: 1 tab daily
Viekira XR *Tab: dasa* 200 mg/*omvi* 8.33 mg/*pari* 50 mg/*rito* 33.33 mg ext-rel (4 weekly cartons, each containing 7 daily dose packs/carton)
Comment: **Viekira XR** is indicated for HCV genotype 1 with mild liver dysfunction (Child-Pugh A). **Viekira XR** is contraindicated for moderate (Child-Pugh B) to severe (Child-Pugh C) liver dysfunction. No adjustment is recommended with mild, moderate, or severe renal dysfunction.

HCV NS5A Inhibitor/HCV NS3/4A Protease Inhibitor/CYP3A Inhibitor PLUS HCV NS5B Polymerase Inhibitor Combination

➤ *ombitasvir/paritaprevir/ritonavir* plus *dasabuvir* (B)
Viekira Pak *ombitasvir/paritaprevir/ritonavir* fixed-dose combination tablet: <12 years: not established; ≥12 years: 2 tablets orally once a day (in the morning); *dasabuvir*: 250 mg orally twice a day (morning and evening)
Tab: omvi 12.5 mg/*pari* 75 mg/*rito* 50 mg plus *Tab:* dasa 250 mg (28 day supply/pck)
Comment: **Viekira Pak** is indicated for mild liver dysfunction (Child-Pugh A). **Viekira Pak** is contraindicated for moderate (Child-Pugh B) to severe (Child-Pugh C) liver dysfunction. No adjustment is recommended with mild, moderate, or severe renal dysfunction.

SOVALDI/HARVONI/RIBAVIRIN COMBINATION TREATMENT REGIMEN

Comment: For this FDA-approved triple therapy regimen, follow the recommended regimen for each individual drug. Patients who are co-infected with hepatitis B are at risk for HBV reactivation during or after treatment with HCV direct-acting retrovirals. Therefore, patients should be screened for current or past HBV infection before starting this triple therapy regimen.

HERPANGINA

ANALGESICS

➤ *acetaminophen* (B) *see Fever page* 136
➤ *tramadol* (C)(IV)(G)
Comment: *Tramadol* is known to be excreted in breast milk. The FDA and the European Medicines Agency (EMA) are investigating the safety of using *tramadol*-containing medications to treat pain in children 12-18 years because of the potential for serious side effects, including slowed or difficult breathing.
Rybix ODT <18 years: not recommended; ≥18 years: initially 100 mg once daily; may increase by 100 mg every 5 days; max 300 mg/day; *CrCl <30 mL/min* or *severe hepatic impairment*: not recommended; *Cirrhosis*: max 50 mg q 12 hours
ODT: 50 mg (mint) (phenylalanine)

Ryzolt <18 years: not recommended; ≥18 years: initially 100 mg once daily; may increase by 100 mg every 5 days; max 300 mg/day; *CrCl <30 mL/min* or *severe hepatic impairment:* not recommended

  Tab: 100, 200, 300 mg ext-rel

Ultram <18 years: not recommended; ≥18 years: 50-100 mg q 4-6 hours prn; max 400 mg/day; *CrCl <30 mL/min:* max 100 mg q 12 hours; *Cirrhosis:* max 50 mg q 12 hours

  Tab: 50*mg

Ultram ER <18 years: not recommended; ≥18 years: initially 100 mg once daily; may increase by 100 mg every 5 days; max 300 mg/day; *CrCl <30 mL/min:* or *severe hepatic impairment:* not recommended

  Tab: 100, 200, 300 mg ext-rel

➤ *tramadol/acetaminophen* (C)(IV)(G) <12 years: contraindicated; 12-<18: use extreme caution; not recommended for children and adolescents with obesity, asthma, obstructive sleep apnea, or other chronic breathing problem, or for post-tonsillectomy/adenoidectomy pain; ≥18 years: 2 tabs q 4-6 hours; max 8 tabs/day; 5 days; *CrCl <30 mL/min:* max 2 tabs q 12 hours; max 4 tabs/day x 5 days

  Ultracet *Tab:* tram 37.5/*acet* 325 mg

Comment: *Tramadol* is known to be excreted in breast milk. The FDA and the European Medicines Agency (EMA) are investigating the safety of using *tramadol*-containing medications to treat pain in children 12-18 years because of the potential for serious side effects, including slowed or difficult breathing.

TOPICAL ANESTHETICS

➤ *lidocaine* viscous soln (B) <4 years: apply 1.25 ml to affected area with cotton-tipped applicator; may repeat after 3 hours; max 8 doses/day; ≥4 years, able to gargle or rinse/spit: 15 ml gargle or rinse/spit; repeat after 3 hours; max 8 doses/day

  Xylocaine 2% Viscous Solution *Viscous soln:* 2% (20, 100, 450 ml)

  Antipyretics *see Fever page 136*

HERPES GENITALIS (HSV TYPE II)

Comment: The following treatment regimens are published in the **2015 CDC Sexually Transmitted Diseases Treatment Guidelines.** Treatment regimens are for patients 18 years-of-age or older only; consult a specialist for treatment of patients less than 18 years-of-age. Treatment regimens are presented in alphabetical order by generic drug name, followed by a listing of brands with dose forms.

RECOMMENDED REGIMENS: FIRST CLINICAL EPISODE

Regimen 1

➤ *acyclovir* <18 years: not established; ≥18 years: 400 mg tid x 7-10 days or 200 mg 5 times/day x 10 days or until clinically resolved

Regimen 2

➤ *acyclovir* cream <18 years: not established; ≥18 years: apply q 3 hours 6 x/day x 7 days

Regimen 3

▷ *famciclovir* <18 years: not established; ≥18 years: 250 mg tid x 7-10 days <u>or</u> until clinically resolved

Regimen 4

▷ *valacyclovir* <18 years: not established; ≥18 years: 1 gm bid x 10 days <u>or</u> until clinically resolved

RECOMMENDED RECURRENT/EPISODIC REGIMENS

Comment: Initiate treatment of recurrent episodes within 1 day of onset of lesions.

Regimen 1

▷ *acyclovir* <18 years: not established; ≥18 years: 200 mg 5 times/day x 5 days

Regimen 2

▷ *famciclovir* <18 years: not established; ≥18 years: 125 mg bid x 5 days

Regimen 3

▷ *valacyclovir* <18 years: not established; ≥18 years: 500 mg bid x 3-5 days <u>or</u> until clinically resolved

SUPPRESSION THERAPY REGIMENS

Regimen 1

▷ *acyclovir* <18 years: not established; ≥18 years: 400 mg bid x 1 year

Regimen 2

▷ *famciclovir* <18 years: not established; ≥18 years: 250 mg bid x 1 year

Regimen 3

▷ *valacyclovir* <18 years: not established; ≥18 years: 500 mg daily x 1 year (for ≤9 recurrences/year) <u>or</u> 1 gm daily x 1 year (for ≥10 recurrences/year)

DAILY SUPPRESSIVE REGIMENS FOR PERSONS WITH HIV

Regimen 1

▷ *acyclovir* <18 years: not established; ≥18 years: 400-800 mg bid-tid

Regimen 2

▷ *famciclovir* <18 years: not established; ≥18 years: 500 mg bid

Regimen 3

▷ *valacyclovir* <18 years: not established; ≥18 years: 500 mg bid

RECURRENT/EPISODIC REGIMENS FOR PERSONS WITH HIV

Regimen 1

▷ *acyclovir* <18 years: not established; ≥18 years: 400 mg tid x 5-10 days

Regimen 2

▷ *famciclovir* <18 years: not established; ≥18 years: 500 mg bid x 5-10 days

Regimen 3

▷ *valacyclovir* <18 years: not established; ≥18 years: 1 gm bid x 5-10 days

DRUG BRANDS AND DOSE FORMS

▷ *acyclovir* (B)(G)
 Zovirax *Cap:* 200 mg; *Tab:* 400, 800 mg
 Zovirax Oral Suspension *Oral susp:* 200 mg/5 ml (banana)
 Zovirax Cream *Crm:* 5% (3, 15 gm); *Oint:* 5% (3, 15 gm)
▷ *famciclovir* (B)(G)
 Famvir *Tab:* 125, 250, 500 mg
▷ *valacyclovir* (B)(G)
 Valtrex *Cplt:* 500, 1,000 mg

HERPES LABIALIS/HERPES FACIALIS (HERPES SIMPLEX VIRUS TYPE I, COLD SORE, FEVER BLISTER)

PRIMARY INFECTION

▷ *acyclovir* (B)(G) <12 years: *see page* 541 *for dose by weight table*; ≥12 years: do not chew, crush, <u>or</u> swallow the buccal tab; apply within 1 hour of symptom onset and before appearance of lesion; apply a single buccal tab to the upper gum region on the affected side and hold in place for 30 seconds
 Sitavig *Buccal tab:* 50 mg
 Comment: Sitavig is contraindicated with allergy to milk protein concentrate.
▷ *valacyclovir* (B) <12 years: not recommended; >2 years: 12 gm q 12 hours x 1 day
 Valtrex *Cplt:* 500, 1,000 mg

SUPPRESSION THERAPY (FOR SIX OR MORE OUTBREAKS/YEAR)

▷ *acyclovir* (B)(G) <2 years: not recommended; ≥2 years, <40 kg: 20 mg/kg 2-5 times/ day x 1 year; >2 years, >40 kg: 200 mg 2-5 times/day x 1 year; *see page* 541 *for dose by weight table*;
 Zovirax *Cap:* 200 mg; *Tab:* 400, 800 mg
 Zovirax Oral Suspension *Oral susp:* 200 mg/5 ml (banana)

TOPICAL ANTIVIRAL THERAPY

▷ *acyclovir* (B)(G) <2 years: not recommended; ≥2 years: apply q 3 hours 6 times/day x 7 days

Zovirax Cream *Crm:* 5% (3, 15 gm); *Oint:* 5% (3, 15 gm)
▷ *docosanol* (B) <12 years: not recommended; ≥12 years: apply and gently rub in 5 times daily until healed
Abreva (OTC) *Crm:* 10% (2 gm)
▷ *penciclovir* (B) <12 years: not recommended; ≥12 years: apply q 2 hours while awake x 4 days
Denavir *Crm:* 1% (2 gm)

TOPICAL ANTIVIRAL/CORTICOSTEROID THERAPY

▷ *acyclovir/hydrocortisone* (B)(G) <12 years: not recommended; ≥12 years: cream apply to affected area 5 x/day x 5 days
Crm: 1% (2, 5 gm)

HERPES ZOSTER (SHINGLES)

ORAL ANTIVIRALS

▷ *famciclovir* (B) <18 years: not recommended; ≥18 years: 500 mg tid x 7 days
Famvir *Tab:* 125, 250, 500 mg
▷ *valacyclovir* (B) <12 years: not recommended; ≥12 years: 1 gm tid x 7 days
Valtrex *Cplt:* 500, 1,000 mg
▷ *acyclovir* (B)(G) <2 years: not recommended; ≥2 years, <40 kg: 20 mg/kg 5 x/day x 7-10 days; >2 years, >40 kg: 800 mg 5 x/day x 7-10 days; *see page* 541 *for dose by weight table;* ≥12 years: 800 mg 5 x/day x 7-10 days
Zovirax *Cap:* 200 mg; *Tab:* 400, 800 mg
Zovirax Oral Suspension *Oral susp:* 200 mg/5 ml (banana)

PROPHYLAXIS AGAINST SECONDARY INFECTION

▷ *silver sulfadiazine* (B)(G) <12 years: not established; ≥12 years: apply bid-qid
Silvadene *Crm:* 1% (20 gm tube; 20, 50, 85, 400, 1,000 gm jar)
Comment: *silver sulfadiazine* is contradicted in sulfa allergy, late pregnancy, within the first 2 months after birth, premature infants.

ANALGESICS

▷ *acetaminophen* (B) *see Fever page* 136
▷ *aspirin* (D) *see Fever page* 137
Comment: *aspirin*-containing medications are contraindicated with history of allergic-type reaction to *aspirin*, children and adolescents with *varicella* or other viral illness, and 3rd trimester pregnancy.
▷ *tramadol* (C)(IV)(G)
Comment: *Tramadol* is known to be excreted in breast milk. The FDA and the European Medicines Agency (EMA) are investigating the safety of using *tramadol*-containing medications to treat pain in children 12-18 years because of the potential for serious side effects, including slowed or difficult breathing.
Rybix ODT <18 years: not recommended; ≥18 years: initially 100 mg once daily; may increase by 100 mg every 5 days; max 300 mg/day; *CrCl <30 mL/min or severe hepatic impairment:* not recommended; *Cirrhosis:* max 50 mg q 12 hours *ODT:* 50 mg (mint) (phenylalanine)

Ryzolt <18 years: not recommended; ≥18 years: initially 100 mg once daily; may increase by 100 mg every 5 days; max 300 mg/day; *CrCl <30 mL/min or severe hepatic impairment:* not recommended
    Tab: 100, 200, 300 mg ext-rel
Ultram <18 years: not recommended; ≥18 years: 50-100 mg q 4-6 hours prn; max 400 mg/day; *CrCl <30 mL/min:* max 100 mg q 12 hours; *Cirrhosis:* max 50 mg q 12 hours
    Tab: 50*mg
Ultram ER <18 years: not recommended; ≥18 years: initially 100 mg once daily; may increase by 100 mg every 5 days; max 300 mg/day; *CrCl <30 mL/min: or severe hepatic impairment:* not recommended
    Tab: 100, 200, 300 mg ext-rel

➤ *tramadol/acetaminophen* (C)(IV)(G) <12 years: contraindicated; 12-<18: use extreme caution; not recommended for children and adolescents with obesity, asthma, obstructive sleep apnea, or other chronic breathing problem, or for post-tonsillectomy/adenoidectomy pain; ≥18 years: 2 tabs q 4-6 hours; max 8 tabs/day; 5 days; *CrCl <30 mL/min:* max 2 tabs q 12 hours; max 4 tabs/day x 5 days
    Ultracet *Tab:* tram 37.5/acet 325 mg

Comment: *Tramadol* is known to be excreted in breast milk. The FDA and the European Medicines Agency (EMA) are investigating the safety of using *tramadol*-containing medications to treat pain in children 12-18 years because of the potential for serious side effects, including slowed or difficult breathing.

Other Oral Analgesics *see Pain page* 298
Postherpetic Neuralgia *see page* 338

SECONDARY INFECTION PROPHYLAXIS

➤ *silver sulfadiazine* (B)(G) <12 years: not established; ≥12 years: apply bid-qid
    Silvadene *Crm:* 1% (20 gm tube; 20, 50, 85, 400, 1,000 gm jar)
Comment: *silver sulfadiazine* is contradicted in sulfa allergy, late pregnancy, within the first 2 months after birth, premature infants.

HICCUPS: INTRACTABLE

➤ *chlorpromazine* (C) <6 months: not recommended; ≥6 months: 0.25 mg/lb orally q 4-6 hours prn or 0.5 mg/lb rectally q 6-8 hours prn; ≥12 years: 25-50 mg tid-qid
    Thorazine *Tab:* 10, 25, 50, 100, 200 mg; *Spansule:* 30, 75, 150 mg sust-rel; *Syr:* 10 mg/5 ml (4 oz; orange custard); *Oral conc:* 30 mg/ml (4 oz); 100 mg/ml (2, 8 oz); *Supp:* 25, 100 mg

HIDRADENITIS SUPPURATIVA

ORAL ANTI-INFECTIVES

➤ *doxycycline* (D)(G) <8 years: not recommended; ≥8 years, <100 lb: 2 mg/lb on first day in 2 divided doses, followed by 1 mg/lb/day in 1-2 divided x 7-14 days; ≥8 years, ≥100 lb: 100 mg bid x 7-14 days; *see page 561 for dose by weight table*

Acticlate *Tab:* 75, 150** mg
Adoxa *Tab:* 50, 75, 100, 150 mg ent-coat
Doryx *Tab:* 50, 75, 100, 150, 200 mg del-rel
Monodox *Cap:* 50, 75, 100 mg
Oracea *Cap:* 40 mg del-rel
Vibramycin *Tab:* 100 mg; *Cap:* 50, 100 mg; *Syr:* 50 mg/5 ml (raspberry-apple) (sulfites); *Oral susp:* 25 mg/5 ml (raspberry)
Vibra-Tab *Tab:* 100 mg film-coat

Comment: *doxycycline* is contraindicated <8 years-of-age, in pregnancy, and lactation (discolors developing tooth enamel). A side effect may be photo-sensitivity (photophobia). Do not take with antacids, calcium supplements, milk or other dairy, or within 2 hours of taking another drug.

➤ *erythromycin base* (B)(G) <45 kg: 30-50 mg in 2-4 divided doses x 7-14 days; ≥45 kg: 1-1.5 gm divided qid x 7-14 days
  Ery-Tab *Tab:* 250, 333, 500 mg ent-coat
  PCE *Tab:* 333, 500 mg

➤ *erythromycin ethylsuccinate* (B)(G) 30-50 mg/kg/day in 4 divided doses x 7-14 days; may double dose with severe infection; max 100 mg/kg/day; *see page 563 for dose by weight table*
  EryPed *Oral susp:* 200 mg/5 ml (100, 200 ml) (fruit); 400 mg/5 ml (60, 100, 200 ml) (banana); *Oral drops:* 200, 400 mg/5 ml (50 ml) (fruit); *Chew tab:* 200 mg wafer (fruit)
  E.E.S. *Oral susp:* 200, 400 mg/5 ml (100 ml) (fruit)
  E.E.S. Granules *Oral susp:* 200 mg/5 ml (100, 200 ml) (cherry)
  E.E.S. 400 Tablets *Tab:* 400 mg

➤ *minocycline* (D)(G) <8 years: not recommended, ≥8 years: 100 mg bid x 7-14 days
  Dynacin *Cap:* 50, 100 mg
  Minocin *Cap:* 50, 75, 100 mg; *Oral susp:* 50 mg/5 ml (60 ml) (custard) (sulfites, alcohol 5%)

Comment: *minocycline* is contraindicated <8 years-of-age, in pregnancy, and lactation (discolors developing tooth enamel). A side effect may be photo-sensitivity (photophobia). Do not give with antacids, calcium supplements, milk or other dairy, or within two hours of taking another drug.

➤ *tetracycline* (D)(G) <8 years: not recommended; ≥8 years, <100 lb: 25-50 mg/kg/day in 4 divided doses x 7-14 days; *see page 574 for dose by weight table*; ≥8 years, ≥100 lb: 250 mg qid or 500 mg tid x 7-14 days
  Achromycin V *Cap:* 250, 500 mg
  Sumycin *Tab:* 250, 500 mg; *Cap:* 250, 500 mg; *Oral susp:* 125 mg/5 ml (100, 200 ml) (fruit) (sulfites)

Comment: *tetracycline* is contraindicated <8 years-of-age, in pregnancy, and lactation (discolors developing tooth enamel). A side effect may be photo-sensitivity (photophobia). Do not give with antacids, calcium supplements, milk or other dairy, or within two hours of taking another drug.

TOPICAL ANTI-INFECTIVES

➤ *clindamycin* (B)(G) apply bid x 7-14 days
  Cleocin T *Pad:* 1% (60/pck; alcohol 50%); *Lotn:* 1% (60 ml); *Gel:* 1% (30, 60 gm); *Soln w. applicator:* 1% (30, 60 ml; alcohol 50%)

HOOKWORM (UNCINARIASIS, CUTANEOUS LARVAE MIGRANS)

ANTHELMINTICS

Comment: Oral bioavailability of anthelmintics is enhanced when administered with a fatty meal (estimated fat content 40 g).

▶ *albendazole* (C) take with a meal; may crush and mix with food; may repeat in 2-3 weeks if needed; <2 years: not recommended; 2-12 years: 400 mg x 3 days; >12 years: 400 mg bid x 5 days
  Albenza *Tab:* 200 mg

▶ *mebendazole* (C) take with a meal; may crush and mix with food; may repeat in 3 weeks if needed; <2 years: not recommended; ≥2 years: 100 mg bid x 3 days
  Emverm *Chew tab:* 100 mg
  Vermox (G) *Chew tab:* 100 mg

▶ *pyrantel pamoate* (C) take with a meal; may open capsule and sprinkle or mix with food; take x 3 days; 11 mg/kg/dose; max 1 gm/dose; <12 lb: not recommended; 25-37 lb: 1/2 tsp/dose; 38-62 lb: 1 tsp/dose; 63-87 lb: 1 tsp/dose; 88-112 lb: 2 tsp/dose; 113-137 lb: 2 tsp/dose; 138-162 lb: 3 tsp/dose; 163-187 lb: 3 tsp/dose; >187 lb: 4 tsp/dose
  Antiminth (OTC) *Cap:* 180 mg; *Liq:* 50 mg/ml (30 ml); 144 mg/ml (30 ml); *Oral susp:* 50 mg/ml (60 ml)
  Pin-X (OTC) *Cap:* 180 mg; *Liq:* 50 mg/ml (30 ml); 144 mg/ml (30 ml); *Oral susp:* 50 mg/ml (30 ml)

HUMAN IMMUNODEFICIENCY VIRUS (HIV) EXPOSURE, ANTIRETROVIRAL PEP/nPEP

Antiretroviral drug brand names and dose forms (*see Anti-HIV Drugs page 511*)
Comment: Antiretroviral prophylactic treatment regimens for occupational HIV exposure (PEP) and non-occupational exposure (nPEP) are referenced from the **2015 CDC Sexually Transmitted Diseases Treatment Guidelines, MMWR,** and NIH available at: https://www.cdc.gov/hiv/pdf/programresources/cdc-hiv-npep-guidelines.pdf

In this section, the 2015 CDC-recommended highly active antiretroviral treatment (HAART) regimens are followed by a listing of the single and combination drugs with dosing regimens and dose forms.

Appendix S is an alphabetical listing of the HIV drugs and dose forms.

For more information on the management of HIV infection in adolescents and ≥18 years, see *Guidelines for the Use of Antiretroviral Agents in HIV-1-Infected Adults and Adolescents:* https://aidsinfo.nih.gov/contentfiles/lvguidelines/adultandadolescentgl.pdf

For specific dosing information in the management of HIV infection in children, see *Guidelines for Use of Antiretroviral Agents in Pediatric HIV Infection:* https://www.aidsinfo.nih.gov/contentfiles/lvguidelines/pediatricguidelines.pdf

Providers should consult, and/refer HIV-infected patients to, a specialist and/or specialty community services for age-appropriate dosing regimens and other specific pediatric considerations.

Initiation of PEP/nPEP with ART as soon as possible increases the likelihood of prophylactic benefit. Treatment regimens must be initiated ≥72 hours following exposure. A 28-day course of ART is recommended for persons with *substantial risk for HIV exposure* (i.e., exposure of vagina, rectum, eye, mouth, or other mucous membrane, non-intact skin, or percutaneous contact with blood, semen, vaginal secretions, breast milk, or any body fluid that is visibly contaminated with blood, when the source is known to be infected with HIV). ART is not recommended for persons with *negligible risk for HIV exposure* (i.e., exposure of vagina, rectum, eye, mouth, or other mucus membrane, intact or non-intact skin, or percutaneous contact with urine, nasal secretions, saliva, sweat, or tears, if not visibly contaminated with blood, regardless of the known or suspected HIV status of the source). There is no evidence indicating any specific antiretroviral medication, or combination of medications is optimal for suppressing local viral replication. There is no evidence to indicate that a 3-drug ART regimen is any more beneficial than a 2-drug regimen. When the source person is available for interview and testing, his or her history of retroviral medication use and most recent/current viral load measurement should be considered when selecting an ART treatment regimen (e.g., to help avoid prescribing an antiretroviral medication to which the source virus is likely to be resistant). Register pregnant patients exposed to antiretroviral agents to the Antiretroviral Pregnancy Registry (APR) at 800-258-4263. The Centers for Disease Control and Prevention recommend that HIV-infected mothers not breastfeed their infants to avoid risking postnatal transmission of HIV infection.

REGIMENS

Non-Nucleoside Reverse Transcriptase Inhibitor (NNRTI)-Based Regimen

➤ *efavirenz* plus (*lamivudine* or *emtricitabine*) plus (*zidovudine* or *tenofovir*)

Protease Inhibitor (PI)-Based Regimens

➤ *lopinavir/ritonavir* (coformulated as **Kaletra**) plus (*lamivudine* or *emtricitabine*) plus *zidovudine*
➤ *darunavir/cobicistat* (coformulated as **Prezcobix**) plus other retroviral agents

ALTERNATIVE REGIMENS

NNRTI-Based Regimen

➤ *efavirenz* plus (*lamivudine* or *emtricitabine*) plus (*abacavir* or *didanosine* or *stavudine*)
Comment: *efavirenz* should be avoided in pregnant females and females of childbearing potential.

Protease Inhibitor-Based Regimens

Regimen 1

➤ *atazanavir* plus (*lamivudine* or *emtricitabine*) plus (*zidovudine* or *stavudine* or *abacavir* or *didanosine*) or (*tenofovir* plus *ritonavir* (100 mg/day)

Regimen 2

➤ *fosamprenavir* plus (*lamivudine* or *emtricitabine*) plus (*zidovudine* or *stavudine*) or (*abacavir* or *tenofovir* or *didanosine*)

Regimen 3

▷ *fosamprenavir/ritonavir* plus (*lamivudine* or *emtricitabine*) plus (*zidovudine* or *stavudine* or *abacavir* or *tenofovir* or *didanosine*)

Regimen 4

▷ *indinavir/ritonavir* plus (*lamivudine* or *emtricitabine*) plus (*zidovudine* or *stavudine* or *abacavir* or *tenofovir* or *didanosine*)
   Comment: Using *ritonavir* with *indinavir* may increase risk for renal adverse events.

Regimen 5

▷ *lopinavir/ritonavir* (coformulated as **Kaletra**) plus (*lamivudine* or *emtricitabine*) plus (*stavudine* or *abacavir* or *tenofovir* or *didanosine*)

Regimen 6

▷ *nelfinavir* plus (*lamivudine* or *emtricitabine*) plus (*zidovudine* or *stavudine* or *abacavir* or *tenofovir* or *didanosine*)

Regimen 7

▷ *saquinavir/ritonavir* plus (*lamivudine* or *emtricitabine*) plus (*zidovudine* or *stavudine* or *abacavir* or *tenofovir* or *didanosine*)

Triple Nucleoside Reverse Transcriptase Inhibitor (NRTI)-Based Regimen

abacavir plus *lamivudine* plus *zidovudine*
Comment: Triple NRTI therapy should be used only when an NNRTI- or PI-based regimen cannot or should not be used.

BRAND NAMES, DOSING, AND DOSE FORMS: SINGLE AGENTS

Integrase Strand Transfer Inhibitor (INSTI)

▷ *dolutegravir* (C) <12 years, <40 kg: not established; ≥12 years, ≥40 kg: *Treatment-naïve or treatment-experienced but INSTI-naïve:* 50 mg once daily; *Treatment-naïve or treatment-experienced or and co-administered with* **efavirenz, FPV/r, TPV/r,** or **rifampin:** 50 mg bid; *INSTI-experienced with certain INSTI-associated resistance substitutions:* 50 mg bid
     Tivicay *Tab:* 10, 25, 50 mg
▷ *raltegravir (as potassium)* (C) <4 weeks: not recommended; ≥4 weeks, 3-11 kg [oral suspension] 3-<4 kg: 20 mg bid; 4-<6 kg: 30 mg bid; 6-<8 kg: 40 mg bid; 8-<11 kg: 60 mg bid; ≥11-<25 kg [oral suspension/chewable tab]: 6 mg/kg/dose bid; see mfr pkg insert for dose by weight table;≥25 kg and unable to swallow tablet use chewable tab; 25-<28 kg: 150 mg bid; 28-<40 kg: 200 mg bid; ≥40 kg: 300 mg bid; 6 years 25 kg, and able to swallow tablets use film-coat tab; 400 mg bid; take with concomitant **rifampin** 800 mg bid; swallow film-coated tablets whole; do not crush or chew
     Isentress *Tab:* 400 mg film-coat; *Chew tab:* 25, 100*mg (orange banana) (phenylalanine)
     Isentress Oral Suspension *Oral susp:* 100 mg/pkt pwdr for oral susp (banana)
   Comment: Oral suspension, chewable tablets and film-coated *raltegravir* tablets are not bioequivalent. Max dose for chewable tablets is 300 mg twice daily. Max dose for film-coated tablets is 400 mg twice daily

Nucleoside Reverse Transcriptase Inhibitors (NRTIs)

▷ *abacavir sulfate* (C)(G) <3 months: not recommended; 3 months-16 years: [tablet/oral solution] 16 mg/kg qd or 8 mg/kg bid; max 300 mg bid; >14 kg: see mfr pkg insert for tablet dosing by weight table; *Mild hepatic impairment:* use oral solution for titration
>> **Ziagen (as sulfate)** *Tab:* 300*mg
>> **Ziagen Oral Solution** *Oral soln:* 20 mg/ml (240 ml) (strawberry-banana)(parabens, propylene glycol)

▷ *didanosine* (C)
>> **Videx EC** <20 kg: not recommended (use oral solution); 20-<25 kg: 200 mg; 25-<60 kg: 250 mg; ≥60 kg: 400 mg; *CrCl 30-59 mL/min:* <60 kg: 125 mg; ≥60 kg: 200 mg; *CrCl 10-29 mL/min:* 125 mg; *CrCl <10 mL/min or dialysis:* <60 kg: use oral solution ≥60 kg: 125 mg; take once daily on an empty stomach; swallow whole, do not crush or chew
>>> *Cap:* 125, 200, 250, 400 mg ent-coat del-rel; *Chew tab:* 25, 50, 100, 150, 200 mg (mandarin orange) (buffered with calcium carbonate and magnesium hydroxide, phenylalanine)
>> **Videx Pediatric Pwdr for Solution** <2 weeks: not recommended; 2 weeks-8 months: 100 mg/m^2 bid; >8 months: 120 mg/m^2 bid; *Renal impairment:* consider reducing dose or increasing dosing interval; take on an empty stomach
>>> *Pwdr for oral soln:* 2, 4 gm (120, 240 ml)

Comment: *didanosine* is contraindicated with concomitant *allopurinol* or *ribavirin*.

▷ *emtricitabine* (B) <3 months: 3 mg/kg oral soln once daily; 3 months-17 years, 6 mg/kg once daily; ≤33 kg: use oral soln, max 240 mg (24 ml); >33 kg: 200 mg cap once daily; max 240 mg/day; ≥18 years: 200 mg once daily; *CrCl 30-49 mL/min:* 200 mg q 48 hours; *CrCl 5-29 mL/min:* 200 mg q 72 hours; *CrCl <15 mL/min or dialysis:* 200 mg q 96 hours
>> **Emtriva** *Cap:* 200 mg
>> **Emtriva Oral Solution** *Oral soln:* 10 mg/ml (170 ml) (cotton candy)

▷ *lamivudine* (C)(G) <3 months: not established; 3 months-16 years: 4 mg/kg oral soln or tab bid; [tab] 14-<20 kg: 150 mg once daily or 75 mg bid; ≥20-<25 kg: 225 mg once daily or 75 mg in the AM and 150 mg in the PM; ≥25 kg: 300 mg once daily or 150 mg bid; max 8 mg/kg once daily or 150 mg bid or 300 mg once daily; >16 years: *CrCl ≥50 mL/min:* 300 mg qd or 150 mg bid; *CrCl >30-50 mL/min:* 150 mg qd; *CrCl 15-29:* first dose 150 mg, then 100 mg once daily; *CrCl 5-14 mL/min:* first dose 150 mg, then 50 mg qd; *CrCl <5 mL/min:* first dose 50 mg, then 25 mg once daily; max 8 mg/kg once daily or 150 mg bid
>> **Epivir** *Tab:* 150*, 300 mg
>> **Epivir Oral Solution** *Oral soln:* 10 mg/ml (240 ml) (strawberry-banana) (sucrose 3 gm/15 ml)

Comment: With renal impairment reduce *lamivudine* dose or extend dosing interval.

▷ *stavudine* (C)(G)birth-13 days: [tablet/oral solution] 0.5 mg/kg q 12 hours; >14 days, <30 kg: [tablet/oral solution] 1 mg/kg q 12 hours; ≥30-<60 kg: 30 mg q 12 hours; ≥60 kg: 40 mg q 12 hours; ≤60 kg: 30 mg q 12 hours; *If peripheral neuropathy develops:* discontinue; *After resolution, ≥60 kg:* may restart at 20 mg q 12 hours; *After resolution, ≤60 kg:* may restart at 15 mg q 12 hours; *if neuropathy returns:* consider permanent discontinuation; *CrCl 10-50 mL/min, ≥60 kg:* 20 mg q 12 hours; *CrCl 10-50 mL/min, ≥60 kg:* 15 mg q 12 hours; *Hemodialysis, ≥60 kg:* 20 mg q 24 hours; *Hemodialysis,* ≤*60 kg:* 15 mg q 24 hours; administer at the same time of day; *Hemodialysis:* administer at the end of dialysis

> **Zerit** *Cap:* 15, 20, 30, 40 mg
> **Zerit for Oral Solution** *Oral soln:* 1 mg/ml pwdr for reconstitution (fruit) (dye-free)

▷ *tenofovir disoproxil fumarate* (C) <2 years: not established; 2-12 years: 8 mg/kg once daily; >12 years, 35 kg: 300 mg once daily; mix oral pwdr with 2-4 oz soft food; max 300 mg once daily; *CrCl 30-49 mL/min:* max 300 mg q 48 hours; *CrCl 10-29:* max 300 mg q 72-96 hours; *Hemodialysis:* max 300 mg once every 7 days or after a total of 12 hours of dialysis; *CrCl <10 mL/min:* not recommended

> **Viread** *Tab:* 150, 200, 250, 300 mg; *Oral pwdr:* 40 mg/g (60 gm w. dosing scoop)

▷ *zidovudine* (C)(G) *Treatment of HIV-1 infection:* 4-<9 kg: 24 mg/kg/day divided bid or tid; ≥9-30 kg: 18 mg/kg/day divided bid or tid; ≥30 kg: 600 mg/day divided bid or tid; *Prevention of maternal-fetal neonatal transmission:* <*12 hours after birth until 6 weeks of age:* [Solution] 2 mg/kg q 6 hours until 6 weeks-of-age; [IV] 1.5 mg/kg infused over 30 minutes q 6 hours until 6 weeks-of-age; max 200 mg q 8 hours; *ESRD/dialysis:* max 100 mg q 6-8 hours; *Vertical transmission, severe anemia,* or *neutropenia:* see mfr pkg insert

> **Retrovir Tablets** *Tab:* 300 mg
> **Retrovir Capsules** *Cap:* 100 mg
> **Retrovir Syrup** *Syrup:* 50 mg/5 ml (strawberry)
> **Retrovir IV** *Vial:* 10 mg/ml after dilution (20 ml) (preservative-free)

Non-Nucleoside Reverse Transcriptase Inhibitors (NNRTIs)

▷ *delavirdine mesylate* (C) <16 years: not established; ≥16 years: 400 mg (4 x 100 mg or 2 x 200 mg) tablets tid in combination with other antiretroviral agents

> **Rescriptor** *Tab:* 100, 200 mg

Comment: The 100 mg **Rescriptor** tablets may be dispersed in water prior to consumption. To prepare a dispersion, add four 100 mg Rescriptor tablets to at least 3 ounces of water, allow to stand for a few minutes, and then stir until a uniform dispersion occurs. The dispersion should be consumed promptly. The glass should be rinsed with water and the rinse swallowed to ensure the entire dose is consumed. The 200 mg tablets should be taken as intact tablets, because they are not readily dispersed in water.

▷ *efavirenz* (D) ≤3 months: not established; >3 months, ≤3.5 kg: [tablet/capsule] 3.5-<5 kg: 100 mg once daily; 5-<7.5 kg: 150 mg once daily; 7.5-<15 kg: 200 mg once daily; 15-<20 kg: 250 mg once daily; 20-<25 kg: 300 mg once daily; 25-<32.5 kg: 350 once daily; 32.5-<40 kg: 400 mg once daily; >40 kg: 600 mg once daily; max 600 mg once daily

Comment: For children who cannot swallow capsules, the capsule contents can be administered with a small amount of food (applesauce, grape jelly, yogurt) or 2 tsp room temperature infant formula using the capsule sprinkle method of administration. See mfr pkg insert for instructions. Tablets should not be crushed or chewed. Administer at bedtime to limit CNS effects. Consider pretreatment with antihistamine to minimize rash.

> **Sustiva** *Tab:* 75, 150, 600, 800 mg; *Cap:* 50, 200 mg

▷ *etravirine* (B) <3 years: not recommended; ≥3 years, >16 kg: 16-< 20 kg: 100 mg bid; 20-<25 kg: 125 mg bid; 25-<30 kg: 150 mg bid; ≥30 kg: 200 mg (1 x 200 mg tablet or 2 x 100 mg tablets) bid following a meal; max 200 mg bid; take following a meal

> **Intelence** *Tab:* 25*, 100, 200 mg

▷ *nevirapine* (B)(G) <6 years: not recommended; 6-<18 years: BSA 0.58-0.83 kg/m²: 200 mg once daily; BSA 0.84-1.16 kg/m²: 300 mg once daily; BSA ≥1.17 kg/m²: 400 mg once daily; max 400 mg once daily; ≥18 years: initially one 200 mg tablet of immediate-release **Viramune** once daily for the first 14 days in combination with other antiretroviral agents; then one 400 mg tablet of **Viramune XR** once daily
Comment: Children must initiate therapy with immediate-release **Viramune** for the first 14 days; ≥15 days: [oral suspension/tablet]: 150 mg/m² once daily for 14 days, then 150 mg/m² bid. The 14-day lead-in period has been found to lessen the frequency of rash.
　　Viramune *Tab:* 200*mg
　　Viramune Oral Suspension *Oral susp:* 50 mg/5 ml (240 ml)
　　Viramune XR *Tab:* 100, 400 mg ext-rel
▷ *rilpivirine* (D) <12 years: not recommended; ≥12 years, >35 kg: 25 mg once daily; *If concomitant* **rifabutin**: 50 mg once daily: *If concomitant* **rifabutin** *stopped:* 25 mg once daily
　　Edurant *Tab:* 25 mg

Nucleoside and Non-Nucleoside Reverse Transcriptase Inhibitor (NRTI/NNRTI) Combinations

▷ **Atripla** (B) *efavirenz/emtricitabine/tenofovir disoproxil fumarate* <12 years: not recommended; ≥12 years, 40 kg: 1 tab once daily preferably at HS; take on an empty stomach; *Concomitant* **rifabutin**: >50 kg: take additional *efavirenz* 200 mg/day
　　Tab: efa 600 mg/*emtri* 200 mg/*teno dis fum* 300 mg
▷ **Complera** (B) *emtricitabine/tenofovir disoproxil fumarate/rilpivirine* <12 years, <35 kg: not established; ≥12 years, ≥35 kg: 1 tab once daily; *CrCl <50 mL/min:* not recommended; *Concomitant* **rifabutin**: take additional **ribavirin** 25 mg qd
　　Tab: emtri 200 mg/*teno dis* 300 mg/*rilpiv* 25 mg

Protease Inhibitors (PIs)

▷ *atazanavir* (B) <3 months: not recommended; ≥3 mos, 5 kg: [oral powder] 5-<15 kg: 200 mg (4 packets) plus *ritonavir* 80 mg once daily; 15-<25 kg: 250 mg (5 packets) plus *ritonavir* 80 mg once daily; ≥25 kg, unable to swallow capsules: 300 mg (6 packets) plus *ritonavir* once daily; 6 yrs, <15 kg: [capsule] 15-<20 kg: 150 mg plus *ritonavir* 100 mg once daily; 20-<40 kg: 200 mg plus *ritonavir* 100 mg once daily; ≥40 kg: 300 mg plus *ritonavir* 100 mg once daily; [capsule]15-<20 kg: 150 mg plus *ritonavir* 100 mg once daily; 20-<40 kg: 200 mg plus *ritonavir* 100 mg once daily; ≥40 kg: 300 mg plus *ritonavir* 100 mg once daily; max dose 400 mg once daily; *Treatment-naïve, ≥40 kg: Recommended regimen:* 300 mg plus *ritonavir* 100 mg once daily; *Unable to tolerate* **ritonavir**: 400 mg once daily; *In combination with* **efavirenz**: 400 mg plus *ritonavir* 100 mg once daily; *Treatment-experienced. ≥40 kg: Recommended regimen:* 300 mg plus *ritonavir* 100 mg once daily; *In combination with both an* H₂-*blocker* or *PPI and* **tenofovir**: 400 mg plus *ritonavir* 100 mg once daily; take with food
　　Reyataz *Cap:* 100, 150, 200, 300 mg; *Oral pwdr:* 50 mg/pkt (30/carton) (phenylalanine)
Comment: Administration of *atazanavir* with *rotinavir* is preferred. Dose for treatment-naïve children ≥13 years-of-age and ≥40 kg unable to tolerate *rotinavir*, administer 400 mg once daily. See mfr pkg insert for special dosing considerations when combining *atazanavir* with other retrovirals.

▷ *darunavir* (C)(G) <3 years: nor recommended; ≥3 years, 10 kg [oral solution/tablet/ capsule] *Treatment-naïve or experienced without **darunavir**-associated substitutions:* 10-<15 kg: 35 mg/kg once daily plus *ritonavir* 7 mg/kg once daily; 15-<30 kg: 600 mg plus *ritonavir* 100 mg once daily; 30-<40 kg: 675 mg plus *ritonavir* 100 mg once daily; ≥40 kg: 800 mg plus *ritonavir* 100 mg once daily; *Treatment-experienced with ≥1 **darunavir**-associated substitution(s):* 10-15 kg: 20 mg/kg bid plus *ritonavir* 3 mg/kg bid; 15-<30 kg: 375 mg plus *ritonavir* 48 mg bid; 30-<40 kg: 450 mg plus *ritonavir* 60 mg bid; ≥40 kg: 600 mg plus *ritonavir* 100 mg bid

    Prezista *Tab:* 75, 150, 600, 800 mg film-coat

    Prezista Oral Suspension *Susp:* 100 mg/ml (strawberry cream)

    Comment: **Prezista** is FDA approved for treatment of HIV-1-infected pregnant females and for the treatment of children >3 years-of-age in combination with *ritonavir* and other antiretrovirals.

    Comment: **Prezista** is FDA approved for treatment of HIV-1-infected pregnant females and for the treatment of children >3 years-of-age in combination with *ritonavir* and other antiretrovirals.

▷ *fosamprenavir* (C)(G) <4 weeks: not recommended; *Protease inhibitor-naïve, ≥4 weeks-18 years or protease inhibitor-experienced:* ≥6 months, <11 kg: 45 mg/kg plus *ritonavir* 7 mg/kg bid; 11-<15 kg: 30 mg/kg plus *ritonavir* 3 mg/kg bid; 15 kg-<20 kg: 23 mg/kg plus *ritonavir* 3 mg/kg bid; ≥20 kg: 18 mg/kg plus *ritonavir* 3 mg/kg bid; *Protease inhibitor-naïve, ≥2 years:* 30 mg/kg bid *without ritonavir:* max dose 700 mg plus *ritonavir* 100 mg bid; *Max dosing: Treatment-naïve:* 1,400 mg bid or 1,400 mg once daily plus *ritonavir* 200 mg once daily or 1,400 mg once daily plus *ritonavir* 100 mg once daily or 700 mg bid plus *ritonavir* 100 mg bid; *Protease inhibitor-experienced:* 700 mg bid plus *ritonavir* 100 mg bid

    Lexiva: *Tab: 700 mg film-coat*

    Lexiva Oral Suspension *Oral susp:* 50 mg/ml (225 ml) (grape-bubble gum-peppermint)

    Comment: *fosamprenavir* 1 ml is equivalent to approximately 43 mg of *amprenavir* 1 ml.

▷ *indinavir sulfate* (C) <18 years: not established (3-18 years, doses of 500 mg/m^2 every 8 hours have been used; see mfr pkg insert); ≥18 years: 800 mg q 8 hours; *Concomitant **rifabutin***: 1 gm q 8 hours and reduce *rifabutin* dose by half; *Hepatic insufficiency or concomitant **ketoconazole**, **itraconazole**, or **delavirdine**:* 600 mg q 8 hours; take with water on an empty stomach or with a light meal

    Crixivan *Cap:* 100, 200, 333, 400 mg

▷ *nelfinavir mesylate* (B) <2 years: not established; 2-13 years: 45-55 mg/kg bid or 25-35 mg/kg tid; take with a meal; max 2,500 mg/day; ≥13 years: 1250 mg (5 x 250 mg tablets or 2 x 625 mg tablets) bid or 750 mg (3 x 250 mg tablets) tid; take with a meal; may dissolve tablets in a small amount of water; max 2500 mg/day

    Viracept *Tab:* 250, 625 mg

    Viracept Oral Powder *Oral pwdr:* 50 mg/g (144 gm) (phenylalanine)

    Comment: The 250 mg **Viracept** tablets are interchangeable with oral powder, the 625 mg tablets are not.

▷ *raltegravir(as potassium)*(B) <4 weeks, <3 kg: not recommended; ≥4 weeks, 3-11 kg: [oral suspension] 3-<4 kg: 20 mg bid; 4-<6 kg: 30 mg bid; 6-<8 kg: 40 mg bid; 8-<11 kg: 60 mg bid; ≥11-<25 kg: [oral suspension/chewable tablet] 6 mg/kg/dose bid; see mfr pkg insert for dosage by weight;≥25 kg and unable to swallow tablet: [chewable tablet]25-<28 kg: 150 mg bid; 28-<40 kg: 200 mg bid; ≥40 kg: 300 mg bid; ≥6 years, ≥25 kg, able to swallow tablets: 400 mg film-coat tablet bid

Comment: Oral suspension, chewable tablets, and film-coated tablets are not bioequivalent. Chewable tablet max dose 300 mg bid. Film-coated tablets max dose 400 mg bid. Oral suspension max dose 100 mg bid.

> Isentress *Tab:* 400 mg film-coat; *Chew tab:* 25, 100*mg (orange-banana) (phenylalanine)

> Isentress Oral Suspension *Oral susp:* 100 mg/pkt pwdr for oral susp (banana)

▶ *ritonavir* (B) <1 month: not recommended; ≥1 month: 350-400 mg/m² bid; initiate at 250 mg/m² bid and titrate upward every 2-3 days by 50 mg/m² bid; max dose 600 mg bid

Comment: Lower doses of *ritonavir* have been used to boost other protease inhibitors but the *ritonavir* doses used for boosting have not been specifically approved in children.

> Norvir *Tab:* 100 mg film-coat; *Gel cap:* 100 mg (alcohol)

> Norvir Oral Solution *Oral soln:* 80 mg/ml, 600 mg/7.5 ml (8 oz) (pepper-mint-caramel) (alcohol)

> Comment: Norvir tablets should be swallowed whole. Take Norvir with meals. Patients may improve the taste of Norvir Oral Solution by mixing with chocolate milk, Ensure, or Advera within one hour of dosing. Dose reduction of Norvir is necessary when used with other protease inhibitors (*atazanavir, darunavir, fosamprenavir, saquinavir,* and *tipranavir*). Patients who take the 600 mg gel cap bid may experience more gastrointestinal side effects such as nausea, vomiting, abdominal pain, or diarrhea when switching from the gel cap to the tablet because of greater maximum plasma concentration (Cmax) achieved with the tablet. These adverse events (gastrointestinal or paresthesias) may diminish as treatment is continued.

▶ *saquinavir mesylate* (B) <16 years: not established; ≥16 years: 1 gm bid plus *ritona-vir* 100 mg bid (take both at the same time); *Treatment-naïve or switching from a delavirdine- or rilpivirine-containing regimen:* initially 500 mg bid x 7 days, then increase to 1 gm bid plus *ritonavir* 100 mg bid; take within 2 hours after a meal

> Fortovase *Tab/Cap:* 200 mg

> Invirase *Tab:* 500 mg; *Cap:* 200 mg

▶ *tipranavir* (C) <2 years: not recommended; 2-18 yrs: [capsule/oral solution] 14 mg/kg plus *ritonavir* 6 mg/kg bid or 375 mg/m² plus *ritonavir* 150 mg/m² bid; max 500 mg plus *ritonavir* 200 mg bid

> Aptivus *Gel cap:* 250 mg (alcohol)

> Aptivus Oral Solution *Oral soln:* 100 mg/ml (buttermint-butter toffee) (Vit E 116 IU/ml)

FUSION INHIBITORS—CCR5 CORECEPTOR ANTAGONISTS

▶ *enfuvirtide* (B) <6 years: not established; 6-16 years: administer 2 mg/kg SC bid; max 90 mg SC bid; rotate injection sites

> Fuzeon *Vial:* 90 mg/ml pwdr for SC inj after reconstitution (1 ml, 60 vials/kit) (preservative-free)

▶ *maraviroc* (B) <16 years: not established; ≥16 years: must be administered concomitant with other retrovirals; *Concomitant potent CYP3A inhibitors (with or without a potent CYP3A inducer) including protease inhibitors (except tipranavir/ritonavir), delavirdine, ketoconazole, itraconazole, clarithromycin, other potent CYP3A inhibitors (e.g., nefazodone, telithromycin):* CrCl ≥30 mL/min: 150 mg bid; CrCl <30 mL/min, dialysis: not recommended; *Potent CYP3A inducers (without a potent CYP3A* *inhibitor) including **efavirenz, rifampin, etravirine, carbamazepine, phenobarbital,** and **phenytoin:*** 300 mg bid; *CrCl ≥30 mL/min:* 600 mg bid; *<30 mL/min:* not recommended; *other concomitant agents, including **tipranavir/ritonavir, nevirapine, raltegravir, all NRTIs,** and **enfuvirtide:*** 300 mg bid

> Selzentry *Tab:* 150, 300 mg film-coat

BRAND NAMES, DOSING, AND DOSE FORMS: COMBINATION AGENTS

▷ Atripla (B) *efavirenz/emtricitabine/tenofovir disoproxil fumarate <12 years:* not established; *≥12 years, ≥40 kg:* 1 tablet once daily on an empty stomach; bedtime dosing may improve the tolerability of nervous system symptoms; *CrCl <50 mL/min:* not recommended
> *Tab:* efa 600 mg/emtri 200 mg/teno dis fum 300 mg film-coat

▷ Combivir (C)(G) *lamivudine/zidovudine <12 years:* not recommended; *≥12 years, ≥30 kg:* 1 tablet bid with food
> *Tab:* lami 150 mg/zido 300 mg

▷ Complera (B) *emtricitabine/tenofovir disoproxil fumarate/rilpivirine <12 years, <40 kg:* not recommended; *≥12 years, ≥40 kg:* 1 tablet once daily; *CrCl <50 mL/min:* not recommended
> *Tab:* emtri 200 mg/teno dis 300 mg/rilpiv 25 mg

▷ Descovy (D) *emtricitabine/tenofovir alafenamide <12 years, <35 kg:* not recommended; *≥12 years, ≥35 kg:* 1 tablet once daily with or without food; *CrCl <30 mL/min:* not recommended
> *Tab:* emtri 200 mg/teno ala 25 mg

Comment: Patients with HIV-1 should be tested for the presence of chronic hepatitis B virus (HBV) before initiating antiretroviral therapy. **Descovy** is not approved for the treatment of chronic HBV infection, and the safety and efficacy of **Descovy** have not been established in patients co-infected with HIV-1 and HBV.

▷ Epzicom (B) *abacavir sulfate/lamivudine <25 kg:* use individual components; *≥25 kg:* one tablet once daily; *Mild hepatic impairment or CrCl <50 mL/min:* not recommended
> *Tab:* aba 600 mg/lami 300 mg

▷ Evotaz (B) *atazanavir/cobicistat <18 years:* not established; *≥18 years:* 1 tab once daily
> *Tab:* ataz 600 mg/cobi 300 mg

▷ Genvoya (B) *elvitegravir/cobicistat/emtricitabine/tenofovir alafenamide <12 years:* not established; *≥12 years, ≥35 kg:* 1 tab once daily; *Severe hepatic impairment or CrCl <30 mL/min:* not recommended; take with food
> *Tab:* elvi 150 mg/cobi 150 mg/emtri 200 mg/teno 10 mg

▷ Kaletra, Kaletra Oral Solution(C)(G) *lopinavir/ritonavir* dose calculation is based on the *lopinavir* component; *<14 days:* not recommended; *14 days-6 months:* 16 mg/kg bid; *≥6 months-12 years:* [tablet/capsule/solution] 7-<15 kg: 12 mg/kg bid (13 mg/kg plus *nevirapine*); 15-40 kg: 10 mg/kg bid (11 mg/kg plus *nevirapine*); >40 kg, >12 years: *lopinavir* 400 mg bid (533 mg bid) for patients who are not receiving *nevirapine* or *efavirenz*; **Kaletra** should not be used in combination with NNRTIs in children <6 months-of-age; see mfr pkg insert for BSA-based dosing; swallow whole, do not crush or chew; take with or without food
> *Tab:* Kaletra 100/25 lopin 100 mg/riton 25 mg
> Kaletra 200/50 lopin 200 mg/riton 50 mg *Oral soln:* lopin 80 mg/riton 20 mg per ml, lopin 400 mg/riton 500 mg per 5 ml (160 ml) (cotton candy) (alcohol 42.4%)

➢ **Odefsey (D)** *emtricitabine/rilpivirine/tenofovir alafenamide* <12 years, <35 kg: not established; ≥12 years: 1 tab once daily with food; *CrCl <30 mL/min:* not recommended
> *Tab:* emtri 200 mg/*rilpi* 25 mg/*teno alafen* 25 mg

➢ **Prezcobix (C)** *darunavir/cobicistat* <18 years: not recommended; ≥18 years: 1 tab once daily; *Treatment-naïve and treatment-experienced with no* **darunavir** *resistance-associated substitution:* 800 mg once daily <u>plus</u> **ritonavir** 100 mg once daily; *Treatment-experienced with at least one* **darunavir** *resistance associated substitution:* 600 mg bid <u>plus</u> **ritonavir** 100 mg bid; take with food; *CrCl <70 mL/min:* not recommended
> *Tab:* darun 800 mg/*cobi* 150 mg

➢ **Stribild (B)(G)** *elvitegravir/cobicistat/emtricitabine/tenofovir disoproxil fumarate* <18 years: not established; ≥18 years: 1 tab once daily; *CrCl <70 mL/min:* not recommended; *if CrCl declines to <50 mL/min during treatment:* discontinue; *Severe hepatic impairment:* not recommended
> *Tab:* elvi 150 mg/*cobi* 150 mg/*emtri* 200 mg/*teno dis fum* 300 mg

➢ **Triumeq (C)(G)** *abacavir sulfate/dolutegravir/lamivudine* <18 years: not established; ≥18 years: 1 tab once daily
> *Tab:* aba 600 mg/*dolu* 50 mg/*lami* 300 mg

➢ **Trizivir (C)(G)** *abacavir sulfate/lamivudine/zidovudine* <40 kg: not recommended; ≥40 kg: 1 tab bid
> *Tab:* aba 300 mg/*lami* 150 mg/*zido* 300 mg

➢ **Truvada (B)** *emtricitabine/tenofovir disoproxil fumarate* <17 kg: not established; 17-<22 kg: 100/150 once daily; 22-<28 kg: 133/200 once daily; 28-35 kg: 167/250 once daily; ≥35 kg: 200/300 once daily
> *Tab:* **Truvada 100/150** emt 100 mg/*teno* 150 mg
> **Truvada 133/200** emt 133 mg/*teno* 200 mg
> **Truvada 167/250** emt 167 mg/*teno* 250 mg
> **Truvada 200/300** emt 200 mg/*teno* 300 mg

Comment: **Truvada** is indicated for treatment of HIV-1 infection and pre-exposure prophylaxis (PrEP) to reduce the risk of sexually acquired HIV-1 in high-risk patients ≥18 years-of-age in combination with safe sex practices.

☐ HUMAN PAPILLOMAVIRUS (HPV, VENEREAL WART)

PROPHYLAXIS

Comment: Administer IM in deltoid. Administer a 3-dose series; 1st dose females (10-25 years-of-age) and males (9-15 years-of-age); 2nd dose: 1-2 months after first dose; 3rd dose: 6 months after first dose. HPV vaccination is indicated for the prevention of cervical, vulvar, vaginal, and anal cancers. Register pregnant patients exposed to **Gardasil** by calling 800-986-8999.

➢ *bivalent human papillomavirus types 16 and 18 vaccine, aluminum adsorbed* (B) <10 years: not applicable; ≥10 years: administer in the deltoid; 1st dose 0.5 ml IM on elected date; then, 2nd dose 0.5 ml IM 1 month later; then, 3rd dose 0.5 ml IM 6 months after the first dose (5 months after 2nd dose)
> **Cervarix**
> *Vial:* susp for IM inj (single dose; prefilled syringe) (preservative-free)

▷ *quadrivalent human papillomavirus types 6, 11, 16, and 18 vaccine, recombinant, aluminum adsorbed* (B) <9 years: not applicable; ≥9 years: administer in the deltoid or upper thigh; 1st dose 0.5 ml IM on elected date; then, 2nd dose 0.5 ml IM 2 months later; then, 3rd dose 0.5 ml IM 6 months after the first dose (4 months after 2nd dose)
    Gardasil
        Vial: susp for IM inj (single dose; prefilled syringe w. needles or tip caps) (preservative-free)

▷ *quadrivalent human papillomavirus types 6, 11, 16, 18, 31, 33, 45, 52, and 58 vaccine, recombinant, aluminum adsorbed* (B) <9 years: not applicable; 9-26 years-of-age: administer in the deltoid or thigh; 1st dose 0.5 ml IM on elected date; then, 2nd dose 0.5 ml IM 2 months later; then, 3rd dose 0.5 ml IM 6 months after the 1st dose (4 months after 2nd dose)
    Gardasil 9
        Vial: susp for IM inj (0.5 ml single dose; prefilled syringe w. needles or tip caps) (preservative-free)

TREATMENT

see **Wart: Venereal** *page 449*

HYPERHIDROSIS (PERSPIRATION, EXCESSIVE)

▷ *aluminum chloride* (NE) 20% solution apply q HS; wash treated area the following morning; after 1-2 treatments, may reduce frequency to 1-2 times/week
    Drysol *Soln:* 35, 60 ml (alcohol 93%) cont-rel
Comment: Apply to clean dry skin (e.g., underarms). Do not apply to broken, irritated, or recently shaved skin.

HYPERHOMOCYSTEINEMIA

Comment: Elevated homocysteine is associated with cognitive impairment, vascular dementia, and dementia of the Alzheimer's type.

HOMOCYSTEINE-LOWERING NUTRITIONAL SUPPLEMENTS

▷ *L-methylfolate calcium (as metafolin)/pyridoxyl 5-phosphate/methyl-cobalamin* (NE) <12 years: not recommended; ≥12 years: take 1 cap daily
    Metanx *Cap: metafo* 3 mg/*pyrid* 35 mg/*methyl* 2 mg (gluten-free, yeast-free, lactose-free)
Comment: **Metanx** is indicated as adjunct treatment of endothelial dysfunction and/or hyperhomocysteinemia in patients who have lower extremity ulceration.

▷ *L-methylfolate calcium (as metafolin)/methylcobalamin/N-acetylcysteine* (NE) <12 years: not recommended; ≥12 years: take 1 cap daily
    Cerefolin *Cap: metafo* 5.6 mg/*methyl* 2 mg/*N-ace* 600 mg (gluten-free, yeast-free, lactose-free)
Comment: **Cerefolin** is indicated in the dietary management of patients treated for early memory loss, with emphasis on those at risk for neurovascular oxidative stress, hyperhomocysteinemia, mild to moderate cognitive impairment with or without vitamin B_{12} deficiency, vascular dementia, or Alzheimer's disease.

▭ HYPERKALEMIA (POTASSIUM EXCESS)

HYPERKALEMIA CATION EXCHANGE RESINS

Comment: Normal serum K$^+$ range is approximately 3.5-5.5 mEq/L. Hyperkalemia is associated with cardiac dysrhythmias and metabolic acidosis. Risk factors include kidney disease, heart failure, and drugs that inhibit the renin-angiotensin-aldosterone system (RAAS) including ACEIs, ARBs, direct renin inhibitors, and aldosterone antagonists. Cation exchange resins are not for emergency treatment of life-threatening hyperkalemia, severe constipation, bowel obstruction or impaction. May cause GI irritability, ulceration, necrosis, sodium retention, hypocalcemia, hypomagnesemia, fecal impaction, ischemic colitis. Avoid non-absorbable cation-donating antacids and laxatives (e.g., *magnesium hydroxide, aluminum hydroxide*). Concomitant sorbitol should be avoided because it may cause intestinal necrosis.

▶ *patiromer sorbitex calcium* (B) <18 years: not established; ≥18 years: initially 8.4 gm once daily; adjust dosage as prescribed based on potassium concentration and target range; may increase dosage at 1-week (or longer) intervals in increments of 8.4 gm; max dose 25.2 gm once daily; prepare immediately prior to administration; do not take in dry form; administer with food; measure 1/3 cup of water and pour half into a glass; then add **Veltassa** and stir; add the remaining water and stir well; the powder will not dissolve and the mixture will look cloudy; add more water as needed for desired consistency; do not heat or mix with heated food or fluids

Veltassa *Pkt:* 8, 4, 16.8, 25.2 gm pwdr for oral susp, 30 single-use pkts/carton

Comment: Take **Veltassa** at least 3 hours before or 3 hours after any other medicine taken by mouth. Store packets in the refrigerator. It stored at room temperature, product must be used within 3 months.

▶ *sodium polystyrene sulfonate* (C)(G) Use 1 gm/1 mEq of K$^+$ as basis of calculation; see mfr literature

Kayexalate *Susp:* 15 gm 1-4 times daily; *Rectal Enema:* 30-50 gm in 100 ml every 6 hours

▭ HYPERPARATHYROIDISM

▶ *calcifediol* (C)(G) <18 years: not established; ≥18 years: 1 cap daily

Rayaldee *Cap:* 30 mcg ext-rel

Comment: **Rayaldee** is indicated for the prevention and treatment of secondary hyperparathyroidism associated with chronic kidney disease (CKD), stage 3 or 4 and serum total 25-hydroxyvitamin D levels <30 mg/mL.

▶ *paricalcitol* (C)(G) <18 years: not established; ≥18 years: administer 0.04-1 mcg/kg (2.8-7 mcg) IV bolus, during dialysis, no more than every other day; may be increased by 2-4 mcg every 2-4 weeks; monitor serum calcium and phosphorus during dose adjustment periods; if Ca x P >75, immediately reduce dose or discontinue until these levels normalize; discard unused portion of single-use vials immediately

Zemplar *Vial:* 2, 5 mcg/ml soln for inj

Comment: **Zemplar** is indicated for the prevention and treatment of secondary hyperparathyroidism associated with chronic kidney disease, stage 5.

HYPERPHOSPHATEMIA

PHOSPHATE BINDERS

Comment: Monitor for development of hypercalcemia. Normal serum PO_4^- is 2.5-4.5 mg/dL and normal serum calcium is 8.5-10.5 mg/dL.

➤ *calcium acetate* (C)(G) <12 years: not established; ≥12 years: initially 2 tabs or caps with each meal; then, titrate gradually to keep serum phosphate at <6 mg/dL; usual maintenance is 3-4 tabs or caps with each meal

    PhosLo *Tab:* 667 mg; *Cap:* 667 mg

➤ *lanthanum carbonate* (C) <12 years: not established; ≥12 years: initially 750 mg to 1.5 gm per day in divided doses; take with meals; titrate at 2-3-week intervals in increments of 750 mg/day based on serum phosphate; usual range 1.5-3 gm/day; usual max 3,750 mg/day

    Fosrenol *Chew tab:* 250, 500, 750 mg; 1 g

➤ *sevelamer* (C) <12 years: not established; ≥12 years: for patients not taking a phosphate binder, take tid with meals; swallow whole; titrate by 1 tab per meal at 1 week intervals to keep serum phosphorus 3.5-5.5 mg/dL; switching from calcium acetate to *sevelamer*, see mfr pkg insert. *Serum phosphorus* >5.5 to >7.5 mg/dL: 800 mg tid; *Serum phosphorus* 7.5-9: 1.2-1.6 gm tid

    Renagel *Tab:* 400, 800 mg
    Renvela *Tab:* 800 mg

 ## HYPERPIGMENTATION

Comment: Depigmenting agents may be used for hyperpigmented skin conditions including chloasma, melasma, freckles, senile lentigines. Limit treatments to small areas at one time. Sunscreen ≥30 SPF recommended.

➤ *hydroquinone* (C)(G) apply sparingly to affected area and rub in bid

    Lustra *Crm:* 4% (1, 2 oz) (sulfites)
    Lustra AF *Crm:* 4% (1, 2 oz) (sunscreen, sulfites)

➤ *monobenzone* (C) apply sparingly to affected area and rub in bid-tid; depigmentation occurs in 1-4 months

    Benoquin *Crm:* 20% (1.25 oz)

➤ *tazarotene* (X)(G) <12 years: not recommended; ≥12 years: apply daily at HS

    Avage Cream *Crm:* 0.1% (30 gm)
    Tazorac Cream *Crm:* 0.05, 0.1% (15, 30, 60 gm)
    Tazorac Gel *Gel:* 0.05, 0.1% (30, 100 gm)

➤ *tretinoin* (C) <12 years: not recommended; ≥12 years: apply daily at HS

    Avita *Crm/Gel:* 0.025% (20, 45 gm)
    Renova *Crm:* 0.02% (40 gm); 0.05% (40, 60 gm)
    Retin-A Cream *Crm:* 0.025, 0.05, 0.1% (20, 45 gm)
    Retin-A Gel *Gel:* 0.01, 0.025% (15, 45 gm) (alcohol 90%)
    Retin-A Liquid *Liq:* 0.05% (28 ml) (alcohol 55%)
    Retin-A Micro *Microspheres:* 0.04, 0.1% (20, 45 gm)

COMBINATION AGENTS

➤ *hydroquinone/fluocinolone/tretinoin* (C) <12 years: not recommended; ≥12 years: apply sparingly to affected area and rub in daily at HS

Tri-Luma *Crm: hydro* 4%/*fluo* 0.01%/*tretin* 0.05% (30 gm) (parabens, sulfites)

▷ *hydroquinone/padimate O/oxybenzone/octyl methoxycinnamate* (C) <12 years: not recommended; ≥12 years: apply sparingly to affected area and rub in bid
Glyquin *Crm:* 4% (1 oz jar)

▷ *hydroquinone/ethyl dihydroxypropyl PABA/dioxybenzone/oxybenzone* (C) <12 years: not recommended; ≥12 years: apply sparingly to affected area and rub in bid; max 2 months
Solaquin *Crm: hydro* 2%/*PABA* 5%/*dioxy* 3%/*oxy* 2% (1 oz) (sulfites)

▷ *hydroquinone/padimate/dioxybenzone/oxybenzone* (C) <12 years: not recommended; ≥12 years: apply sparingly to affected area and rub in bid; max 2 months
Solaquin Forte *Crm: hydro* 4%/*pad* 0.5%/*dioxy* 3%/*oxy* 2% (1 oz) (sunscreen, sulfites)

▷ *hydroquinone/padimate/dioxybenzone* (C) <12 years: not recommended; ≥12 years: apply sparingly to affected area and rub in bid; max 2 months
Solaquin Forte *Gel: hydro* 4%/*pad* 0.5%/*dioxy* 3% (1 oz) (alcohol, sulfites)

HYPERPROLACTINEMIA

DOPAMINE RECEPTOR AGONIST

▷ *dostinex* (B)(G) <12 years: not established; ≥12 years: initial therapy is 0.25 mg twice a week; may increase by 0.25 mg twice weekly up to 1 mg twice a week according to the patient's serum prolactin level; dose increases should not occur more than every 4 weeks; after a normal serum prolactin level has been maintained for 6 months, may be discontinued, with periodic monitoring of serum prolactin level to determine if/when treatment should be reinstituted
Cabergoline *Tab:* 0.5 mg
Comment: Cabergoline is indicated to treat hyperprolactinemia disorders due to idiopathic *or* pituitary adenoma.

HYPERTENSION: PRIMARY, ESSENTIAL

see JNC-8 Recommendations page 461

BETA-BLOCKERS: CARDIOSELECTIVE

Comment: Cardioselective beta-blockers are less likely to cause bronchospasm, peripheral vasoconstriction, *or* hypoglycemia than non-cardioselective beta-blockers.

▷ *acebutolol* (B)(G) <12 years: not recommended; ≥12 years: initially 400 mg in 1-2 divided doses; usual range 200-800 mg/day; max 1.2 gm/day in 2 divided doses
Sectral *Cap:* 200, 400 mg

▷ *atenolol* (D)(G) <12 years: not recommended; ≥12 years: initially 50 mg daily; may increase after 1-2 weeks to 100 mg daily; max 100 mg/day
Tenormin *Tab:* 25, 50, 100 mg

▷ *betaxolol* (C) <12 years: not recommended; ≥12 years: initially 10 mg daily; may increase to 20 mg/day after 7-14 days; usual max 20 mg/day
Kerlone *Tab:* 10*, 20 mg

▷ *bisoprolol* (C) <12 years: not recommended; ≥12 years: 5 mg daily; max 20 mg daily
Zebeta *Tab:* 5*, 10 mg

➤ *metoprolol succinate* (C)(G) <12 years: not recommended; ≥12 years: initially
12.5-25 mg in a single dose daily; increase weekly if needed; reduce if symptomatic
bradycardia occurs; max 400 mg/day
  Toprol-XL *Tab:* 25*, 50*, 100*, 200*mg ext-rel
➤ *metoprolol tartrate* (C)(G) <12 years: not recommended; ≥12 years: initially 25-50
mg bid; increase weekly if needed; max 400 mg/day
  Lopressor *Tab:* 25, 37.5, 50, 75, 100 mg
➤ *nebivolol* (C)(G) <12 years: not recommended; ≥12 years: initially 5 mg daily; may
increase at 2 week intervals; max 40 mg/day
  Bystolic *Tab:* 2.5, 5, 10, 20 mg

BETA-BLOCKERS: NON-CARDIOSELECTIVE

Comment: Non-cardioselective beta-blockers are more likely to cause bronchospasm,
peripheral vasoconstriction, and/or hypoglycemia than cardioselective beta-blockers.
➤ *nadolol* (C)(G) <12 years: not recommended; ≥12 years: initially 40 mg daily; usual
maintenance 40-80 mg daily; max 320 mg/day
  Corgard *Tab:* 20*, 40*, 80*, 120*, 160*mg
➤ *penbutolol* (C) <12 years: not recommended; ≥12 years: 20 mg once daily
  Levatol *Tab:* 20*mg
➤ *pindolol* (B)(G) <12 years: not recommended; ≥12 years: initially 5 mg bid; may
increase after 3-4 weeks in 10 mg increments; max 60 mg/day
  Pindolol *Tab:* 5, 10 mg
  Visken *Tab:* 5, 10 mg
➤ *propranolol* (C)(G)
  Inderal <12 years: initially 1 mg/kg/day; usual range 2-4 mg/kg/day in 2 divided
  doses; max 16 mg/kg/day; ≥12 years: initially 40 mg bid; usual maintenance
  120-240 mg/day; max 640 mg/day
    Tab: 10*, 20*, 40*, 60*, 80*mg
  Inderal LA <12 years: not recommended; ≥12 years: initially 80 mg daily in a
  single dose; increase q 3-7 days; usual range 120-160 mg/day; max 320 mg/day
  in a single dose
    Cap: 60, 80, 120, 160 mg sust-rel
  InnoPran XL <12 years: not recommended; ≥12 years: initially 80 mg q HS;
  max 120 mg/day
    Cap: 80, 120 mg ext-rel
➤ *timolol* (C)(G) <12 years: not recommended; ≥12 years: initially 10 mg bid; increase
weekly if needed; usual maintenance 20-40 mg/day; max 60 mg/day in 2 divided doses
  Blocadren *Tab:* 5, 10*, 20*mg

BETA-BLOCKER: (NON-CARDIOSELECTIVE)/ALPHA-1 BLOCKER COMBINATIONS

➤ *carvedilol* (C)
  Coreg <1 years: not recommended; ≥1 years: initially 6.25 mg bid; may increase
  at 1-2-week intervals to 12.5 mg bid; max 25 mg bid
    Tab: 3.125, 6.25, 12.5, 25 mg
  Coreg CR <18 years: not recommended; ≥18 years: initially 20 mg once daily
  for 2 weeks; may increase at 1-2-week intervals; max 80 mg once daily
    Tab: 10, 20, 40, 80 mg cont-rel
➤ *carteolol* (C) <12 years: not recommended; ≥12 years: initially 2.5 mg daily, gradually increase to 5 or 10 mg daily; usual maintenance 2.5-5 mg daily

      Cartrol
        Tab: 2.5, 5 mg
➤ *labetalol* (C)(G) <12 years: not recommended; ≥12 years: initially 100 mg bid; increase after 2-3 days if needed; usual maintenance 200-400 mg bid; max 2.4 gm/day
        Normodyne *Tab:* 100*, 200*, 300 mg
        Trandate *Tab:* 100*, 200*, 300*mg

DIURETICS

Thiazide Diuretics

➤ *chlorthalidone* (B)(G) <12 years: not established; ≥12 years: initially 15 mg daily; may increase to 30 mg once daily based on clinical response; max 45-60 mg/day
        Chlorthalidone *Tab:* 25, 50 mg **Thalitone** *Tab:* 15 mg
➤ *chlorothiazide* (B)(G) <6 months: up to 15 mg/lb/day in 2 divided doses; ≥6 months-<12 years: 10 mg/lb/day in 2 divided doses; ≥12 0.5-1 gm/day in a single <u>or</u> divided doses; max 2 gm/day
        Diuril *Tab:* 250*, 500*mg; *Oral susp:* 250 mg/5 ml (237 ml)
➤ *hydrochlorothiazide* (B)(G)
        Esidrix <12 years: not recommended; ≥12 years: 25 mg once daily; usual max 100 mg/day 25-100 mg once daily
          Tab: 25, 50, 100 mg
        Hydrochlorothiazide <12 years: not recommended; ≥12 years: 12.5 mg once daily; usual max 50 mg/day
          Tab: 25*, 50*mg
        Microzide <12 years: not recommended; ≥12 years: 12.5 mg once daily; usual max 50 mg/day
          Cap: 12.5 mg
➤ *polythiazide* (C) <12 years: not recommended; ≥12 years: 2-4 mg once daily
        Renese *Tab:* 1, 2, 4 mg

Potassium-Sparing Diuretics

➤ *amiloride* (B)(C) <12 years: not recommended; ≥12 years: initially 5 mg; may increase to 10 mg; max 20 mg
        Midamor *Tab:* 5 mg
➤ *spironolactone* (D)(G) <12 years: not recommended; ≥12 years: initially 50-100 mg in a single <u>or</u> divided doses; titrate at 2-week intervals
        Aldactone *Tab:* 25, 50*, 100*mg
➤ *triamterene* (B) <12 years: not recommended; ≥12 years: 100 mg bid; max 300 mg
        Dyrenium *Cap:* 50, 100 mg

Loop Diuretics

➤ *bumetanide* (C)(G) <18 years: not recommended; ≥18 years: 0.5-2 mg daily; may repeat at 4-5-hour intervals; max 10 mg/day
        Bumex *Tab:* 0.5*, 1*, 2*mg
    Comment: *bumetanide* is contraindicated with sulfa drug allergy.
➤ *ethacrynic acid* (B)(G) ≤1 month: not recommended; >1 month-12 years: initially 25 mg/day; then adjust dose in 25 mg increments; >12 years: max 50-200 mg once daily
        Edecrin *Tab:* 25, 50 mg

▷ *ethacrynate sodium* (B)(G) <1 month: not recommended; ≥1 month-12 years: use the smallest effective dose; initially 25 mg; then careful stepwise increments in dosage of 25 mg to achieve effective maintenance; ≥12 years: administer smallest dose required to produce gradual weight loss (about 1-2 pounds per day); onset of diuresis usually occurs at 50-100 mg in children ≥12 years; after diuresis has been achieved, the minimally effective dose (usually 50-200 mg/day) may be administered on a continuous or intermittent dosage schedule; dose titrations are usually in 25-50 mg increments to avoid derangement electrolyte and water excretion; the patient should be weighed under standard conditions before and during administration of *ethacrynate sodium;* the following schedule may be helpful in determining the lowest effective dose; *Day 1:* 50 mg once daily after a meal; *Day 2:* 50 mg bid after meals, if necessary; *Day 3:* 100 mg in the morning and 50-100 mg following the afternoon or evening meal, depending upon response to the morning dose; a few patients may require initial and maintenance doses as high as 200 mg bid; these higher doses, which should be achieved gradually, are most often required in patients with severe, refractory edema

    Sodium Edecrin *Vial:* 50 mg single dose

    Comment: **Sodium Edecrin** is more potent than more commonly used loop and thiazide diuretics. Treatment of the edema associated with congestive heart failure, cirrhosis of the liver, and renal disease, including the nephrotic syndrome, short-term management of ascites due to malignancy, idiopathic edema, and lymphedema, short-term management of hospitalized pediatric patients, other than infants, with congenital heart disease or the nephrotic syndrome. IV **Sodium Edecrin** is indicated when a rapid onset of diuresis is desired, for example, in acute pulmonary edema or when gastrointestinal absorption is impaired or oral medication is not practical.

▷ *furosemide* (C)(G) <12 years: not recommended; ≥12 years: initially 40 mg bid

    Lasix *Tab:* 20, 40*, 80 mg; *Oral Soln:* 10 mg/ml (2, 4 oz w. dropper)

    Comment: *furosemide* is contraindicated with sulfa drug allergy.

▷ *torsemide* (B) <12 years: not recommended; ≥12 years: 5 mg once daily; may increase to 10 mg once daily

    Demadex *Tab:* 5*, 10*, 20*, 100*mg

Other Diuretics

▷ *indapamide* (B) <12 years: not recommended; ≥12 years: initially 1.25 mg once daily; may titrate dosage upward q 4 weeks if needed; max 5 mg/day

    Lozol *Tab:* 1.25, 2.5 mg

    Comment: *indapamide* is contraindicated with sulfa drug allergy.

▷ *metolazone* (B) <12 years: not recommended; ≥12 years: 2.5-5 mg qd

    Zaroxolyn

      Tab: 2.5, 5, 10 mg

    Comment: *metolazone* is contraindicated with sulfa drug allergy.

DIURETIC COMBINATIONS

▷ *amiloride/hydrochlorothiazide* (B)(G) <12 years: not recommended; ≥12 years: initially 1 tab daily; may increase to 2 tabs/day in a single or divided doses

    Moduretic *Tab:* amil 5 mg/hydro 50 mg*

▷ *spironolactone/hydrochlorothiazide* (D)(G)

    Aldactazide 25 <12 years: not recommended; ≥12 years: usual maintenance 50-100 mg in a single or divided doses

Tab: spiro 25 mg/*hctz* 25 mg

Aldactazide 50 <12 years: not recommended; ≥12 years: usual maintenance 50-100 mg in a single <u>or</u> divided doses

Tab: spiro 50 mg/*hydro* 50 mg

▷ *triamterene/hydrochlorothiazide* (C)(G)

Dyazide <12 years: not recommended; ≥12 years: 1-2 caps once daily

Cap: triam 37.5 mg/*hctz* 25 mg

Maxzide <12 years: not recommended; ≥12 years: 1 tab once daily

Tab: triam 75 mg/*hctz* 50 mg*

Maxzide-25 <12 years: not recommended; ≥12 years: 1-2 tabs once daily

Tab: triam 37.5 mg/*hctz* 25 mg*

ANGIOTENSIN CONVERTING ENZYME INHIBITORS (ACEIs)

Comment: Black patients receiving ACEI monotherapy have been reported to have a higher incidence of angioedema compared to non-Blacks. Non-Blacks have a greater decrease in BP when ACEIs are used compared to Black patients.

▷ *benazepril* (D)(G) <12 years: not recommended; ≥12 years: initially 10 mg daily; usual maintenance 20-40 mg/day in 1-2 divided doses; usual max 80 mg/day

Lotensin *Tab:* 5, 10, 20, 40 mg

▷ *captopril* (D)(G) <12 years: not recommended; ≥12 years: initially 25 mg bid-tid; after 1-2 weeks increase to 50 mg bid-tid

Capoten *Tab:* 12.5*, 25*, 50*, 100*mg

▷ *enalapril* (D) <12 years: not recommended; ≥12 years: initially 5 mg daily; usual dosage range 10-40 mg/day; max 40 mg/day

Epaned Oral Solution *Oral soln:* 1 mg/ml (150 ml) (mixed berry)

Vasotec (G) *Tab:* 2.5*, 5*, 10, 20 mg

▷ *fosinopril* (D) <6 years, <50 kg: not recommended; ≥6-12 years, >50 kg: 5-10 mg once daily; ≥12 years: initially 10 mg daily; usual maintenance 20-40 mg/day in a single <u>or</u> divided doses; max 80 mg/day

Monopril *Tab:* 10*, 20, 40 mg

▷ *lisinopril* (D)

Prinivil <6 years, <50 kg: not recommended; ≥6-12 years: initially 10 mg once daily; usual range 20-40 mg/day

Tab: 5*, 10*, 20*, 40 mg

Qbrelis Oral Solution <6 years, GFR <30 mL/min: not recommended; ≥6-12 years, GFR >30 mL/min: initially 0.07 mg/kg, max 5 mg; adjust according to BP up to a max 0.61 mg/kg (40 mg) once daily; administer as a single dose once daily

Oral soln: 1 mg/ml (150 ml)

Zestril <12 years: not recommended; ≥12 years: initially 10 mg daily; usual range 20-40 mg/day

Tab: 2.5, 5*, 10, 20, 30, 40 mg

▷ *moexipril* (D) <12 years: not recommended; ≥12 years: initially 7.5 mg daily; usual range 15-30 mg/day in 1-2 divided doses; max 30 mg/day

Univasc *Tab:* 7.5*, 15*mg

▷ *perindopril* (D) <12 years: not recommended; ≥12 years: 2-8 mg daily-bid; max 16 mg/day

Aceon *Tab:* 2*, 4*, 8*mg

▷ *quinapril* (D) <12 years: not recommended; ≥12 years: initially 10 mg once daily; usual maintenance 20-80 mg daily in 1-2 divided doses
    Accupril *Tab:* 5*, 10, 20, 40 mg
▷ *ramipril* (D)(G) <12 years: not recommended; ≥12 years: initially 2.5 mg bid; usual maintenance 2.5-20 mg in 1-2 divided doses
    Altace *Tab/Cap:* 1.25, 2.5, 5, 10 mg
▷ *trandolapril* (C; D in 2nd, 3rd) <12 years: not recommended; ≥12 years: initially 1-2 mg once daily; adjust at 1-week intervals; usual range 2-4 mg in 1-2 divided doses; max 8 mg/day
    Mavik *Tab:* 1*, 2, 4 mg

ANGIOTENSIN II RECEPTOR BLOCKERS (ARBs)

▷ *azilsartan medoxomil* (D) <12 years: not recommended; ≥12 years: *Monotherapy, not volume depleted:* 80 mg once daily; *Volume-depleted (concomitant high-dose diuretic):* initially 40 mg once daily
    Edarbi *Tab:* 40, 80 mg
▷ *candesartan* (D)(G) <12 years: not recommended; ≥12 years: initially 16 mg daily; range 8-32 mg in 1-2 divided doses
    Atacand *Tab:* 4, 8, 16, 32 mg
▷ *eprosartan* (D)(G) <12 years: not recommended; ≥12 years: initially 400 mg bid <u>or</u> 600 mg once daily; max 800 mg/day
    Teveten *Tab:* 400, 600 mg
▷ *irbesartan* (D)(G) <12 years: not recommended; ≥12 years: initially 150 mg daily; titrate up to 300 mg
    Avapro *Tab:* 75, 150, 300 mg
▷ *losartan* (D)(G) <12 years: not recommended; ≥12 years: initially 50 mg daily; max 100 mg/day
    Cozaar *Tab:* 25, 50, 100 mg
▷ *olmesartan medoxomil* (D)(G) <6 years: not recommended; ≥6-16 years: 20-35 kg: initially 10 mg once daily; after 2 weeks, may increase to max 20 mg once daily; ≥6-16 years: >35 kg: initially 20 mg once daily; after 2 weeks, may increase to max 40 mg once daily; ≥16 years: initially 20 mg once daily; after 2 weeks, may increase to 40 mg once daily
    Benicar *Tab:* 5, 20, 40 mg
▷ *telmisartan* (D)(G) <12 years: not recommended; ≥12 years: initially 40 mg once daily
    Micardis *Tab:* 20, 40, 80 mg
▷ *valsartan* (D)(G) <12 years: not recommended; ≥12 years: initially 80 mg once daily; may increase to 160 <u>or</u> 320 mg once daily after 2-4 weeks; usual range 80-320 mg/day
    Diovan *Tab:* 40*, 80, 160, 320 mg

CALCIUM CHANNEL BLOCKERS (CCBs)

Benzothiazepines

▷ *diltiazem* (C)(G)
    Cardizem <12 years: not established; ≥12 years: initially 30 mg qid; may increase gradually every 1-2 days; max 360 mg/day in divided doses
    Tab: 30, 60, 90, 120 mg

Cardizem CD <12 years: not established; ≥12 years: initially 120-180 mg daily; adjust at 1-2-week intervals; max 480 mg/day
    Cap: 120, 180, 240, 300, 360 mg ext-rel
Cardizem LA <12 years: not established; ≥12 years: initially 180-240 mg daily; titrate at 2-week intervals; max 540 mg/day
    Tab: 120, 180, 240, 300, 360, 420 mg ext-rel
Cardizem SR <12 years: not established; ≥12 years: initially 60-120 mg bid; adjust at 2-week intervals; max 360 mg/day
    Cap: 60, 90, 120 mg sust-rel
Cartia XT <12 years: not established; ≥12 years: initially 180 or 240 mg once daily; max 540 mg once daily
    Cap: 120, 180, 240, 300 mg ext-rel
Dilacor XR <12 years: not established; ≥12 years: initially 180 or 240 mg in AM; usual range 180-480 mg/day; max 540 mg/day
    Cap: 120, 180, 240 mg ext-rel
Tiazac (G) <12 years: not established; ≥12 years: initially 120-240 mg daily; adjust at 2-week intervals; usual max 540 mg/day
    Cap: 120, 180, 240, 300, 360, 420 mg ext-rel
➤ *diltiazem maleate* (C) <12 years: not recommended; ≥12 years: initially 120-180 mg daily; adjust at 2-week intervals; usual range 120-480 mg daily
    Tiamate *Cap:* 120, 180, 240 mg ext-rel

Dihydropyridines

➤ *amlodipine* (C) <12 years: not established; ≥12 years: initially 5 mg once daily; max 10 mg/day
    Norvasc *Tab:* 2.5, 5, 10 mg
➤ *clevidipine butyrate* (C) <18 years: not recommended; ≥18 years: administer by IV infusion; initially 1-2 mg/hour; double dose at 90-second intervals until BP approaches goal; then titrate slower; adjust at 5-10-minute intervals; maintenance 4-6 mg/hour; usual max, 16-32 mg/hour; do not exceed 1,000 ml (21 mg/hour for 24 hours) due to lipid load
    Cleviprex *Vial:* 0.5 mg/ml soln for IV infusion (single use, 50, 100 ml) (lipids)
    Comment: **Cleviprex** is indicated to reduce blood pressure when oral therapy is not feasible or desirable. **Cleviprex** is contraindicated with egg or soy allergy.
➤ *felodipine* (C)(G) <12 years: not recommended; ≥12 years: initially 5 mg daily; usual range 2.5-10 mg daily; adjust at 2-week intervals; max 10 mg/day
    Plendil *Tab:* 2.5, 5, 10 mg ext-rel
➤ *isradipine* (C)
    DynaCirc <12 years: not recommended; ≥12 years: initially 2.5 mg bid; adjust in increments of 5 mg/day at 2-4-week intervals; max 20 mg/day
        Cap: 2.5, 5 mg
    DynaCirc CR <12 years: not recommended; ≥12 years: initially 5 mg daily; adjust in increments of 5 mg/day at 2-4-week intervals; max 20 mg/day
        Tab: 5, 10 mg cont-rel
➤ *nicardipine* (C)(G)
    Cardene <18 years: not recommended; ≥18 years: initially 20 mg tid; adjust at intervals of at least 3 days; max 120 mg/day
        Cap: 20, 30 mg
    Cardene SR <12 years: not recommended; ≥12 years: 30-60 mg bid
        Cap: 30, 45, 60 mg sust-rel

▷ *nifedipine* (C)(G)

 Adalat <12 years: not recommended; ≥12 years: initially 10 mg tid; usual range 10-20 mg tid; max 180 mg/day
  Cap: 10, 20 mg
 Adalat CC <12 years: not recommended; ≥12 years: initially 10 mg tid; usual range 10-20 mg tid; max 180 mg/day
  Cap: 30, 60, 90 mg ext-rel
 Afeditab CR <12 years: not recommended; ≥12 years: initially 30 mg once daily; titrate over 7-14 days; max 90 mg/day
  Cap: 30, 60 mg ext-rel
 Procardia <12 years: not recommended; ≥12 years: initially 10 mg tid; titrate over 7-14 days: max 30 mg/dose and 180 mg/day in divided doses
  Cap: 10, 20 mg
 Procardia XL <12 years: not recommended; ≥12 years: initially 30-60 mg daily; titrate over 7-14 days; max dose 90 mg/day
  Tab: 30, 60, 90 mg ext-rel

▷ *nisoldipine* (C)

 Sular <12 years: not recommended; ≥12 years: initially 20 mg daily; may increase by 10 mg weekly; usual maintenance 20-40 mg/day; max 60 mg/day
  Tab: 10, 20, 30, 40 mg ext-rel

Diphenylalkylamines

▷ *verapamil* (C)(G)

 Calan <12 years: not recommended; ≥12 years: 80-120 mg tid; may titrate up; usual max 360 mg in divided doses
  Tab: 40, 80*, 120*mg
 Calan SR <12 years: not recommended; ≥12 years: initially 120 mg in the AM; may titrate up; max 480 mg/day in divided doses
  Cplt: 120, 180*, 240*mg sust-rel
 Covera HS <12 years: not recommended; ≥12 years: initially 180 mg q HS; titrate to 240 mg; then to 360 mg; then to 480 mg if needed
  Tab: 180, 240 mg ext-rel
 Isoptin <12 years: not recommended; ≥12 years: initially 80-120 mg tid
  Tab: 40, 80, 120 mg
 Isoptin SR <12 years: not recommended; ≥12 years: initially 120-180 mg in the AM; may increase to 240 mg in the AM; then 180 mg q 12 hours or 240 mg in the AM and 120 mg in the PM; then 240 mg q 12 hours
  Tab: 120, 180*, 240*mg sust-rel
 Verelan <12 years: not recommended; ≥12 years: initially 240 mg once daily; adjust in 120 mg increments; max 480 mg/day
  Cap: 120, 180, 240, 360 mg sust-rel
 Verelan PM <12 years: not recommended; ≥12 years: initially 200 mg q HS; may titrate upward to 300 mg; then 400 mg if needed
  Cap: 100, 200, 300 mg ext-rel

ALPHA-1 ANTAGONISTS

Comment: Educate the patient regarding potential side effects of hypotension when taking an alpha-1 antagonist, especially with first dose ("first dose effect"). Start at lowest dose and titrate upward.

▶ *doxazosin* (C)(G) <12 years: not recommended; ≥12 years: initially 1 mg once daily at HS; increase dose slowly every 2 weeks if needed; max 16 mg/day
Cardura *Tab:* 1*, 2*, 4*, 8*mg **Cardura XL** *Tab:* 4, 8 mg

▶ *prazosin* (C)(G) <12 years: not recommended; ≥12 years: first dose at HS, 1 mg bid-tid; increase dose slowly; usual range 6-15 mg/day in divided doses; max 20-40 mg/day
Minipress *Cap:* 1, 2, 5 mg

▶ *terazosin* (C) <12 years: not recommended; ≥12 years: 1 mg q HS, then increase dose slowly; usual range 1-5 mg q HS; max 20 mg/day
Hytrin *Cap:* 1, 2, 5, 10 mg

CENTRAL ALPHA-AGONISTS

▶ *clonidine* (C)
Catapres <12 years: not recommended; ≥12 years: initially 0.1 mg bid; usual range 0.2-0.6 mg/day in divided doses; max 2.4 mg/day; *Tab:* 0.1*, 0.2*, 0.3*mg
Catapres-TTS <12 years: not recommended; ≥12 years: 0.1 mg patch weekly; increase after 1-2 weeks if needed; max 0.6 mg/day
Patch: 0.1, 0.2 mg/day (12/carton); 0.3 mg/day (4/carton)
Kapvay (G) <12 years: not recommended; ≥12 years: initially 0.1 mg bid; usual range 0.2-0.6 mg/day in divided doses; max 2.4 mg/day; *Tab:* 0.1, 0.2 mg
Nexiclon XR <12 years: not recommended; ≥12 years: initially 0.18 mg (2 ml) suspension or 0.17 mg tab once daily; usual max 0.52 mg (6 ml suspension) once daily
Tab: 0.17, 0.26 mg ext-rel; *Oral susp:* 0.09 mg/ml ext-rel (4 oz)

▶ *guanabenz* (C)(G) <12 years: not recommended; ≥12 years: initially 4 mg bid; may increase by 4-8 mg/day every 1-2 weeks; max 32 mg/day
Tab: 4, 8 mg

▶ *guanfacine* (B)(G) <12 years: not recommended; ≥12 years: initially 1 mg/day q HS; may increase to 2 mg/day q HS; usual max 3 mg/day
Tenex *Tab:* 1, 2 mg

▶ *methyldopa* (B)(G) <12 years: initially 10 mg/kg/day in 2-4 divided doses; max 65 mg/kg/day or 3 gm/day, whichever is less; ≥12 years: initially 250 mg bid-tid; titrate at 2-day intervals; usual maintenance 500 mg/day to 2 gm/day; max 3 gm/day
Aldomet *Tab:* 125, 250, 500 mg; *Oral susp:* 250 mg/5 ml (473 ml)

ALDOSTERONE RECEPTOR BLOCKER

▶ *eplerenone* (B) <12 years: not recommended; ≥12 years: 25-50 mg daily; may increase to 50 mg bid; max 100 mg/day
Inspra *Tab:* 25, 50 mg
Comment: Contraindicated with concomitant potent CYP3A4 inhibitors. Risk of hyperkalemia with concomitant ACE-I or ARB. Monitor serum potassium at baseline, 1 week, and 1 month. Caution with serum Cr >2 mg/dL (male) or >1.8 mg/dL (female) and/or *CrCl <50 mL/min*, and DM with proteinuria.

PERIPHERAL ADRENERGIC BLOCKER

▶ *guanethidine* (C) <12 years: not recommended; ≥12 years: initially 10 mg daily; may adjust dose at 5-7 day intervals; usual range 25-50 mg/day

Ismelin *Tab:* 10, 25 mg

DIRECT RENIN INHIBITOR

▷ *aliskiren* (D) <18 years: not recommended; ≥18 years: initially 150 mg once daily; max 300 mg/day
Tekturna *Tab:* 150, 300 mg

PERIPHERAL VASODILATORS

▷ *hydralazine* (C)(G) <12 years: initially 0.75 mg/kg/day in 4 divided doses; increase gradually over 3-4 weeks; max 7.5 mg/kg/day or 2,000 mg/day; ≥12 years: initially 10 mg qid x 2-4 days; then increase to 25 mg qid for remainder of 1st week; then increase to 50 mg qid; max 300 mg/day
Tab: 10, 25, 50, 100 mg
▷ *minoxidil* (C) <12 years: initially 0.2 mg/kg daily; may increase in 50%-100% increments every 3 days; usual range 0.25-1 gm/kg/day; max 50 mg/day; ≥12 years: initially 5 mg daily; may increase at 3-day intervals to 10 mg/day, then 20 mg/day, then 40 mg/day; usual range 10-40 mg/day; max 100 mg/day
Loniten *Tab:* 2.5*, 10*mg

ACEI/DIURETIC COMBINATIONS

▷ *benazepril*/*hydrochlorothiazide* (D)
Lotensin HCT <12 years: not recommended; ≥12 years: 1 tab once daily; titrate individual components
Tab: Lotensin HCT 5/6.25 *benaz* 5 mg/*hctz* 6.25 mg*
Lotensin HCT 10/12.5 *benaz* 10 mg/*hctz* 12.5 mg*
Lotensin HCT 20/12.5 *benaz* 20 mg/*hctz* 12.5 mg*
Lotensin HCT 20/25 *benaz* 20 mg/*hctz* 25 mg*
▷ *captopril*/*hydrochlorothiazide* (D)(G)
Capozide <12 years: not recommended; ≥12 years: 1 tab once daily; titrate individual components
Tab: Capozide 25/15 *capt* 25 mg/*hctz* 15 mg*
Capozide 25/25 *capt* 25 mg/*hctz* 25 mg*
Capozide 50/15 *capt* 50 mg/*hctz* 15 mg*
Capozide 50/25 *capt* 50 mg/*hctz* 25 mg*
▷ *enalapril*/*hydrochlorothiazide* (D)
Vaseretic <12 years: not recommended; ≥12 years: 1 tab once daily; titrate individual components
Tab: Vaseretic 5/12.5 *enal* 5 mg/*hctz* 12.5 mg
Vaseretic 10/25 *enal* 10 mg/*hctz* 25 mg
▷ *lisinopril*/*hydrochlorothiazide* (D)
Prinzide <12 years: not recommended; ≥12 years: 1 tab once daily; titrate individual components
Tab: Prinzide 10/12.5 *lis* 10 mg/*hctz* 12.5 mg
Prinzide 20/12.5 *lis* 20 mg/*hctz* 12.5 mg
Prinzide 20/25 *lis* 20 mg/*hctz* 25 mg
Zestoretic <12 years: not recommended; ≥12 years: 1 tab once daily; titrate individual components; *CrCl <40 mL/min:* not recommended
Tab: Zestoretic 10/12.5 *lis* 10 mg/*hctz* 12.5 mg
Zestoretic 20/12.5 *lis* 20 mg/*hctz* 12.5 mg*

            Zestoretic 20/25 *lis* 20 mg/*hctz* 25 mg
▷ *moexipril/hydrochlorothiazide* (D)
    Uniretic <12 years: not recommended; ≥12 years: 1 tab once daily; titrate individual components
        Tab: **Uniretic 7.5/12.5** *moex* 7.5 mg/*hctz* 12.5 mg*
            Uniretic 15/12.5 *moex* 15 mg/*hctz* 12.5 mg*
            Uniretic 15/25 *moex* 15 mg/*hctz* 25 mg*
▷ *quinapril/hydrochlorothiazide* (D)
    Accuretic <12 years: not recommended; ≥12 years: 1 tab once daily; titrate individual components
        Tab: **Accuretic 10/12.5** *quin* 10 mg/*hctz* 12.5 mg*
            Accuretic 20/12.5 *quin* 20 mg/*hctz* 12.5 mg*
            Accuretic 20/25 *quin* 20 mg/*hctz* 25 mg*

ARB/DIURETIC COMBINATIONS

▷ *azilsartan/chlorthalidone* (D)
    Edarbyclor <18 years: not recommended; ≥18 years: 1 tab once daily; titrate individual components
        Tab: **Edarbyclor 40/12.5** *azil* 40 mg/*chlor* 12.5 mg
            Edarbyclor 40/25 *azil* 40 mg/*chlor* 25 mg
▷ *candesartan/hydrochlorothiazide* (D) <12 years: not recommended; ≥12 years: 1 tab once daily; titrate individual components
    Atacand HCT
        Tab: **Atacand HCT 16/12.5** *cande* 16 mg/*hctz* 12.5 mg
            Atacand HCT 32/12.5 *cande* 32 mg/*hctz* 12.5 mg
▷ *eprosartan/hydrochlorothiazide* (D)
    Teveten HCT <12 years: not recommended; ≥12 years: 1 tab once daily; titrate individual components
        Tab: **Teveten HCT 600/12.5** *epro* 600 mg/*hctz* 12.5 mg
            Teveten HCT 600/25 *epro* 600 mg/*hctz* 25 mg
▷ *irbesartan/hydrochlorothiazide* (D)
    Avalide <12 years: not recommended; ≥12 years: 1 tab once daily; titrate individual components
        Tab: **Avalide 150/12.5** *irbes* 150 mg/*hctz* 12.5 mg
            Avalide 300/12.5 *irbes* 300 mg/*hctz* 12.5 mg
▷ *losartan/hydrochlorothiazide* (D)(G)
    Hyzaar <12 years: not recommended; ≥12 years: 1 tab once daily; titrate individual components
        Tab: **Hyzaar 50/12.5** *losar* 50 mg/*hctz* 12.5 mg
            Hyzaar 100/12.5 *losar* 100 mg/*hctz* 12.5 mg
            Hyzaar 100/25 *losar* 100 mg/*hctz* 25 mg
▷ *olmesartan medoxomil/hydrochlorothiazide* (D)(G)
    Benicar HCT <12 years: not recommended; ≥12 years: 1 tab once daily; titrate individual components
        Tab: **Benicar HCT 20/12.5** *olme* 20 mg/*hctz* 12.5 mg
            Benicar HCT 40/12.5 *olme* 40 mg/*hctz* 12.5 mg
            Benicar HCT 40/25 *olme* 40 mg/*hctz* 25 mg
▷ *telmisartan/hydrochlorothiazide* (D)(G)
    Micardis HCT <12 years: not recommended; ≥12 years: 1 tab once daily; titrate individual components

    Tab: **Micardis HCT 40/12.5** *telmi* 40 mg/*hctz* 12.5 mg
           Micardis HCT 80/12.5 *telmi* 80 mg/*hctz* 12.5 mg
           Micardis HCT 80/25 *telmi* 80 mg/*hctz* 25 mg

➤ *valsartan/hydrochlorothiazide* (D)

    Diovan HCT <12 years: not recommended; ≥12 years: 1 tab once daily; titrate individual components

    Tab: **Diovan HCT 80/12.5** *vals* 80 mg/*hctz* 12.5 mg
           Diovan HCT 160/12.5 *vals* 160 mg/*hctz* 12.5 mg
           Diovan HCT 160/25 *vals* 160 mg/*hctz* 25 mg
           Diovan HCT 320/12.5 *vals* 320 mg/*hctz* 12.5 mg
           Diovan HCT 320/25 *vals* 320 mg/*hctz* 25 mg

CENTRAL ALPHA-AGONIST/DIURETIC COMBINATIONS

➤ *clonidine/chlorthalidone* (C)

    Combipres <12 years: not recommended; ≥12 years: 1 tab daily-bid

    Tab: **Combipres 0.1** *clon* 0.1 mg/*chlorthal* 15 mg*
           Combipres 0.2 *clon* 0.2 mg/*chlorthal* 15 mg*
           Combipres 0.3 *clon* 0.3 mg/*chlorthal* 15 mg*

➤ *methyldopa/hydrochlorothiazide* (C)(G)

    Aldoril <12 years: not recommended; ≥12 years: initially **Aldoril 15** bid-tid <u>or</u> **Aldoril 25** bid; titrate individual components

    Tab: **Aldoril 15** *meth* 250 mg/*hctz* 15 mg
           Aldoril 25 *meth* 250 mg/*hctz* 25 mg
           Aldoril D30 *meth* 500 mg/*hctz* 30 mg
           Aldoril D50 *meth* 500 mg/*hctz* 50 mg

BETA-BLOCKER (CARDIOSELECTIVE)/DIURETIC COMBINATIONS

➤ *atenolol/chlorthalidone* (D)(G)

    Tenoretic <12 years: not recommended; ≥12 years: initially *tenoretic* 50 mg once daily; may increase to *tenoretic* 100 mg once daily

    Tab: **Tenoretic 50/25** *aten* 50 mg/*chlor* 25 mg*
           Tenoretic 100/25 *aten* 100 mg/*chlor* 25 mg

➤ *bisoprolol/hydrochlorothiazide* (C)

    Ziac <12 years: not recommended; ≥12 years: initially one 2.5/6.25 mg tab daily; adjust at 2 week intervals; max two 10/6.25 mg tabs daily

    Tab: **Ziac 2.5** *biso* 2.5 mg/*hctz* 6.25 mg
           Ziac 5 *biso* 5 mg/*hctz* 6.25 mg
           Ziac 10 *biso* 10 mg/*hctz* 6.25 mg

➤ *metoprolol succinate/hydrochlorothiazide* (C)

    Lopressor HCT <12 years: not recommended; ≥12 years: titrate individual components

    Tab: **Lopressor HCT 50/25** *meto succ* 50 mg/*hctz* 25 mg*
           Lopressor HCT 100/25 *meto succ* 100 mg/*hctz* 25 mg*
           Lopressor HCT 100/50 *meto succ* 100 mg/*hctz* 50 mg*

➤ *metoprolol succinate/ext-rel hydrochlorothiazide* (C)

    Dutoprol <12 years: not established; ≥12 years: titrate individual components; may titrate to max 200/25 mg once daily

    Tab: **Dutoprol 25/12.5** *meto succ* 25 mg/*ext-rel hctz* 12.5 mg
           Dutoprol 50/12.5 *meto succ* 50 mg/*ext-rel hctz* 12.5 mg

Dutoprol 100/12.5 *meto succ* 100 mg/*ext-rel hctz* 12.5 mg

BETA-BLOCKER (NON-CARDIOSELECTIVE)/DIURETIC COMBINATIONS

▷ *nadolol/bendroflumethiazide* (C)
    Corzide <12 years: not recommended; ≥12 years: titrate individual components
        Tab: **Corzide 40/5** *nado* 40 mg/*bend* 5 mg*
            Corzide 80/5 *nado* 80 mg/*bend* 5 mg*
▷ *propranolol/hydrochlorothiazide* (C)(G)
    Inderide <12 years: not recommended; ≥12 years: titrate individual components
        Tab: **Inderide 40/25** *prop* 40 mg/*hctz* 25 mg*
            Inderide 80/25 prop 80 mg/hctz 25 mg*
            Inderide LA titrate individual components
        Cap: **Inderide LA 80/50** *prop* 80 mg/*hctz* 50 mg sust-rel
            Inderide LA 120/50 *prop* 120 mg/*hctz* 50 mg sust-rel
            Inderide LA 160/50 *prop* 160 mg/*hctz* 50 mg sust-rel
▷ *timolol/hydrochlorothiazide* (C)
    Timolide <12 years: not recommended; ≥12 years: usual maintenance 2 tabs/
    day in a single <u>or</u> 2 divided doses
        Tab: *timo* 10 mg/*hctz* 25 mg

BETA-BLOCKER (CARDIOSELECTIVE)/ARB COMBINATION

▷ *nebivolol/valsartan* (X) <12 years: not recommended; ≥12 years: 1 tab daily; may
    initiate when inadequately controlled on ***nebivolol*** 10 mg <u>or</u> ***valsartan*** 80 mg
        Byvalson *Tab:* *nebi* 5 mg/*val* 80 mg

ALPHA-1 ANTAGONIST/DIURETIC COMBINATIONS

▷ *prazosin/polythiazide* (C)
    Minizide <12 years: not recommended; ≥12 years: titrate individual
    components
        Cap: **Minizide 1** *praz* 1 mg/*poly* 0.5 mg
            Minizide 2 *praz* 2 mg/*poly* 0.5 mg
            Minizide 5 *praz* 5 mg/*poly* 0.5 mg

PERIPHERAL ADRENERGIC BLOCKER/HCTZ COMBINATIONS

▷ *guanethidine/hydrochlorothiazide* (C)
    Esimil <12 years: not recommended; ≥12 years: titrate individual components
        Tab: **Esimil 10/25** *guan* 1 mg/*hctz* 25 mg

ACEI/CCB COMBINATIONS

▷ *amlodipine/benazepril* (D)
    Lotrel <12 years: not recommended; ≥12 years: titrate individual components
        Cap: **Lotrel 2.5/10** *amlo* 2.5 mg/*benaz* 10 mg
            Lotrel 5/10 *amlo* 5 mg/*benaz* 10 mg
            Lotrel 5/20 *amlo* 5 mg/*benaz* 20 mg
            Lotrel 10/20 *amlo* 10 mg/*benaz* 20 mg
            Lotrel 5/40 *amlo* 5 mg/*benaz* 40 mg
            Lotrel 10/40 *amlo* 10 mg/*benaz* 40 mg

▷ *amlodipine/perindopril* (D)
  Prolastin <12 years: not recommended; ≥12 years: titrate individual components
    Cap: **Prolastin 2.5/3.5** *amlo* 2.5 mg/*peri* 3.5 mg
      Prolastin 5/7 *amlo* 5 mg/*peri* 7 mg
      Prolastin 5/14 *amlo* 5 mg/*peri* 14 mg
▷ *enalapril/diltiazem* (D)
  Teczem <12 years: not recommended; ≥12 years: titrate individual components
    Tab: **Teczem** *enal* 5 mg/*dil* 180 mg ext-rel
▷ *enalapril/felodipine* (D)
  Lexxel <12 years: not recommended; ≥12 years: initially 1 tab daily; after 1-2 weeks may increase to 2 tabs/day; titrate individual components
    Tab: **Lexxel 5/2.5** *enal* 5 mg/*felo* 2.5 mg ext-rel
      Lexxel 5/5 *enal* 5 mg/*felo* 5 mg ext-rel
▷ *perindopril/amlodipine* (D)
  Prestalia <12 years: not recommended; ≥12 years: titrate individual components; max 14/10 once daily
    Tab: **Prestalia 3.5/2.5** *peri* 3.5 mg/*amlo* 2.5 mg
      Prestalia 7/5 *peri* 7 mg/*amlo* 5 mg
      Prestalia 14/10 *peri* 14 mg/*amlo* 10 mg
▷ *trandolapril/verapamil* (D)
  Tarka <12 years: not recommended; ≥12 years: titrate individual components
    Tab: **Tarka 1/240** *tran* 1 mg/*ver* 240 mg ext-rel
      Tarka 2/180 *tran* 2 mg/*ver* 180 mg ext-rel
      Tarka 2/240 *tran* 2 mg/*ver* 240 mg ext-rel
      Tarka 4/240 *tran* 4 mg/*ver* 240 mg ext-rel

DRI/HCTZ COMBINATIONS

▷ *aliskiren/hydrochlorothiazide* (D) <12 years: not recommended; ≥12 years: initially *aliskiren* 150 mg once daily; max *aliskiren* 300 mg/day
  Tekturna HCT
    Tab: **Tekturna HCT 150/12.5** *alisk* 150 mg/*hctz* 12.5 mg
      Tekturna HCT 150/25 *alisk* 150 mg/*hctz* 25 mg
      Tekturna HCT 300/12.5 *alisk* 300 mg/*hctz* 12.5 mg
      Tekturna HCT 300/25 *alisk* 300 mg/*hctz* 25 mg

DRI/ARB COMBINATIONS

▷ *aliskiren/valsartan* (D)
  Valturna <12 years: not recommended; ≥12 years: initially 150/160 once daily; may increase to max 300/320 once daily
    Tab: **Valturna 150/160** *alisk* 150 mg/*vals* 160 mg
      Valturna 300/320 *alisk* 300 mg/*vals* 320 mg

DRI/CCB COMBINATIONS

▷ *aliskiren/amlodipine* (D)
  Tekamlo <12 years: not recommended; ≥12 years: initially 150/5 once daily; may increase to max 300/10 once daily

    Tab: **Tekamlo 150/5** *alisk* 150 mg/*amlo* 5 mg
          Tekamlo 150/10 *alisk* 150 mg/*amlo* 10 mg
          Tekamlo 300/5 *alisk* 300 mg/*amlo* 5 mg
          Tekamlo 300/10 *alisk* 300 mg/*amlo* 10 mg

DRI/CCB/HCTZ COMBINATIONS

▷ *aliskiren/amlodipine/hydrochlorothiazide* (D)
    Amturnide <12 years: not recommended; ≥12 years: initially 150/5/12.5 once
    daily; may increase to max 300/10/25 once daily
        Tab: **Amturnide 150/5/12.5** *alisk* 150 mg/*amlo* 5 mg/*hctz* 12.5 mg
            Amturnide 300/5/12.5 *alisk* 300 mg/*amlo* 5 mg/*hctz* 12.5 mg
            Amturnide 300/5/25 *alisk* 300 mg/*amlo* 5 mg/*hctz* 25 mg
            Amturnide 300/10/25 *alisk* 300 mg/*amlo* 10 mg/*hctz* 25 mg

HYPERTENSION

ARB/CCB COMBINATIONS

▷ *amlodipine/valsartan medoxomil* (D)(G)
    Exforge <12 years: not recommended; ≥12 years: 1 tab daily; titrate individual
    components at 1-week intervals; max 10/320 daily
        Tab: **Exforge 5/160** *amlo* 5 mg/*vals* 160 mg
            Exforge 5/320 *amlo* 5 mg/*vals* 320 mg
            Exforge 10/160 *amlo* 10 mg/*vals* 160 mg
            Exforge 10/320 *amlo* 10 mg/*vals* 320 mg
▷ *amlodipine/olmesartan* (D)(G)
    Azor <12 years: not recommended; ≥12 years: titrate individual components
        Tab: **Azor 5/20** *amlo* 5 mg/*olme* 20 mg
            Azor 10/20 *amlo* 10 mg/*olme* 20 mg
            Azor 5/40 *amlo* 5 mg/*olme* 40 mg
            Azor 10/40 *amlo* 10 mg/*olme* 40 mg
▷ *telmisartan/amlodipine* (D)
    Twynsta <12 years: not recommended; ≥12 years: initially 40/5 once daily;
    titrate at 1 week intervals; max 80/10 once daily
        Tab: **Twynsta 40/5** *telmi* 40 mg/*amlo* 5 mg
            Twynsta 40/10 *telmi* 40 mg/*amlo* 10 mg
            Twynsta 80/5 *telmi* 80 mg/*amlo* 5 mg
            Twynsta 80/10 *telmi* 80 mg/*amlo* 10 mg

ARB/CCB/HCTZ COMBINATIONS

▷ *amlodipine/valsartan medoxomil/hydrochlorothiazide* (D)(G)
    Exforge HCT: <12 years: not recommended; ≥12 years: initially 5/160/12.5 once
    daily; may titrate at 1-week intervals to max 10/320/25 once daily
        Tab: **Exforge HCT 5/160/12.5** *amlo* 5 mg/*vals* 160 mg/*hctz* 12.5 mg
            Exforge HCT 5/160/25 *amlo* 5 mg/*vals* 160 mg/*hctz* 25 mg
            Exforge HCT 10/160/12.5 *amlo* 10 mg/*vals* 160 mg/*hctz* 12.5 mg
            Exforge HCT 10/160/25 *amlo* 10 mg/*vals* 160 mg/*hctz* 25 mg
            Exforge HCT 10/320/25 *amlo* 10 mg/*vals* 320 mg/*hctz* 25 mg

▷ *olmesartan medoxomil/amlodipine/hydrochlorothiazide* (D)(G)

Tribenzor: <12 years: not recommended; ≥12 years: initially 40/5/12.5 once daily; may titrate at 1-week intervals to max 40/10/25 daily

Tab: **Tribenzor 40/5/12.5** *olme* 40 mg/*amlo* 5 mg/*hctz* 12.5 mg
Tribenzor 40/5/25 *olme* 40 mg/*amlo* 5 mg/*hctz* 25 mg
Tribenzor 40/10/12.5 *olme* 40 mg/*amlo* 10 mg/*hctz* 12.5 mg
Tribenzor 40/10/25 *olme* 40 mg/*amlo* 10 mg/*hctz* 25 mg

OTHER COMBINATION AGENTS

▷ *clonidine/chlorthalidone* (C)

Clorpres <12 years: not recommended; ≥12 years: initially 0.1/15 once daily; may titrate to max 0.3/15 bid

Tab: **Clorpres 0.1/15** *clon* 0.1 mg/*chlor* 15 mg
Clorpres 0.2/15 *clon* 0.2 mg/*chlor* 15 mg
Clorpres 0.3/15 *clon* 0.3 mg/*chlor* 15 mg

▷ *reserpine/hydroflumethiazide* (C)

Salutensin <12 years: not recommended; ≥12 years: initially 1.25/25 once daily; may titrate to 1.25/25 bid <u>or</u> 1.25/50 once daily

Tab: **Salutensin 1.25/25** *enal* 1.25 mg/*hydro* 25 mg
Salutensin 1.25/50: *enal* 1.25 mg/*hydro* 50 mg

ANTIHYPERTENSION/ANTILIPID COMBINATIONS

CCB/Statin Combinations

▷ *amlodipine/atorvastatin* (X)

Caduet <10 years: not established; ≥10 years (female post menarche) select according to blood pressure and lipid values; titrate *amlodipine* over 7-14 days; titrate *atorvastatin* according to monitored lipid values; max *amlodipine* 10 mg/day and max *atorvastatin* 80 mg/day; refer to contraindications and precautions for CCB and statin therapy

Tab: **Caduet 2.5/10** *amlo* 2.5 mg/*ator* 10 mg
Caduet 2.5/20 *amlo* 2.5 mg/*ator* 20 mg
Caduet 5/10 *amlo* 5 mg/*ator* 10 mg
Caduet 5/20 *amlo* 5 mg/*ator* 20 mg
Caduet 5/40 *amlo* 5 mg/*ator* 40 mg
Caduet 5/80 *amlo* 5 mg/*ator* 80 mg
Caduet 10/10 *amlo* 10 mg/*ator* 10 mg
Caduet 10/20 *amlo* 10 mg/*ator* 20 mg
Caduet 10/40 *amlo* 10 mg/*ator* 40 mg
Caduet 10/80 *amlo* 10 mg/*ator* 80 mg

HYPERTHYROIDISM

▷ *methimazole* (D) <12 years: initially 0.4 mg/kg/day in 3 divided doses; maintenance 0.2 mg/kg/day <u>or</u> 1/2 initial dose; ≥12 years: initially 15-60 mg/day in 3 divided doses; maintenance 5-15 mg/day

Tapazole *Tab:* 5*, 10*mg

Comment: *methimazole* potentiates anticoagulants. Contraindicated in nursing mothers.

➤ *propylthiouracil (ptu) (D)(G)*

Propyl-Thyracil <6 years: not recommended; ≥6-10 years: initially 50-150 mg/day or 5-7 mg/kg/day in 3 divided doses; >10 years: initially 150-300 mg/day or 5-7 mg/kg/day in 3 divided doses; *maintenance:* 0.2 mg/kg/day or 1/2-2/3 of initial dose; initially 100-900 mg/day in 3 divided doses; maintenance usually 50-600 mg/day in 2 divided doses

Tab: 50*mg

Comment: Preferred agent in pregnancy. Side effects include dermatitis, nausea, agranulocytosis, and hypothyroidism. Should be taken regularly for 2 years. Do not discontinue abruptly.

BETA-ADRENERGIC BLOCKER

➤ *propranolol (C)(G)*

Inderal <12 years: not recommended; ≥12 years: 40-240 mg once daily
Tab: 10*, 20*, 40*, 60*, 80*mg
Inderal LA <12 years: not recommended; ≥12 years: initially 80 mg daily in a single dose; increase q 3-7 days; usual range 120-160 mg/day; max 320 mg/day in a single dose
Cap: 60, 80, 120, 160 mg sust-rel
InnoPran XL <12 years: not recommended; ≥12 years: initially 80 mg q HS; max 120 mg/day
Cap: 80, 120 mg ext-rel

HYPERTRIGLYCERIDEMIA

OMEGA 3-FATTY ACID ETHYL ESTERS

Comment: *Vascepa*, *Lovaza*, and **Epanova** are indicated for the treatment of TG ≥500 mg/dL.

➤ *icosapent ethyl (omega 3-fatty acid ethyl ester of EPA) (C)* <18 years: not recommended; ≥18 years: 2 caps bid with food; max 4 gm/day; swallow whole, do not crush or chew
Vascepa *sgc:* 1 gm (α-tocopherol 4 mg/cap)
➤ *omega 3-fatty acid ethyl esters (C)(G)* <18 years: not recommended; ≥18 years: 2 gm bid or 4 gm daily; swallow whole, do not crush or chew
Lovaza *Gelcap:* 1 gm (α-tocopherol 4 mg/cap) **(C)** take 2-4 *gel caps* (2-4 gm) daily without regard to meals
Epanova *Gelcap:* 1 gm

ISOBUTYRIC ACID DERIVATIVE

➤ *gemfibrozil (C)(G)*

Lopid <12 years: not recommended; ≥12 years: 600 mg bid 30 minutes before AM and PM meals
Tab: 600*mg

FIBRATES (FIBRIC ACID DERIVATIVES)

➤ *fenofibrate (C)* take with meals; adjust at 4-8-week intervals; discontinue if inadequate response after 2 months; lowest dose or contraindicated with renal impairment

Antara <12 years: not recommended; ≥12 years: 43-130 mg once daily; max 130 mg/day
> *Cap:* 43, 87, 130 mg

FibriCor <12 years: not recommended; ≥12 years: 30-105 mg once daily; max 105 mg/day
> *Tab:* 30, 105 mg

TriCor (G) <12 years: not recommended; ≥12 years: 48-145 mg once daily; max 145 mg/day
> *Tab:* 48, 145 mg

TriLipix (G) <12 years: not recommended; ≥12 years: 45-135 mg once daily; max 135 mg/day
> *Cap:* 45, 135 mg del-rel

Lipofen (G) <12 years: not recommended; ≥12 years: 50-150 mg once daily; max 150 mg/day
> *Cap:* 50, 150 mg

Lofibra <12 years: not recommended; ≥12 years: 67-200 mg daily; max 200 mg/day
> *Tab:* 67, 134, 200 mg

NICOTINIC ACID DERIVATIVES

Comment: Contraindicated in liver disease. Decrease total cholesterol, LDL-C, and TG; increase HDL-C. Before initiating and at 4-6 weeks, 3 months, and 6 months of therapy, check fasting lipid profile <u>or</u> as indicated by manufacturer, LFT, glucose, and uric acid. Significant side effect of transient skin flushing. Take with food and take *aspirin* 325 mg 30 minutes before dose to decrease flushing.

▷ *niacin* (C)

Niaspan <12 years: not recommended; ≥12 years: 375 mg daily for 1st week; then, 500 mg daily for 2nd week; then, 750 mg daily for 3rd week; then, 1 gm daily for weeks 4-7; may increase by 500 mg q 4 weeks; usual range 1-3 gm/day
> *Tab:* 500, 750, 1,000 mg ext-rel

Slo-Niacin <12 years: not recommended; ≥12 years: 250 mg <u>or</u> 500 mg <u>or</u> 750 mg q AM <u>or</u> HS
> *Tab:* 250, 500, 750 mg cont-rel

HMG-COA REDUCTASE INHIBITORS

▷ *atorvastatin* (X)(G) <10 years: not recommended; ≥10 years (female post menarche): initially 10 mg daily; usual range 10-80 mg daily
> **Lipitor** *Tab:* 10, 20, 40, 80 mg

▷ *fluvastatin* (X)(G) <18 years: not recommended; ≥18 years: initially 20-40 mg q HS; usual range 20-80 mg/day
> **Lescol** *Cap:* 20, 40 mg
> **Lescol XL** *Tab:* 80 mg ext-rel

▷ *lovastatin* (X) <10 years: not recommended; 10-17 years: initially 10-20 mg daily at evening meal; may increase at 4 week intervals; max 40 mg daily; *Concomitant fibrates, niacin,* <u>or</u> *CrCl <40 mL/min:* usual max 20 mg/day initially 20 mg daily at evening meal; may increase at 4 week intervals; max 80 mg/day in a single <u>or</u> divided doses; *Concomitant fibrates,* **niacin,** <u>or</u> *CrCl <40 mL/min:* usual max 20 mg/day

Mevacor *Tab:* 10, 20, 40 mg
➤ *pravastatin* (X)(G) <8 years: not recommended; 8-13 years: 20 mg q HS; 14-17 years: 40 mg q HS; >17 years: initially 10-20 mg q HS; usual range 10-80 mg/day; may start at 40 mg/day
Pravachol *Tab:* 10, 20, 40, 80 mg
➤ *rosuvastatin* (X)(G) <10 years: not recommended; 10-17 years: 5-20 mg q HS; >17 years: initially 20 mg q HS; usual range 5-40 mg/day; adjust at 4 week intervals; max 20 mg q HS
Crestor *Tab:* 5, 10, 20, 40 mg
➤ *simvastatin* (X)(G) <10 years: not recommended; 10-17 years: initially 10 mg q HS; may increase at 4 week intervals; >17 years: initially 20 mg q HS; usual range 5-80 mg/day; adjust at 4 week intervals; max 40 mg q HS
Zocor *Tab:* 5, 10, 20, 40, 80 mg

NICOTINIC ACID DERIVATIVE/HMG-COA REDUCTASE INHIBITOR

➤ *niacin/lovastatin* (X) Advicor <18 years: not recommended; ≥18 years: take 1 tab once daily
Tab: **Advicor 500 mg/20 mg** *niac* 500 mg ext-rel/*lova* 20 mg
Advicor 750 mg/20 mg *niac* 750 mg ext-rel/*lova* 20 mg
Advicor 1,000 mg/20 mg *niac* 1,000 mg ext-rel/*lova* 20 mg

HYPOCALCEMIA

Comment: Hypocalcemia resulting in metabolic bone disease may be secondary to hyperparathyroidism, pseudoparathyroidism, and chronic renal disease. Normal serum Ca++ range is approximately 8.5-12 mg/dL. Signs and symptoms of hypocalcemia include confusion, increased neuromuscular excitability, muscle spasms, paresthesias, hyperphosphatemia, positive Chvostek's sign, and positive Trousseau's sign. Signs and symptoms of hypercalcemia include fatigue, lethargy, decreased concentration and attention span, frank psychosis, anorexia, nausea, vomiting, constipation, bradycardia, heart block, shortened QT interval. Foods high in calcium include almonds, broccoli, baked beans, salmon, sardines, buttermilk, turnip greens, collard greens, spinach, pumpkin, rhubarb, and bran. Recommended daily calcium intake: 1-3 years: 700 mg; 4-8 years: 1,000 mg; 9-18 years: 1,300 mg; >18 years: 1,000 mg; pregnancy or nursing: 1,000-1,300 mg. Recommended daily vitamin D intake: >1 year: 600 IU; The American Academy of Rheumatology (AAR) recommends the following daily doses for anyone on a chronic oral corticosteroid regimen: Calcium 1,200-1,500 mg/day and vitamin D 800-1,000 IU/day.

CALCIUM SUPPLEMENTS

Comment: Take *calcium* supplements after meals to avoid gastric upset. Dosages of *calcium* over 2,000 mg/day have not been shown to have any additional benefit. *Calcium* decreases *tetracycline* absorption. *Calcium* absorption is decreased by corticosteroids.
➤ *calcitonin-salmon* (C)
Miacalcin 200 units (1 spray intranasally) once daily; alternate nostrils each day
Nasal spray: 14 dose (2 ml)

Miacalcin injection 100 units/day SC <u>or</u> IM
  Vial: 2 ml
▷ *calcium carbonate* (C)(OTC)(G)
  Rolaids chew 2 tabs bid; max 14 tabs/day
    Tab: calcium carbonate: 550 mg
  Rolaids Extra Strength chew 2 tabs bid; max 8 tabs/day
    Tab: 1,000 mg
  Tums chew 2 tabs bid; max 16 tabs/day
    Tab: 500 mg
  Tums Extra Strength chew 2 tabs bid; max 10 tabs/day
    Tab: 750 mg
  Tums Ultra chew 2 tabs bid; max 8 tabs/day
    Tab: 1,000 mg
  Os-Cal 500 (OTC) 1-2 tab bid-tid
    Tab: elemental calcium carbonate 500 mg
▷ *calcium carbonate/vitamin D* (C)(G)
  Os-Cal 250+D (OTC) 1-2 tabs tid
    Tab: elemental calcium carbonate 250 mg/*vit d* 125 IU
  Os-Cal 500+D (OTC) 1-2 tabs bid-tid
    Tab: elemental calcium carbonate 500 mg/*vit d* 125 IU
  Viactiv (OTC) 1 tab tid
    Chew tab: elemental calcium 500 mg/*vit d and vit a* 100 IU/*Vit k* 40 mEq
▷ *calcium citrate*
  Citracal (OTC) 1-2 tabs bid
    Tab: elemental calcium citrate 200 mg
▷ *calcium citrate/vitamin D* (C)(G)
  Citracal+D (OTC) 1-2 cplts bid
    Cplt: elemental calcium citrate 315 mg/*vit d* 200 IU
  Citracal 250+D (OTC) 1-2 tabs bid
    Tab: elemental calcium citrate 250 mg/*vit d* 62.3 IU

VITAMIN D ANALOGS

Comment: Concurrent *vitamin D* supplementation is contraindicated for patients taking *calcitriol* or *doxercalciferol* due to the risk of *vitamin D* toxicity. Symptoms of hypervitaminosis D: hypercalcemia, hypercalciuria, elevated creatinine, erythema multiforme, hyperphosphatemia. Maintain adequate daily calcium and fluid intake. Keep serum calcium times phosphate (Ca x P) product below 70. Monitor serum calcium (esp. during dose titration), phosphorus, other lab values (see literature for frequency)

▷ **calcitriol (C)(G)** <12 years: *Predialysis:* <3 years: 10-15 ng/kg per day; ≥3 years: initially 0.25 mcg daily; may increase to 0.5mcg daily; *Dialysis:* not recommended; *Hypoparathyroidism:* initially 0.25 mcg daily in the AM; may increase by 0.25 mcg day at 2-4 week intervals; usual maintenance: (1-5 years): 0.25-0.75 mcg daily; (≥6 years): 0.5-2 mcg daily; *Pseudohypoparathyroidism:* (<6 years): insufficient data, see mfr pkg insert; ≥12 years: *Predialysis:* initially 0.25 mcg daily; may increase to 0.5mcg daily *Dialysis:* initially 0.25 mcg daily; may increase by 0.25 mcg daily at 4-8 week intervals; usual maintenance: 0.5-1 mcg daily. *Hypoparathyroidism:* initially 0.25 mcg q AM; may increase by 0.25 mcg/day at 4-8 week intervals; usual maintenance 0.5-2 mcg/day

Rocaltrol *Cap:* 0.25, 0.5 mcg
Rocaltrol Solution *Soln:* 1 mcg/ml (15 ml, single-use dispensers)
Comment: *calcitriol* is indicated for the treatment of secondary hyperparathyroidism and resultant metabolic bone disease in predialysis patients (CrCl 15-55 mL/min), hypocalcemia and resultant metabolic bone disease in patients on chronic renal dialysis, hypocalcemia in hypoparathyroidism, and pseudohypoparathyroidism.

➤ *doxercalciferol* (C)(G) <12 years: not established; ≥12 years: *Dialysis:* initially 10 mcg 3 x/week at dialysis; adjust to maintain intact parathyroid hormone (iPTH) between 150-300 pg/mL; if iPTH is not lowered by 50% and fails to reach target range, may increase by 2.5 mcg at 8-week intervals; max 20 mcg 3 x/week; if iPTH <100 pg/mL, suspend for 1 week, then resume at a dose that is at least 2.5 mcg lower; *Predialysis:* initially 1mcg once daily; may increase by 0.5 mcg at 2 week intervals to target iPTH levels; max 3.5 mcg/day

Hectorol *Cap:* 0.25, 0.5, 1, 2.5 mcg
Comment: Oral **Hectorol** is indicated for the treatment of secondary hyperparathyroidism in patients with chronic kidney disease (CKD) on dialysis; *Predialysis stage 3 or 4 CKD:* use oral form only.

Hectoral Injection <12 years: not recommended; ≥12 years: 4 mcg 3 x weekly after dialysis; adjust dose to maintain intact parathyroid hormone (iPTH) between 150-300 pg/mL; if iPTH is not lowered by 50% and fails to reach target range, may increase by 1-2 mcg at 8 week intervals; max 18 mcg/week; if iPTH <100 pg/mL, suspend for 1 week, then resume at a dose that is at least 1 mcg lower

Vial: 2 mcg/ml (1, 2 ml single dose; 2 ml multidose)
Comment: **Hectorol Injection** is indicated for the treatment of secondary hyperparathyroidism in patients with chronic kidney disease (CKD) on dialysis.

➤ *paricalcitol* (C)(G) <18 years: not established; ≥18 years: administer 0.04-1 mcg/kg (2.8-7 mcg) IV bolus, during dialysis, no more than every other day; may be increased by 2-4 mcg/dose every 2-4 weeks; monitor serum calcium and phosphorus during dose adjustment periods; if Ca x P >75, immediately reduce dose or discontinue until these levels normalize; discard unused portion of single-use vials immediately

Zemplar *Vial:* 2, 5 mcg/ml soln for inj
Comment: *paricalcitol* is indicated for the prevention and treatment of secondary hyperparathyroidism associated with chronic kidney disease (CKD) stage 5.

BIOENGINEERED REPLICA OF HUMAN PARATHYROID HORMONE

➤ *bioengineered replica of human parathyroid hormone* (C) before starting, confirm 25-hydroxyvitamin D stores are sufficient; if insufficient, replace to sufficient levels per standard of care; confirm serum calcium is above 7.5 mg/dL; the goal of treatment is to achieve serum calcium within the lower half of the normal range; administer SC into the thigh once daily; alternate thighs; initially, 50 mcg/day; when initiating, decrease dose of active vitamin D by 50%, if serum calcium is above 7.5 mg/dL; monitor serum calcium levels every 3 to 7 days after starting or adjusting dose and when adjusting either active vitamin D or calcium supplements dose. Abrupt interruption or discontinuation of **Natpara** can result in severe hypocalcemia. Resume treatment with, or increase the dose of, an active form of vitamin D and calcium supplements. Monitor for signs and symptoms of hypocalcemia and monitor serum calcium levels, In the case of a missed dose, the next **Natpara** dose should be administered as soon as reasonably feasible and additional exogenous calcium should be taken in the event of hypocalcemia.

Natpara *Soln for inj:* 25, 50, 75, 100 mcg (2/pkg) multiple dose, dual-chamber glass cartridge containing a sterile powder and diluent

Comment: **Natpara** is indicated as an adjunct to calcium and vitamin D in patients with hypoparathyroidism. Because of a potential risk of osteosarcoma, use **Natpara** only in patients who cannot be well-controlled on calcium and active forms of vitamin D alone and for whom the potential benefits are considered to outweigh the potential risk. Avoid use of **Natpara** in patients who are at increased baseline risk for osteosarcoma, such as patients with Paget's disease of bone or unexplained elevations of alkaline phosphatase, pediatric and patients ≥18 years with open epiphyses, patients with hereditary disorders predisposing to osteosarcoma or patients with a prior history of external beam or implant radiation therapy involving the skeleton. Because of the risk of osteosarcoma, **Natpara** is available only through a restricted program under a Risk Evaluation and Mitigation Strategy (REMS) at www .natparaREMS.com

HYPOKALEMIA

Comment: Normal serum K^+ range is approximately 3.5-5.5 mEq/L. Signs and symptoms of hypokalemia include neuromuscular weakness, muscle twitching and cramping, hyporeflexia, postural hypotension, anorexia, nausea and vomiting, depressed ST segments, flattened T waves, and cardiac tachyarrhythmias. Signs and symptoms of hyperkalemia include peaked T waves, elevated ST segment, and widened QRS complexes.

PROPHYLAXIS

Comment: Usual dose range is 8-10 mEq/day.

TREATMENT OF HYPOKALEMIA: NON-EMERGENCY (K^+<3.5 mEq/L)

Comment: Usual dose range 40-120 mEq/day in divided doses. Solutions are preferred; potentially serious GI side effects may occur with tablet formulations <u>or</u> when taken on an empty stomach.

POTASSIUM SUPPLEMENTS

Comment: Potassium supplements should be taken with food. Solutions are the preferred form. Extended-release and sustained-release forms should be swallowed whole; do not crush <u>or</u> chew. Potassium supplementation is indicated for hypokalemia including that caused by diuretic use, and digitalis intoxication without atrioventricular (AV) block.

▷ *potassium* (C)(G) <12 years: not established; ≥12 years:

    KCL Solution Oral soln: 10% (30 ml unit dose, 50/case)

    K-Dur (as chloride) *Tab:* 10, 20* mEq sust-rel

    K-Lor for Oral Solution (as chloride) *Pkts* for reconstitution: 20 mEq/pkt (fruit)

    Klor-Con/25 (as chloride) *Pkts* for reconstitution: 25 mEq/pkt

Klor-Con/EF 25 (as bicarbonate) *Pkts* for reconstitution: 25 mEq/pkt (effervescent) (fruit)

Klor-Con Extended-Release (as chloride) *Tab:* 8, 10 mEq ext-rel

Klor-Con M (as chloride) *Tab:* 10, 15*, 20* mEq ext-rel

Klor-Con Powder (as chloride) 20, 25 mEq *Pkts* for reconstitution: (30/carton) (fruit)

Klorvess (as bicarbonate and citrate) *Tab:* 20 mEq effervescent for solution; *Granules:* 20 mEq/pkt effervescent for solution; *Oral liq:* 20 mEq/15 ml (16 oz)

Klotrix (as chloride) *Tab:* 10 mEq sust-rel

K-Lyte (as bicarbonate and citrate) *Tab:* 25 mEq effervescent for solution (lime, orange)

K-Lyte/CL (as chloride) *Tab:* 25 mEq effervescent for solution (citrus, fruit)

K-Lyte/CL 50 (as chloride) *Tab:* 50 mEq effervescent for solution (citrus, fruit)

K-Lyte/DS (as bicarbonate and citrate) *Tab:* 50 mEq effervescent for solution (lime, orange)

K-Tab (as chloride) *Tab:* 10 mEq sust-rel

Micro-K (as chloride) *Cap:* 8, 10 mEq sust-rel

Potassium Chloride Extended Release Caps *Cap:* 8, 10 mEq ext-rel

Potassium Chloride Sust-Rel Tabs *Tab/Cap:* 10 mEq sust-rel

Potassium Chloride ER *Tab:* 8 mEq (600 mg), 10 mEq (750 mg)

HYPOMAGNESEMIA

Comment: Normal serum Mg^{++} range is approximately 1.2-2.6 mEq/L. Signs and symptoms of hypomagnesemia include confusion, disorientation, hallucinations, hyperreflexia, tetany, convulsions, tachyarrhythmia, positive Chvostek's sign, and positive Trousseau's sign. Signs and symptoms of hypermagnesemia include drowsiness, lethargy, muscle weakness, hypoactive reflexes, slurred speech, bradycardia, hypotension, convulsions, and cardiac arrhythmias.

MAGNESIUM SUPPLEMENTS

▷ *magnesium* (B) <12 years: not established; ≥12 years: 2 tabs daily
  Slow-Mag *Tab:* 64 mg (as chloride)/110 mg (as carbonate)
▷ *magnesium oxide* (B) <12 years: not established; ≥12 years: 1 tab daily
  Mag-Ox 400 *Tab:* 400 mg

HYPOPARATHYROIDISM

VITAMIN D ANALOGS

Comment: Concurrent vitamin D supplementation is contraindicated for patients taking *calcitriol* **or** *doxercalciferol* owing to the risk of vitamin D toxicity.

▷ *calcitriol* (C) <12 years: initially 0.25 mcg q AM; may increase by 0.25 mcg/day at 4 to 8 week intervals; usual maintenance 0.5-2 mcg/day; ≥12 years: initially 0.25 mcg daily; may increase by 0.25 mcg/day at 2-4-week intervals; usual maintenance (1-6 years) 0.25-0.75 mcg/day, (≥6 years) 0.5-2 mcg/day
  Rocaltrol *Cap:* 0.25, 0.5 mcg
  Rocaltrol Solution *Soln:* 1 mcg/ml (15 ml, single-use dispensers)

➢ *doxercalciferol* (C) <12 years: initially 0.25 mcg q AM; may increase by 0.25 mcg/day at 4-8-week intervals; usual maintenance 0.5-2 mcg/day; ≥12 years: initially 0.25 mcg daily; may increase by 0.25 mcg/day at 2-4-week intervals; usual maintenance (1-6 years) 0.25-0.75 mcg/day, (≥6 years) 0.5-2 mcg/day
    Hectorol *Cap:* 0.25, 0.5 mcg
➢ *teriparatide* (C) <12 years: not recommended; ≥12 years: 20 mcg SC daily in the thigh or abdomen; may treat for up to 2 years
    Forteo Multidose Pen *Multidose pen:* 250 mcg/ml (3 ml)
    Comment: **Forteo** is indicated for the treatment of osteoporosis in females who are at high risk for fracture and to increase bone mass in males with primary or hypogonadal osteoporosis who are at high risk for fracture.

BIOENGINEERED REPLICA OF HUMAN PARATHYROID HORMONE

➢ *bioengineered replica of human parathyroid hormone* (C) <12 years: not established; ≥12 years: initially inject mg IM into the thigh once daily; when initiating, decrease dose of active vitamin D by 50% if serum calcium is above 7.5 mg/dL; monitor serum calcium levels every 3-7 days after starting or adjusting dose and when adjusting either active vitamin D or calcium supplements dose
    Natpara *Soln for inj:* 25, 50, 75, 100 mcg (2/pkg) multiple dose, dual-chamber glass cartridge containing a sterile powder and diluent
    Comment: **Natpara** is indicated as an adjunct to calcium and vitamin D in patients with parathyroidism.

HYPOPHOSPHATASIA (OSTEOMALACIA, RICKETS)

Comment: Hypophosphatasia (HPP) is an inborn error of metabolism marked by abnormally low serum alkaline phosphatase activity and phosphoethanolamine in the urine. It is manifested by osteomalacia in older adolescents and rickets in infants and children. It is most severe in infants under 6 months-of-age. With congenital absence of alkaline phosphatase, an enzyme essential to the calcification of bone tissue, complications include vomiting, growth retardation, and often death in infancy. Surviving children have numerous skeletal abnormalities and dwarfism.
➢ *asfotase alfa* (NE) 6 mg/kg/week SC, administered as 2 mg/kg or 1 mg/kg 6 x/week; max 9 mg/kg/week SC administered as 3 mg/kg 3 x/week
    Strensiq *Vial:* 18 mg/0.45 ml, 28 mg/0.7 ml, 40 mg/ml, 80 mg/0.8 ml for SC inj, single use (1, 12/carton) (preservative-free)
    Comment: **Strensiq** is the first FDA-approved (2015) treatment for perinatal, infantile, and juvenile onset HPP. Prior to the availability of **Strensiq**, there was no effective treatment and patient prognosis was very poor.

HYPOTENSION: NEUROGENIC, ORTHOSTATIC

ALPHA-1 AGONIST

➢ *midodrine* (C)(G) <12 years: not recommended; ≥12 years: 10 mg tid at 3-4-hour intervals; take while upright; take last dose at least 4 hours before bedtime
    ProAmatine *Tab:* 2.5*, 5*, 10*mg

SYNTHETIC AMINO ACID PRECURSOR OF NOREPINEPHRINE

▷ *droxidopa* (C) <12 years: not recommended; ≥12 years: initially 100 mg, taken 3 times/day, upon arising in the morning, at midday, and in the late afternoon at least 3 hours prior to bedtime (to reduce the potential for supine hypertension during sleep); administer with or without; swallow whole; titrate to symptomatic response, in increments of 100 mg tid every 24-48 hours; max 600 mg tid (max total 1,800 mg/day)

Northera *Cap:* 100, 200, 300 mg

Comment: Northera is indicated for the treatment of orthostatic dizziness, lightheadedness, or feeling about to black out in patients ≥18 years-of-age with symptomatic neurogenic orthostatic hypotension (NOH) caused by primary autonomic failure (Parkinson's disease [PD], multiple system atrophy [MSA], and pure autonomic failure), dopamine beta-hydroxylase deficiency, and non-diabetic autonomic neuropathy. Effectiveness beyond 2 weeks of treatment has not been established. The continued effectiveness of **Northera** should be assessed. Administering **Northera** in combination with other agents that increase blood pressure (e.g., norepinephrine, ephedrine, midodrine, triptans) would be expected to increase the risk for supine hypertension.

HYPOTHYROIDISM

Comment: Take thyroid replacement hormone in the morning on an empty stomach. Start thyroid hormone replacement at 25 mcg/day. Target TSH is 0.4-5.5 mIU/L; target T4 is 4.5-12.5 ng/L. Signs and symptoms of thyroid toxicity include tachycardia, palpitations, nervousness, chest pain, heat intolerance, and weight loss.

ORAL THYROID HORMONE SUPPLEMENTS

T3

▷ *liothyronine* (A) initially 5 mcg/day; may increase by 5 mcg/day every 3-4 days; *Cretinism:* maintenance dose: <1 year: 20 mcg/day; 1-3 years: 50 mcg/day; >3 years: initially 25 mcg daily; may increase by 25 mcg every 1-2 weeks as needed; usual maintenance 25-75 mcg/day

Cytomel *Tab:* 5, 25, 50 mcg

T4

▷ *levothyroxine* (A)(G)

Levoxyl <6 months: 8-10 mcg/kg/day; 6-12 months: 6-8 mcg/kg/day; >1-5 years: 5-6 mcg/kg/day; 6-12 years: 4-5 mcg/kg/day; >12 years: initially 25-100 mcg/day; increase by 25 mcg/day q 2-3 weeks as needed; maintenance 100-200 mcg/day

Tab: 25*, 50* (dye-free), 75*, 88*, 100*, 112*, 125*, 137*, 150*, 175*, 200*, 300*mcg

Synthroid <6 months: 8-10 mcg/kg/day; 6-12 months: 6-8 mcg/kg/day; >1-5 years: 5-6 mcg/kg/day; 6-12 years: 4-5 mcg/kg/day; >12 years: initially 50 mcg/day; increase by 25 mcg/day q 2-3 weeks as needed; max 300 mcg/day

Tab: 25*, 50* (dye-free), 75*, 88*, 100*, 112*, 125*, 137*, 150*, 175*, 200*, 300*mcg

Unithroid 0-3 months: 10-15 mcg/kg/day; 3-6 months: 8-10 mcg/kg/day; 6-12 months: 6-8 mcg/kg/day; 1-5 years: 5-6 mcg/kg/day; 6-12 years: 4-5 mcg/kg/day; >12 years: 2-3 mcg/kg/day; *Growth and puberty complete:* initially 50 mcg/day; increase by 25 mcg/day q 2-3 weeks as needed; max 300 mcg/day

Tab: 25*, 50* (dye-free), 75*, 88*, 100*, 112*, 125*, 150*, 175*, 200*, 300*mcg

T3/T4 Combination

➤ *liothyronine/levothyroxine* (A) <6 months: 4.6-6 mcg/kg/day; 6-12 months: 3.6-4.8 mcg/kg/day; >1-5 years: 3-3.6 mcg/kg/day; 6-12 years: 2.4-3 mcg/kg/day; >12 years: 1.2-1.8 mcg/kg/day; *Growth and puberty complete:* initially 15-30 mg/day; increase by 15 mg/day q 2-3 weeks to target goal; usual maintenance 60-120 mg/day

Armour Thyroid Tab *Tab:* per grain: T3 9 mcg/T4 38 mcg: 1/4, 1/2, 1, 1, 2, 3*, 4*, 5* gr; 15, 30, 60, 90, 120, 180*, 240*, 300*mg

Thyrolar *Tab: per grain:* T3 12.5 mcg/T4 50 mcg: 1/4, 1/5, 1, 2, 3 gr

PARENTERAL THYROID HORMONE SUPPLEMENT

➤ *levothyroxine sodium* (A)(G) <12 years: not recommended; ≥12 years: 1/2 oral dose by IV or IM and titrate; *Myxedema Coma:* 200-500 mcg IV x 1 dose; may administer 100-300 mcg (or more) IV on second day if needed; then 50-100 mcg IV daily; switch to oral form as soon as possible

T4 *Vial:* 100, 200, 500 mcg (pwdr for IM or IV administration after reconstitution)

☐ IDIOPATHIC PULMONARY FIBROSIS (IPF)

➤ *nintedanib* (D) <12 years: not established; ≥12 years: 150 mg bid, 12 hours apart; max 300 mg/day; take with food at the same time each day

Ofev *Cap:* 100, 150 mg

Comment: Monitor liver enzymes. If elevated LFTs (3 < AST/ALT <5 x ULN) without severe liver damage, interrupt therapy or reduce dose to 100 mg bid. When liver enzymes return to baseline, restart at 100 mg bid and titrate up.

➤ *pirfenidone* (C) <12 years: not established; ≥12 years: *Days 1-7:* 1 cap tid; *Days 8-14:* 2 caps tid; *Days 15 and ongoing:* 3 caps tid; max 9 caps/day; take with food at the same time each day

Esbriet *Gelcap:* 267 mg

☐ IMPETIGO CONTAGIOSA (INDIAN FIRE)

Comment: The most common infectious organisms are *Staphylococcus aureus* and *Streptococcus pyogenes*.

TOPICAL ANTI-INFECTIVES

➤ *mupirocin* (B)(G) apply to lesions bid; apply to walls of nares bid

Bactroban *Oint:* 2% (22 gm); *Crm:* 2% (15, 30 gm)

Centany *Oint:* 2% (15, 30 gm)

ORAL ANTI-INFECTIVES

▷ *amoxicillin* (B)(G) <40 kg (88 lb): 20-40 mg/kg/day in 3 divided doses x 10 days or 25-45 mg/kg/day in 2 divided doses x 10 days; *see page 543 for dose by weight table;* ≥40 kg: 500-875 mg bid or 250-500 mg tid x 10 days

    Amoxil *Cap:* 250, 500 mg; *Tab:* 875*mg; *Chew tab:* 125, 200, 250, 400 mg (cherry-banana-peppermint) (phenylalanine); *Oral susp:* 125, 250 mg/5 ml (80, 100, 150 ml) (strawberry); 200, 400 mg/5 ml (50, 75, 100 ml) (bubble gum); *Oral drops:* 50 mg/ml (30 ml) (bubble gum)

    Moxatag *Tab:* 775 mg ext-rel

    Trimox *Tab:* 125, 250 mg; *Cap:* 250, 500 mg; *Oral susp:* 125, 250 mg/5 ml (80, 100, 150 ml) (raspberry-strawberry)

▷ *amoxicillin/clavulanate* (B)(G)

    Augmentin <40 kg: 40-45 mg/kg/day divided tid x 10 days or 90 mg/kg/day divided bid x 10 days; *see page 545 for dose by weight table;* ≥40 kg: 500 mg tid or 875 mg bid x 10 days

        Tab: 250, 500, 875 mg; *Chew tab:* 125, 250 mg (lemon-lime); 200, 400 mg (cherry-banana) (phenylalanine); *Oral susp:* 125 mg/5 ml (banana), 250 mg/5 ml (75, 100, 150 ml) (orange); 200, 400 mg/5 ml (50, 75, 100 ml) (orange) (phenylalanine)

    Augmentin ES-600 <3 months: not recommended; ≥3 months, <40 kg: 90 mg/kg/day divided q 12 hours x 10 days; *see page 546 for dose by weight table;* ≥40 kg: not recommended

        Oral susp: 600 mg/5 ml (50, 75, 100, 125, 150, 200 ml) (strawberry cream) (phenylalanine)

    Augmentin XR <16 years: use other forms; ≥16 years: 2 tabs q 12 hours x 7-10 days

        Tab: 1000*mg ext-rel

▷ *azithromycin* (B)(G) <12 years: 12 mg/kg/day x 5 days; *see page 548 for dose by weight table;* max 500 mg/day; ≥12 years: 500 mg x 1 dose on day 1, then 250 mg daily on days 2-5 or 500 mg daily x 3 days or **Zmax** 2 gm in a single dose

    Zithromax *Tab:* 250, 500, 600 mg; *Oral susp:* 100 mg/5 ml (15 ml); 200 mg/5 ml (15, 22.5, 30 ml) (cherry); *Pkt:* 1 gm for reconstitution (cherry-banana)

    Zithromax Tri-pak *Tab:* 3 x 500 mg tabs/pck

    Zithromax Z-pak *Tab:* 6 x 250 mg tabs/pck

    Zmax *Oral susp:* 2 gm ext-rel for reconstitution (cherry-banana) (148 mg Na$^+$)

▷ *cefaclor* (B)(G) <1 month: not recommended; 1 month-12 years: 20-40 mg/kg divided bid x 10 days; *see page 549 for dose by weight table;* max 1 gm/day; >12 years: 250-500 mg q 8 hours x 10 days; max 2 gm/day

    Tab: 500 mg; *Cap:* 250, 500 mg; *Susp:* 125 mg/5 ml (75, 150 ml) (strawberry); 187 mg/5 ml (50, 100 ml) (strawberry); 250 mg/5 ml (75, 150 ml) (strawberry); 375 mg/5 ml (50, 100 ml) (strawberry)

    Cefaclor Extended Release <16 years: not recommended; ≥16 years: 500 mg bid x 10 days (clinically equivalent to 250 mg immed-rel caps tid); swallow whole; take with meals

        Tab: 375, 500 mg ext-rel

▷ *cefadroxil* <12 years: 30 mg/kg/day in 2 divided doses x 10 days; *see page 550 for dose by weight table;* ≥12 years: 1-2 gm in a single or 2 divided doses x 10 days

    Duricef *Cap:* 500 mg; *Tab:* 1 g; *Oral susp:* 250 mg/5 ml (100 ml); 500 mg/5 ml (75, 100 ml) (orange-pineapple)

▷ *cefpodoxime proxetil* **(B)** <2 months: not recommended; 2 months-12 years: 10 mg/kg/day (max 400 mg/dose) <u>or</u> 5 mg/kg/day bid (max 200 mg/dose) x 10 days; *see page 553 for dose by weight table;* >12 years: 200 mg bid x 10 days

▷ *cefprozil* **(B)** ≤6 months: not recommended; 6 months-12 years: 7.5 mg/kg bid x 10 days; *see page 554 for dose by weight table;* >12 years: 250-500 mg bid <u>or</u> 500 mg daily x 10 days 500 mg bid x 10 days

   Cefzil *Tab:* 250, 500 mg; *Oral susp:* 125, 250 mg/5 ml (50, 75, 100 ml) (bubble gum) (phenylalanine)

▷ *ceftaroline fosamil* **(B)** administer by IV infusion after reconstitution every 12 hours x 5-14 days; *CrCl >50 mL/min:* 600 mg; *CrCl >30-<50 mL/min:* 400 mg; *CrCl >1 5-<30 mL/min:* 300 mg; ESRD: 200 mg

   Teflaro *Vial:* 400, 600 mg

▷ *cefuroxime axetil* **(B)(G)** <12 years: 15 mg/kg bid x 10 days; *see page 556 for dose by weight table;* ≥12 years: 250-500 mg bid x 10 days

   Ceftin *Tab:* 250, 500 mg; *Oral susp:* 12, 250 mg/5 ml (50, 100 ml) (tutti-frutti)

▷ *cephalexin* **(B)(G)** <12 years: 25-50 mg/kg/day in 4 divided doses x 10 days; *see page 557 for dose by weight table;* ≥12 years: 250-500 mg qid <u>or</u> 500 mg bid x 10 days

   Keflex *Cap:* 250, 333, 500, 750 mg; *Oral susp:* 125, 250 mg/5 ml (100, 200 ml) (strawberry)

▷ *clarithromycin* **(C)(G)** <6 months: not recommended; ≥6 months-12 years: 7.5 mg/kg bid x 7 days; *see page 558 for dose by weight table;* >12 years: 500 mg <u>or</u> 500 mg ext-rel daily x 7 days

   Biaxin *Tab:* 250, 500 mg

   Biaxin Oral Suspension *Oral susp:* 125, 250 mg/5 ml (50, 100 ml) (fruit punch)

   Biaxin XL *Tab:* 500 mg ext-rel

▷ *dicloxacillin* **(B)(G)** <12 years: 12.5-25 mg/kg/day in 4 divided doses x 10 days; *see page 560 for dose by weight table;* ≥12 years: 500 mg q 6 hours x 10 days

   Dynapen *Cap:* 125, 250, 500 mg; *Oral susp:* 62.5 mg/5 ml (80, 100, 200 ml)

▷ *erythromycin base* **(B)(G)** <45 kg: 30-50 mg in 2-4 divided doses x 7-10 days; ≥45 kg: 250 mg qid, <u>or</u> 333 mg tid, <u>or</u> 500 mg bid x 7-10 days

   Ery-Tab *Tab:* 250, 333, 500 mg ent-coat

   PCE *Tab:* 333, 500 mg

▷ *erythromycin ethylsuccinate* **(B)(G)** 30-50 mg/kg/day in 4 divided doses x 7-10 days; may double dose with severe infection; max 100 mg/kg/day <u>or</u> 400 mg qid; *see page 563 for dose by weight table*

   EryPed *Oral susp:* 200 mg/5 ml (100, 200 ml) (fruit); 400 mg/5 ml (60, 100, 200 ml) (banana); *Oral drops:* 200, 400 mg/5 ml (50 ml) (fruit); *Chew tab:* 200 mg wafer (fruit)

   E.E.S. *Oral susp:* 200, 400 mg/5 ml (100 ml) (fruit)

   E.E.S. Granules *Oral susp:* 200 mg/5 ml (100, 200 ml) (cherry)

   E.E.S. 400 Tablets *Tab:* 400 mg

▷ *loracarbef* **(B)** <12 years: 15 mg/kg/day in 2 divided doses x 10 days; *see page 560 for dose by weight table;* ≥12 years: 200 mg bid x 10 days

   Lorabid *Pulvule:* 200, 400 mg; *Oral susp:* 100 mg/5 ml (50, 100 ml); 200 mg/5 ml (50, 75, 100 ml) (strawberry bubble gum)

▷ *penicillin g (benzathine)* **(B)** <12 years: <60 lb: 300,000-600,000 units IM x 1 dose; ≥60 lb: 900,000 units x 1 dose; ≥12 years: 1.2 million units IM x 1 dose

   Bicillin L-A *Cartridge-needle unit:* 600,000 units (1 ml); 1.2 million units (2 ml)

▷ *penicillin g (benzathine/procaine)* (B)(G) <30 lb: 600,000 units IM x 1 dose; 30-60 lb: 900,000-1.2 million units IM x 1 dose; ≥12 years: 2.4 million units IM x 1 dose
  Bicillin C-R *Cartridge-needle unit:* 600,000 units (1 ml); 1.2 million units (2 ml); 2.4 million units (4 ml)
▷ *penicillin v potassium* (B) <12 years: 25-75 mg/kg day divided q 6-8 hours x 3 days; *see page 572 for dose by weight table;* ≥12 years: 250-500 mg q 6 hours x 10 days
  Pen-VK *Tab:* 250, 500 mg; *Oral soln:* 125 mg/5 ml (100, 200 ml); 250 mg/5 ml (100, 150, 200 ml)

INCONTINENCE: FECAL

Comment: Treatment of fecal incontinence in patients who have failed conservative therapy (e.g., diet, fiber therapy, antimotility agents).
▷ *dextranomer microspheres/sodium hyaluronate* (NE) <18 years: not recommended; ≥18 years: *Pretreatment:* bowel preparation using enema (required) and prophylactic antibiotics (recommended) prior to injection; *Treatment:* inject slowly into the deep submucosal layer in the proximal part of the high pressure zone of the anal canal about 5 mm above the dentate line; 4 x 1 ml injections in the following order: posterior, left lateral, anterior, right lateral; keep needle in place 15-30 seconds to minimize leakage; use a new needle for each syringe and injection site; *Post-treatment:* avoid hot baths and physical activity during first 24 hours; avoid antidiarrheal drugs, sexual intercourse, and strenuous activity for 1 week; avoid anal manipulation for 1 month; *Retreatment:* may repeat if needed with max 4 ml, no sooner than 4 weeks after the first injection; point of injection should be made in between initial injection sites (i.e., shifted 1/8 of a turn)
  Solesta *dex micro* 50 mg/*sod hyal* 15 mg per ml; *Syringe:* 1 ml (4 w. needles)

INCONTINENCE: URINARY (STRESS INCONTINENCE/ OVERACTIVE BLADDER/ATONIC BLADDER)

See **Enuresis** *page 133*
▷ *pseudoephedrine* (C)(G) 30-60 mg tid
  Sudafed (OTC) *Tab:* 30 mg; *Liq:* 15 mg/5 ml (1, 4 oz)

VASOPRESSIN

▷ *desmopressin acetate (DDAVP)* (B)(G)
  DDAVP <6 years: not recommended; ≥6 years: 0.5 mg daily or q HS prn; ≥12 years: usual dosage 0.1-1.2 mg/day in 2-3 divided doses; 0.2 mg q HS prn for nocturnal enuresis
    Tab: 0.1*, 0.2*mg
  DDAVP Rhinal Tube <6 years: not recommended; ≥6 years: 10 mcg or 0.1 ml of soln each nostril (20 mcg total dose) q HS prn; max 40 mcg total dose
    Rhinal tube: 0.1 mg/ml (2.5 ml)

BETA-3 ADRENERGIC AGONIST

▷ *mirabegron* (C) <12 years: not established; ≥12 years: initially 25 mg once daily; max 50 mg once daily; *Severe renal impairment:* 25 mg once daily
  Myrbetriq *Tab:* 25, 50 mg ext-rel

MUSCARINIC RECEPTOR ANTAGONISTS

➤ *fesoterodine* (C)(G) <12 years: not recommended; ≥12 years: 4 mg daily; max 8 mg/day
>>Toviaz *Tab:* 4, 8 mg ext-rel
➤ *tolterodine tartrate* (C)(G) <12 years: not established; ≥12 years: **Detrol** 2 mg bid; may decrease to 1 mg bid
>>*Tab:* 1, 2 mg
>>**Detrol LA** 2-4 mg once daily
>>*Cap:* 2, 4 mg ext-rel

ANTISPASMODIC/ANTICHOLINERGICS

➤ *darifenacin* (C) <12 years: not recommended; ≥12 years: not recommended; ≥12 years: 7.5-15 mg daily with liquid; max 15 mg/day
>>**Enablex** *Tab:* 7.5, 15 mg ext-rel
➤ *dicyclomine* (B)(G) <12 years: not recommended; ≥12 years: 10-20 mg qid
>>**Bentyl** *Tab:* 20 mg; *Cap:* 10 mg; *Syr:* 10 mg/5 ml (16 oz)
➤ *flavoxate* (B) <12 years: not recommended; ≥12 years: 100-200 mg tid-qid
>>**Urispas** *Tab:* 100 mg
➤ *hyoscyamine* (C)(G)
>>**Anaspaz** <2 years: not recommended; 2-12 years: 0.0625-0.125 mg q 4 hours prn; max 0.75 mg/day; >12 years: 1-2 tabs q 4 hours prn; max 12 tabs/day
>>>*Tab:* 0.125*
>>**Levbid** <12 years: not recommended; ≥12 years: 1-2 tabs q 12 hours prn; max 4 tabs/day
>>>*Tab:* 0.375*mg ext-rel
>>**Levsin** <6 years: not recommended; 6-12 years: 1 tab q 4 hours prn; >12 years: 1-2 tabs q 4 hours prn; max 12 tabs/day
>>>*Tab:* 0.125*mg;
>>**Levsin Drops** <12 years: 3.4 kg: 4 drops q 4 hours prn; max 24 drops/day; 5 kg: 5 drops q 4 hours prn; max 30 drops/day; 7 kg: 6 drops q 4 hours prn; max 36 drops/day; 10 kg: 8 drops q 4 hours prn; max 40 drops/day; ≥12 years: 1-2 ml q 4 hours prn; max 60 ml/day
>>>*Oral drops:* 0.125 mg/ml (15 ml) (orange) (alcohol 5%)
>>**Levsin Elixir** <12 years: <10 kg: use drops; 10-19 kg: 1.25 ml q 4 hours prn; 20-39 kg: 2.5 ml q 4 hours prn; 40-49 kg: 3.75 ml q 4 hours prn; ≥50 kg: 5 ml q 4 hours prn; ≥12 years: 5-10 ml q 4 hours prn
>>>*Elix:* 0.125 mg/5 ml (16 oz) (orange) (alcohol 20%)
>>**Levsinex SL** <2 years: not recommended; 2-12 years: 1 tab q 4 hours; max 6 tabs/day; >12 years:
>>>*Tab:* 0.125 mg sublingual; ≥12 years: 1-2 tabs q 4 hours SL or PO; max 12 tabs/day
>>**Levsinex Timecaps** <2 years: not recommended; 2-12 years: 1 cap q 12 hours; max 2 caps/day; >12 years: 1-2 caps q 12 hours; may adjust to 1 cap q 8 hours
>>>*Cap:* 0.375 mg time-rel
>>**NuLev** <2 years: not recommended; 2-12 years: dissolve 1 tab on tongue, with or without water, q 4 hours prn; max 6 tabs/day; >12 years: dissolve 1-2 tabs on tongue, with or without water, q 4 hours prn; max 12 tabs/day
>>>*ODT:* 0.125 mg (mint; phenylalanine)

▷ *oxybutynin chloride* (B)

Ditropan <5 years: not recommended; 5-12 years: 5 mg bid; max 15 mg/day; >12 years: 5 mg bid-tid; max 20 mg/day

Tab: 5*mg; *Syr:* 5 mg/5 ml

Ditropan XL <6 years: not recommended; ≥6 years: initially 5 mg once daily; may increase weekly in 5 mg increments as needed; max 20 mg/day; ≥12 years: initially 5 mg daily; may increase weekly in 5 mg increments as needed; max 30 mg/day

Tab: 5, 10, 15 mg ext-rel

GelniQUE 3 mg Pump: <6 years: not recommended; ≥6 years: apply 3 pumps (84 mg) once daily to clean dry intact skin on the abdomen, upper arm, shoulders, or thighs; rotate sites; wash hands; avoid washing application site for 1 hour after application

Gel: 3% (92 g, metered pump dispenser) (alcohol)

GelniQUE 1 gm Sachet: <6 years: not recommended; ≥6 years: apply 1 gm gel (1 sachet) once daily to dry intact skin on abdomen, upper arms/shoulders, or thighs; rotate sites; wash hands; avoid washing application site for 1 hour after application

Gel: 10%, 1 gm/sachet (30/carton) (alcohol)

Oxytrol Transdermal Patch (OTC) <12 years: not established; ≥12 years: apply patch to clean dry area of the abdomen, hip, or buttock; one patch twice weekly; rotate sites

Transdermal patch: 3.9 mg/day

▷ *propantheline* (C) <12 years: not recommended; ≥12 years: 15-30 mg tid

Pro-Banthine *Tab:* 7.5, 15 mg

▷ *solifenacin* (C)(G) <12 years: not recommended; ≥12 years: 5-10 mg daily

VESIcare *Tab:* 5, 10 mg

▷ *trospium chloride* (C)(G)

Sanctura <6 years: not recommended; ≥6 years: 20 mg twice daily; ≥75 years: *CrCl ≤30 mL/min:* 20 mg once daily

Tab: 20 mg

Sanctura XR <6 years: not recommended; ≥6 years: 60 mg daily in the morning

Cap: 60 mg ext-rel

Comment: Take *trospium chloride* on an empty stomach.

OVERFLOW INCONTINENCE/ATONIC BLADDER

▷ *bethanechol* (C) <12 years: not recommended; ≥12 years: 10-30 mg tid

Urecholine *Tab:* 5, 10, 25, 50 mg

INFLUENZA (FLU)

Comment: With the exception of **Flucelvax**, flu vaccine is contraindicated with allergy to egg or chicken proteins, or egg products. All flu vaccines are contraindicated with allergy to latex, active infection, acute respiratory disease, active neurological disorder; history of Guillain-Barre syndrome. Have epinephrine 1:1,000 on hand. Flu vaccine is contraindicated for children under 18 years-of-age who are taking aspirin and/or an aspirin-containing product due to the risk of developing Reye's syndrome. Under 1 year of age, administer flu vaccine in the vastus lateralis. Over 1 year of age, administer flu vaccine in the deltoid. Flu vaccine formulations change annually. Administer flu vaccine 1 month before flu season. Spray may be administered earlier.

PROPHYLAXIS (NASAL SPRAY)

▷ *trivalent, live attenuated influenza vaccine, types a and b* (C) ≤5 years: not recommended; ≥5 years: 1 spray each nostril
> Never vaccinated with **FluMist**: 5-8 years: 2 divided doses 46-74 days apart.
> Previously vaccinated with **FluMist**: 5-8 years: 1 spray each nostril
> **FluMist Nasal Spray** 0.5 ml spray annually
>> *Nasal spray:* 0.5 ml (0.25 ml/spray) (10/carton) (preservative-free)

PROPHYLAXIS (INJECTABLE)

▷ *quadrivalent inactivated influenza subvirion vaccine, types a and b* (C) <3 years: not recommended; ≥3 years: 0.5 ml IM annually
> **Fluarix Quadrivalent** *Prefilled syringes:* 0.5 ml (10/carton; preservative-free, latex-free)

▷ *trivalent inactivated influenza subvirion vaccine, types A and B*
> **Afluria** (B) <5 years: not recommended; 5-8 years: 1-2 doses/season at least 4 weeks apart; >9 years: 1 dose/season
> Comment: Contraindicated with allergy to egg or chicken protein, neomycin, polymyxin, or history of life-threatening reaction to any previous fly vaccine.
> **Fluarix** (B) 0.5 ml IM annually; <3 years: not recommended; 3-9 years (previously unvaccinated or vaccinated for the first time last season with one dose of flu vaccine): 2 doses per season at least 1 month apart; 3-9 years (previously vaccinated with two doses of flu vaccine); and >9 years: 1 dose per season
>> *Prefilled syringe:* 0.5 ml single dose (5/carton) (may contain trace amounts of hydrocortisone, gentamicin; preservative-free)
> Comment: Contraindicated with allergy to egg protein.
> **Flublok** <18 years: not recommended; ≥18 years: 0.5 ml IM in the deltoid annually
>> *Vial:* 0.5 ml single dose (10/carton) (preservative-free, egg protein-free, antibiotic-free, latex-free)
> Comment: **Flublok** is a cell culture-derived vaccine and, therefore, is an alternative to the traditional egg-based vaccines. Contains 3 times the amount of active ingredient in traditional flu vaccines
> **Flucelvax** <18 years: not established; ≥18 years: 0.5 ml IM annually
>> *Prefilled syringes:* 0.5 ml (10/carton; preservative-free, latex-free)
> Comment: **Flucelvax** is a cell culture-derived vaccine and, therefore, is an alternative to the traditional egg-based vaccines.
> **FluLaval** (C) <3 years: not established; 3-8 years, *never received the vaccine:* 2 doses/season administered at least 4 weeks apart; 3-8 years, *vaccinated in a previous season:* 1-2 doses/season administered at least 4 weeks apart; ≥9 years: one dose/season; a single dose is 0.5 ml; all ages, administer IM in the deltoid
>> *Vial:* 5 ml multi-dose (10 doses)
> Comment: Contraindicated with allergy to egg protein.
> **FluShield** <6 months: not recommended; *Never vaccinated:* <9 years: 2 doses at least 4 weeks apart; 9-12 years: same as adult; *Previously vaccinated:* 6-35 months: 0.25 ml IM x 1 dose; 3-8 years: 0.5 ml IM annually
> **Fluzone** 0.5 ml IM annually
>> *Vial:* 5 ml (thimerosal)
> Comment: Contraindicated with allergy to egg protein, or history of life-threatening reaction to any previous flu vaccine.

Fluzone Preservative-Free: Adult Dose <6 months: not recommended; *Not previously vaccinated:* 6 months-8 years: 0.25 ml IM; repeat in 1 month; *Previously vaccinated:* 6-35 months: 0.25 ml IM x 1 dose; ≥3 years: 0.5 ml IM annually
Prefilled syringe: 0.5 ml (10/carton) (preservative-free, trace thimerosal)
Fluzone Preservative-Free: Pediatric Dose <6 months: not recommended; *Not previously vaccinated:* 6 months-8 years: 0.25 ml IM; repeat in 1 month; *Previously vaccinated:* 6-35 months: 0.25 ml IM x 1 dose; ≥3 years: 0.5 ml IM (use **Fluzone for Adult**). All ages: administer in the deltoid
  Prefilled syringe: 0.5 ml (10/carton; preservative-free; trace thimerosal)
Comment: Contraindicated with allergy to egg protein, or history of life-threatening reaction to any previous flu vaccine.

PROPHYLAXIS AND TREATMENT

Neuraminidase Inhibitors

Comment: Effective for influenza type A and B. Indicated for treatment of uncomplicated acute illness in patients who have been symptomatic for no more than 2 days; therefore, start within 2 days of symptom onset <u>or</u> exposure. Indicated for influenza prophylaxis in patients ≥3 months of age.

▷ *oseltamivir phosphate* **(C)(G)** *Prophylaxis:* <1 year: not recommended; 1-12 years: <15 kg: 30 mg once daily x 10 days; 16-23 kg: 45 mg once daily x 10 days; 24-40 kg: 60 mg once daily x 10 days; >40 kg: 75 mg daily for at least 7 days and up to 6 weeks for community outbreak; *Treatment:* <1 year: not recommended; 1-12 years: <15 kg: 30 mg bid x 5 days; 16-23 kg: 45 mg bid x 5 days; 24-40 kg: 60 mg bid x 5 days; >40 kg: 75 mg bid x 5 days; initiate treatment only if symptomatic <2 days
  Tamiflu *Cap:* 30, 45, 75 mg; *Oral susp:* 6 mg/ml pwdr for reconstitution (60 ml w. oral dispenser) (tutti-frutti)
  Comment: **Tamiflu** is effective for influenza type A and B.

▷ *zanamivir* **(C)** <7 years: not recommended; ≥7 years: 2 inhalations (10 mg) bid x 5 days
  Relenza Inhaler *Inhaler:* 5 mg/inh blister; 4 blisters/Rotadisk (5 Rotadisks/carton w. 1 inhaler)
  Comment: **Relenza Inhaler** is effective for influenza type A and B. Use caution with asthma.
  Antipyretics *see Fever page 138*

INSECT BITE/STING

TOPICAL ANESTHETIC

▷ *lidocaine* 3% cream **(B)** apply bid-tid prn; reduce dosage commensurate with age, body weight, and physical condition
  LidaMantle *Crm:* 3% (1 oz)
Oral Prescription Drugs for the Management of Allergy, Cough, and Cold Symptoms *see page 523*
Topical Corticosteroids *see page 494*
Parenteral Corticosteroids *see page 499*
Oral Corticosteroids *see page 498*

OTHER AGENTS

▷ *epinephrine* (C)(G) <12 years: 0.01 ml/kg SC; ≥12 years: 1:1,000 0.3-0.5 ml

TETANUS PROPHYLAXIS

▷ *tetanus toxoid* vaccine (C)(G) 0.5 ml IM x 1 dose if previously immunized
Vial: 5 Lf units/0.5 ml (0.5, 5 ml); *Prefilled syringe:* 5 Lf units/0.5 ml (0.5 ml) (For
patients not previously immunized *see* **Tetanus** page 398)

INSOMNIA

MELATONIN RECEPTOR AGONIST

▷ *ramelteon* (C)(IV) <12 years: not recommended; ≥12 years: 8 mg within 30 minutes
of bedtime; delayed effect if taken with a meal
Rozerem *Tab:* 8 mg

NON-BENZODIAZEPINES

▷ *eszopiclone* (pyrrolopyrazine) (C)(IV)(G) <18 years: not recommended; ≥18 years:
1-3 mg; max 3 mg/day x 1 month; do not take if unable to sleep for at least 8 hours
before required to be active again; delayed effect if taken with a meal
Lunesta *Tab:* 1, 2, 3 mg
▷ *zaleplon* (imidazopyridine) (C)(IV) <12 years: not recommended; ≥12 years: 5-10
mg at HS or after going to bed if unable to sleep; do not take if unable to sleep for at
least 4 hours before required to be active again; max 20 mg/day x 1 month; delayed
effect if taken with a meal
Sonata *Cap:* 5, 10 mg (tartrazine)
Comment: **Sonata** is indicated for the treatment of insomnia when a middle-of-
the-night awakening is followed by difficulty returning to sleep.
▷ *zolpidem* oral solution spray (imidazopyridine hypnotic) (C)(IV) <12 years: not
recommended; ≥12 years: 2 actuations (10 mg) immediately before bedtime;
Debilitated, or *hepatic impairment:* 2 actuations (5 mg); max 2 actuations (10 mg)
ZolpiMist *Oral soln spray:* 5 mg/actuation (60 metered actuations) (cherry)
Comment: The lowest dose of *zolpidem* in all forms is recommended for females as
drug elimination is slower than in males.
▷ *zolpidem* tabs (pyrazolopyrimidine hypnotic) (B)(IV)(G) <18 years: not recommended; ≥18 years: 5-10 mg or 6.25-12.5 ext-rel q HS prn; max 12.5 mg/day x 1
month; do not take if unable to sleep for at least 8 hours before required to be active
again; delayed effect if taken with a meal
Ambien *Tab:* 5, 10 mg
Ambien CR *Tab:* 6.25, 12.5 mg ext-rel
Comment: The lowest dose of *zolpidem* in all forms is recommended for females as
drug elimination is slower than in men.
▷ *zolpidem* sublingual tabs (imidazopyridine hypnotic) (C)(IV) <18 years: not
recommended; ≥18 years: dissolve 1 tab under the tongue; allow to disintegrate
completely before swallowing; take only once per night and only if at least 4 hours
of bedtime remain before planned time for awakening
Edluar *SL Tab:* 5, 10 mg
Intermezzo *SL Tab:* 1.75, 3.5 mg

Comment: **Intermezzo** is indicated for the treatment of insomnia when a middle-of-the-night awakening is followed by difficulty returning to sleep. The lowest dose of *zolpidem* in all forms is recommended for females as drug elimination is slower than in males.

OREXIN RECEPTOR ANTAGONIST

▷ *suvorexant* (C)(IV) <12 years: not recommended; ≥12 years: use lowest effective dose; take 30 minutes before bedtime; do not take if unable to sleep for ≥7 hours, max 20 mg
Belsomra *Tab:* 5, 10, 15, 20 mg (30/blister pck)

BENZODIAZEPINES

▷ *estazolam* (X)(IV)(G) <18 years: not recommended; ≥18 years: initially 1 mg q HS prn; may increase to 2 mg q HS
ProSom *Tab:* 1*, 2*mg
▷ *flurazepam* (X)(IV)(G) <15 years: not recommended; ≥15 years: 30 mg q HS prn; *Debilitated:* 15 mg
Dalmane *Cap:* 15, 30 mg
▷ *temazepam* (X)(IV)(G) <18 years: not recommended; ≥18 years: 7.5-30 mg q HS prn; short term, 7-10 days; max 30 mg; max 1 month
Restoril *Cap:* 7.5, 15, 22.5, 30 mg
▷ *triazolam* (X)(IV) <18 years: not recommended; ≥18 years: 0.125-0.25 mg q HS prn; short term, 7-10 days; max 0.5 mg; max 1 month
Halcion *Tab:* 0.125, 0.25*mg

BENZODIAZEPINES

▷ *pentobarbital* (D)(II)(G) <12 years: not recommended; ≥12 years: 50 <u>or</u> 100 mg
Nembutal 100 mg q HS prn
Cap: 50, 100 mg
Nembutal Suppository one supp q HS prn; <2 months: not recommended; 2-12 months (10-20 lb): 30 mg supp; >1 year-4 years (21-40 lb): 30 <u>or</u> 60 mg supp; 5-12 years (41-80 lb): 60 mg supp; >12-14 years (81-110 lb): 60 <u>or</u> 120 mg supp; >14 years: 120 <u>or</u> 200 mg supp q HS prn
Rectal supp: 30, 60, 120, 200 mg

ORAL H1 RECEPTOR AGONIST (1ST GENERATION ANTIHISTAMINE)

▷ *doxepin* (C) <12 years: not recommended; ≥12 years: 3-6 mg q HS prn; *Hepatic impairment, tendency to urinary retention:* initially 3 mg
Silenor *Tab:* 3, 6 mg

ANALGESIC/1ST GENERATION ANTIHISTAMINE COMBINATIONS

▷ *acetaminophen/diphenhydramine* (B)
Excedrin PM (OTC) <12 years: not recommended; ≥12 years: 2 tabs q HS prn
Tab/Gel tab: acet 500 mg/*diphen* 38 mg
Tylenol PM (OTC) <12 years: not recommended; ≥12 years: 2 caps q HS prn
Tab/Cap/Gel cap: acet 500 mg/*diphen* 25 mg
Tricyclic Antidepressants *see* **Depression** *page* 99

INTERSTITIAL CYSTITIS

Comment: Avoid peppers and spicy food, citrus, vinegar, caffeine (e.g., coffee, tea, cola), alcohol, carbonated beverages, and other GU tract irritants.

MANAGEMENT OF PAIN AND URINARY URGENCY

Acetaminophen for IV Infusion *see Pain page 296*
Oral Prescription NSAIDs *see page 490*

▶ *phenazopyridine* (B)(G) 12 years: not recommended; ≥12 years: 95-200 mg q 6 hours prn; max 2 days

> **AZO Standard, Prodium, Uristat (OTC)** *Tab:* 95 mg
> **AZO Standard Maximum Strength (OTC)** *Tab:* 97.5 mg
> **Pyridium, Urogesic** *Tab:* 100, 200 mg *phenazopyridine* (B)(G) 190-200 mg tid; max 2 days
> **Azo Standard (OTC)** *Tab:* 95 mg
> **Azo Standard Maximum Strength (OTC)** *Tab:* 97.5 mg
> **Pyridium** *Tab:* 100, 200 mg ent-coat
> **Uristat (OTC)** *Tab:* 95 mg
> **Urogesic** *Tab:* 100, 200 mg

▶ *hyoscyamine* (C)(G)

> **Anaspaz** <2 years: not recommended; 2-12 years: 0.0625-0.125 mg q 4 hours prn; max 0.75 mg/day; >12 years: 1-2 tabs q 4 hours prn; max 12 tabs/day
> *Tab:* 0.125*mg
> **Levbid** <12 years: not recommended; ≥12 years: 1-2 tabs q 12 hours prn; max 4 tabs/day
> *Tab:* 0.375*mg ext-rel
> **Levsin** <6 years: not recommended; 6-12 years: 1 tab q 4 hours prn; ≥12 years: 1-2 tabs q 4 hours prn; max 12 tabs/day
> *Tab:* 0.125*mg
> **Levsin Drops** <3 kg: not recommended: 3.4 kg: 4 drops q 4 hours prn; max 24 drops/day; 5 kg: 5 drops q 4 hours prn; max 30 drops/day; 7 kg: 6 drops q 4 hours prn; max 36 drops/day; 10 kg: 8 drops q 4 hours prn; max 40 drops/day; >10 kg: 1-2 ml q 4 hours prn; max 60 ml/day
> *Oral drops:* 0.125 mg/ml (15 ml) (orange) (alcohol 5%)
> **Levsin Elixir** <10 kg: use drops; 10-19 kg: 1.25 ml q 4 hours prn; 20-39 kg: 2.5 ml q 4 hours prn; 40-49 kg: 3.75 ml q 4 hours prn; ≥50 kg: 5 ml q 4 hours prn
> *Elix:* 0.125 mg/5 ml (16 oz) (orange) (alcohol 20%)
> **Levsinex SL** <2 years: not recommended; 2-12 years: 1 tab q 4 hours; max 6 tabs/day; >12 years: 1-2 tabs q 4 hours SL or PO; max 12 tabs/day
> *SL tab:* 0.125 mg
> **Levsinex Timecaps** <2 years: not recommended; 2-12 years: 1 cap q 12 hours; max 2 caps/day; >12 years: 1-2 caps q 12 hours; may adjust to 1 cap q 8 hours
> *Cap:* 0.375 mg time-rel
> **NuLev** <2 years: not recommended; 2-12 years: dissolve 1 tab on tongue, with or without water, q 4 hours prn; max 6 tabs/day; >12 years: dissolve 1-2 tabs on tongue, with or without water, q 4 hours prn; max 12 tabs/day
> *ODT:* 0.125 mg (mint) (phenylalanine)

▷ *methenamine/na phosphate monobasic/phenyl salicylate/methylene blue/hyoscy-amine sulfate* (C) <6 years: not recommended; ≥6 years: individualize dose (see mfr pkg insert)

> **Uribel** *Cap:* meth 118 mg/*sod phos* 40.8 mg/*phenyl sal* 36 mg/*meth blue* 10 mg/*hyoscy* 0.12 mg

▷ *methenamine/phenyl salicylate/methylene blue/benzoic acid/atropine sulfate/hyos-cyamine sulfate* (C)(G) <6 years: not recommended; ≥6 years: 2 tabs qid

> **Urised** *Tab:* meth 40.8 mg/*phenyl sal* 18.1 mg/*meth blue* 5.4 mg/*benz acid* 4.5 mg/*atro sul* 0.03 mg/*hyoscy* 0.03 mg

> **Comment:** **Urised** imparts a blue-green color to urine which may stain fabrics.

▷ *oxybutynin chloride* (B)

> **Ditropan** <5 years: not recommended; 5-12 years: 5 mg bid; max 15 mg/day; ≥12 years: 5 mg bid-tid; max 20 mg/day
>> *Tab:* 5*mg; *Syr:* 5 mg/5 ml
>
> **Ditropan XL** <12 years: not recommended; ≥12 years: initially 5 mg daily; may increase weekly in 5 mg increments as needed; max 30 mg/day
>> *Tab:* 5, 10, 15 mg ext-rel

▷ *pentosan* (B) <16 years: not recommended; ≥16 years: 100 mg tid; re-evaluate at 3 and 6 months

> **Elmiron** *Cap:* 100 mg

URINARY TRACT ANALGESIA

▷ *phenazopyridine* (B)(G) <12 years: not recommended; ≥12 years: 95-200 mg q 6 hours prn; max 2 days

> **AZO Standard, Prodium, Uristat** (OTC) *Tab:* 95 mg
> **AZO Standard Maximum Strength** (OTC) *Tab:* 97.5 mg
> **Pyridium, Urogesic** *Tab:* 100, 200 mg
> **Azo Standard** (OTC) *Tab:* 95 mg
> **Azo Standard Maximum Strength** (OTC) *Tab:* 97.5 mg
> **Pyridium** *Tab:* 100, 200 mg ent-coat
> **Uristat** (OTC) *Tab:* 95 mg
> **Urogesic** *Tab:* 100, 200 mg

> **Comment:** *Phenazopyridine* imparts an orange-red color to urine which may stain fabrics.

▷ *propantheline* (C) <12 years: not recommended; ≥12 years: 15-30 mg tid

> **Pro-Banthine** *Tab:* 7.5, 15 mg

▷ *tolterodine tartrate* (C)(G)

> **Detrol** <12 years: not recommended; ≥12 years: 2 mg bid; may decrease to 1 mg bid
>> *Tab:* 1, 2 mg
>
> **Detrol XL** 2-4 mg daily
>> *Cap:* 2, 4 mg ext-rel

ANTICHOLINERGIC/SEDATIVE COMBINATION

▷ *chlordiazepoxide/clidinium* (D)(IV) <12 years: not recommended; ≥12 years: 1-2 caps ac and HS; max 8 caps/day

> **Librax** *Cap:* chlor 5 mg/*clid* 2.5 mg

TRICYCLIC ANTIDEPRESSANTS (TCAs)

Comment: Co-administration of SSRIs and TCAs requires extreme caution.
▶ *amitriptyline* (C)(G) <12 years: not recommended; ≥12 years: 10-20 mg q HS
    Tab: 10, 25, 50, 75, 100, 150 mg
▶ *amoxapine* (C) <12 years: not recommended; ≥12 years: initially 50 mg bid-tid;
    after 1 week may increase to 100 mg bid-tid; usual effective dose 200-300 mg/day; if
    total dose exceeds 300 mg/day, give in divided doses (max 400 mg/day); may give as
    a single bedtime dose (max 300 mg q HS)
    Tab: 25, 50, 100, 150 mg
▶ *clomipramine* (C)(G) <10 years: not recommended; 10-<16 years: initially 25 mg
    daily in divided doses; gradually increase; max 3 mg/kg or 100 mg, whichever is
    smaller;>16 years: initially 25 mg daily in divided doses; gradually increase to 100 mg
    during first 2 weeks; max 250 mg/day; total maintenance dose may be given at HS
    Anafranil Cap: 25, 50, 75 mg
▶ *desipramine* (C)(G) <12 years: not recommended; ≥12 years: 100-200 mg/day in
    single or divided doses; max 300 mg/day
    Norpramin Tab: 10, 25, 50, 75, 100, 150 mg
▶ *doxepin* (C)(G) <12 years: not recommended; ≥12 years: 75 mg/day; max 150 mg/day
    Cap: 10, 25, 50, 75, 100, 150 mg; Oral conc: 10 mg/ml (4 oz w. dropper)
▶ *imipramine* (C)(G) <12 years: not recommended; ≥12 years:
    Tofranil <12 years: not recommended; ≥12 years: adolescents initially 30-40 mg
    daily (max 100 mg/day); if maintenance dose exceeds 75 mg daily, may switch
    to Tofranil PM for divided or bedtime dose
       Tab: 10, 25, 50 mg
    Tofranil PM initially 75 mg daily 1 hour before HS; max 200 mg
       Cap: 75, 100, 125, 150 mg
▶ *nortriptyline* (D)(G) <12 years: not recommended; ≥12 years: initially 25 mg tid-
    qid; max 150 mg/day
    Pamelor Cap: 10, 25, 50, 75 mg; Oral soln: 10 mg/5 ml (16 oz)
▶ *protriptyline* (C) <12 years: not recommended; ≥12 years: initially 5 mg tid; usual
    dose 15-40 mg/day in 3-4 divided doses; max 60 mg/day
    Vivactil Tab: 5, 10 mg
▶ *trimipramine* (C) <12 years: not recommended; ≥12 years: initially 75 mg/day in
    divided doses; max 200 mg/day
    Surmontil Cap: 25, 50, 100 mg

INTERTRIGO

Comment: Intertrigo is an irritation and rash secondary to adjacent skin surfaces
rubbing together. Treatment is dependent on symptoms and presence of infection.
Topical Corticosteroids see page 494
Topical Antifungals see Tinea Corporis page 400
Topical Anti-infectives see Skin Infection: Bacterial page 386

IRITIS: ACUTE

▶ *loteprednol etabonate* (C) <12 years: not recommended; ≥12 years: 1-2 drops qid;
    may increase to 1 drop hourly as needed
    Lotemax Ophthalmic Solution Ophth soln: 0.3% (2.5, 5, 10, 15 ml)

➤ *prednisone acetate* (**C**) <12 years: not recommended; ≥12 years: 1 drop q 1 hour x 24-48 hours, then 1 drop q 2 hours while awake x 24-48 hours, then 1 drop bid-qid until resolved

    Pred Forte *Ophth soln:* 1% (1, 5, 10, 15 ml)

IRON OVERLOAD

IRON CHELATING AGENTS

➤ *deferasirox* (*tridentate ligand*) (**C**)(**G**) <2 years: not recommended; ≥2 years: initially 20 mg/kg/day; titrate; may increase 5-10 mg/kg q 3-6 months based on serum ferritin trends; max 30 mg/kg/day

    Exjade *Tab for oral soln:* 125, 250, 500 mg
    Jadenu *Tab:* 90, 180, 360 mg film-coat

Comment: *deferasirox* is an orally active chelator selective for iron. It is indicated for the treatment of chronic iron overload due to blood transfusions (transfusional hemosiderosis). Monitor serum ferritin monthly. Consider interrupting therapy if serum ferritin falls below 500 mcg/L. Take *deferasirox* (**Jadenu**, **Exjade**) on an empty stomach. Completely disperse tablet(s) for oral solution in 3.5 oz liquid if dose is ≤1 gm or 7 oz liquid if dose is ≥1 gm.

➤ *succimer* (**C**) <12 years: not recommended; ≥12 years: initially 10 mg/kg q 8 hours x 5 days; then, reduce frequency to every 12 hours x 14 more days; allow at least 14 days between courses unless blood lead levels indicate need for prompt treatment

    Chemet *Cap:* 100 mg

Comment: **Chemet** *is* indicated for the treatment of lead poisoning when blood lead level 45 mcg/dL. Treatment for more than 3 consecutive weeks is not recommended. Monitor hydration, renal, and hepatic function.

IRRITABLE BOWEL SYNDROME WITH CONSTIPATION (IBS-C)

Bulk-Producing Agents, Laxatives, Stool Softeners *see Constipation* page 87

GUANYLATE CYCLASE-C AGONIST

➤ *linaclotide* (**C**) <6 years: not recommended; 6-17 years: avoid; >17 years: 290 mcg once daily; take on an empty stomach at least 30 minutes before the first meal of the day; swallow whole

    Linzess *Cap:* 72, 145, 290 mcg

Comment: May open **Linzess** cap and sprinkle on applesauce or in water for administration

➤ *lubiprostone* (**C**) <18 years: not recommended; ≥18 years: 8 mcg bid; take with food and water; *Severe hepatic impairment (Child-Pugh Class C):* 8 mcg once daily

    Amitiza *Cap:* 8, 24 mcg

IRRITABLE BOWEL SYNDROME WITH DIARRHEA (IBS-D)

Bulk-Producing Agents *see Constipation page* 87

CONSTIPATING AGENTS

➤ *difenoxin/atropine* (C) <12 years: not recommended; ≥12 years: 2 tabs, then 1 tab after each loose stool <u>or</u> 1 tab q 3-4 hours as needed; max 8 tab/day x 2 days
   Motofen *Tab:* difen 1 mg/atro 0.025 mg

➤ *diphenoxylate/atropine* (C)(G) <2 years: not recommended; 2-12 years: initially 0.3-0.4 mg/kg/day in 4 divided doses; >12 years: 2 tabs <u>or</u> 10 ml qid
   Lomotil *Tab:* difen 2.5 mg/atro 0.025 mg; *Liq:* difen 2.5 mg/atro 0.025 mg per 5 ml (2 oz)

➤ *eluxadoline* (NA)(IV) <12 years: not established; ≥12 years: 100 mg bid; 75 mg bid if unable to tolerate 100 mg, <u>or</u> without a gall bladder, <u>or</u> mild-to-moderate hepatic impairment, <u>or</u> receiving concomitant OATP1B1 inhibitors
   Viberzi 4 mg initially, then 2 mg after each loose stool; max 16 mg/day
   Tab: 75, 100 mg film-coat

Comment: *eluxadoline* is a mu-opioid receptor agonist. It is contraindicated with biliary obstruction, Sphincter of Oddi disease <u>or</u> dysfunction, alcohol abuse <u>or</u> addiction, pancreatitis, pancreatic duct obstruction, severe hepatic impairment, and mechanical GI obstruction.

➤ *loperamide* (B)(G)
   Imodium (OTC) <5 years: not recommended; ≥5 years: 4 mg initially, then 2 mg after each loose stool; max 16 mg/day
   Cap: 2 mg
   Imodium A-D (OTC) <2 years: not recommended; 2-5 years (24-47 lb): 1 mg up to tid x 2 days; 6-8 years (48-59 lb): 2 mg initially, then 1 mg after each loose stool; max 4 mg/day x 2 days; 9-11 years (60-95 lb): 2 mg initially, then 1 mg after each loose stool; max 6 mg/day x 2 days; ≥12 years: 4 mg initially, then 2 mg after each loose stool; usual max 8 mg/day x 2 days
   Cplt: 2 mg; *Liq:* 1 mg/5 ml (2, 4 oz)

➤ *loperamide/simethicone* (B)(G)
   Imodium Advanced (OTC) <6 years: not recommended; 6-8 years: 1 tab chewed after loose stool, then 1/2 after next loose stool; max 2 tabs/day; 9-11 years: 1 tab chewed after loose stool, then 1/2 after next loose stool; max 3 tabs/day; ≥12 years: 2 tabs chewed after loose stool, then 1 after the next loose stool; max 4 tabs/day
   Chew tab: lop 2 mg/sim 125 mg

5-HT3 RECEPTOR ANTAGONIST

➤ *alosetron* (B)(G) <12 years: not recommended; ≥12 years: initially 0.5 mg bid; may increase to 1 mg bid after 4 weeks if starting dose is tolerated but inadequate
   Lotronex *Tab:* 0.5, 1 mg

ANTISPASMODIC/ANTICHOLINERGIC COMBINATIONS

➤ *dicyclomine* (B)(G) <12 years: not recommended; ≥12 years: initially 20 mg bid-qid; may increase to 40 mg qid PO; usual IM dose 80 mg/day divided qid; do not use IM route for more than 1-2 days

> Bentyl *Tab:* 20 mg; *Cap:* 10 mg; *Syr:* 10 mg/5 ml (16 oz); *Vial:* 10 mg/ml (10 ml); *Amp:* 10 mg/ml (2 ml)

▷ *methscopolamine bromide* (B) <12 years: not recommended; ≥12 years: 1 tab q 6 hours prn

Pamine *Tab:* 2.5 mg
Pamine Forte *Tab:* 5 mg

ANTICHOLINERGICS

▷ *hyoscyamine* (C)(G)

Anaspaz <2 years: not recommended; 2-12 years: 0.0625-0.125 mg q 4 hours prn; max 0.75 mg/day; >12 years: 1-2 tabs q 4 hours prn; max 12 tabs/day
Tab: 0.125*mg

Levbid <12 years: not recommended; ≥12 years: 1-2 tabs q 12 hours prn; max 4 tabs/day
Tab: 0.375*mg ext-rel

Levsin <6 years: not recommended; 6-12 years: 1 tab q 4 hours prn; >12 years: 1-2 tabs q 4 hours prn; max 12 tabs/day
Tab: 0.125*mg

Levsinex SL <2 years: not recommended; 2-12 years: 1 tab q 4 hours; max 6 tabs/day; >12 years: 1-2 tabs q 4 hours SL <u>or</u> PO; max 12 tabs/day
Tab: 0.125 mg sublingual

Levsinex Timecaps <2 years: not recommended; 2-12 years: 1 cap q 12 hours; max 2 caps/day; >12 years: 1-2 caps q 12 hours; may adjust to 1 cap q 8 hours
Cap: 0.375 mg time-rel

NuLev <2 years: not recommended; 2-12 years: dissolve 1 tab on tongue, with <u>or</u> without water, q 4 hours prn; max 6 tabs/day; >12 years: dissolve 1-2 tabs on tongue, with <u>or</u> without water, q 4 hours prn; max 12 tabs/day
ODT: 0.125 mg (mint; phenylalanine)

▷ *simethicone* (C)(G) 0.3 ml qid pc and HS

Mylicon Drops (OTC) *Oral drops:* 40 mg/0.6 ml (30 ml)

▷ *phenobarbital/hyoscyamine/atropine/scopolamine* (C)(IV)(G)

Donnatal <12 years: not recommended; ≥12 years: 1-2 tabs ac and HS
Tab: pheno 16.2 mg/*hyo* 0.1037 mg/*atro* 0.0194 mg/*scop* 0.0065 mg

Donnatal Elixir <12 years: not recommended; ≥12 years: 1-2 tsp ac and HS 20 lb: 1 ml q 4 hours <u>or</u> 1.5 ml q 6 hours; 30 lb: 1.5 ml q 4 hours <u>or</u> 2 ml q 6 hours; 50 lb: 1/2 tsp q 4 hours <u>or</u> 3/4 tsp q 6 hours; 75 lb: 3/4 tsp q 4 hours <u>or</u> 1 tsp q 6 hours; 100 lb: 1 tsp q 4 hours <u>or</u> 1 tsp q 6 hours
Elix: pheno 16.2 mg/*hyo* 0.1037 mg/*atro* 0.0194 mg/*scop* 0.0065 mg per 5 ml (4, 16 oz)

Donnatal Extentabs <12 years: not recommended; ≥12 years: 1 tab q 12 hours
Tab: pheno 48.6 mg/*hyo* 0.3111 mg/*atro* 0.0582 mg/*scop* 0.0195 mg ext-rel

ANTICHOLINERGIC/SEDATIVE COMBINATION

▷ *chlordiazepoxide/clidinium* (D)(IV) <12 years: not recommended; ≥12 years: 1-2 caps ac and HS: max 8 caps/day

Librax *Cap: chlor* 5 mg/*clid* 2.5 mg

TRICYCLIC ANTIDEPRESSANTS (TCAS)

Comment: Co-administration of SSRIs and TCAs requires extreme caution.

➤ *amitriptyline* (C)(G) <12 years: not recommended; ≥12 years: 10-20 mg q HS
    Tab: 10, 25, 50, 75, 100, 150 mg
➤ *amoxapine* (C) <12 years: not recommended; ≥12 years: initially 50 mg bid-tid;
    after 1 week may increase to 100 mg bid-tid; usual effective dose 200-300 mg/day; if
    total dose exceeds 300 mg/day, give in divided doses (max 400 mg/day); may give as
    a single bedtime dose (max 300 mg q HS)
    Tab: 25, 50, 100, 150 mg
➤ *clomipramine* (C)(G) <10 years: not recommended; 10-16 years: initially 25 mg
    daily in divided doses; gradually increase; max 3 mg/kg <u>or</u> 100 mg, whichever is
    smaller; >16 years: initially 25 mg daily in divided doses; gradually increase to 100
    mg during first 2 weeks; max 250 mg/day; total maintenance dose may be given at
    HS
    Anafranil *Cap:* 25, 50, 75 mg
➤ *desipramine* (C)(G) <12 years: not recommended; ≥12 years: 100-200 mg/day in
    single <u>or</u> divided doses; max 300 mg/day
    Norpramin *Tab:* 10, 25, 50, 75, 100, 150 mg
➤ *doxepin* (C)(G) <12 years: not recommended; ≥12 years: 75 mg/day; max 150 mg/
    day
    Cap: 10, 25, 50, 75, 100, 150 mg; *Oral conc:* 10 mg/ml (4 oz w. dropper)
➤ *imipramine* (C)(G) <12 years: not recommended; ≥12 years:
    Tofranil initially 75 mg daily (max 200 mg); adolescents initially 30-40 mg daily
    (max 100 mg/day); if maintenance dose exceeds 75 mg daily, may switch to
    Tofranil PM for divided <u>or</u> bedtime dose
        Tab: 10, 25, 50 mg
    Tofranil PM initially 75 mg daily 1 hour before HS; max 200 mg
    Cap: 75, 100, 125, 150 mg
➤ *nortriptyline* (D)(G) <12 years: not recommended; ≥12 years: initially 25 mg tid-
    qid; max 150 mg/day
    Pamelor *Cap:* 10, 25, 50, 75 mg; *Oral soln:* 10 mg/5 ml (16 oz)
➤ *protriptyline* (C) <12 years: not recommended; ≥12 years: initially 5 mg tid; usual
    dose 15-40 mg/day in 3-4 divided doses; max 60 mg/day
    Vivactil *Tab:* 5, 10 mg
➤ *trimipramine* (C) <12 years: not recommended; ≥12 years: initially 75 mg/day in
    divided doses; max 200 mg/day
    Surmontil *Cap:* 25, 50, 100 mg

JUVENILE IDIOPATHIC ARTHRITIS (JIA), POLYARTICULAR JUVENILE IDIOPATHIC ARTHRITIS (PJIA), SYSTEMIC JUVENILE IDIOPATHIC ARTHRITIS (SJIA)

Acetaminophen for IV Infusion *see Pain page* 296
Oral Prescription NSAIDs *see page* 490
Other Oral Analgesics *see Pain page* 298
Topical/Transdermal NSAIDs *see Pain page* 298
Parenteral Corticosteroids *see page* 499
Oral Corticosteroids *see page* 498
Topical Analgesic and Anesthetic Agents *see page* 488

TOPICAL ANALGESICS

➤ *capsaicin* cream **(B)(G)** <2 years: not recommended; 2-12 years: apply sparingly to intact skin bid prn; >12 years: apply tid-qid prn

> **Axsain** *Crm:* 0.075% (1, 2 oz)
> **Capsin (OTC)** *Lotn:* 0.025, 0, 075% (59 ml)
> **Capzasin-P (OTC)** *Crm:* 0.025% (1.5 oz); *Lotn:* 0.025% (2 oz)
> **Capzasin-HP (OTC)** *Crm:* 0.075% (1.5 oz); *Lotn:* 0.075% (2 oz)
> **Dolorac** *Crm:* 0.025% (28 gm)
> **Double Cap (OTC)** *Crm:* 0.05% (2 oz)
> **R-Gel** *Gel:* 0.025% (15, 30 gm)
> **Zostrix (OTC)** *Crm:* 0.025% (0.7, 1.5, 3 oz)
> **Zostrix HP (OTC)** *Emol crm:* 0.075% (1, 2 oz)

Comment: Provides some relief by 1-2 weeks; optimal benefit may take 4-6 weeks. Avoid contact with mucous membranes.

ORAL SALICYLATES

➤ *indomethacin* **(C)** <14 years: usually not recommended; >2 years, if risk warranted: 1-2 mg/kg/day in divided doses; max 3-4 mg/kg/day (or 150-200 mg/day, whichever is less); <14 years, ER cap not recommended; ≥14 years: initially 25 mg bid or tid, increase as needed at weekly intervals by 25-50 mg/day; max 200 mg/day

> *Cap:* 25, 50 mg; *Susp;* 25 mg/5 ml (pineapple-coconut, mint) (alcohol 1%);
> *Supp:* 50 mg; *ER Cap:* 75 mg ext-rel

Comment: *indomethacin* is indicated only for acute painful flares. Administer with food and/or antacids. Use lowest effective dose for shortest duration.

➤ *methotrexate* **(X)** <2 years: not recommended; 2-12 years: 10 mg/m² once weekly; max 20 mg/m²; >12 years: 7.5 mg x 1 dose per week or 2.5 mg x 3 at 12 hour intervals once a week; max 20 mg/week; therapeutic response begins in 3-6 weeks; administer *methotrexate* injection SC only into the abdomen or thigh

> **Rasuvo** *Autoinjector:* 7.5 mg/0.15 ml, 10 mg/0.20 ml, 12.5 mg/0.25 ml, 15 mg/0.30 ml, 17.5 mg/0.35 ml, 20 mg/0.40 ml, 22.5 mg/0.45 ml, 25 mg/0.50 ml, 27.5 mg/0.55 ml, 30 mg/0.60 ml (solution concentration for SC injection is 50 mg/ml)
> **Rheumatrex** *Tab:* 2.5*mg (5, 7.5, 10, 12.5, 15 mg/week, 4/card unit dose pack)
> **Trexall** *Tab:* 5*, 7.5*, 10*, 15*mg (5, 7.5, 10, 12.5, 15 mg/week, 4/card unit dose pack)

Comment: *methotrexate* (MTX) is contraindicated with immunodeficiency, blood dyscrasias, alcoholism, and chronic liver disease.

Interleukin-6 Receptor Antagonist

➤ *tocilizumab* **(B)** <2 years: not recommended; ≥2 years: weight-based dosing according to *SJIA: ≥30 kg:* 8 mg/kg SC every 2 weeks; *<30 kg:* 12 mg/kg SC every 2 weeks; *IV Infusion:* administer over 1 hour; do not administer as bolus or IV push; *PJIA, and SJIA, ≥30 kg:* dilute to 100 mL in 0.9% or 0.45% NaCl. *PJIA and SJIA, <30 kg:* dilute to 50 mL in 0.9% or 0.45% NaCl; ≥18 years: whether used in combination with DMARDs or as monotherapy, the recommended IV infusion starting dose is 4 mg/kg IV every 4 weeks followed by an increase to 8 mg/kg IV every 4 weeks based on clinical response; Max 800 mg per infusion in RA patients; *SC Administration:* ≥100 kg: 162 mg SC once weekly on the same day; <100 kg: 162 mg SC every other week on the same day followed by an increase according to clinical response

Actemra *Vial:* 80 mg/4 ml, 200 mg/10 ml, 400 mg/20 ml, single-use, for IV infusion after dilution; *Prefilled syringe:* 162 mg (0.9 ml, single-dose)

Comment: *tocilizumab* is an interleukin-6 receptor-α inhibitor indicated for use in moderate-to-severe rheumatoid arthritis (RA) that has not responded to conventional therapy, and also for some subtypes of juvenile idiopathic arthritis (JIA). **Actemra** may be used alone or in combination with **methotrexate** and in RA, other DMARDs may be used. Monitor patient for dose related laboratory changes including elevated LFTs, neutropenia, and thrombocytopenia. **Actemra** should not be initiated in patients with an absolute neutrophil count (ANC) below 2000 per mm3, platelet count below 100,000 per mm3, or who have ALT or AST above 1.5 times the upper limit of normal (ULN). Registration in the Pregnancy Exposure Registry (1-877-311-8972) is encouraged for monitoring pregnancy outcomes in women exposed to **Actemra** during pregnancy. The limited available data with **Actemra** in pregnant women are not sufficient to determine whether there is a drug-associated risk for major birth defects and miscarriage. Monoclonal antibodies, such as *tocilizumab*, are actively transported across the placenta during the third trimester of pregnancy and may affect immune response in the infant exposed *in utero*. It is not known whether *tocilizumab* passes into breast milk; therefore, breastfeeding is not recommended while using **Actemra**.

JUVENILE RHEUMATOID ARTHRITIS (JRA)

Acetaminophen for IV Infusion *see Pain page 296*
Oral Prescription NSAIDs *see page 490*
Other Oral Analgesics *see Pain page 298*
Topical/Transdermal NSAIDs *see Pain page 298*
Parenteral Corticosteroids *see page 499*
Oral Corticosteroids *see page 498*
Topical Analgesic and Anesthetic Agents *see page 488*
Juvenile Idiopathic Arthritis (JIA), Polyarticular Juvenile Idiopathic Arthritis (PJIA), Systemic Juvenile Idiopathic Arthritis *see page 242*

TOPICAL ANALGESICS

▶ *capsaicin* cream **(B)(G)** <2 years: not recommended; 2-12 years: apply sparingly to intact skin bid prn; >12 years: apply tid-qid prn
    Axsain *Crm:* 0.075% (1, 2 oz)
    Capsin (OTC) *Lotn:* 0.025, 0,075% (59 ml)
    Capzasin-P (OTC) *Crm:* 0.025% (1.5 oz); *Lotn:* 0.025% (2 oz)
    Capzasin-HP (OTC) *Crm:* 0.075% (1.5 oz); *Lotn:* 0.075% (2 oz)
    Dolorac *Crm:* 0.025% (28 gm)
    Double Cap (OTC) *Crm:* 0.05% (2 oz)
    R-Gel *Gel:* 0.025% (15, 30 gm)
    Zostrix (OTC) *Crm:* 0.025% (0.7, 1.5, 3 oz)
    Zostrix HP (OTC) *Emol crm:* 0.075% (1, 2 oz)

Comment: Provides some relief by 1-2 weeks; optimal benefit may take 4-6 weeks. Avoid contact with mucous membranes.

ORAL SALICYLATE

▶ *indomethacin* **(C)** <14 years: usually not recommended; ≥2 years, if risk warranted: 1-2 mg/kg/day in divided doses; max 3-4 mg/kg/day (or total

150-200 mg/day, whichever is less); ≤14 years, ER cap not recommended; ≥14 years: initially 25 mg bid-tid, increase as needed at weekly intervals by 25-50 mg/day; max 200 mg/day

> *Cap: 25, 50 mg; Susp: 25 mg/5 ml (pineapple-coconut, mint; alcohol 1%); Supp: 50 mg; ER Cap: 75 mg ext-rel*

Comment: *indomethacin* is indicated only for acute painful flares. Administer with food and/or antacids. Use lowest effective dose for shortest duration.

▷ *methotrexate* (X) <2 years: not recommended; 2-12 years: 10 mg/m² once weekly; max 20 mg/m²; >12 years: 7.5 mg x 1 dose per week or 2.5 mg x 3 at 12-hour intervals once a week; max 20 mg/week; therapeutic response begins in 3-6 weeks; administer *methotrexate* injection SC only into the abdomen or thigh

> **Rasuvo** *Autoinjector:* 7.5 mg/0.15 ml, 10 mg/0.20 ml, 12.5 mg/0.25 ml, 15 mg/0.30 ml, 17.5 mg/0.35 ml, 20 mg/0.40 ml, 22.5 mg/0.45 ml, 25 mg/0.50 ml, 27.5 mg/0.55 ml, 30 mg/0.60 ml (solution concentration for SC injection is 50 mg/ml)
> **Rheumatrex** *Tab:* 2.5*mg (5, 7.5, 10, 12.5, 15 mg/week, 4/card unit-of-use dose pack)
> **Trexall** *Tab:* 5*, 7.5*, 10*, 15*mg (5, 7.5, 10, 12.5, 15 mg/week, 4/card unit-of-use dose pack)

Comment: *methotrexate* (MTX) is contraindicated with immunodeficiency, blood dyscrasias, alcoholism, and chronic liver disease.

INTERLEUKIN-6 RECEPTOR ANTAGONIST

▷ *tocilizumab* (B) <2 years: not recommended; ≥2 years: weight-based dosing according to *SJIA:* ≥*30 kg:* 8 mg/kg SC every 2 weeks; <*30 kg:* 12 mg/kg SC every 2 weeks; *IV Infusion:* administer over 1 hour; do not administer as bolus or IV push; *PJIA, and SJIA, ≥30 kg:* dilute to 100 mL in 0.9% or 0.45% NaCl. *PJIA and SJIA, <30 kg:* dilute to 50 mL in 0.9% or 0.45% NaCl; ≥18 years: whether used in combination with DMARDs or as monotherapy, the recommended IV infusion starting dose is 4 mg/kg IV every 4 weeks followed by an increase to 8 mg/kg IV every 4 weeks based on clinical response; Max 800 mg per infusion in RA patients; *SC Administration:* ≥*100 kg:* 162 mg SC once weekly on the same day; <*100 kg:* 162 mg SC every other week on the same day followed by an increase according to clinical response

> **Actemra** *Vial:* 80 mg/4 ml, 200 mg/10 ml, 400 mg/20 ml, single-use, for IV infusion after dilution; *Prefilled syringe:* 162 mg (0.9 ml, single-dose)

Comment: *tocilizumab* is an interleukin-6 receptor-α inhibitor indicated for use in moderate-to-severe rheumatoid arthritis (RA) that has not responded to conventional therapy, and also for some subtypes of juvenile idiopathic arthritis (JIA). **Actemra** may be used alone or in combination with *methotrexate* and in RA, other DMARDs may be used. Monitor patient for dose related laboratory changes including elevated LFTs, neutropenia, and thrombocytopenia. **Actemra** should not be initiated in patients with an absolute neutrophil count (ANC) below 2000 per mm3, platelet count below 100,000 per mm3, or who have ALT or AST above 1.5 times the upper limit of normal (ULN). Registration in the Pregnancy Exposure Registry (1-877-311-8972) is encouraged for monitoring pregnancy outcomes in women exposed to **Actemra** during pregnancy. The limited available data with **Actemra** in pregnant women are not sufficient to determine whether there is a drug-associated risk for major birth defects and miscarriage. Monoclonal antibodies, such as *tocilizumab*, are actively transported across the placenta during the third trimester of pregnancy and may affect immune response in the infant exposed *in utero*. It is not known whether **tocilizumab** passes into breast milk; therefore, breastfeeding is not recommended while using **Actemra**.

KERATITIS/KERATOCONJUNCTIVITIS: HERPES SIMPLEX

▷ *ganciclovir* (C) <2 years: not recommended; ≥2 years: instill 1 drop 5 times per day (every 3 hours) while awake until corneal ulcer heals; then 1 drop tid x 7 days
Zirgan *Ophth gel:* 0.15% (5 gm)(benzalkonium chloride)
▷ *idoxuridine* (C) instill 1 drop q 1 hour during day and every other hour at night <u>or</u> 1 drop every minute for 5 minutes and repeat q 4 hours during day and night
Herplex *Ophth soln:* 0.1% (15 ml)
▷ *trifluridine* (C) <6 years: not recommended; ≥6 years: instill 1 drop q 2 hours while awake (max 9 drops/day until re-epithelialization; then 1 drop q 4 hours x 7 more days (at least 5 drops/day); max 21 days
Viroptic *Ophth soln:* 1% (7.5 ml) (thimerosal)
▷ *vidarabine* (C) <2 years: not recommended; ≥2 years: apply 1/2 inch in lower conjunctival sac 5 times/day q 3 hours until re-epithelialization occurs, then bid x 7 more days
Vira-A *Ophth oint:* 3% (3.5 gm)

KERATITIS/KERATOCONJUNCTIVITIS: VERNAL

OPHTHALMIC MAST CELL STABILIZERS

Comment: Contact lens wear is contraindicated
▷ *cromolyn sodium* (B) <4 years: not recommended; ≥4 years: 1-2 drops 4-6 times/day
Crolom, Opticrom *Ophth soln:* 4% (10 ml) (benzalkonium chloride)
▷ *lodoxamide tromethamine* (B) <2 years: not recommended; ≥2 years: 1-2 drops qid; max 3 months
Alomide *Ophth susp:* 0.1% (10 ml)

LABYRINTHITIS

▷ *meclizine* (B) <12 years: not recommended; ≥12 years: 25 mg tid
Antivert *Tab:* 12.5, 25, 50*mg
Bonine (OTC) *Cap:* 15, 25, 30 mg; *Tab:* 12.5, 25, 50 mg; *Chew tab/Film-coat tab:* 25 mg
Dramamine II (OTC) *Tab:* 25*mg
Zentrip *Strip:* 25 mg orally disintegrating
▷ *promethazine* (C)(G) <2 years: not recommended; 2-12 years 12.5-25 mg q 4-6 hours prn; >12 years: 25-50 mg q 4-6 hours prn
Phenergan *Tab:* 12.5*, 25*, 50 mg; *Plain syr:* 6.25 mg/5 ml; *Fortis syr:* 25 mg/5 ml; *Rectal supp:* 12.5, 25, 50 mg
Comment: *promethazine* is contraindicated in children with uncomplicated nausea, dehydration, Reye's syndrome, history of sleep apnea, asthma, and lower respiratory disorders in children. **Promethazine** lowers the seizure threshold in children, may cause cholestatic jaundice, anticholinergic effects, extrapyramidal effects, and potentially fatal respiratory depression.

➤ *scopolamine* (C) <12 years: not recommended; ≥12 years: 1 patch behind ear; each patch is effective for 3 days; apply a new patch on behind the opposite ear every 4th day

   Transderm Scop *Transdermal patch:* 1.5 mg (4/carton)

LACTOSE INTOLERANCE

➤ *lactase* enzyme (NE) 9,000 FCC units taken with dairy food; adjust based on abatement of symptoms; usual max 18,000 units/dose

   Lactaid Drops (OTC) 5-7 drops to each quart of milk and shake gently; may increase to 10-15 drops if needed; hydrolyzes 70%-99% of lactose at refrigerator temperature in 24 hours

   Oral drops: 1,250 units/5 gtts (7 ml w. dropper)

   Lactaid Extra (OTC) *Cplt:* 4,500 FCC units

   Lactaid Fast ACT (OTC) *Cplt:* 9,000 FCC units; *Chew tab:* 9,000 FCC units (vanilla twist)

   Lactaid Original (OTC) *Cplt:* 3,000 FCC units

   Lactaid Ultra (OTC) *Cplt:* 9,000 FCC units; *Chew tab:* 9,000 FCC units (vanilla twist)

LARVA MIGRANS: CUTANEOUS/VISCERAL

➤ *thiabendazole* (C) dosing is bid, is based on weight in pounds, and must be taken with meals; <30 lbs: consult mfr pkg insert; 30 lbs: 250 mg bid; 50 lbs: 500 mg bid; 75 lbs: 750 mg bid; 100 lbs: 1 gm bid; 125 lbs: 1.25 gm bid: ≥150 lbs: 1.5 gm bid; max 3 gm/day; *Cutaneous larva migrans:* treat x 2 days; *Visceral larva migrans:* treat x 7 days

   Mintezol *Chew tab:* 500*mg (orange); *Oral susp:* 500 mg/5 ml (120 ml) (orange)

Comment: *thiabendazole* is not for prophylaxis. May impair mental alertness.

LEAD POISONING

Comment: Chelation therapy for lead poisoning requires maintenance of adequate hydration, close monitoring of renal and hepatic function, and monitoring for neutropenia; discontinue therapy at first sign of toxicity. Contraindicated with severe renal disease or anuria.

CHELATING AGENTS

➤ *deferoxamine mesylate* (C) <3 months: not recommended; ≥3 months: initially 1 gm IM, followed by 500 mg IM every 4 hours x 2 doses; then repeat every 4-12 hours if needed; max 6 gm/day

   Desferal *Vial:* 250 mg/ml after reconstitution (500 mg)

➤ *edetate calcium disodium (EDTA)* (B) administer IM or IV; use IM route of administration for children and overt lead encephalopathy; *Serum lead level:* 20-70 mcg/dL: 1 gm/m² per day; *IV:* infuse over 8-12 hours; *IM:* divided doses q 8-12 hours; Treat for 5 days; then stop for 2-4 days; may repeat if serum lead level is >70 mcg/dL

   Calcium Disodium Versenate *Amp:* 200 mg/ml (5 ml)

➤ *succimer* (C) <12 months: not recommended; ≥12 months: *Serum lead level:* >45 mcg/dL: initially 10 mg/kg (or 350 mg/m²) every 8 hours for 5 days; then reduce frequency to every 12 hours for 14 more days; allow at least 14 days between courses unless serum lead levels indicate a need for more prompt treatment; for more than 3 consecutive weeks not recommended; may swallow caps whole or put contents onto a small amount of soft food or a spoon and swallow, followed by a fruit drink

Chemet *Cap:* 100 mg

LEG CRAMPS: NOCTURNAL, RECUMBENCY

▶ *quinine sulfate* **(C)(G)** <16 years: not recommended; ≥16 years: 1 tab or cap q HS
　　Qualaquin *Tab:* 260 mg; *Cap:* 260, 300, 325 mg

Comment: If hypokalemia is the cause of leg cramps, treat with potassium supplementation (*see page 222*).

LEISHMANIASIS: CUTANEOUS, MUCOSAL, VISCERAL

Comment: The leishmanial parasite species addressed in this section are: **cutaneous leishmaniasis** (due to *Leishmania braziliensis, Leishmania guyanensis, Leishmania panamensis*), **mucosal leishmaniasis** (due to *Leishmania braziliensis*), and **visceral leishmaniasis** (due to *Leishmania donovani*). The weight-based treatment for adults and adolescents is the same for each of the species, the anti-leishmanial drug *miltefosone* (**Impavido**). Contraindications to this drug include pregnancy, lactation, and Sjogren-Larsson-Syndrome. The contraindication in pregnancy is due to embryo-fetal toxicity, teratogenicity, and fetal death. Obtain a serum or urine pregnancy test for females of reproductive potential and advise females to use effective contraception during therapy and for 5 months following treatment. Breastfeeding is contraindicated while taking this drug and for 5 months following termination of breastfeeding. Potential ASEs include loss of appetite, abdominal pain, nausea, vomiting, diarrhea, headache, dizziness, pruritis, somnolence, elevated liver transaminases, bilirubin, and serum creatinine and thrombocytopenia. *miltefosine* is associated with impaired fertility in females and males in animal studies. To report a suspected adverse reaction to this drug, call 888-550-6060 or the FDA at 800-FDA-1088 or visit www.fda.gov/medwatch.

▶ *miltefosine* **(D)(G)** <12 years, <30 kg (60 lbs): not established: ≥12 years: 30-44 kg: one cap bid x 28 consecutive days; >45 kg: one cap tid x 28 consecutive days; take with a full meal
　　Impavido *Cap:* 50 mg

LISTERIOSIS

▶ *erythromycin base* **(B)(G)** <45 kg: 30-40 mg/kg/day in 4 divided doses x 10 days; ≥45 kg: 500 mg qid x 10 days
　　Ery-Tab *Tab:* 250, 333, 500 mg ent-coat
　　PCE *Tab:* 333, 500 mg

▶ *erythromycin ethylsuccinate* **(B)(G)** 30-50 mg/kg/day in 4 divided doses x 10 days; may double dose with severe infection; max 100 mg/kg/day or 400 mg qid; *see page 563 for dose by weight table*
　　EryPed *Oral susp:* 200 mg/5 ml (100, 200 ml) (fruit); 400 mg/5 ml (60, 100, 200 ml; banana); *Oral drops:* 200, 400 mg/5 ml (50 ml) (fruit); *Chew tab:* 200 mg wafer (fruit)

E.E.S. *Oral susp:* 200, 400 mg/5 ml (100 ml) (fruit)
E.E.S. Granules *Oral susp:* 200 mg/5 ml (7.5 ml) (thimerosal)
E.E.S. 400 Tablets *Tab:* 400 mg

LOW BACK STRAIN

Acetaminophen for IV Infusion *see **Pain** page* 296
Oral Prescription NSAIDs *see page* 490
Other Oral Analgesics *see **Pain** page* 298
Topical/Transdermal NSAIDs *see **Pain** page* 298
Parenteral Corticosteroids *see page* 499
Oral Corticosteroids *see page* 498
Topical Analgesic and Anesthetic Agents *see page* 488

LYME DISEASE (ERYTHEMA CHRONICUM MIGRANS)

Comment: The bite of the deer tick (*Ixodes scapularis*) carries the *Borrelia burgdorferi* organism causing Lyme disease. Proper removal of the tick, and early diagnosis and treatment are essential to effective management of this disease.

STAGE 1

▶ *amoxicillin* (B)(G) <40 kg (88 lb): 20-40 mg/kg/day in 3 divided doses x 10 days or 25-45 mg/kg/day in 2 divided doses x 10 days; *see page 543 for dose by weight table;* ≥40 kg: 500-875 mg bid or 250-500 mg tid x 10 days
　　Amoxil *Cap:* 250, 500 mg; *Tab:* 875*mg; *Chew tab:* 125, 200, 250, 400 mg (cherry-banana-peppermint) (phenylalanine); *Oral susp:* 125, 250 mg/5 ml (80, 100, 150 ml) (strawberry); 200, 400 mg/5 ml (50, 75, 100 ml) (bubble gum); *Oral drops:* 50 mg/ml (30 ml) (bubble gum)
　　Moxatag *Tab:* 775 mg ext-rel
　　Trimox *Tab:* 125, 250 mg; *Cap:* 250, 500 mg; *Oral susp:* 125, 250 mg/5 ml (80, 100, 150 ml) (raspberry-strawberry)
▶ *cefuroxime axetil* (B)(G) <3 months: not recommended; ≥3 months-12 years: 15 mg/kg bid x 20 days; ≥12 years: 500 mg bid x 20 days
　　Ceftin *Tab:* 250, 500 mg; *Oral susp:* 125, 250 mg/5 ml (50, 100 ml) (tutti-frutti)
▶ *clarithromycin* (C)(G) <6 months: not recommended; ≥6 months-12 years: 7.5 mg/kg bid x 7-14 days; *see page 544 for dose by weight table;* >12 years: 500 mg bid or 500 mg ext-rel daily x 7-14 days
　　Biaxin *Tab:* 250, 500 mg
　　Biaxin Oral Suspension *Oral susp:* 125, 250 mg/5 ml (50, 100 ml)
　　Biaxin XL *Tab:* 500 mg ext-rel
▶ *doxycycline* (D)(G) <8 years: not recommended; ≥8 years, ≤100 lb: 2 mg/lb on first day in 2 divided doses, followed by 1 mg/lb/day in 1-2 divided doses x 14-21 days; ≥8 years, >100 lb: 100 mg bid x 7-14 days; *see page 545 for dose by weight table*
　　Acticlate *Tab:* 75, 150** mg
　　Adoxa *Tab:* 50, 75, 100, 150 mg ent-coat
　　Doryx *Tab:* 50, 75, 100, 150, 200 mg del-rel
　　Monodox *Cap:* 50, 75, 100 mg
　　Oracea *Cap:* 40 mg del-rel

Vibramycin *Tab:* 100 mg; *Cap:* 50, 100 mg; *Syr:* 50 mg/5 ml (raspberry-apple) (sulfites); *Oral susp:* 25 mg/5 ml (raspberry)

Vibra-Tab *Tab:* 100 mg film-coat

Comment: *doxycycline* is contraindicated <8 years-of-age, in pregnancy, and lactation (discolors developing tooth enamel). A side effect may be photosensitivity (photophobia). Do not take with antacids, calcium supplements, milk or other dairy, or within 2 hours of taking another drug.

▶ *minocycline* **(D)(G)** <8 years: not recommended; ≥8 years, ≤100 lb: 2 mg/lb on first day in 2 divided doses, followed by 1 mg/lb q 12 hours x 9 more days; ≥8 years, >100 lb: Arestin 200 mg on first day; then 100 mg q 12 hours x 9 more days

Dynacin *Cap:* 50, 100 mg

Minocin *Cap:* 50, 75, 100 mg; *Oral susp:* 50 mg/5 ml (60 ml) (custard) (sulfites, alcohol 5%)

Comment: *minocycline* is contraindicated <8 years-of-age, in pregnancy, and lactation (discolors developing tooth enamel). A side effect may be photo-sensitivity (photophobia). Do not give with antacids, calcium supplements, milk or other dairy, or within two hours of taking another drug.

▶ *tetracycline* **(D)(G)** <8 years: not recommended; ≥8 years, ≤100 lb: 25-50 mg/kg/day in 4 divided doses x 7 days; *see page 574 for dose by weight table*, ≥8 years, >100 lb: 250-500 mg qid ac x 21 days

Achromycin V *Cap:* 250, 500 mg

Sumycin *Tab:* 250, 500 mg; *Cap:* 250, 500 mg; *Oral susp:* 125 mg/5 ml (100, 200 ml) (fruit) (sulfites)

Comment: *tetracycline* is contraindicated <8 years-of-age, in pregnancy, and lactation (discolors developing tooth enamel). A side effect may be photosensitivity (photophobia). Do not give with antacids, calcium supplements, milk or other dairy, or within two hours of taking another drug.

☐ LYMPHADENITIS

Comment: Therapy should continue for no less than 5 days after resolution of symptoms.

▶ *amoxicillin/clavulanate* **(B)(G)**

Augmentin <40 kg: 40-45 mg/kg/day divided tid x 10 days or 90 mg/kg/day divided bid x 10 days; *see page 545 for dose by weight table;* ≥40 kg: 500 mg tid or 875 mg bid x 10 days

Tab: 250, 500, 875 mg; *Chew tab:* 125, 250 mg (lemon-lime); 200, 400 mg (cherry-banana) (phenylalanine); *Oral susp:* 125 mg/5 ml (banana), 250 mg/5 ml (75, 100, 150 ml) (orange); 200, 400 mg/5 ml (50, 75, 100 ml) (orange) (phenylalanine)

Augmentin ES-600 <3 months: not recommended; ≥3 months, <40 kg: 90 mg/kg/day divided q 12 hours x 10 days; *see page 546 for dose by weight table;* ≥40 kg: not recommended

Oral susp: 600 mg/5 ml (50, 75, 100, 125, 150, 200 ml) (strawberry cream) (phenylalanine)

Augmentin XR <16 years: use other forms; ≥16 years: 2 tabs q 12 hours x 7-10 days

Tab: 1000*mg ext-rel

▷ *cephalexin* **(B)(G)** <12 years: 25-50 mg/kg/day in 4 divided doses x 10 days; *see page 557 for dose by weight table;* ≥12 years: 500 mg bid x 10 days
  Keflex *Cap:* 250, 333, 500, 750 mg; *Oral susp:* 125, 250 mg/5 ml (100, 200 ml) (strawberry)
▷ *dicloxacillin* **(B)** <12 years: 12.5-25 mg/kg/day in 4 divided doses x 10 days; *see page 560 for dose by weight table;* ≥12 years: 500 mg q 6 hours x 10 days
  Dynapen *Cap:* 125, 250, 500 mg; *Oral susp:* 62.5 mg/5 ml (80, 100, 200 ml)

LYMPHOGRANULOMA VENEREUM

Comment: The following treatment regimens are published in the **2015 CDC Sexually Transmitted Diseases Treatment Guidelines**. This section contains treatment regimens for patients ≥18 years only; consult a specialist for treatment of patients < 18 years-of-age. Treatment regimens are presented in alphabetical order by generic drug name, followed by brands and dose forms. Treat all sexual contacts. Persons with both LGV and HIV infection should receive the same treatment regimens as those who are HIV-negative; however, prolonged treatment may be required and delay in resolution of symptoms may occur.

RECOMMENDED REGIMEN
Regimen 1

▷ *doxycycline* 100 mg bid x 21 days

ALTERNATIVE REGIMEN
Regimen 1

▷ *erythromycin base* **(B)(G)** 500 mg qid x 21 days *or* *erythromycin ethylsuccinate* 400 mg qid x 21 days

RECOMMENDED REGIMENS FOR THE MANAGEMENT OF SEXUAL CONTACTS

Comment: LGV is caused by *C. trachomatis* serovars L1, L2, *or* L3. Persons who have had sexual contact with a patient who has LGV within 60 days before onset of the patient's symptoms should be examined, tested for urethral *or* cervical chlamydial infection, and treated with a chlamydia regimen.

Regimen 1

▷ *azithromycin* 1 gm in a single dose

Regimen 2

▷ *doxycycline* 100 mg bid x 7 days

DRUG BRANDS AND DOSE FORMS

▷ *azithromycin* **(B)(G)**
  Zithromax *Tab:* 250, 500, 600 mg; *Oral susp:* 100 mg/5 ml (15 ml); 200 mg/5 ml (15, 22.5, 30 ml) (cherry); *Pkt:* 1 gm for reconstitution (cherry-banana)

    Zithromax Tri-pak *Tab:* 3 x 500 mg tabs/pck
    Zithromax Z-pak *Tab:* 6 x 250 mg tabs/pck
    Zmax *Oral susp:* 2 gm ext-rel for reconstitution (cherry-banana) (148 mg Na$^+$)

▶ *doxycycline* (D)(G) <8 years: not recommended; ≥8 years, ≤100 lb: 2 mg/lb on first day in 2 divided doses, followed by 1 mg/lb/day in 1-2 divided doses; ≥8 years, >100 lb: 40-100 mg bid; *see page 561 for dose by weight table*
    Acticlate *Tab:* 75, 150** mg
    Adoxa *Tab:* 50, 75, 100, 150 mg ent-coat
    Doryx *Tab:* 50, 75, 100, 150, 200 mg del-rel
    Monodox *Cap:* 50, 75, 100 mg
    Oracea *Cap:* 40 mg del-rel
    Vibramycin *Tab:* 100 mg; *Cap:* 50, 100 mg; *Syr:* 50 mg/5 ml (raspberry-apple) (sulfites); *Oral susp:* 25 mg/5 ml (raspberry)
    Vibra-Tab *Tab:* 100 mg film-coat

Comment: *doxycycline* is contraindicated <8 years-of-age, in pregnancy, and lactation (discolors developing tooth enamel). A side effect may be photo-sensitivity (photophobia). Do not take with antacids, calcium supplements, milk or other dairy, or within 2 hours of taking another drug.

▶ *erythromycin base* (B)(G)
    Ery-Tab *Tab:* 250, 333, 500 mg ent-coat
    PCE *Tab:* 333, 500 mg

▶ *erythromycin ethylsuccinate* (B)(G)
    EryPed *Oral susp:* 200 mg/5 ml (100, 200 ml) (fruit); 400 mg/5 ml (60, 100, 200 ml) (banana); *Oral drops:* 200, 400 mg/5 ml (50 ml) (fruit); *Chew tab:* 200 mg wafer (fruit)
    E.E.S. *Oral susp:* 200, 400 mg/5 ml (100 ml) (fruit)
    E.E.S. Granules *Oral susp:* 200 mg/5 ml (100, 200 ml) (cherry)
    E.E.S. 400 Tablets *Tab:* 400 mg

MALARIA (*PLASMODIUM FALCIPARUM, PLASMODIUM VIVAX*)

▶ *doxycycline* (D)(G) *Treatment:* <8 years: not recommended; ≥8 years, ≤100 lb: 2 mg/lb on first day in 2 divided doses, followed by 1 mg/lb/day in 1-2 divided doses; ≥8 years, >100 lb: 100 mg daily; *Prophylaxis:* initiate 1-2 days prior to travel; take during travel; continue for 4 weeks after leaving the endemic area; *see page 561 for dose by weight table*
    Acticlate *Tab:* 75, 150** mg
    Adoxa *Tab:* 50, 75, 100, 150 mg ent-coat
    Doryx *Tab:* 50, 75, 100, 150, 200 mg del-rel
    Monodox *Cap:* 50, 75, 100 mg
    Oracea *Cap:* 40 mg del-rel
    Vibramycin *Tab:* 100 mg; *Cap:* 50, 100 mg; *Syr:* 50 mg/5 ml (raspberry-apple) (sulfites); *Oral susp:* 25 mg/5 ml (raspberry)
    Vibra-Tab *Tab:* 100 mg film-coat

Comment: *doxycycline* is contraindicated <8 years-of-age, in pregnancy, and lactation (discolors developing tooth enamel). A side effect may be photo-sensitivity (photophobia). Do not take with antacids, calcium supplements, milk or other dairy, or within 2 hours of taking another drug.

▷ *minocycline* (D)(G) *Treatment:* <8 years: not recommended; ≥8 years, ≤100 lb: 2 mg/lb on first day in 2 divided doses, followed by 1 mg/lb q 12 hours x 9 more days; ≥8 years, >100 lb: 100 mg daily; *Prophylaxis:* initiate 1-2 days prior to travel; take during travel; continue for 4 weeks after leaving the endemic area

Dynacin *Cap:* 50, 100 mg

Minocin *Cap:* 50, 75, 100 mg; *Oral susp:* 50 mg/5 ml (60 ml) (custard) (sulfites, alcohol 5%)

Comment: *minocycline* is contraindicated <8 years-of-age, in pregnancy, and lactation (discolors developing tooth enamel). A side effect may be photo-sensitivity (photophobia). Do not give with antacids, calcium supplements, milk or other dairy, or within 2 hours of taking another drug.

▷ *tetracycline* (D)(G) *Treatment:* <8 years: not recommended; ≥8 years, ≤100 lb: 25-50 mg/kg/day in 4 divided doses; *see page 574 for dose by weight table;* ≥8 years, >100 lb: 250 mg once daily; *Prophylaxis:* initiate 1-2 days prior to travel; take during travel; continue for 4 weeks after leaving the endemic area

Achromycin V *Cap:* 250, 500 mg

Sumycin *Tab:* 250, 500 mg; *Cap:* 250, 500 mg; *Oral susp:* 125 mg/5 ml (100, 200 ml) (fruit) (sulfites)

Comment: *tetracycline* is contraindicated <8 years-of-age, in pregnancy, and lactation (discolors developing tooth enamel). A side effect may be photo-sensitivity (photophobia). Do not give with antacids, calcium supplements, milk or other dairy, or within 2 hours of taking another drug.

ANTIMALARIALS

▷ *quinine sulfate* (C)(G) <16 years: not recommended; ≥16 years: 1 tab or cap every 8 hours x 7 days

Tab: 260 mg; *Cap:* 260, 300, 325 mg

Qualaquin *Cap:* 324 mg

Comment: **Qualaquin** is indicated in the treatment of uncomplicated *P. falciparum* malaria (including chloroquine-resistant strains).

▷ *atovaquone* (C)(G) <12 years: see mfr pkg insert for weight-based dosing table; ≥12 years: take as a single dose with food or a milky drink at the same time each day; repeat dose if vomited within 1 hour; *Prophylaxis:* 1,500 mg once daily; *Treatment:* 750 mg bid x 21 days

Mepron *Susp:* 750 mg/5 ml (210 ml) (citrus)

▷ *atovaquone/proguanil* (C)(G) take as a single dose with food or a milky drink at the same time each day; repeat dose if vomited within 1 hour; *Prophylaxis:* daily dose starting 1-2 days before entering endemic area, during stay, and for 7 days after return; <5 kg: not recommended; 5-20 kg: 1 ped tab; 21-30 kg: 2 ped tabs; 31-40 kg: 3 ped tabs; ≥40 kg: 1 adult tab; *Treatment (acute, uncomplicated):* a single dose once daily x 3 days; <5 kg: not recommended; 5-8 kg: 2 ped tabs; 9-10 kg: 3 ped tabs; 11-20 kg: 1 adult tab; 21-30 kg: 2 adult tabs; 31-40 kg: 3 adult tabs; >40 kg: 4 adult tabs

Malarone *Tab: atov* 250 mg/*prog* 100 mg

Malarone Pediatric *Tab: atov* 62.5 mg/*prog* 25 mg

Comment: *atovaquone* is antagonized by *tetracycline* and *metoclopramide*. Concomitant *rifampin* is not recommended (may elevate LFTs).

▷ *chloroquine* (C)(G) *Prophylaxis:* <12 years: 8.35 mg/kg (max 500 mg); ≥12 years: 500 mg; a single dose once weekly (on the same day of each week); start 2 weeks prior to exposure, continue while in the endemic area, and continue 4 weeks after departure; *Treatment:* *<12 years:* initially 16.7 mg/kg (max 1 gm); then 8.35 mg/kg (max 500 mg) 6 hours, 24 hours, and 48 hours after initial dose, or initially 6.25 mg/kg IM; may repeat in 6 hours; max 12.5 mg/kg/day; ≥12 years: initially 1 gm; then 500 mg 6 hours, 24 hours, and 48 hours after initial dose or initially 200-250 mg IM; may repeat in 6 hours; max 1 gm in first 24 hours; continue to 1.875 gm in 3 days

    Aralen *Tab:* 500 mg; *Amp:* 50 mg/ml (5 ml)

➤ *hydroxychloroquine* **(C)(G)** *Prophylaxis:* *<12 years:* 6.45 mg/kg (max 400 mg); ≥12 years: 400 mg; dose once weekly(on the same day of each week); start weeks prior to arrival, continue while in endemic area, and continue for 4 weeks after departure; *Treatment:* *<12 years:* initially 12.9 mg/kg (max 800 mg); then 6.45 mg/kg (max 400 mg) at 6 hours, 24 hours, and 48 hours after initial dose; ≥12 years: initially 800 mg; then 400 mg at 6 hours, 24 hours, and 48 hours after initial dose

    Plaquenil *Tab:* 200 mg

➤ *mefloquine* **(C)** *Prophylaxis:* *<6 months:* not recommended; ≥6 months-12 years: 3-5 mg/kg (max 250 mg); ≥12 years: 250 mg; dose once weekly (on the same day of each week); start 1 week prior to exposure, continue while in the endemic area, and continue for 4 weeks after departure; *Treatment:* ≥6 months-12 years: 25-50 mg/kg as a single dose (max 250 mg); ≥12 years: 1,250 mg as a single dose

    Lariam *Tab:* 250*mg

Comment: *mefloquine* is contraindicated with active or recent history of depression, generalized anxiety disorder, psychosis, schizophrenia or any other psychiatric disorder or history of convulsions.

MASTITIS (BREAST ABSCESS)

ANTI-INFECTIVES

➤ *amoxicillin/clavulanate* **(B)(G)**
    Augmentin <40 kg: 40-45 mg/kg/day divided tid x 10 days or 90 mg/kg/day divided bid x 10 days; *see page 545 for dose by weight table;* ≥40 kg: 500 mg tid or 875 mg bid x 10 days
        Tab: 250, 500, 875 mg; *Chew tab:* 125, 250 mg (lemon-lime); 200, 400 mg (cherry-banana) (phenylalanine); *Oral susp:* 125 mg/5 ml (banana), 250 mg/5 ml (75, 100, 150 ml) (orange); 200, 400 mg/5 ml (50, 75, 100 ml) (orange) (phenylalanine)
    Augmentin ES-600 <3 months: not recommended; ≥3 months, <40 kg: 90 mg/kg/day divided q 12 hours x 10 days; *see page 546 for dose by weight table;* ≥40 kg: not recommended
        Oral susp: 600 mg/5 ml (50, 75, 100, 125, 150, 200 ml) (strawberry cream) (phenylalanine)
    Augmentin XR <16 years: use other forms; ≥16 years: 2 tabs q 12 hours x 7-10 days
        Tab: 1000*mg ext-rel
➤ *cefaclor* **(B)(G)** <1 month: not recommended; 1 month-12 years: 20-40 mg/kg divided bid x 10 days; *see page 549 for dose by weight table;* max 1 gm/day; >12 years: 250-500 mg q 8 hours x 10 days; max 2 gm/day
        Tab: 500 mg; *Cap:* 250, 500 mg; *Susp:* 125 mg/5 ml (75, 150 ml) (strawberry); 187 mg/5 ml (50, 100 ml) (strawberry); 250 mg/5 ml (75, 150 ml) (strawberry); 375 mg/5 ml (50, 100 ml) (strawberry)

Cefaclor Extended Release <16 years: not recommended; ≥16 years: 500 mg bid x 10 days; (clinically equivalent to 250 mg immed-rel caps tid); swallow whole; take with meals
Tab: 375, 500 mg ext-rel

▶ *ceftriaxone* (B)(G) <12 years: 50 mg/kg IM daily; continue 2 days after signs of infection have disappeared; ≥12 years: 1-2 grams IM daily; continue 2 days after signs of infection have disappeared; max 4 gm/day
Rocephin *Vial:* 250, 500 mg; 1, 2 g

▶ *cephalexin* (B)(G) <12 years: 25-50 mg/kg/day in 4 divided doses x 10 days; *see page 557 for dose by weight table;* ≥12 years: 500 mg bid x 10 days
Keflex *Cap:* 250, 333, 500, 750 mg; *Oral susp:* 125, 250 mg/5 ml (100, 200 ml) (strawberry)

▶ *clindamycin* (B)(G) <12 years: not recommended; ≥12 years: 300 mg tid x 10 days
Cleocin *Cap:* 75 (tartrazine), 150 (tartrazine), 300 mg
Cleocin Pediatric Granules *Oral susp:* 75 mg/5 ml (100 ml) (cherry)

▶ *erythromycin base* (B)(G) <45 kg: 30-40 mg/kg/day in 4 divided doses x 10 days; ≥45 kg: 250-500 mg qid x 10 days
Ery-Tab *Tab:* 250, 333, 500 mg ent-coat
PCE *Tab:* 333, 500 mg

MELASMA/CHLOASMA

SKIN DEPIGMENTING AGENTS

▶ *hydroquinone* (C) <12 years: not recommended; ≥12 years: apply a thin film to clean dry affected areas bid; discontinue if lightening does not occur after 2 months
Lustra *Crm:* hydro 4% (1, 2 oz) (sulfites)
Lustra AF *Crm:* hydro 4% (1, 2 oz) (sunscreens, sulfites)

▶ *hydroquinone/fluocinolone acetonide/tretinoin* (C) <12 years: not recommended; ≥12 years: apply a thin film to clean dry affected areas once daily at least 30 minutes before bedtime
Tri-Luma *Crm:* hydro 4%/*fluo acet* 0.01%/*tret* 0.05% (30 gm) (sulfites, parabens)

MENIERE'S DISEASE

▶ *diazepam* (D)(IV)(G) <6 months: not recommended; ≥6 months: initially 1-2.5 mg tid-qid; may increase gradually
Diastat *Rectal gel delivery system:* 2.5 mg
Diastat AcuDial *Rectal gel delivery system:* 10, 20 mg
Valium *Tab:* 2*, 5*, 10* mg
Valium Intensol Oral Solution *Conc oral soln:* 5 mg/ml (30 ml w. dropper) (alcohol 19%)
Valium Oral Solution *Oral soln:* 5 mg/5 ml (500 ml) (wintergreen spice)

▶ *dimenhydrinate* (B) <2 years: not recommended; 2-6 years: 12.5-25 mg q 6-8 hours; max 75 mg/day; >6-11 years: 25-50 mg q 6-8 hours; max 150 mg/day; >11 years: 50 mg q 4-6 hours
Dramamine (OTC) *Tab:* 50* mg; *Chew tab:* 50 mg (phenylalanine, tartrazine); *Liq:* 12.5 mg/5 ml (4 oz)

➤ *diphenhydramine* (B)(G)
  Benadryl (OTC) <2 years: not recommended; 2-6 years: 6.25 mg q 4-6 hours;
  max 37.5 mg/day; >6-12 years: 12.5-25 mg q 4-6 hours; max 150 mg/day; >12
  years: 25-50 mg q 6-8 hours; max 100 mg/day
  Chew tab: 12.5 mg (grape) (phenylalanine); *Liq:* 12.5 mg/5 ml (4, 8 oz); *Cap:* 25
  mg; *Tab:* 25 mg; *Dye-free soft gel:* 25 mg;
  Dye-free liq: 12.5 mg/5 ml (4, 8 oz)
➤ *diphenhydramine* injectable (B)(G)
  Benadryl Injectable <12 years: *See mfr pkg insert:* 1.25 mg/kg up to 25 mg IM x 1
  dose; then q 6 hours prn; ≥12 years: 25-50 mg IM immediately; then q 6 hours prn
  Vial: 50 mg/ml (1 ml single use); 50 mg/ml (10 ml multi-dose); *Amp:* 10 mg/ml
  (1 ml); *Prefilled syringe:* 50 mg/ml (1 ml)
➤ *hydroxyzine* (C)(G) <6 years: 50 mg/day divided qid; 6-12 years: 50-100 mg/day
  divided qid; >12 years: 50-100 mg qid; max 600 mg/day
  Atarax *Tab:* 10, 25, 50, 100 mg; *Syr:* 10 mg/5 ml (alcohol 0.5%)
  Vistaril *Cap:* 25, 50, 100 mg; *Oral susp:* 25 mg/5 ml (4 oz) (lemon)
➤ *meclizine* (B)(G)
  Antivert <12 years: not recommended; ≥12 years: *Tab:* 12.5, 25, 50*mg; *Amp:*
  50 mg/ml (1 ml); *Vial:* 50 mg/ml (1 ml single use); 50 mg/ml (10 ml multidose)
  Bonine (OTC) <12 years: not recommended; ≥12 years: *Cap:* 15, 25, 30 mg;
  Tab: 12.5, 25, 50 mg; *Chew tab/Film-coat tab:* 25 mg
  Dramamine II <12 years: not recommended; ≥12 years: 25 mg bid; max 50 mg/day
    Tab: 25*mg
  Zentrip *Strip:* 25 mg orally disintegrating
➤ *promethazine* (C) <2 years: not recommended; 2-12 years: 0.5 mg/lb or 6.25-25 mg
  q 4-6 hours PO or rectally; >12 years: 12.5-25 q 4-6 hours PO or rectally
  Phenergan *Tab:* 12.5*, 25*, 50 mg; *Plain syr:* 6.25 mg/5 ml; *Fortis syr:* 25 mg/5
  ml; *Rectal supp:* 12.5, 25, 50 mg
Comment: *promethazine* is contraindicated in children with uncomplicated nausea,
dehydration, Reye's syndrome, history of sleep apnea, asthma, and lower respiratory
disorders in children. *Promethazine* lowers the seizure threshold in children, may
cause cholestatic jaundice, anticholinergic effects, extrapyramidal effects, and
potentially fatal respiratory depression.
➤ *scopolamine* transdermal patch (C) <12 years: not recommended; ≥12 years: 1
  patch behind ear; each patch is effective for 3 days; change patch every 4th day;
  alternate sides
  Transderm Scop *Patch:* 1.5 mg (4/carton)

MENINGITIS (*NEISSERIA MENINGITIDIS*)

PROPHYLAXIS

Comment: Meningitis vaccine is a 3-dose series (0, 2, 6 month schedule) indicated for
persons aged ≥10-25 years. Have epinephrine 1:1,000 readily available and monitor for
15 minutes post-dose of meningitis vaccine.
➤ *Meningococcal group b vaccine [recombinant, absorbed]* <10 years: not established;
  ≥10 years: 1st dose 0.5 ml IM in the deltoid; 2nd dose 0.5 ml IM 2 months later; 3rd
  dose 0.5 ml IM 6 months after the first dose;
  Bexsero *Susp for IM inj:* 0.5 ml single-dose prefilled syringes (1, 10/carton)

Trumenba *Susp for IM inj:* 0.5 ml single-dose prefilled syringes (5, 10/carton)

▶ *Neisseria meningitides oligosaccharide conjugate* quadrivalent meningococcal vaccine **(B)** contains *Corynebacterium diphtheria* CRM197 protein; 10 mcg of Group A + 5 mcg each of Group C, Y, and W-135 + 32.7-64.1 mcg of diphtheria CRM197 protein per 0.5 ml pwdr for reconstitution; <2 months: not established; 2 months: administer 4-dose series at 2, 4, 6, and 12 months; 7-23 months: administer 3-dose series with 2nd dose administered in the 2nd year of life and at least 3 months after the 1st dose; ≥2 years: 0.5 ml IM once; 2-5 years, continued high risk: may administer 2nd dose 2 months after the 1st dose

Menveo *Vial multidose:* 5 doses/vial (MenA conjugate component pwdr for reconstitution + 1 vial liquid MenCWY conjugate component for reconstitution) (preservative-free)

▶ *Neisseria meningitidis polysaccharides* vaccine **(C)**

Menactra administer in the deltoid only; <9 months: not recommended; *Primary vaccination:* 9-23 months: 0.5 ml administered as a 2-dose series 3 months apart; ≥24 months: 0.5 ml IM once; *Booster vaccination:* ≥15 years: 0.5 ml IM once for those at continued risk if at least 4 years have elapsed since the prior dose

Single-dose prefilled tip-lock syringe: 4 mcg each of group A, C, Y, and W-135 per 0.5 ml soln (preservative-free)

Comment: Latex allergy is a contraindication to **Menactra.**

Menomune-A/C/Y/W-135 <2 years: not recommended (except ≥3 months of age as short-term protection against group A); ≥2 years: same as adult; if at high risk, may revaccinate children first vaccinated ≤4 years-of-age after 2-3 years (older children after 3-5 years)

Vial (single dose): 50 mcg each of group A, C, Y, and W-135 per 0.5 ml (pwdr for SC inj after reconstitution; preservative-free diluent); *Vial (multidose):* 50 mcg each of group A, C, Y, and W-130 per 0.5 ml (pwdr for SC inj after reconstitution [10 doses/vial] [thimerosal-preserved diluent])

Comment: Use precaution with latex allergy.

MENOMETRORRHAGIA: IRREGULAR HEAVY MENSTRUAL BLEEDING/MENORRHAGIA: HEAVY CYCLICAL MENSTRUAL BLEEDING

ANTIFIBRINOLYTIC AGENT

▶ *tranexamic acid* **(B)(G)** <18 years: not recommended; ≥18 years: 1,300 mg tid; treat for up to 5 days during menses; *Normal renal function (SCr ≤1.4 mg/dL):* 1,300 mg tid; *SCr ≥1.4-2.8 mg/dL:* 1,300 mg bid; *SCr ≥2.8-5.7 mg/dL:* 1,300 mg once daily; *SCr ≥5.7 mg/dL:* 650 mg once daily

Lysteda *Tab:* 650 mg

INJECTABLE PROGESTERONE ONLY CONTRACEPTIVES

Combined Oral Contraceptives *see page* 476

Intrauterine Devices *see page* 487

▶ *medroxyprogesterone* **(X)(G)** *Pre-menarche:* not applicable; administer IM in the deltoid or hip; do not massage site; administer first dose within 5 days of onset of normal menses, within 5 days postpartum if not breastfeeding, or at 6 weeks postpartum if breastfeeding exclusively; do not use for >2 years unless other methods are inadequate

Depo-Provera 150 mg deep IM q 3 months
Vial: 150 mg/ml (1 ml)
Prefilled syringe: 150 mg/ml

Depo-SubQ Provera 104 mg SC q 3 months
Prefilled syringe: 104 mg/ml (0.65 ml) (parabens)

Comment: Contraindications to injectable progesterone include: thromboembolic disorders, cerebral vascular disease, breast cancer, significant hepatic disease, undiagnosed vaginal bleeding, pregnancy.

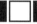

MITRAL VALVE PROLAPSE (MVP)

► *propranolol* (C)(G)
Inderal <12 years: not recommended; ≥12 years: initially 10 mg bid; usual range 160-320 mg/day in divided doses
Tab: 10*, 20*, 40*, 60*, 80*mg
Inderal LA <12 years: not recommended; ≥12 years: initially 80 mg daily in a single dose; increase q 3-7 days; usual range 120-160 mg/day; max 320 mg/day in a single dose
Cap: 60, 80, 120, 160 mg sust-rel
InnoPran XL <12 years: not recommended; ≥12 years: initially 80 mg q HS; max 120 mg/day
Cap: 80, 120 mg ext-rel

MONONUCLEOSIS (MONO)

ANALGESICS

► *acetaminophen* (B) *see Fever page* 137
Acetaminophen for IV Infusion *see page* 296
Other Oral Analgesics *see Pain page* 298
Parenteral Corticosteroids *see page* 499
Oral Corticosteroids *see page* 498
► *prednisone* (C) initially 40-80 mg/day, then taper off over 5-7 days
Comment: Corticosteroids recommended in patients with significant pharyngeal edema.

MOTION SICKNESS

► *dimenhydrinate* (B)(OTC) <2 years: not recommended; 2-6 years: 12.5-25 mg; max 75 mg/day; start 1 hour before travel; may repeat q 6-8 hours; 6-11 years: 25-50 mg; max 150 mg/day; start 1 hour before travel; may repeat q 6-8 hours; ≥12 years 50-100 mg q 4-6 hours; start 1 hour before travel; max 400 mg/day
Dramamine
Tab: 50*mg; *Chew tab:* 50 mg (phenylalanine, tartrazine); *Liq:* 12.5 mg/5 ml (4 oz)

▷ *meclizine* (B)(G) 12 years: not recommended; ≥12 years: 25-50 mg 1 hour before travel; may repeat q 24 hours as needed; max 50 mg/day
  Antivert *Tab:* 12.5, 25, 50*mg
  Bonine (OTC) *Cap:* 15, 25, 50 mg; *Tab:* 12.5, 25, 50 mg; *Chew tab/Film-coat tab:* 25 mg
  Dramamine II (OTC) *Tab:* 25 mg
  Zentrip *Strip:* 25 mg orally-disint

▷ *prochlorperazine* (C)(G) 12 years: not recommended; ≥12 years:
  Compazine 5-10 mg q 4 hours prn
    Tab: 5 mg; *Syr:* 5 mg/5 ml (4 oz; fruit); *Rectal supp:* 2.5, 5, 25 mg
  Compazine Spansule 15 mg q AM or 10 mg q 12 hours prn
    Spansules: 10, 15 mg sust-rel

▷ *promethazine* (C)(G) <12 years: not recommended; ≥12 years: 12.5-25 mg 30-60 minutes before travel; may repeat in 8-12 hours
  Phenergan *Tab:* 12.5*, 25*, 50 mg; *Plain syr:* 6.25 mg/5 ml; *Fortis syr:* 25 mg/5 ml; *Rectal supp:* 12.5, 25, 50 mg
  Comment: *promethazine* is contraindicated in children with uncomplicated nausea, dehydration, Reye's syndrome, history of sleep apnea, asthma, and lower respiratory disorders in children. *Promethazine* lowers the seizure threshold in children, may cause cholestatic jaundice, anticholinergic effects, extrapyramidal effects, and potentially fatal respiratory depression.

▷ *scopolamine* (C) <12 years: not recommended; ≥12 years:
  Scopace 0.4-0.8 mg 1 hour before travel; may repeat in 8 hours
    Tab: 0.4 mg
  Transderm Scop 1 patch behind ear at least 4 hours before travel; each patch is effective for 3 days; apply a new patch on the 4th day on the opposite side
    Transdermal patch: 1.5 mg (4/carton)

MULTIPLE SCLEROSIS (MS)

NICOTINIC ACID RECEPTOR AGONIST

▷ *dimethyl fumarate* (C) <18 years: not recommended; ≥18 years: initially 120 mg bid x 7 days; then maintenance 240 mg bid
  Tecfidera *Cap:* 120, 240 mg del-rel; *Starter Pack:* 14 x 120 mg, 46 x 240 mg
  Comment: The mechanism by which *dimethyl fumarate* (DMF) exerts its therapeutic effect in multiple sclerosis is unknown. DMF and the metabolite, *monomethyl fumarate* (MMF), have been shown to activate the nuclear factor (erythroid-derived 2)-like 2 (Nrf2) pathway in vitro and in vivo in animals and humans. The Nrf2 pathway is involved in the cellular response to oxidative stress. MMF has been identified as a nicotinic acid receptor agonist in vitro.

POTASSIUM CHANNEL BLOCKER

▷ *dalfampridine* (C)(G) <18 years: not recommended; ≥18 years: 10 mg q 12 hours
  Ampyra *Tab:* 10 mg ext-rel
  Comment: *dalfampridine* is indicated to improve walking speed.

PYRIMIDINE SYNTHESIS INHIBITOR (DMARD)

▷ *teriflunomide* (X) <18 years: not recommended; ≥18 years: 7 mg or 14 mg once daily

Aubagio *Tab:* 7, 14 mg

Comment: Contraindicated with severe hepatic impairment and females of childbearing potential not using reliable contraception. Co-administer *teriflunomide* with the DMARD *leflunomide* (**Arava**).

IMMUNOMODULATORS

Comment: The role of immunomodulators in the treatment of MS is to slow the progression of physical disability and to decrease frequency of clinical exacerbations.

▷ *alemtuzumab* (C) <18 years: not recommended; ≥18 years: administer two treatment courses: *First treatment course:* 12 mg/day x 5 days (total 60 mg); *Second treatment course:* 12 months later, administer 12 mg/day x 3 days (total 36 mg); complete all immunizations 6 weeks prior to the first treatment; premedicate with 1,000 mg methylprednisolone or equivalent immediately prior to the first 3 treatment days in each treatment course

Lemtrada *Vial:* 12 mg/1.2 ml soln for IV infusion, single-use vial

Comment: **Lemtrada** is indicated for the treatment of patients with relapsing forms of MS. Because of its safety profile, the use of **Lemtrada** should generally be reserved for patients who have had an inadequate response to two or more drugs indicated for the treatment of MS. **Lemtrada REMS** is a restricted distribution program, which allows early detection and management of some of the serious risks associated with its use.

▷ *fingolimod* (C) <18 years: not recommended; ≥18 years: 0.5 mg once daily

Gilenya *Cap:* 0.5 mg

Comment: First-dose monitoring for bradycardia. In the first 2 weeks, first-dose monitoring is recommended after an interruption of 1 day or more. During weeks 3 and 4, first-dose monitoring is recommended after an interruption of more than 7 days.

▷ *glatiramer acetate* (B)(G) <18 years: not recommended; ≥18 years: 20-40 mg SC daily

Copaxone *Prefilled syringe:* 20, 40 mg/ml (mannitol, preservative-free)

▷ *interferon beta-1a* (C) <18 years: not recommended; ≥18 years:

Avonex 30 mcg IM weekly; rotate sites; may titrate to reduce flu-like symptoms; may use concurrent analgesics/antipyretics on treatment days; *Titration Schedule:* 7.5 mcg week 1; 15 mcg week 2; 22.5 mcg week 3; 30 mcg week 4 and ongoing

Vial: 30 mcg/vial pwdr for reconstitution (single dose w. diluent, 4 vials/kit) (albumin [human], preservative-free); *Prefilled syringe:* 30 mcg single dose (0.5 ml) (4/dose pck)

Rebif, administer SC 3x/week (at least 48 hours apart and preferably in the late afternoon or evening); increase over 4 weeks to usual dose 22-44 mcg 3x/week; *Titration Schedule (22 mcg prescribed dose):* 4.4 mcg weeks 1 & 2; 11 mcg weeks 3 & 4; 22 mcg weeks 5 and ongoing; *Titration Schedule (44 mcg prescribed dose):* 8.8 mcg weeks 1 & 2; 22 mcg weeks 3 & 4; 44 mcg weeks 5 and ongoing

Prefilled syringe: 22, 44 mcg/0.5 ml w. needle (12/carton) (albumin [human], preservative-free); (titration pack, 6 doses of 8.8 mcg [0.2 ml] w. needle per carton) (albumin [human], preservative-free)

Comment: Only prefilled syringes (**Rebif**) can be used to titrate to the 22 mcg prescribed dose. Prefilled syringes or autoinjectors (**Rebif Rebidose**) can be used to titrate to the 44 mcg prescribed dose.

Rebif Rebidose administer SC 3x/week (at least 48 hours apart and preferably in the late afternoon or evening) after titration to 22 mcg or 44 mcg; *Titration Schedule: see* **Rebif**.

> *Prefilled autoinjector:* 22, 44 mcg/0.5 ml (0.5 ml, 12/carton) (titration pack, 6 doses of 8.8 mcg [0.2 ml] per carton) (albumin [human], preservative-free)

Comment: Only prefilled syringes (**Rebif**) can be used to titrate to the 22 mcg prescribed dose. Prefilled syringes or autoinjectors (**Rebif Rebidose**) can be used to titrate to the 44 mcg prescribed dose.

▷ *interferon beta-1b* (C) <18 years: not recommended; ≥18 years:

Actimmune *BSA ≤0.5 m²*: 1.5 mcg/kg SC in a single dose 3 times weekly; *BSA ≥0.5 m²*: 50 mgc/m² SC in a single dose 3 times weekly

> *Vial:* 100 mcg/0.5 ml single dose for SC injection

Betaseron, Extavia 0.0625 mg (0.25 ml) SC every other day; increase over 6 weeks to 0.25 mg (1 ml) SC every other day

> *Vial:* 0.3 mg/vial pwdr for reconstitution (single-dose w. prefilled diluents syringes) (albumin [human], mannitol, preservative-free)

▷ *natalizumab* (C) a <18 years: not recommended; ≥18 years: administer 300 mg by IV infusion over 1 hour every 4 weeks; monitor during infusion and for 1 hour post-infusion

Tysabri *Vial:* 300 mg/15 ml (15 ml)

MUMPS (INFECTIOUS PAROTITIS)

PROPHYLAXIS

▷ *measles, mumps, rubella, live, attenuated, neomycin vaccine* (C) MMR II 25 mcg SC (preservative-free)

Comment: Contraindications: hypersensitivity to *neomycin* or eggs, primary or acquired immune deficiency, immunosuppressant therapy, bone marrow or lymphatic malignancy, and pregnancy (within 3 months after vaccination).

see **Childhood Immunizations** *page 473*
Parenteral Corticosteroids *see page 499*
Oral Corticosteroids *see page 498*
Antipyretics *see Fever page 138*

MUSCLE STRAIN

Comment: Usual length of treatment for acute injury is approximately 5 days.
Acetaminophen for IV Infusion *see Pain page 296*
Narcotic Analgesics *see Pain page 308*
Parenteral Corticosteroids *see page 499*
Oral Corticosteroids *see page 498*

SKELETAL MUSCLE RELAXANTS

▷ *baclofen* (C)(G) <12 years: not recommended; ≥12 years: 5 mg tid; titrate up by 5 mg every 3 days to 20 mg tid; max 80 mg/day

Lioresal *Tab:* 10*, 20* mg

Comment: *baclofen* is indicated for muscle spasm pain and chronic spasticity associated with multiple sclerosis and spinal cord injury or disease. Potential for seizures or hallucinations on abrupt withdrawal.

➤ *carisoprodol* (C)(G) <12 years: not recommended; ≥12 years: 1 tab tid or qid
　　Soma *Tab:* 350 mg

➤ *chlorzoxazone* (NE)(G) <12 years: not recommended; ≥12 years: 1 caplet qid; max 750 mg qid
　　Parafon Forte DSC *Cplt:* 500*mg

➤ *cyclobenzaprine* (B)(G) <15 years: not recommended; ≥15 years: 10 mg tid; usual range 20-40 mg/day in divided doses; max 60 mg/day x 2-3 weeks or 15 mg ext-rel once daily; max 30 mg ext-rel/day x 2-3 weeks
　　Amrix *Cap:* 15, 30 mg ext-rel
　　Fexmid *Tab:* 7.5 mg
　　Flexeril *Tab:* 5, 10 mg

➤ *dantrolene* (C) <12 years: 0.5 mg/kg daily x 7 days; then 0.5 mg/kg tid x 7 days; then 1 mg/kg tid x 7 days; then 2 mg/kg tid; max 100 mg qid; ≥12 years: 25 md daily x 7 days; then 25 mg tid x 7 days; then 50 mg tid x 7 days; max 100 mg qid
　　Dantrium *Tab:* 25, 50, 100 mg

Comment: *dantrolene* is indicated for chronic spasticity associated with multiple sclerosis and spinal cord injury or disease.

➤ *diazepam* (C)(IV) <6 months: not recommended; >6 months-12 years: initially 1-2.5 mg bid-qid; may increase gradually; ≥12 years: 2-10 mg bid-qid; may increase gradually
　　Diastat *Rectal gel delivery system:* 2.5 mg
　　Diastat AcuDial *Rectal gel delivery system:* 10, 20 mg
　　Valium *Tab:* 2, 5, 10 mg
　　Valium Intensol Oral Solution *Conc oral soln:* 5 mg/ml (30 ml w. dropper) (alcohol 19%)
　　Valium Oral Solution *Oral soln:* 5 mg/5 ml (500 ml) (wintergreen spice)

➤ *metaxalone* (B) <12 years: not recommended; ≥12 years: 1 tab tid-qid
　　Skelaxin *Tab:* 800*mg

➤ *methocarbamol* (C)(G) <16 years: not recommended; ≥16 years: initially 1.5 gm qid x 2-3 days; maintenance, 750 mg every 4 hours or 1.5 gm 3 times daily; max 8 gm/day
　　Robaxin *Tab:* 500 mg
　　Robaxin 750 *Tab:* 750 mg
　　Robaxin Injection 10 ml IM or IV; max 30 ml/day; max 3 days; max 5 ml/gluteal injection q 8 hours; max IV rate 3 ml/min
　　　　Vial: 100 mg/ml (10 ml)

➤ *nabumetone* (C) <12 years: not recommended; ≥12 years: initially 1,000 mg as a single dose; titrate as needed; may split dose bid; max 2,000 mg/day
　　Relafen *Tab:* 500, 750 mg
　　Relafen 500 *Tab:* 500 mg

➤ *orphenadrine citrate* (C)(G) <12 years: not recommended; ≥12 years: 1 tab bid
　　Norflex *Tab:* 100 mg sust-rel

➤ *tizanidine* (C) <12 years: not recommended; ≥12 years: 1-4 mg q 6-8 hours; max 36 mg/day
　　Zanaflex *Tab:* 2*, 4**mg; *Cap:* 2, 4, 6 mg

SKELETAL MUSCLE RELAXANT/NSAID COMBINATIONS

Comment: *aspirin*-containing medications are contraindicated with history of allergic type reaction to *aspirin*, children and adolescents with *Varicella* or other viral illness, and 3rd trimester pregnancy.

➤ *carisoprodol/aspirin* (C)(III)(G) <12 years: not recommended; ≥12 years: 1-2 tabs qid

Soma Compound *Tab: caris* 200 mg/*asp* 325 mg (sulfites)

➤ *meprobamate/aspirin* (D)(IV) <12 years: not recommended; ≥12 years: 1-2 tabs tid or qid

Equagesic *Tab: mepro* 200 mg/*asp* 325*mg

SKELETAL MUSCLE RELAXANT/NSAID/CAFFEINE COMBINATIONS

➤ *orphenadrine/aspirin/caffeine* (D)(G) <12 years: not recommended; ≥12 years:

Norgesic 1-2 tabs tid-qid

Tab: orphen 25 mg/*asp* 385 mg/*caf* 30 mg

Norgesic Forte 1 tab tid or qid; max 4 tabs/day

Tab: orphen 50 mg/*asp* 770 mg/*caf* 60*mg

SKELETAL MUSCLE RELAXANT/NSAID/CODEINE COMBINATIONS

➤ *carisoprodol/aspirin/codeine* (D)(III)(G) <12 years: contraindicated; 12-<18: use extreme caution; not recommended for children and adolescents with obesity, asthma, obstructive sleep apnea, or other chronic breathing problem, or for post-tonsillectomy/adenoidectomy pain; ≥18 years:

Soma Compound w. Codeine 1-2 tabs qid

Tab: caris 200 mg/*asp* 325 mg/*cod* 16 mg (sulfites)

Comment: *Codeine* is known to be excreted in breast milk. <12 years: not recommended; 12-<18: use extreme caution; not recommended for children and adolescents with asthma or other chronic breathing problem. The FDA and the European Medicines Agency (EMA) are investigating the safety of using *codeine* containing medications to treat pain, cough and colds, in children 12-<18 years because of the potential for serious side effects, including slowed or difficult breathing.

TOPICAL/TRANSDERMAL NSAIDs

➤ *capsaicin* cream (B)(G) <2 years: not recommended; 2-12 years: apply sparingly to intact skin bid prn; >12 years: apply tid-qid prn

Axsain *Crm:* 0.075% (1, 2 oz)

Capsin (OTC) *Lotn:* 0.025, 0,075% (59 ml)

Capzasin-P (OTC) *Crm:* 0.025% (1.5 oz); *Lotn:* 0.025% (2 oz)

Capzasin-HP (OTC) *Crm:* 0.075% (1.5 oz); *Lotn:* 0.075% (2 oz)

Dolorac *Crm:* 0.025% (28 gm)

Double Cap (OTC) *Crm:* 0.05% (2 oz)

R-Gel *Gel:* 0.025% (15, 30 gm)

Zostrix (OTC) *Crm:* 0.025% (0.7, 1.5, 3 oz)

Zostrix HP (OTC) *Emol crm:* 0.075% (1, 2 oz)

Comment: Provides some relief by 1-2 weeks; optimal benefit may take 4-6 weeks. Avoid contact with mucous membranes.

▷ *capsaicin* 8% patch **(B)** <18 years: not recommended; ≥18 years: apply up to 4 patches for one 60-minute application to clean dry skin; may prep area with topical anesthetic; wear non-latex gloves; patches may be cut to size/shape; treatment may be repeated every 3 months; remove with cleansing gel after treatment

Qutenza *Patch:* 8% 1640 mcg/cm (179 mg; 1 or 2 patches, each w. 1-50 gm tube cleansing gel/carton)

▷ *diclofenac epolamine transdermal patch* **(C; D ≥30 wks)** <12 years: not recommended; ≥12 years: apply one patch to affected area bid; remove during bathing; avoid non-intact skin

Flector Patch *Patch:* 180 mg/patch (30/carton)

ORAL NSAIDs

▷ *diclofenac* **(C)** <18 years: not recommended; ≥18 years: take on empty stomach; 35 mg tid; *Hepatic impairment:* use lowest dose

Zorvolex *Gelcap:* 18, 35 mg

▷ *diclofenac sodium* **(C)** <18 years: not recommended; ≥18 years:

Voltaren 50 mg bid-qid or 75 mg bid or 25 mg qid with an additional 25 mg at HS if necessary

Tab: 25, 50, 75 mg ent-coat

Voltaren XR 100 mg once daily; rarely, 100 mg bid may be used

Tab: 100 mg ext-rel

For an expanded list of **Oral Prescription NSAIDs** *see page* 490

ORAL NSAIDS/PPI COMBINATIONS

▷ *esomeprazole/naproxen* **(C; not for use in 3rd)(G)** <18 years: not recommended; ≥18 years: 1 tab bid; use lowest effective dose for the shortest duration; swallow whole; take at least 30 minutes before a meal

Vimovo *Tab: nap* 375 mg/*eso* 20 mg ext-rel; *nap* 500 mg/*eso* 20 mg ext-rel

Comment: **Vimovo** is indicated to improve signs/symptoms, and risk of gastric ulcer in patients at risk of developing NSAID-associated gastric ulcer.

COX-2 INHIBITORS

Comment: Cox-2 inhibitors are contraindicated with history of asthma, urticaria, and allergic-type reactions to *aspirin*, other NSAIDs, and sulfonamides, 3rd trimester of pregnancy, and coronary artery bypass graft (CABG) surgery.

▷ *celecoxib* **(C)(G)** <18 years: not recommended; ≥18 years: 100-400 mg bid; max 800 mg/day

Celebrex *Cap:* 50, 100, 200, 400 mg

▷ *meloxicam* **(C)(G)**

Mobic <2 years, <60 kg: not recommended; ≥2, >60 kg: 0.125 mg/kg; max 7.5 mg once daily; ≥18 years: initially 7.5 mg once daily; max 15 mg once daily; *Hemodialysis:* max 7.5 mg/day

Tab: 7.5, 15 mg; *Oral susp:* 7.5 mg/5 ml (100 ml) (raspberry)

Vivlodex <18 years: not established; ≥18 years: initially 5 mg qd; may increase to max 10 mg/day; *Hemodialysis:* max 5 mg/day

Cap: 5, 10 mg

TOPICAL/TRANSDERMAL NSAIDs

▷ *capsaicin* cream (B)(G) <2 years: not recommended; 2-12 years: apply sparingly to intact skin bid prn; >12 years: apply tid-qid prn

Axsain *Crm:* 0.075% (1, 2 oz)
Capsin (OTC) *Lotn:* 0.025, 0,075% (59 ml)
Capzasin-P (OTC) *Crm:* 0.025% (1.5 oz); *Lotn:* 0.025% (2 oz)
Capzasin-HP (OTC) *Crm:* 0.075% (1.5 oz); *Lotn:* 0.075% (2 oz)
Dolorac *Crm:* 0.025% (28 gm)
Double Cap (OTC) *Crm:* 0.05% (2 oz)
R-Gel *Gel:* 0.025% (15, 30 gm)
Zostrix (OTC) *Crm:* 0.025% (0.7, 1.5, 3 oz)
Zostrix HP (OTC) *Emol crm:* 0.075% (1, 2 oz)

Comment: Provides some relief by 1-2 weeks; optimal benefit may take 4-6 weeks. Avoid contact with mucous membranes.

▷ *capsaicin* 8% patch (B) <18 years: not recommended; ≥18 years: apply sparingly to intact skin tid-qid prn; apply up to 4 patches for one 60-minute application to clean dry skin; may prep area with topical anesthetic; wear non-latex gloves; patches may be cut to size/shape; treatment may be repeated every 3 months; remove with cleansing gel after treatment

Qutenza *Patch:* 8% 1640 mcg/cm (179 mg; 1 or 2 patches, each w. 1-50 gm tube cleansing gel/carton)

▷ *diclofenac epolamine transdermal patch* (C; D ≥30 wks) <12 years: not recommended; ≥12 years: apply sparingly tid-qid prn apply one patch to affected area bid; remove during bathing; avoid non-intact skin

Flector Patch *Patch:* 180 mg/patch (30/carton)

▷ *diclofenac sodium* (C; D ≥30 wks)(G) <18 years: not established; ≥18 years:

Pennsaid 1.5% in 10 drop increments, dispense and rub into front, side, and back of knee; usually; 40 drops (40 mg) qid
Topical soln: 1.5% (150 ml)
Pennsaid 2% apply 2 pump actuations (40 mg) and rub into front, side, and back of knee bid
Topical soln: 2% (20 mg/pump actuation, 112 gm)

Comment: **Pennsaid** <12 years: not recommended; ≥12 years: indicated for the treatment of pain associated with osteoarthritis of the knee

Solaraze Gel *Gel:* 3% (50 gm) (benzyl alcohol)

Comment: Contraindicated with *aspirin* allergy. As with other NSAIDs, **Solaraze Gel** should be avoided in late pregnancy (≥30 weeks) because it may cause premature closure of the ductus arteriosus.

Voltaren Gel apply qid; avoid non-intact skin
Gel: 1% (100 gm)

Comment: *diclofenac* is contraindicated with *aspirin* allergy. As with other NSAIDs, **Voltaren Gel** should be avoided in late pregnancy (≥30 weeks) because it may cause premature closure of the ductus arteriosus.

TOPICAL/TRANSDERMAL LIDOCAINE

▷ *lidocaine* transdermal patch (C)(G) <12 years: not recommended; ≥12 years: apply one patch to affected area for 12 hours (then off for 12 hours); remove during bathing; avoid non-intact skin

Lidoderm *Patch:* 5% (10 cm x 14 cm; 30/carton)

NARCOLEPSY

STIMULANTS

▶ *amphetamine sulfate* (C)(II)
> **Evekeo** <6 years: not recommended; 6-12 years: initially 5 mg once or twice daily at the same time(s) each day; may increase by 5 mg/day at weekly intervals; max 40 mg/day; >12 years: initially 10 mg once or twice daily at the same time(s) each day; may increase by 10 mg/day at weekly intervals; max 40 mg/day
> *Tab:* 5, 10 mg

▶ *armodafinil* (C)(IV)(G) <17 years: not recommended; ≥17 years: *OSAHS:* 50-250 mg once daily in the AM; *SWSD:* 150 mg 1 hour before starting shift; reduce dose with severe hepatic impairment
> **Nuvigil** *Tab:* 50, 150, 200, 250 mg

▶ *dextroamphetamine sulfate* (C)(II)(G) <3 years: not recommended; 3-5 years: 2.5 mg daily; may increase by 2.5 mg daily at weekly intervals if needed; 6-12 years: initially 5 mg daily-bid; may increase by 5 mg/day at weekly intervals; usual max 40 mg/day; >12 years: initially 10 mg daily; may increase by mg/day at weekly intervals; max 40 mg/day; initially start with 10 mg daily; increase by 10 mg at weekly intervals if needed; may switch to daily dose with sust-rel spansules when titrated
> **Dexedrine** *Tab:* 5*mg (tartrazine)
> **Dexedrine Spansule** *Cap:* 5, 10, 15 mg sust-rel
> **Dextrostat** *Tab:* 5, 10 mg (tartrazine)

▶ *dextroamphetamine saccharate/dextroamphetamine sulfate/amphetamine aspartate/amphetamine sulfate* (C)(II)(G)
> **Adderall** <6 years: not indicated; 6-12 years: initially 5 mg daily; may increase weekly by 5 mg/day; usual max 40 mg/day in 2-3 divided doses; >12 years: initially 10 mg daily; may increase weekly by 10 mg/day; usual max 60 mg/day in 2-3 divided doses; first dose on awakening and then q 4-6 hours prn
> *Tab:* 5**, 7.5**, 10**, 12.5**, 15**, 20**, 30**mg
> **Adderall XR** <6 years: not recommended; 6-12 years: initially 10 mg daily in the AM; may increase by 10 mg weekly; max 30 mg/day; >12 years: initially 10 mg daily; may increase to 20 mg/day after 1 week; max 30 mg/day; do not chew; may sprinkle on applesauce
> *Cap:* 5, 10, 15, 20, 25, 30 mg ext-rel
> **Comment: Adderall** is also indicated to improve wakefulness in patients with SWSD and OSAHS.

▶ *dexmethylphenidate* (C)(II)(G) <6 years: not recommended; ≥6 years:
> **Focalin** initially 2.5 mg bid; allow at least 4 hours between doses; may increase at 1 week intervals; max 40 mg/day
> *Tab:* 2.5, 5, 10*mg (dye-free)
> **Focalin XR** 20-40 mg q AM; max 40 mg/day
> *Tab:* 5, 10, 15, 20, 30, 40 mg ext-rel (dye-free)

▶ *methamphetamine* (C)(II)(G)
> **Desoxyn** Gradumet <6 years: not recommended; ≥6 years: initially 5 mg daily bid; may increase by 5 mg/day at weekly intervals; usual effective dose; 20-25 mg/day
> *Tab:* 5, 10, 15 mg sust-rel

▶ *methylphenidate (regular-acting)* (C)(II)(G)

Methylin, Methylin Chewable, Methylin Oral Solution <6 years: not recommended; ≥6 years-12 years: initially 5 mg twice daily before breakfast and lunch; may increase 5-10 mg/week; max 60 mg/day; >12 years: usual dose 20-30 mg/day in 2-3 divided doses 30-45 minutes before a meal; may increase to 60 mg/day

Tab: 5, 10*, 20*mg; *Chew tab:* 2.5, 5, 10 mg (grape) (phenylalanine); *Oral soln:* 5, 10 mg/5 ml) (grape)

Ritalin <6 years: not recommended; ≥6-12 years: years: initially 5 mg bid ac (before breakfast and lunch); may gradually increase by 5-10 mg at weekly intervals as needed; max 60 mg/day; >12 years: 10-60 mg/day in 2-3 divided doses 30-45 minutes ac; max 60 mg/day

Tab: 5, 10*, 20*mg

▷ *methylphenidate (long-acting)* (C)(II)

Concerta <6 years: not recommended; ≥6 years: initially 18 mg q AM; may increase in 18 mg increments as needed; max 54 mg/day; do not crush <u>or</u> chew

Tab: 18, 27, 36, 54 mg sust-rel

Metadate CD (G) <6 years: not recommended; 6-12 years: initially 20 mg daily; may gradually increase by 20 mg/day at weekly intervals as needed; max 60 mg/day; >12 years: 1 cap daily in the AM; may sprinkle on food; do not crush <u>or</u> chew

Cap: 10, 20, 30, 40, 50, 60 mg immed- and ext-rel beads

Metadate ER <6 years: not recommended; ≥6 years-12 years: use in place of regular-acting *methylphenidate* when the 8-hour dose of **Metadate-ER** corresponds to the titrated 8-hour dose of regular-acting *methylphenidate*: >12 years: 1 tab daily in the AM; do not crush <u>or</u> chew

Tab: 10, 20 mg ext-rel (dye-free)

Ritalin LA <6 years: not recommended; ≥6 years: use in place of regular-acting *methylphenidate* when the 8-hour dose of **Ritalin LA** corresponds to the titrated 8-hour dose of regular-acting *methylphenidate*; 1 cap daily in the AM; max 60 mg/day

Cap: 10, 20, 30, 40 mg ext-rel (immed- and ext-rel beads)

Ritalin SR <6 years: not recommended; ≥6 years: use in place of regular-acting *methylphenidate* when the 8-hour dose of **Ritalin SR** corresponds to the titrated 8-hour dose of regular-acting *methylphenidate*; max 60 mg/day

Tab: 20 mg sust-rel (dye-free)

▷ *methylphenidate (transdermal patch)* (C)(II)(G) <6 years: not recommended; ≥6 years: initially 10 mg patch daily in the AM; may increase by 5-10 mg/week; max 60 mg/day

Transdermal patch: 10, 15, 20, 30 mg

▷ *modafinil* (C)(IV)(G) <17 years: not recommended; ≥17 years: 100-200 mg q AM; max 400 mg/day

Provigil *Tab:* 100, 200*mg

Comment: **Provigil** also promotes wakefulness in patients with SWSD and excessive sleepiness due to OSAHS.

▷ *pemoline* (B)(IV) <6 years: not recommended; ≥6 years: 18.75-112.5 mg/day; usually start with 37.5 mg in AM; increase weekly by 18.75 mg/day if needed; max 112.5 gm/day

Cylert *Tab:* 18.75*, 37.5*, 75*mg

Cylert Chewable *Chew tab:* 37.5*mg

Comment: Monitor baseline serum ALT and repeat every 2 weeks thereafter.

➤ *sodium oxybate* (B) <16 years: not recommended; ≥16 years: take dose at bedtime while in bed and repeat 2.5-4 hours later; titrate to effect; initially 4.5 grams/night in 2 divided doses; may increase by 1.5 gm/night in 2 divided doses; max 9 gm/night

    Xyrem *Oral soln:* 100, 200*mg

    Comment: Xyrem is used to reduce the number of cataplexy attacks (sudden loss of muscle strength) and reduce daytime sleepiness in patients with narcolepsy. Contraindicated with *alcohol* or CNS depressant (may impair consciousness; may lead to respiratory depression, coma, or death). Prepare both doses prior to bedtime and do not attempt to get out of bed after taking the first dose. Place both doses within reach at the bedside. Set the bedside clock to awaken for the second dose. Dilute each dose in 60 ml (1/4 cup, 4 tbsp) water in child resistant dosing containers. Food significantly reduces the bioavailability of *sodium oxybate*; take at least 2 hours after ingesting food.

NAUSEA/VOMITING

PROPHYLAXIS (FOR PREVENTION OF MOTION SICKNESS AND POST-OP NAUSEA AND VOMITING)

Anticholinergic Agents

➤ *scopolamine* (C)

    Scopace <12 years: not recommended; ≥12 years: 0.4-0.8 mg 1 hour before travel; may repeat in 8 hours

    Tab: 0.4 mg

    Transderm Scop <12 years: not recommended; ≥12 years: 1 patch behind ear at least 4 hours before travel; each patch is effective for 3 days; apply a new patch every 4th day to the opposite side

    Transdermal patch: 1.5 mg (4/carton)

MILD NAUSEA

➤ *phosphorylated carbohydrate* solution (C)(G) 1-2 tbsp q 15 minutes until nausea subsides; max 5 doses/day

    Emetrol (OTC) *Soln:* dextrose 1.87 gm/fructose 1.87 gm/phosphoric acid 21.5 mg per 5 ml (4, 8, 16 oz)

Cannabinoids

Comment: Cannabinoids potentiate CNS depression with benzodiazepines, barbiturates, alcohol, and other CNS depressants, and other psychoactive substances, may affect and be affected by other drugs that are highly protein bound (e.g., sympathomimetics, anticholinergics, TCAs), antagonizes theophylline, and phenothiazines may potentiate cannabinoid effects without additional toxicities.

➤ *dronabinol* (C)(III) initially 5 mg/m^2 1-3 hours before chemotherapy; then q 2-4 hours prn; max 4-6 doses/day, 15 mg/m^2

    Marinol *Cap:* 2.5, 5, 10 mg (sesame seed oil)

➤ *nabilone* (C)(II) 1-2 mg bid; max 6 mg/day in 3 divided doses; initially 1-3 hours before chemotherapy; may give 1-2 mg the night before chemo; may continue 48 hours after each chemo cycle

    Cesamet *Cap:* 1 mg (sesame seed oil)

Antihistamines

▷ *meclizine* (C)(G) <12 years: 5 mg/kg/day in 4 divided doses; max 300 mg/day; ≥12 years: *Travel:* 25-50 mg 1 hour prior to travel; repeat every 24 hours; *Vertigo of vestibular origin:* 25-100 mg/day in divided doses

Antivert *Tab:* 12.5, 25, 50*mg; *Amp:* 50 mg/ml (1 ml); *Vial:* 50 mg/ml (1 ml single use); 50 mg/ml (10 ml multidose)

Bonine (OTC) *Cap:* 15, 25, 50 mg; *Tab:* 12.5, 25, 50 mg; *Chew tab/Film-coat tab:* 25 mg

Dramamine II (OTC) *Tab:* 25 mg

Zentrip *Strip:* 25 mg orally-disint

MODERATE TO SEVERE NAUSEA

Phenothiazines

▷ *chlorpromazine* (C)(G) <6 months: not recommended; ≥6 months-12 years: 0.25 mg/lb orally q 4-6 hours prn or 0.5 mg/lb rectally q 6-8 hours prn; ≥12 years: 10-25 mg PO q 4 hours prn or 50-100 mg rectally q 6-8 hours prn

Thorazine *Tab:* 10, 25, 50, 100, 200 mg; *Spansule:* 30, 75, 150 mg sust-rel; *Syr:* 10 mg/5 ml (4 oz; orange custard); *Conc:* 30 mg/ml (4 oz); 100 mg/ml (2, 8 oz); *Supp:* 25, 100 mg

▷ *perphenazine* (C) <12 years: not recommended; ≥12 years: 0.4-0.8 mg 1 hour before travel; may repeat in 8 hours 5 mg IM (may repeat in 6 hours) or 8-16 mg/day PO in divided doses; max 15 mg/day IM; max 24 mg/day PO

Trilafon *Tab:* 2, 4, 8, 16 mg; *Oral conc:* 16 mg/5 ml (118 ml); *Amp:* 5 mg/ml (1 ml)

▷ *prochlorperazine* (C)(G)

Compazine <2 years or <20 lb: not recommended; 20-29 lb: 2.5 mg daily bid prn; max 7.5 mg/day; 30-39 lb: 2.5 mg bid-tid prn; max 10 mg/day; 40-85 lb: 2.5 mg tid or 5 mg bid prn; max 15 mg/day; ≥85 lbs: 5-10 mg tid-qid prn; usual max 40 mg/day

Tab: 5, 10 mg; *Syr:* 5 mg/5 ml (4 oz) (fruit)

Compazine Suppository <2 years or <20 lb: not recommended; 20-29 lb: 2.5 mg daily-bid prn; max 7.5; mg/day; 30-39 lb: 2.5 mg bid-tid prn; max 10 mg/day; 40-85 lb: 2.5 mg tid or 5 mg bid prn; max 15 mg/day; ≥85 lbs: 25 mg rectally bid prn; usual max 50 mg/day

Rectal supp: 2.5, 5, 25 mg

Compazine Injectable <2 years or <20 lb: not recommended; ≥2 years-12 years, ≥20 lb: 0.06 mg/kg x 1 dose; ≥12 years: 5-10 mg tid or qid prn

Vial: 5 mg/ml (2, 10 ml)

Compazine Spansule <12 years: not recommended; ≥12 years: 0.4-0.8 mg 1 hour before travel; may repeat in 8 hours 15 mg q AM prn or 10 mg q 12 hours prn; usual max 40 mg/day

Spansule: 10, 15 mg sust-rel

▷ *promethazine* (C) <2 years: not recommended; 2-12 years: 0.5 mg/lb or 6.25-25 mg q 4-6 hours PO or rectally; >12 years: 12.5-25 q 4-6 hours PO or rectally **Phenergan** *Tab:* 12.5*, 25*, 50 mg; *Plain syr:* 6.25 mg/5 ml; *Fortis syr:* 25 mg/5 ml; *Rectal supp:* 12.5, 25, 50 mg

Comment: *promethazine* is contraindicated in children with uncomplicated nausea, dehydration, Reye's syndrome, history of sleep apnea, asthma, and lower respiratory disorders in children. *Promethazine* lowers the seizure threshold in children, may cause cholestatic jaundice, anticholinergic effects, extrapyramidal effects, and potentially fatal respiratory depression.

Substance P/Neurokinin 1 Receptor Antagonist

▷ *aprepitant* (B)(G) <6 months: years: not recommended; ≥6 months-12 years: use oral suspension (see mfr pkg insert for dose by weight); >12 years: administer with corticosteroid and 5-HT-3 receptor antagonist; *Day 1 of chemotherapy cycle:* 125 mg 1 hour prior to chemotherapy *Day 2 &3:* 80 mg in the morning

Emend *Cap:* 40, 80, 125 mg (2 x 80 mg bifold pck; 1 x 25 mg/2 x 80 mg trifold pck); *Oral susp:* 125 mg pwdr for oral suspension, single dose pouch w dispenser; *Vial:* 150 mg pwdr for reconstitution and IV infusion

5-HT-3 Receptor Antagonists

Comment: The selective 5-HT-3 receptor antagonists indicated for prevention of nausea and vomiting associated with moderately to highly emetogenic chemotherapy.

▷ *dolasetron* (B) <2 years: not recommended; 2-16 years: 1.8 mg/kg; >16 years: administer 100 mg IV over 30 seconds, 30 min prior to administration of chemotherapy or 2 hours before surgery; max 100 mg/dose

Anzemet *Tab:* 50, 100 mg; *Amp:* 12.5 mg/0.625 ml; *Prefilled carpuject syringe:* 12.5 mg (0.625 ml); *Vial:* 100 mg/5 ml (single use); *Vial:* 500 mg/25 ml (multidose)

▷ *granisetron*

Kytril (B) <2 years: not recommended; 2-12 years: years: 10 mcg/kg; >12 years: administer IV over 30 seconds, 30 min prior to administration of chemotherapy; max 1 dose/week

Tab: 1 mg; *Oral soln:* 2 mg/10 ml (30 ml; orange); *Vial:* 1 mg/ml (1 ml single dose; preservative-free); 1 mg/ml (4 ml multidose) (benzyl alcohol)

Sancuso (B) <18: not recommended; ≥18 years: apply 1 patch 24-48 hours before chemo; remove 24 hours (minimum) to 7 days (maximum) after completion of treatment

Transdermal patch: 3.1 mg/day

Sustol (NE) <18: not established; ≥18 years: administer SC over 20-30 seconds (due to drug viscosity) on Day 1 of chemotherapy and not more frequently than once every 7 days; *CrCl 30-59 mL/min:* repeat dose no more than every 14th day; *CrCl <30 mL/min:* not recommended; for patients receiving MEC, the recommended *dexamethasone* dosage is 8 mg IV on *Day 1*; for patients receiving AC combination chemotherapy regimens, the recommended *dexamethasone* dosage is 20 mg IV on *Day 1*, followed by 8 mg PO bid on *Days 2*, 3 and 4; if **Sustol** is administered with an NK1 receptor antagonist, see that drug's mfr pkg insert for the recommended *dexamethasone* dosing

Syringe: 10 mg/0.4 ml ext-rel; prefilled single dose/kit

Comment: At least 60 minutes prior to administration, remove the **Sustol** kit from refrigeration, activate a warming pouch, and wrap the syringe in the warming pouch for 5-6 minutes to warm it to room temperature.

▷ *ondansetron* (C)(G) <4 years: not recommended; 4-11 years, moderately emetogenic chemotherapy: 4 mg q 4 hours x 3 doses beginning 30 min prior to start; then 4 mg q 8 hours x 1-2 days following; >11 years: use oral forms: *Highly emetogenic chemotherapy:* 24 mg x 1 dose 30 min prior to start of single-day chemotherapy;

Moderately emetogenic chemotherapy: 8 mg q 8 hours x 2 doses beginning 30 minutes prior to start of chemotherapy; then 8 mg q 12 hours x 1-2 days following

Zofran *Tab:* 4, 8, 24 mg

Zofran ODT *ODT:* 4, 8 mg (strawberry) (phenylalanine)

Zofran Oral Solution *Oral soln:* 4 mg/5 ml (50 ml) (strawberry) (phenylalanine); *Parenteral form:* see mfr pkg insert

Zofran Injection *Vial:* 2 mg/ml (2 ml single dose); 2 mg/ml (20 ml multidose); 32 mg/50 ml (50 ml multidose); *Prefilled syringe:* 4 mg/2 ml, single use (24/carton)

Zuplenz Oral Soluble Film: 4, 8 mg oral-dis (10/carton) (peppermint)

▷ *palonosetron* (B)(G) <1 month: not recommended; 1 month-17 years: 20 mcg/kg; max 1.5 mg single dose; infuse over 15 minutes beginning 30 minutes prior to administration of chemo; >17 years: *Chemotherapy:* administer 0.25 mg IV over 30 seconds, 30 min prior to administration of chemo; max 1 dose/week or 1 cap 1 hour before chemo; *Post-op:* administer 0.075 mg IV over 10 seconds immediately before induction of anesthesia

Aloxi *Vial (single use):* 0.075 mg/1.5 ml; 0.25 mg/5 ml (mannitol)

ANTI-DOPAMINERGIC (PROMOTILITY) AGENTS

▷ *metoclopramide* (B)(G) <12 years: not established; ≥12 years: 10 mg 30 minutes before each meal and at HS for 2-8 weeks

Metozolv ODT *ODT:* 5, 10 mg (mint)

Reglan *Tab:* 5, 10*mg

Comment: *metoclopramide* is contraindicated when stimulation of GI motility may be dangerous. Observe for tardive dyskinesia and Parkinsonism. Avoid concomitant drugs which may cause an extrapyramidal reaction (e.g., phenothiazines, *haloperidol*).

SUBSTANCE P/NEUROKININ-1(NK-1) RECEPTOR ANTAGONIST

▷ *rolapitant* (NE) <18 years: not established; ≥18 years: take 180 mg in a single dose 1-2 hours before chemotherapy treatment; administer in combination with dexamethasone and 5-HT3 receptor antagonist

Varubi *Tab:* 90 mg film-coat

Comment: Varubi is indicated in combination with other antiemetic agents in patients ≥18 years for the prevention of delayed nausea and vomiting associated with emetogenic cancer chemotherapy.

SUBSTANCE P/NEUROKININ-1 (NK-1) RECEPTOR ANTAGONIST/5-HT-3 RECEPTOR ANTAGONIST COMBINATION

▷ *netupitant/palonosetron* (C) <18 years: not established; ≥18 years: take one cap approximately 1 hour prior to chemotherapy; administer in combination with dexamethasone 12 mg 30 minutes prior to chemotherapy on Day 1; then 8 mg orally on Days 2-4

Akynzeo *Gelcap: netu* 300 mg/*palo* 0.5 mg

Comment: Akynzeo is indicated in combination with other antiemetic agents in patients ≥18 years: for the prevention of delayed nausea and vomiting associated with highly emetogenic cancer chemotherapy.

NERVE AGENT POISONING

▷ *atropine sulfate* (NE)(G) <15 lb: not recommended; ≥15-40 lb: 0.5 mg IM; ≥40-90 lb: 1 mg IM; >90 lb: 2 mg IM
   AtroPen *Pen (single use):* 0.5, 1, 2 mg (0.5 ml)

NON-24 SLEEP–WAKE DISORDER

Comment: For other drug options (stimulants, sedative hypnotics), *see* **Insomnia** *page* 234, **Sleepiness: Excessive, Shift Work Sleep Disorder** *page* 390

MELATONIN RECEPTOR AGONIST

▷ *tasimelteon* (C) <12 years: not established; ≥12 years: 1 gel cap before bedtime at the same time every night; do not take with food
   Hetlioz *Gel cap:* 20 mg

OREXIN RECEPTOR ANTAGONIST

▷ *suvorexant* (C)(IV) <12 years: not established; ≥12 years: use lowest effective dose; take 30 minutes before bedtime; do not take if unable to sleep for ≥7 hours; max 20 mg
   Belsomra *Tab:* 5, 10, 15, 20 mg (30/blister pck)

OBESITY

Comment: Target BMI is 25-30 (≤27 preferred).

STIMULANTS

▷ *amphetamine sulfate* (C)(II) <12 years: not recommended; ≥12 years: initially 5 mg 30-60 minutes before meals; usually up to 30 mg/day
   Evekeo *Tab:* 5, 10 mg

LIPASE INHIBITOR

▷ *orlistat* (X)(G) <12 years: not recommended; ≥12 years: 1 cap tid 1 hour before or during each main meal containing fat
   Alli (OTC) *Cap:* 60 mg
   Xenical *Cap:* 120 mg
   Comment: For use when BMI >30 kg/m² or BMI >27 kg/m² in the presence of other risk factors (i.e., HTN, DM, dyslipidemia).

ANOREXIGENICS

Sympathomimetics

Comment: ASEs of sympathomimetics include hypertension, tachycardia, restlessness, insomnia, and dry mouth.
▷ *benzphetamine* (X)(III) <12 years: not recommended; ≥12 years: initially 25-50 mg daily in the mid-morning or mid-afternoon; may increase to bid-tid as needed
   Didrex *Tab:* 50*mg

➤ *naltrexone/bupropion* (X)(G) <18 years: not recommended; ≥18 years: swallow whole; avoid high-fat meals; initially 10 mg bid; evaluate weight loss after 12 weeks; discontinue if less than 5% weight loss

Contrave *Tab:* nal 8 mg/*bup* 900 mg ext-rel

➤ *methamphetamine* (C)(II) <12 years: not recommended; ≥12 years: 10-15 mg q AM

Desoxyn *Tab:* 5, 10, 15 mg sust-rel

➤ *phendimetrazine* (C)(III)

Bontril PDM <12 years: not recommended; ≥12 years: 35 mg bid-tid 1 hour ac; may reduce to 17.5 mg (1/2 tab)/dose; max 210 mg/day in 3 divided doses

Tab: 35*mg

Bontril Slow-Release <12 years: not recommended; ≥12 years: 105 mg in the AM 30-60 minutes before breakfast

Cap: 105 mg slow-rel

➤ *phentermine* (C)(IV)

Adipex-P (G) <16 years: not recommended; ≥16 years: 1 cap <u>or</u> tab before breakfast <u>or</u> 1/2 tab bid ac

Cap: 37.5 mg; *Tab:* 37.5*mg

Fastin (G) <16 years: not recommended; ≥16 years: 1 cap before breakfast

Cap: 30 mg

Ionamin (G) <16 years: not recommended; ≥16 years: cap before breakfast <u>or</u> 10-14 hours prior to HS

Cap: 15, 30 mg

Suprenza ODT (X)(IV) <16 years: not recommended; ≥16 years: dissolve 1 tab on top of tongue once daily in the morning, with <u>or</u> without food; use lowest effective dose

Tab: 15, 30, 37.5 mg orally-disint

Comment: *phentermine* is contraindicated with history of cardiovascular disease (e.g., coronary artery disease, stroke, arrhythmias, congestive heart failure, uncontrolled hypertension, during <u>or</u> within 14 days following the administration of an MAOI, hyperthyroidism, glaucoma, agitated states, history of drug abuse, pregnancy, nursing).

Sympathomimetic/Antiepileptic Combination

➤ *phentermine/topiramate ext-rel* (X)(IV)(G) <16 years: not established; ≥16 years: initially 3.75 mg/23 mg daily in the AM x 14 days; then, increase to 7.5 mg/46 mg and evaluate weight loss on this dose after 12 weeks; if ≤3% weight loss from baseline, discontinue <u>or</u> increase dose to 11.25 mg/69 mg x 14 days; then, increase to 15 mg/92 mg and evaluate weight loss on this dose after 12 weeks; if ≤5% weight loss from baseline, discontinue by taking a dose every other day for at least one week prior to stopping; max 7.5 mg/46 mg for moderate to severe renal impairment <u>or</u> moderate hepatic impairment.

Qsymia

Cap: **Qsymia 3.75/23:** *phen* 3.75 mg/*topir* 23 mg ext-rel

Qsymia 7.5/46: *phen* 7.5 mg/*topir* 46 mg ext-rel

Qsymia 11.25/69: *phen* 11.25 mg/*topir* 69 mg ext-rel

Qsymia 15/92: *phen* 15 mg/*topir* 92 mg ext-rel

Comment: Side effects include hypertension, tachycardia, restlessness, insomnia, and dry mouth. Contraindicated with glaucoma, hyperthyroidism, and within 14 days of taking an MAOI. **Qsymia 3.75/23** and **Qsymia 11.25/69** are for titration purposes only.

Serotonin 2C Receptor Agonist

▷ *lorcaserin* (X)(G) <18 years: not recommended; ≥18 years: 10 mg bid; discontinue if 5% weight loss is not achieved by week 12

Belviq *Tab:* 10 mg film-coat

Comment: **Belviq** is indicated as an adjunct to a reduced-calorie diet and increased physical activity for chronic weight management in patients ≥18 years with an initial body mass index (BMI) of 30 kg/m^2 or greater (obese) or 27 kg/m^2 or greater (overweight) in the presence of at least one weight-related comorbid condition (e.g., hypertension, dyslipidemia, type 2 diabetes). Serotonin 2C receptor agonists interact with serotonergic drugs (selective serotonin reuptake inhibitors [SSRIs], serotonin-norepinephrine reuptake inhibitors [SNRIs], monoamine oxidase inhibitors [MAOIs], triptans, *bupropion, dextromethorphan, St. John's wort*); therefore, use with extreme caution due to the risk of *serotonin syndrome.*

GLUCAGON-LIKE PEPTIDE-1 (GLP-1) RECEPTOR AGONIST

▷ *liraglutide* (C) <18 years: not recommended; ≥18 years: administer SC in the upper arm, abdomen, or thigh once daily; escalate dose gradually over 5 weeks to 3 mg SC daily; *Week 1:* 0.6 mg SC daily; *Week 2:* 1.2 mg SC daily; *Week 3:* 1.8 mg SC daily; *Week 4:* 2.4 mg SC daily; *Week 5:* 3 mg SC daily

Saxenda Soln for SC inj: 6 mg/ml multidose prefilled pen (3 ml; 3, 5 pens/carton)

Comment: **Saxenda** is indicated as an adjunct to a reduced-calorie diet and increased physical activity for chronic weight management in patients ≥18 years with an initial body mass index (BMI) of 30 kg/m^2 or greater (obese) or 27 kg/m^2 or greater overweight) in the presence of at least one weight-related comorbid condition (e.g., hypertension, dyslipidemia, type 2 diabetes). Not indicated for treatment of T2DM. Do not use with **Victoza**, other GLP-1 receptor agonists, or insulin. Contraindicated with personal or family history of medullary thyroid carcinoma (MTC) and multiple endocrine neoplasia syndrome (MENS) type 2. Monitor for signs/symptoms pancreatitis. Discontinue if gastroparesis, renal, or hepatic impairment.

▮ OBSESSIVE-COMPULSIVE DISORDER (OCD)

SELECTIVE SEROTONIN REUPTAKE INHIBITORS (SSRIS)

Comment: Co-administration of SSRIs with TCAs requires extreme caution. Concomitant use of MAOIs and SSRIs is absolutely contraindicated. Avoid other serotonergic drugs. A potentially fatal adverse event is *serotonin syndrome*, caused by serotonin excess. Milder symptoms require HCP intervention to avert severe symptoms that can be rapidly fatal without urgent/emergent medical care. Symptoms include restlessness, agitation, confusion, hallucinations, tachycardia, hypertension, dilated pupils, muscle twitching, muscle rigidity, loss of muscle coordination, diaphoresis, diarrhea, headache, shivering, piloerection, hyperpyrexia, cardiac arrhythmias, seizures, loss of consciousness, coma, death. Abrupt withdrawal or interruption of treatment with an antidepressant medication is sometimes associated with an *antidepressant discontinuation syndrome*, which may be mediated by gradually tapering the drug over a period of two weeks or longer, depending on the dose strength and length of treatment. Common symptoms of the *serotonin discontinuation syndrome* include flu-like symptoms (nausea, vomiting, diarrhea, headaches, sweating), sleep disturbances (insomnia, nightmares, constant sleepiness), mood disturbances (dysphoria, anxiety, agitation), cognitive disturbances (mental confusion, hyperarousal), sensory and movement disturbances (imbalance, tremors, vertigo, dizziness, electric-shock-like sensations in the brain, often described by sufferers as "brain zaps").

▷ *fluoxetine* (C)(G)

Prozac <8 years: not recommended; 8-17 years: initially 10 mg/day; may increase after 1 week to 20 mg/day; range 20-60 mg/day; range for lower weight children, 20-30 mg/day; ≥17 years: initially 20 mg daily; may increase after 1 week; doses >20 mg/day should be divided into AM and noon doses; max 80 mg/day

Cap: 10, 20, 40 mg; *Tab:* 30*, 60*mg; *Oral soln:* 20 mg/5 ml (4 oz) (mint)

Prozac Weekly <12 years: not recommended; ≥12 years: following daily *fluoxetine* therapy at 20 mg/day for 13 weeks, may initiate **Prozac Weekly** 7 days after the last 20 mg *fluoxetine* dose

Cap: 90 mg ent-coat del-rel pellets

▷ *fluvoxamine* (C)(G)

Luvox <8 years: not recommended; 8-17 years: initially 25 mg q HS; adjust in 25 mg increments q 4-7 days; usual range 50-200 mg/day; over 50 mg/day, divide into 2 doses giving the larger dose at HS; >17 years: initially 50 mg q HS; adjust in 50 mg increments at 4-7 day intervals; range 100-300 mg/day; over 100 mg/day, divide into 2 doses giving the larger dose at HS

Tab: 25, 50*, 100*mg

Luvox CR <18 years: not recommended; ≥18 years: initially 100 mg once daily at HS; may increase by 50 mg increments at 1 week intervals; max 300 mg/day; swallow whole

Cap: 100, 150 mg ext-rel

▷ *paroxetine maleate* (D)(G)

Paxil <12 years: not recommended; ≥12 years: initially 20 mg daily in AM; may increase by 10 mg/day at weekly intervals as needed; max 60 mg/day

Tab: 10*, 20*, 30, 40 mg

Paxil CR <12 years: not recommended; ≥12 years: initially 25 mg daily in AM; may increase by 12.5 mg at weekly intervals as needed; max 62.5 mg/day

Tab: 12.5, 25, 37.5 mg cont-rel ent-coat

Paxil Suspension <12 years: not recommended; ≥12 years: initially 20 mg daily in AM; may increase by 10 mg/day at weekly intervals as needed; max 60 mg/day

Oral susp: 10 mg/5 ml (250 ml) (orange)

▷ *sertraline* (C) <6 years: not recommended; 6-12 years: initially 25 mg daily; max 200 mg/day; 13-17 years: initially 50 mg daily; max 200 mg/day; >17 years: initially 50 mg daily; increase at 1 week intervals if needed; max 200 mg daily

Zoloft *Tab:* 15*, 50*, 100*mg; *Oral conc:* 20 mg per ml (60 ml [dilute just before administering in 4 oz water, ginger ale, lemon-lime soda, lemonade, or orange juice]) (alcohol 12%)

TRICYCLIC ANTIDEPRESSANTS (TCAs)

Comment: Co-administration of SSRIs and TCAs requires extreme caution.

▷ *amitriptyline* (C)(G) <12 years: not recommended; ≥12 years: 10-20 mg q HS

Tab: 10, 25, 50, 75, 100, 150 mg

▶ *amoxapine* (C) <12 years: not recommended; ≥12 years: initially 50 mg bid-tid; after 1 week may increase to 100 mg bid-tid; usual effective dose 200-300 mg/day; if total dose exceeds 300 mg/day, give in divided doses (max 400 mg/day); may give as a single bedtime dose (max 300 mg q HS)
   Tab: 25, 50, 100, 150 mg

▶ *clomipramine* (C)(G) <10 years: not recommended; 10-<16 years: initially 25 mg daily in divided doses; gradually increase; max 3 mg/kg or 100 mg, whichever is smaller; ≥16 years: initially 25 mg daily in divided doses; gradually increase to 100 mg during first 2 weeks; max 250 mg/day; total maintenance dose may be given at HS
   Anafranil *Cap:* 25, 50, 75 mg

▶ *desipramine* (C)(G) <12 years: not recommended; ≥12 years: 100-200 mg/day in single or divided doses; max 300 mg/day
   Norpramin *Tab:* 10, 25, 50, 75, 100, 150 mg

▶ *doxepin* (C)(G) <12 years: not recommended; ≥12 years: 75 mg/day; max 150 mg/day
   Cap: 10, 25, 50, 75, 100, 150 mg; *Oral conc:* 10 mg/ml (4 oz w. dropper)

▶ *imipramine* (C)(G) <12 years: not recommended; ≥12 years:
   Tofranil initially 75 mg daily (max 200 mg); adolescents initially 30-40 mg daily (max 100 mg/day); if maintenance dose exceeds 75 mg daily, may switch to **Tofranil PM** for divided or bedtime dose
      Tab: 10, 25, 50 mg
   Tofranil PM initially 75 mg daily 1 hour before HS; max 200 mg
      Cap: 75, 100, 125, 150 mg

▶ *nortriptyline* (D)(G) <12 years: not recommended; ≥12 years: initially 25 mg tid-qid; max 150 mg/day
   Pamelor *Cap:* 10, 25, 50, 75 mg; *Oral soln:* 10 mg/5 ml (16 oz)

▶ *protriptyline* (C) <12 years: not recommended; ≥12 years: initially 5 mg tid; usual dose 15-40 mg/day in 3-4 divided doses; max 60 mg/day
   Vivactil *Tab:* 5, 10 mg

▶ *trimipramine* (C) <12 years: not recommended; ≥12 years: initially 75 mg/day in divided doses; max 200 mg/day
   Surmontil *Cap:* 25, 50, 100 mg

ONYCHOMYCOSIS (FUNGAL NAIL)

ORAL AGENTS

▶ *griseofulvin, microsize* (C)(G) <12 years: <30 lb: 5 mg/lb/day; 30-50 lb: 125-250 mg/day; >50 lb: 250-500 mg/day; 5 mg/lb/day x 4-6 weeks or longer; *see page 568 for dose by weight table*; ≥12 years: 500 mg once daily x 4-6 weeks or longer; max 1 gm/day
   Grifulvin V *Tab:* 250, 500 mg; *Oral susp:* 125 mg/5 ml (120 ml; alcohol 0.02%)

▶ *griseofulvin, ultramicrosize* (C)(G) <2 years: not recommended; 2-12 years: 3.3 mg/lb/day in a single or divided doses x 4-6 weeks or longer; >12 years: 375 mg/day in a single or divided doses x 4-6 weeks or longer
   Gris-PEG *Tab:* 125, 250 mg

▶ *itraconazole* (C)(G) <12 years: not recommended; ≥12 years: 200 mg daily x 12 consecutive weeks for toenails; 200 mg bid x 1 week, off 3 weeks, then 200 mg bid x 1 additional week for fingernails
   Sporanox *Cap:* 100 mg; *Soln:* 10 mg/ml (150 ml) (cherry-caramel)
   Pulse Pack: 100 mg caps (7/pck)

▷ *terbinafine* (B)(G) <12 years: not recommended; ≥12 years: 250 mg daily x 6 weeks
for fingernails; 250 mg daily x 12 weeks for toenails
   Lamisil *Tab:* 250 mg

TOPICAL AGENTS

Comment: File and trim nail while nail is free from drug. Remove unattached infected nail
as frequently as monthly. For use with mild to moderate onychomycosis of the fingernails
and toenails, without lunula involvement due to *Trichophyton rubrum* immunocompetent
patients as part of a comprehensive treatment program. For use on nails and adjacent
skin only. Apply evenly to entire onycholytic nail and surrounding 5 mm of skin daily,
preferably at HS or 8 hours before washing; apply to nail bed, hyponychium, and under
surface of nail plate when it is free of the nail bed; apply over previous coats, then remove
with alcohol once per week; treat for up to 48 weeks. <12 years not recommended.
▷ *ciclopirox* (B)
   Penlac Nail Lacquer *Topical soln (lacquer):* 8% (6.6 ml w. applicator)
▷ *efinaconazole* (C)
   Jublia *Topical soln:* 5% (10 ml w. brush applicator)
▷ *tavaborole* (C)
   Kerydin *Topical soln:* 10% (10 ml w. dropper)

OPHTHALMIA NEONATORUM: CHLAMYDIAL

PROPHYLAXIS

▷ *erythromycin* ophthalmic ointment 0.5-1 cm ribbon into lower conjunctival sac of
each eye x 1 application
   Ilotycin Ophthalmic Ointment *Ophth oint:* 5 mg/g (1/8 oz)
Comment: The following treatment regimens are published in the **2015 CDC Sexually
Transmitted Diseases Treatment Guidelines**. Treatment regimens are presented by
generic drug name first, followed by information about brands and dose forms.

RECOMMENDED REGIMENS

Regimen 1

▷ *erythromycin base* (B)(G) 50 mg/kg/day in 4 doses x 14 days

Regimen 2

▷ *erythromycin ethylsuccinate* (B)(G) 50 mg/kg/day in 4 doses x 14 days

DRUG BRANDS AND DOSE FORMS

▷ *erythromycin base* (B)(G)
   Ery-Tab *Tab:* 250, 333, 500 mg ent-coat
   PCE *Tab:* 333, 500 mg
▷ *erythromycin ethylsuccinate* (B)(G)
   EryPed *Oral susp:* 200 mg/5 ml (100, 200 ml) (fruit); 400 mg/5 ml (60, 100, 200
   ml) (banana); *Oral drops:* 200, 400 mg/5 ml (50 ml) (fruit); *Chew tab:* 200 mg
   wafer (fruit)
   E.E.S. *Oral susp:* 200, 400 mg/5 ml (100 ml) (fruit)
   E.E.S. Granules *Oral susp:* 200 mg/5 ml (100, 200 ml) (cherry)

OPHTHALMIA NEONATORUM: GONOCOCCAL

Comment: The following prophylaxis and treatment regimens for gonococcal conjunctivitis are published in the **2015 CDC Sexually Transmitted Diseases Treatment Guidelines**.

REGIMEN 1

▷ *erythromycin 0.5%* ophthalmic ointment 0.5-1 cm ribbon into lower conjunctival sac of each eye x 1 application

> **Ilotycin Ophthalmic Ointment** *Ophth oint:* 5 mg/g (1/8 oz)

REGIMEN 2

▷ *ceftriaxone* (B)(G) <12 years: 1 gm IM in a single dose; ≥12 years: 25-50 mg/kg IV or IM in a single dose, not to exceed 125 mg

> **Rocephin** *Vial:* 250, 500 mg; 1, 2 g

 OPIOID DEPENDENCE, OPIOID WITHDRAWAL SYNDROME

Comment: Health care Safety labeling for all immediate-release (IR) opioids has been issued by the FDA. The boxed warning includes serious risks of misuse, abuse, addiction, overdose, and death. The dosing section offers clear steps regarding administration and patient monitoring including initial dose, dose changes, and the abrupt cessation of treatment in physical dependence. Chronic maternal use of opioids during pregnancy can lead to potentially life-threatening neonatal opioid withdrawal. The American Pain Society (APS) has released new evidence-based clinical practice guidelines that include 32 recommendations related to post-op pain management in adults and children.

NARCOTIC ANALGESIC

▷ *methadone* (C) <12 years: not established; ≥12 years: *Narcotic detoxification:* 15-40 mg daily in decreasing doses not to exceed 21 days; *Narcotic maintenance:* ≥21 days; see mfr pkg insert

> **Dolophine** *Tab:* 5, 10 mg; *Dispersible tab:* 40 mg (dissolve in 120 ml orange juice or other citrus drink); *Oral conc:* 5, 10 mg/5 ml; 10 mg/10 ml

Comment: *methadone* maintenance is allowed only by approved providers with strict state and federal regulations.

OPIOID ANTAGONIST

▷ *naltrexone* (C)

> **ReVia** <12 years: not established; ≥12 years: 50 mg daily
> *Tab:* 50 mg
> **Vivitrol** <12 years: not established; ≥12 years: 380 mg IM once monthly; alternate buttocks
> *Vial:* 380 mg

OPIOID PARTIAL AGONIST-ANTAGONIST

Comment: **Belbuca, Butrans, Probuphine, and Subutex** maintenance are allowed only by approved providers with strict state and federal regulations. These drugs are potentiated by CYP3A4 inhibitors (e.g, azole antifungals, macrolides, HIV protease inhibitors) and antagonized by CYP3A4 inducers (monitor for opioid withdrawal). Concomitant NNRTIs (e.g., *efavirenz*, *nevirapine*, *etravirine*, *delavirdine*) or PIs (e.g., *atazanavir* with/without *ritonavir*): monitor. Risk of respiratory or CNS depression with concomitant opioid analgesics, general anesthetics, benzodiazepines, phenothiazines, other tranquilizers, sedative/hypnotics, alcohol, or other CNS depressants. Risk of serotonin syndrome with concomitant SSRIs, SNRIs, TCAs, 5-HT3 receptor antagonists, *mirtazapine*, *trazodone*, *tramadol*, MAO inhibitors.

▷ *buprenorphine* (C)(III) <16 years: not established

> Belbuca <12 years: not established; ≥12 years: apply buccal film to inside of cheek; do not chew or swallow; *Opioid naïve:* initially 75 mcg once daily-q 12 hours x at least 4 days; then, increase to 150 mcg q 12 hours; may increase in increments of 150 mcg q 12 hours no sooner than every 4 days; max 900 mcg q 12 hours; see mfr pkg insert for conversion from other opioids; *Severe hepatic impairment or oral mucositis:* reduce initial and titration doses by half

> *Buccal film:* 75, 150, 300, 450, 600, 750, 900 mcg (60/pck) (peppermint)

> **Butrans Transdermal System** <12 years: not established; ≥12 years: apply one patch to clean, dry, hairless, intact skin on the upper outer arm, upper chest, upper back, or side of chest every 7 days; rotate sites and do not reuse a site for at least 21 days; *Opioid naïve or oral morphine <30 mg/day or equivalent:* one 5 mcg/hour patch; *Converting from oral morphine equivalents 30-80 mg/day:* taper current opioids for up to 7 days to ≤30 mg/day oral morphine equivalents before starting; then initiate with 10 mcg/hour patch; may use a short-acting analgesic until efficacy is attained; increase dose only after exposure to previous dose x at least 72 hours; max one 20 mcg/hour patch/week; *Conversion from higher opioid doses:* not recommended

> *Transdermal patch:* 5, 7.5, 10, 15, 20 mcg/hour (4/pck)

> **Probuphine** <16 years: not established; ≥16 years: initiate when stable on *buprenorphine* ≤8 mg/day; insertion site is the inner side of the upper arm; 4 implants are intended to be in place for 6 months; remove the implants by the end of the 6th month and insert four new implants on the same day in the contralateral arm; if a new implant is not inserted on the same day as removal of a previous implant, maintain the patient on the previous dose of transmucosal *buprenorphine* (i.e., the dose from which the patient was transferred to **Probuphine** treatment).

> *Subdermal implant:* 74.2 mg of *buprenorphine* (equivalent to 80 mg of *buprenorphine hcl*)

> Comment: Health care providers who prescribe, perform insertions, and/or perform removals of **Probuphine** must successfully complete a live training program, and demonstrate procedural competency prior to inserting or removing the implants. Further information: www.ProbuphineREMS.com or 844-859-6341.

> **Subutex (G)** <12 years: not established; ≥12 years: 8 mg in a single dose on day 1; then 16 mg in a single dose on day 2; target dose is 16 mg/day in a single dose; dissolve under tongue; do not chew or swallow whole

> *SL tab (lemon-lime) or SL film (lime):* 2, 8 mg (30/pck)

OPIOID PARTIAL AGONIST-ANTAGONIST/OPIOID ANTAGONIST

Comment: **Bunavail**, **Suboxone**, **Sucartonone**, *Troxyca ER,* and **Zubsolv** maintenance are allowed only by approved providers with strict state and federal regulations.

▷ *buprenorphine/naloxone* (C)(III)

Bunavail <16 years: not recommended; ≥16 years: administer one buccal film once daily at the same time each day; target dose is 8.4/1.4 once daily; place the side of the **Bunavail** film with the text (BN2, BN4, or BN6) against the inside of the cheek; press and hold the film in place for 5 seconds; maintenance is usually 2.1/0.3 to 12.6/2.1 once daily

SL film:

Bunavail 2.1/0.3 *bup* 2.1 mg/*nal* 0.3 mg (lime) (30/carton)
Bunavail 4.2/0.7 *bup* 4.2 mg/*nal* 0.7 mg (lime) (30/carton)
Bunavail 6.3/1 *bup* 6.3 mg/*nal* 1 mg (lime) (30/carton)

Comment: A **Bunavail** 4.2/0.7 mg buccal film provides equivalent *buprenorphine* exposure to a **Sucartonone** 8/2 mg sublingual tablet.

Suboxone (G) <12 years: not recommended; ≥12 years: adjust dose in increments/decrements of 2 mg/0.5 mg or 4 mg/1 mg once daily *buprenorphine/ naloxone*, based on the patient's daily dose of *buprenorphine*, to a level that suppresses opioid withdrawal signs and symptoms; *Recommended target dosage:* 16 mg/4 mg as a single daily dose; *Maintenance dose:* generally in the range of 4 mg/1 mg to 24 mg/6 mg per day; higher once daily doses have not been demonstrated to provide any clinical advantage

SL tab, SL film:

Suboxone 2/0.5 *bup* 2 mg/*nal* 0.5 mg (lime) (30/bottle)
Suboxone 8/2 *bup* 8 mg/*nal* 2 mg (lime) (30/bottle)

Sucartonone <12 years: not recommended; ≥12 years: adjust in 2-4 mg of *buprenorphine*/day in a single dose; usual range is 4-24 mg/day in a single dose; target dose is 6 mg/day in a single dose; dissolve under tongue; do not chew or swallow whole *SL film* (lime):

Sucartonone 2/0.5 *bup* 2 mg/*nal* 0.5 mg (30/pck)
Sucartonone 4/1 *bup* 4 mg/*nal* 1 mg (30/pck)
Sucartonone 8/2 *bup* 8 mg/*nal* 2 mg (30/pck)
Sucartonone 12/3 *bup* 12 mg/*nal* 3 mg (30/pck)

Zubsolv <16 years: not recommended; ≥16 years: initial induction with *buprenorphine* sublingual tabs; administer as a single dose once daily; titrate dose in increments of 1.4/0.36 or 2.9/0.72 per day; recommended target dose is 11.4/2.9 per day; usual max 17.2/4.2 per day

SL tab:

Zubsolv 1.4/0.36 *bup* 1.4 mg/*nal* 0.36 mg
Zubsolv 2.9/0.72 *bup* 2.9 mg/*nal* 0.71 mg
Zubsolv 5.7/1.4 *bup* 5.7 mg/*nal* 1.4 mg
Zubsolv 8.6/2.1 *bup* 8.6 mg/*nal* 2.1 mg
Zubsolv 11.4/2.9 *bup* 11.4 mg/*nal* 2.9 mg

Comment: One **Subutex** 5.7/1.4 SL tab is bioequivalent to one **Sucartonone** 8/2 SL film.

▷ *oxycodone/naloxone* (C)(II) <18 years: not recommended; ≥18 years: *Opioid-naïve and opioid non-tolerant:* initially 10 mg/1.2 mg q 12 hours; *Opioid-tolerant:* single doses greater than 40 mg/4.8 mg, or a total daily dose greater than 80 mg/9.6 mg are only for use in patients for whom tolerance to an opioid of comparable potency has been established; swallow whole, or sprinkle contents on applesauce and swallow immediately without chewing

Troxyca ER

Cap: **Troxyca ER 10/1.2** *oxy 10 mg/nalox 1.2 mg ext-rel*

Troxyca ER 20/1.2 *oxy 20 mg/nalox 2.4 mg ext-rel*
Troxyca ER 30/1.2 *oxy 30 mg/nalox 3.6 mg ext-rel*
Troxyca ER 40/1.2 *oxy 40 mg/nalox 4.8 mg ext-rel*
Troxyca ER 60/1.2 *oxy 60 mg/nalox 7.2 mg ext-rel*
Troxyca ER 80/1.2 *oxy 80 mg/nalox 9.6 mg ext-rel*

Comment: Opioid-tolerant patients are those taking, for one week or longer, at least 60 mg oral *morphine* per day, 25 mcg transdermal *fentanyl* per hour, 30 mg oral *oxycodone* per day, 8 mg oral *hydromorphone* per day, 25 mg oral *oxymorphone* per day, 60 mg oral *hydrocodone* per day, or an equianalgesic dose of another opioid.

OPIOID-INDUCED CONSTIPATION (OIC)

▶ *lubiprostone* (C) <18 years: not established; ≥18 years: swallow whole; take with food and water; initially 24 mcg bid; *Moderate hepatic impairment (Child Pugh Class B):* 16 mg bid; *Severe hepatic impairment (Child Pugh Class C):* 8 mg bid
    Amitiza *Cap:* 8, 24 mg

▶ *methylnaltrexone bromide* (C) <18 years: not established; ≥18 years: one oral dose or one weight-based SC dose every other day as needed; max one dose per 24 hours; administer SC inject into the upper arm, abdomen, or thigh; rotate sites
    Chronic Non-cancer Pain: 450 mg po once daily in the morning (take with water on an empty stomach at least 30 minutes before the first meal of the day) or 12 mg SC once daily in the morning; *Severe Hepatic Impairment:* <38 kg: 0.075 mg/kg; 38-<62 kg: 4 mg (0.2 ml); 62-114 kg: 6 mg (0.3 ml); >114 kg: 0.075 mg/kg
    Advanced Illness, Receiving Palliative Care: <38 kg: 0.15 mg/kg; 38-<62 kg: 8 mg (0.4 ml); 62-114 kg: 12 mg (0.6 ml); >114 kg: 0.15 mg/kg; *Moderate and Severe Renal Impairment (CrCl<60 mL/min):* <38 kg: 0.075 mg/kg; 38-<62 kg: 4 mg (0.2 ml); 62-114 kg: 6 mg (0.3 ml); >114 kg: 0.075 mg/kg
    Relistor *Tab:* 150 mg film-coat; *Vial:* 12 mg single-dose (0.6 ml, 7/carton); *Prefilled syringe:* 8 mg (0.4 ml), 12 mg (0.6 ml) (7/carton)

Comment: *methylnaltrexone* is a selective antagonist of opioid binding at the mu-opioid receptor. As a quaternary amine, the ability of *methylnaltrexone* to cross the blood-brain barrier is restricted. This allows *methylnaltrexone* to function as a peripherally-acting muopioid receptor antagonist in tissues such as the gastrointestinal tract, thereby decreasing the constipating effects of opioids without impacting opioid-mediated analgesic effects on the central nervous system. The pre-filled syringe is only for patients who require a **Relistor** injection dose of 8 mg or 12 mg. Use the vial for patients who require other doses. **Relistor** is contraindicated with known or suspected GI obstruction and patients at increased risk of recurrent obstruction, due to the potential for gastrointestinal perforation. Be within close proximity to toilet facilities once **Relistor** is administered. Discontinue all maintenance laxative therapy prior to initiation. Laxative(s) can be used as needed if there is a suboptimal response after three days. Discontinue if treatment with the opioid pain medication is also discontinued. Safety and effectiveness of **Relistor** have not been established in pediatric patients. Avoid concomitant use with other opioid antagonists because of the potential for additive effects of opioid receptor antagonism and increased risk of opioid withdrawal symptoms (sweating, chills, diarrhea, abdominal pain, anxiety, and yawning). Advise females of reproductive potential, who become pregnant or are planning to become pregnant, that the use of **Relistor** during pregnancy may precipitate opioid withdrawal in a fetus due to the undeveloped blood-brain barrier. Breastfeeding is not recommended during treatment.

➤ *naloxegol* (C) <18 years: not established; ≥18 years: swallow whole; take on an empty stomach; initially 25 mg once daily in the AM; discontinue other laxatives; *CrCl <60 mL/min:* 12.5 mg

Movantik *Tab:* 12.5, 25 mg

OPIOID OVERDOSE

OPIOID ANTAGONISTS

➤ *nalmefene* (B) <12 years: not recommended; ≥12 years: initially 0.25 mcg/kg IV, IM, <u>or</u> SC, then incremental doses of 0.25 mcg/kg at 2-5 minute intervals; cumulative max 1 mcg/kg; if opioid dependency suspected use 0.1 mg/70 kg initially and then proceed as usual if no response in 2 minutes

Revex *Amp:* 100 mcg/1 ml (1 ml); 1 mg/ml (2 ml)

➤ *naloxone* (B)(G) <12 years: 0.01 mg/kg initially, repeat in 2-3 minutes at 0.1 mg/kg if response inadequate; ≥12 years: 0.4-2 mg; repeat in 2-3 minutes if no response

Evzio *Prefilled autoinjector:* 0.4 mg/0.4 ml IM/SC only

Narcan *Vial/Amp:* 0.4 mg/ml (1 ml), 1 mg/ml (2 ml); *Prefilled syringe:* 0.4 mg ml (1 ml), 1 mg/ml (2 ml) IV, IM, <u>or</u> SC (parabens-free)

Comment: If the electronic voice instruction system does not operate properly, **Evzio** will still deliver the intended dose of *naloxone* when used according to the printed instructions on the flat surface of the autoinjector label. **Evzio** cannot be administered IV. Due to the short duration of action of naloxone, as compared to opioids which are longer acting, monitoring of the patient is critical as the opioid reversal effects of naloxone may wear off before the effects of the opioid.

Narcan Nasal Spray position supine with head tilted back; 1 spray in one nostril; if an additional dose is needed, spray into the opposite nostril

Nasal spray: 4 mg/0.1 ml, single dose, single use (2 blister pcks, each w a single nasal spray/carton)

OSGOOD–SCHLATTER DISEASE

Acetaminophen for IV Infusion *see* **Pain** *page 296*
Oral Prescription NSAIDs *see page 490*
Other Oral Analgesics *see* **Pain** *page 298*
Topical/Transdermal NSAIDs *see* **Pain** *page 298*
Parenteral Corticosteroids *see page 499*
Oral Corticosteroids *see page 498*
Topical Analgesic and Anesthetic Agents *see page 488*

OSTEOARTHRITIS

Acetaminophen for IV Infusion *see* **Pain** *page 296*
Oral Prescription NSAIDs *see page 490*
Other Oral Analgesics *see* **Pain** *page 298*
Topical/Transdermal NSAIDs *see* **Pain** *page 298*
Parenteral Corticosteroids *see page 499*

Oral Corticosteroids *see page* 498
Topical Analgesic and Anesthetic Agents *see page* 488

TOPICAL ANALGESICS

➤ *capsaicin* cream (B)(G) <2 years: not recommended; 2-12 years: apply sparingly to
intact skin bid prn; >12 years: apply tid-qid prn
> **Axsain** *Crm:* 0.075% (1, 2 oz)
> **Capsin** (OTC) *Lotn:* 0.025, 0,075% (59 ml)
> **Capzasin-P** (OTC) *Crm:* 0.025% (1.5 oz); *Lotn:* 0.025% (2 oz)
> **Capzasin-HP** (OTC) *Crm:* 0.075% (1.5 oz); *Lotn:* 0.075% (2 oz)
> **Dolorac** *Crm:* 0.025% (28 gm)
> **Double Cap** (OTC) *Crm:* 0.05% (2 oz)
> **R-Gel** *Gel:* 0.025% (15, 30 gm)
> **Zostrix** (OTC) *Crm:* 0.025% (0.7, 1.5, 3 oz)
> **Zostrix HP** (OTC) *Emol crm:* 0.075% (1, 2 oz)

Comment: Provides some relief by 1-2 weeks; optimal benefit may take 4-6 weeks.
Avoid contact with mucous membranes.

ORAL SALICYLATE

➤ *indomethacin* (C) <14 years: usually not recommended; ≥2 years, if risk warranted:
1-2 mg/kg/day in divided doses; max 3-4 mg/kg/day (<u>or</u> 150-200 mg/day, whichever is less); <14 years, ER cap not recommended; ≥14 years: initially 25 mg bid to
tid, increase as needed at weekly intervals by 25-50 mg/day; max 200 mg/day
> *Cap:* 25, 50 mg; *Susp;* 25 mg/5 ml (pineapple-coconut, mint) (alcohol 1%);
> *Supp:* 50 mg; *ER Cap:* 75 mg ext-rel

Comment: *indomethacin* is indicated only for acute painful flares. Administer with
food <u>and/or</u> antacids. Use lowest effective dose for shortest duration.

ORAL NSAIDs

See more **Oral NSAIDs** *page* 490
➤ *diclofenac* (C) <18 years: not recommended; ≥18 years: take on empty stomach; 35
mg tid; *Hepatic impairment:* use lowest dose
> **Zorvolex** *Gelcap:* 18, 35 mg
➤ *diclofenac sodium* (C) <18 years: not recommended; ≥18 years:
> **Voltaren** 50 mg bid to qid <u>or</u> 75 mg bid <u>or</u> 25 mg qid with an additional 25 mg
> at HS if necessary
> *Tab:* 25, 50, 75 mg ent-coat
> **Voltaren XR** 100 mg once daily; rarely, 100 mg bid may be used
> *Tab:* 100 mg ext-rel

ORAL NSAIDs PLUS PPI

➤ *esomeprazole/naproxen* (C; not for use in 3rd)(G) <18 years: not recommended;
≥18 years: 1 tab bid; use lowest effective dose for the shortest duration; swallow
whole; take at least 30 minutes before a meal
> **Vimovo** *Tab: nap* 375 mg/*eso* 20 mg ext-rel; *nap* 500 mg/*eso* 20 mg ext-rel
> Comment: **Vimovo** is indicated to improve signs/symptoms, and risk of gastric
> ulcer in patients at risk of developing NSAID-associated gastric ulcer.

COX-2 INHIBITORS

Comment: Cox-2 inhibitors are contraindicated with history of asthma, urticaria, and allergic-type reactions to *aspirin*, other NSAIDs, and sulfonamides, 3rd trimester of pregnancy, and coronary artery bypass graft (CABG) surgery.

➤ *celecoxib* (C)(G) <18 years: not recommended; ≥18 years: 100-400 mg daily bid; max 800 mg/day

Celebrex *Cap:* 50, 100, 200, 400 mg

➤ *meloxicam* (C)(G)

Mobic <2 years, <60 kg: not recommended; ≥2, >60 kg: 0.125 mg/kg; max 7.5 mg once daily; ≥18 years: initially 7.5 mg once daily; max 15 mg once daily; *Hemodialysis:* max 7.5 mg/day

Tab: 7.5, 15 mg; *Oral susp:* 7.5 mg/5 ml (100 ml) (raspberry)

Vivlodex <18 years: not established; ≥18 years: initially 5 mg qd; may increase to max 10 mg/day; *Hemodialysis:* max 5 mg/day

Cap: 5, 10 mg

INTRA-ARTICULAR INJECTION

➤ *sodium hyaluronate* (B) <12 years: not recommended; using strict aseptic technique, administer by intra-articular injection (into the synovial space) once weekly for the prescribed number of weeks (see mfr pkg insert); after preparing the injection site and attaining local analgesia, remove joint synovial fluid or effusion prior to injection

Gelsyn-3 *Syringe:* 8.4 mg/ml (2 ml) prefilled

Hyalgan *Vial:* 20 mg (2 ml); *Prefilled syringe:* 20 mg (2 ml)

Hylan *Syringe:* 48 mg/6 ml (6 ml) prefilled

Synvisc One *Syringe:* 46 mg/6 ml (6 ml) prefilled

OSTEOPOROSIS

Comment: Prior to initiating, or concomitant prescribing, corticosteroids in patients at risk for, or diagnosed with, osteoporosis, referral to the following ACR guidelines is recommended: Guidelines on Prevention & Treatment of Glucocorticoid-induced Osteoporosis [press release]. Atlanta, GA. American College of Rheumatology; June 7, 2017. https://www.rheumatology.org/About-Us/Newsroom/Press-Releases/ID/812/ACR-Releases-Guideline-on-Prevention-Treatment-of-Glucocorticoid-Induced-Osteoporosis. Indications for bone density screening include: personal history of fragility fracture, presence of high serum markers of bone resorption, smoker, height >67 inches, weight <125 lb, taking a steroid, GnRH agonist, or antiseizure drug, immobilization, hyperthyroidism, post transplantation, malabsorption syndrome, hyperparathyroidism, prolactinemia. Foods high in calcium include almonds, broccoli, baked beans, salmon, sardines, buttermilk, turnip greens, collard greens, spinach, pumpkin, rhubarb, and bran. *Recommended daily calcium intake:* 1-3 years: 700 mg; 4-8 years: 1,000 mg; 9-18 years: 1,300 mg; >18 years: 1,000 mg; pregnancy or nursing: 1,000-1,300 mg.

CALCIUM SUPPLEMENTS

Comment: Take *calcium* supplements with meals to avoid gastric upset. Dosages of calcium over 2000 mg/day have not demonstrated any additional benefit. *Calcium* decreases *tetracycline* absorption. *Calcium* absorption is decreased by corticosteroids.

▷ *calcitonin-salmon* (C)

> **Fortical** 200 IU intranasally daily; alternate nostrils each day
> > *Nasal spray:* 200 IU/actuation (30 doses, 3.7 ml)
>
> **Miacalcin Nasal Spray** 200 IU spray in one nostril once daily; alternate nostrils each day
> > *Nasal spray:* 200 IU/actuation (30 doses, 3.7 ml)
>
> **Miacalcin Injection** 100 units SC <u>or</u> IM every other day
> > *Vial:* 200 units/ml (2 ml)

Comment: Supplement diet with calcium (1 gm/day) and vitamin D (400 IU/day).

▷ *calcium carbonate* (C)(OTC)(G)

> **Rolaids** chew 2 tabs bid; max 14 tabs/day
> > *Chew tab:* 550 mg
>
> **Rolaids Extra Strength** chew 2 tabs bid; max 8 tabs/day
> > *Chew tab:* 1000 mg
>
> **Tums** chew 2 tabs bid; max 16 tabs/day
> > *Chew tab:* 500 mg
>
> **Tums Extra Strength** chew 2 tabs bid; max 10 tabs/day
> > *Chew tab:* 750 mg
>
> **Tums Ultra** chew 2 tabs bid; max 8 tabs/day
> > *Chew tab:* 1000 mg
>
> **Os-Cal 500 (OTC)** 1-2 tab bid to tid
> > *Chew tab:* elemental calcium carbonate 500 mg

▷ *calcium carbonate/vitamin d* (C)(G)

> **Os-Cal 250+D (OTC)** 1-2 tab tid
> > *Tab:* elemental calcium carbonate 250 mg/*vit d* 125 IU
>
> **Os-Cal 500+D (OTC)** 1-2 tab bid-tid
> > *Tab:* elemental calcium carbonate 500 mg/*vit d* 125 IU
>
> **Viactiv (OTC)** 1 tab tid
> > *Chew tab:* elemental calcium 500 mg/*vit d* 100 IU/*vitamin k* 40 mcg

▷ *calcium citrate* (C)(G)

> **Citracal (OTC)** 1-2 tabs bid
> > *Tab:* elemental calcium citrate 200 mg

▷ *calcium citrate/vitamin d* (C)(G)

> **Citracal +D (OTC)** 1-2 cplts bid
> > *Cplt:* elemental calcium citrate 315 mg/*vit d* 200 IU
>
> **Citracal 250+D (OTC)** 1-2 tabs bid
> > *Tab:* elemental calcium citrate 250 mg/*vit d* 62.3 IU

VITAMIN D ANALOGS

Comment: Concurrent *vitamin D* supplementation is contraindicated for patients taking *calcitriol* <u>or</u> *doxercalciferol* due to the risk of *vitamin D* toxicity.

▷ *calcitriol* (C) <12 years: *Predialysis:* <3 years: 10-15 ng/kg/day; ≥3 years: initially 0.25 mcg daily; may increase to 0.5 mcg/day; *Dialysis:* not recommended; *Hypoparathyroidism:* initially 0.25 mcg daily; may increase by 0.25 mcg/day at 2-4 week intervals; usual maintenance (1-5 years) 0.25-0.75 mcg/day, (>6 years) 0.5-2 mcg/day; ≥12 years: *Predialysis:* initially 0.25 mcg daily; may increase to 0.5 mcg daily; *Dialysis:* initially 0.25 mcg daily; may increase by 0.25 mcg/day at 4-8 week intervals; usual maintenance 0.5-1 mcg/day; *Hypoparathyroidism:* initially 0.25 mcg q AM; may increase by 0.25 mcg/day at 4- to 8-week intervals; usual maintenance 0.5-2 mcg/day

Rocaltrol *Cap:* 0.25, 0.5 mcg
Rocaltrol Solution *Soln:* 1 mcg/ml (15 ml, single-use dispensers)
▷ *doxercalciferol* (C) <12 years: initially 0.25 mcg daily; may increase by 0.25 mcg; 0.25 mcg/day at 2-4 week intervals; usual maintenance (1-5 years) 0.25-0.75 mcg/day, (≥6 years) 0.5-2 mcg/day; ≥12 weeks: initially 0.25 mcg q AM; may increase by 0.25 mcg/day at 4-8 week intervals; usual maintenance 0.5-2 mcg/day
　　Hectorol *Cap:* 0.25, 0.5 mcg

BISPHOSPHONATES (CALCIUM MODIFIERS)

Comment: bisphosphonates should be swallowed whole in the AM with 6-8 oz of plain water 30 minutes before first meal, beverage, or other medications of the day. Monitor serum alkaline phosphatase. Contraindications include abnormalities of the esophagus which delay esophageal emptying such as stricture or achalasia, inability to stand or sit upright for at least 30 minutes post-dose, patients at risk of aspiration, and hypocalcemia. Co-administration of bisphosphonates and *calcium*, antacids, or oral medications containing multivalent cations will interfere with absorption of the biphosphonate. Therefore, instruct patients to wait at least half hour after taking the biphosphonate before taking any other oral medications.
▷ *alendronate (as sodium)* (C) <12 years: not recommended; ≥12 years: take once weekly, in the AM, 30 minutes before the first food, beverage, or medication of the day; do not lie down (remain upright) for at least 30 minutes and after the first food of the day; *CrCl <35 mL/min:* not recommended
　　Binosto dissolve the effervescent tab in 4 oz (120 ml) of plain, room temperature, water (not mineral or flavored); wait 5 minutes after the effervescence has subsided, then stir for 10 seconds, then drink
　　　Tab: 70 mg effervescent for buffered solution (4, 12/carton) (strawberry)
　　Fosamax (G) swallow tab whole; dosing regimens are the same for males and females; *Prevention:* 5 mg once daily or 35 mg once weekly; *Treatment:* 10 mg once daily or 70 mg once weekly
　　　Tab: 5, 10, 35, 40, 70 mg
▷ *alendronate/cholecalciferol (vit d3)* (C)(G) <12 years: not recommended; ≥12 years: take 1 tab once weekly, in the AM, with plain water (not mineral) 30 minutes before the first food, beverage, or medication of the day; do not lie down (remain upright) for at least 30 minutes and after the first food of the day
　　Fosamax Plus D
　　　Tab: **Fosamax Plus D 70/2800:** *alen* 70 mg/*chole* 2,800 IU
　　　　Fosamax Plus D 70/5600: *alen* 70 mg/*chole* 5,600 IU
▷ *ibandronate (as monosodium monohydrate)* (C)(G) <18 years: not recommended; ≥18 years:
　　Boniva take 2.5 mg once daily or 150 mg once monthly on the same day; take in the AM, with plain water (not mineral) 60 minutes before the first food, beverage, or medication of the day; do not lie down (remain upright) for at least 30 minutes and after the first food of the day
　　　Tab: 2.5, 150 mg
　　Boniva Injection administer 3 mg every 3 months by IV bolus over 15-30 seconds; if dose is missed, administer as soon as possible; then every 3 months from the date of the last dose
　　　Prefilled syringe: 3 mg/3 ml (5 ml)
　　Comment: **Boniva Injection** must be administered by a health care professional.

➤ *risedronate (as sodium)* (C)(G) take in the AM; swallow whole with a full glass of plain water (not mineral); do not lie down (remain upright) for 30 minutes afterward

> **Actonel** <12 years: not recommended; ≥12 years: take at least 30 minutes before any food <u>or</u> drink; *Females:* 5 mg once daily <u>or</u> 35 mg once weekly <u>or</u> 75 mg on two consecutive days monthly <u>or</u> 150 mg once monthly; *Males:* 35 mg once weekly
>> *Tab:* 5, 30, 35, 75, 150 mg

> **Atelvia** <12 years: not recommended; ≥12 years: 35 mg once weekly immediately after breakfast
>> *Tab:* 35 mg del-rel

➤ *risedronate/calcium* (C) <12 years: not recommended; ≥12 years: 1 x 5 mg *risedronate* tab weekly <u>plus</u> 1 x 500 mg *calcium* tab on days 2-7 weekly

> **Actonel with Calcium** *Tab:* risedronate 5 mg <u>and</u> *Tab:* calcium 500 mg (4 *risedronate* tabs + 30 *calcium* tabs/pck)

➤ *zoledronic acid* (D)(G)

> **Reclast** <12 years: not recommended; ≥12 years: administer 5 mg via IV infusion over at least 15 minutes mg once a year (for osteoporosis) <u>or</u> once every 2 years (for osteopenia <u>or</u> prophylaxis)
>> *Bottle:* 5 mg/100 ml (single dose)

> **Comment:** **Reclast** is indicated for the treatment of postmenopausal osteoporosis in females who are at high risk for fracture and to increase bone mass in men with primary <u>or</u> hypogonadal osteoporosis who are at high risk for fracture. Administered by a health care professional. Contraindicated in hypocalcemia. **Zometa** *Bottle:* 4 mg/5 ml administer 4 mg via IV infusion over at least 15 minutes every 3-4 weeks; optimal duration of treatment not known
>> *Vial:* 4 mg/5 ml (single dose)

> **Comment:** **Zometa** is indicated for the treatment of hypercalcemia of malignancy. The safety and efficacy of **Zometa** in the treatment of hypercalcemia associated with hyperparathyroidism <u>or</u> with other non-tumor-related conditions has not been established.

SELECTIVE ESTROGEN RECEPTOR MODULATOR (SERMs)

➤ *raloxifene* (X)(G) <12 years: not recommended; ≥12 years: 60 mg once daily

> **Evista** *Tab:* 60 mg

> **Comment:** Contraindicated in females who have history of, <u>or</u> current, venous thrombotic event.

HUMAN PARATHYROID HORMONE

➤ *teriparatide* (C) <12 years: not recommended; ≥12 years: 20 mcg SC daily in the thigh <u>or</u> abdomen; may treat for up to 2 years

> **Forteo Multidose Pen** *Multidose pen:* 250 mcg/ml (3 ml)

> **Comment:** **Forteo** is indicated for the treatment of postmenopausal osteoporosis in females who are at high risk for fracture and to increase bone mass in men with primary <u>or</u> hypogonadal osteoporosis who are at high risk for fracture.

BIOENGINEERED REPLICA OF HUMAN PARATHYROID HORMONE

➤ *bioengineered replica of human parathyroid hormone* (C) <12 years: not recommended; ≥12 years: initially inject mg IM into the thigh once daily; when initiating, decrease dose of active *vitamin D* by 50% if serum *calcium* is above 7.5 mg/dL;

monitor serum *calcium* levels every 3 to 7 days after starting or adjusting dose and when adjusting either active *vitamin D* or *calcium* supplements dose

>   **Natpara** *Soln for inj:* 25, 50, 75, 100 mcg (2/pkg) multidose, dual-chamber glass cartridge containing a sterile powder and diluent

>   Comment: **Natpara** is indicated as adjunct to *calcium* and *vitamin D* in patients with parathyroidism.

OSTEOCLAST INHIBITOR (RANKL INHIBITOR)

▷ *denosumab* (X) <12 years: not recommended; ≥12 years: for SC injection 60 mcg SC once every 6 months in the upper arm, abdomen, or upper thigh

>   **Prolia** *Vial/Pen:* 60 mg/ml (1 ml) single dose

>   Comment: **Prolia** is indicated for the treatment of postmenopausal osteoporosis in females who are at high risk for fracture defined as a history of osteoporotic fracture, or multiple risk factors for fracture, or patients who have failed or are intolerant to other therapy. Administered by a health care professional. Contraindicated in hypocalcemia.

HUMAN PARATHYROID HORMONE RELATED PEPTIDE (PTHRP [1-34]) ANALOG

▷ *abaloparatide* 80 mcg (40 mcl) SC once daily

>   **Tymlos** *Pen:* 80 mcg/40 mcl (1.56 ml, 2,000 mcg/ml) (30 doses) preassembled, single-patient use, disposable w/glass cartridge

Comment: **Tymlos** is a bone building agent for the treatment of postmenopausal women with osteoporosis at high risk for fracture. **Tymlos** is not indicated for use in females of reproductive potential. There are no human data with use in pregnant women to inform any drug associated risks and animal reproduction studies with *abaloparatide* have not been conducted. There is no information on the presence of *abaloparatide* in human milk, the effects on the breastfed infant, or the effects on milk production; however, breastfeeding is not recommended while using **Tymlos**. **Tymlos** is not recommended for use in pediatric patients with open epiphyses or hereditary disorders predisposing to osteosarcoma because of an increased baseline risk of osteosarcoma. **Tymlos** may cause hypercalciuria. It is unknown whether **Tymlos** may exacerbate urolithiasis in patients with active or a history of urolithiasis. If active urolithiasis or pre-existing hypercalciuria is suspected, measurement of urinary calcium excretion should be considered. No dosage adjustment is required for patients any degree of renal impairment. Currently, there are no specific drug-drug interaction studies.

OTITIS EXTERNA

OTIC ANALGESIC

▷ *antipyrine/benzocaine/zinc acetate dihydrate* (C) fill ear canal with solution; then insert a cotton plug into meatus; may repeat every 1-2 hours prn

>   **Otozin** *Otic soln:* antipyr 5.4%/benz 1%/zinc1% per ml (10 ml w. dropper)

OTIC ANTI-INFECTIVE

▷ *chloroxylenol/pramoxine* (C) <1 year: not recommended; 1-12 years: 5 drops bid x 10 days; >12 years: 4-5 drops tid x 5-10 days

PramOtic *Otic drops: chlorox/pramox* (5 ml w. dropper)
➤ *finafloxacin* (C) <1 year: not recommended; ≥1 year: 4-5 drops tid x 5-10 days
Xtoro *Otic soln:* 0.3% (5, 8 ml)
➤ *ofloxacin* (C)(G) <1 year: not recommended; 1-12 years: 5 drops bid x 10 days; >12 years: 10 drops bid x 10 days
Floxin Otic *Otic soln:* 0.3% (5, 10 ml w. dropper; 0.25 ml, 5 drop singles, 20/carton)
Comment: Floxin Otic is indicated for patients ≥18 years with perforated tympanic membranes and pediatric patients with PE tubes.

OTIC ANTI-INFECTIVE/CORTICOSTEROID COMBINATIONS

➤ *chloroxylenol/pramoxine/hydrocortisone* (C) <12 years: 3 drops tid-qid x 5-10 days; ≥12 years: 4 drops tid-qid x 5-10 days
Cortane B, *Otic soln: chlo* 1 mg/*pram* 10 mg/*hydro* 10 mg per ml (10 ml w. dropper)
Comment: Cortane B Aqueous may be used to saturate a cotton wick.
➤ *ciprofloxacin/hydrocortisone* (C) <1 year: not recommended; ≥1 year: 3 drops bid x 7 days
Cipro HC Otic *Otic susp: cipro* 0.2%/*hydro* 1% (10 ml w. dropper)
➤ *ciprofloxacin/dexamethasone* (C) <6 months: not recommended; ≥6 months: 4 drops bid x 7 days
Ciprodex *Otic susp: cipro* 0.3%/*dexa* 1% (7.5 ml)
Comment: Ciprodex is indicated for the treatment of otitis media in pediatric patients with tympanostomy tubes.
➤ *colistin/neomycin/hydrocortisone/thonzonium* (C) <12 years: 4 drops tid-qid x 5-10 days; ≥12 years: 5 drops tid or qid x 5-10 days
Coly-Mycin S *Otic susp:* 5, 10 ml
Cortisporin-TC Otic *Otic susp: colis* 3 mg/*neo* 3.3 mg/*hydro* 10 mg/*thon* 0.5 mg per ml (10 ml w. dropper) (thimerosal)
➤ *polymyxin b/neomycin/hydrocortisone* (C) <12 years: 3 drops tid-qid; max 10 days; 4 drops tid-qid; ≥12 years: max 10 days
Cortisporin Otic Suspension *Otic susp: poly b* 10,000 u/*neo* 3.5 mg/*hydro* 10 mg per 5 ml (10 ml w. dropper)
Cortisporin Otic Solution *Otic soln: poly b* 10000 u/*neo* 3.5 mg/*hydro* 10 mg per 5 ml (10 ml w. dropper)

OTIC ASTRINGENTS

➤ *acetic acid 2% in aluminum sulfate* (C) 4-6 drops q 2-3 hours
Domeboro Otic *Otic soln:* 60 ml w. dropper
➤ *acetic acid/propylene glycol/benzethonium chloride/sodium acetate* (C) 3-5 drops q 4-6 hours
VoSol *Otic soln: acet* 2% (15, 30 ml)
➤ *acetic acid/propylene glycol/hydrocortisone/benzethonium chloride/sodium acetate* (C) 3-5 drops q 4-6 hours
VoSol HC *Otic soln: acet* 2%/*hydro* 1% (10 ml)

OTIC ANESTHETIC/ANALGESIC COMBINATIONS

➤ *antipyrine/benzocaine/glycerine* (C) fill ear canal and insert cotton plug; may repeat q 1-2 hours

A/B Otic *Otic soln:* 15 ml w. dropper
▶ *benzocaine* (C) <1 year: not recommended; ≥1 year: 4-5 drops q 1-2 hours
Americaine Otic *Otic soln:* 20% (15 ml w. dropper)
Benzotic *Otic soln:* 20% (15 ml w. dropper)

SYSTEMIC ANTI-INFECTIVES

Comment: Used for severe disease or with culture.
▶ *amoxicillin/clavulanate* (B)(G)
Augmentin <40 kg: 40-45 mg/kg/day divided tid x 10 days or 90 mg/kg/day divided bid x 10 days; *see page 545 for dose by weight table;* ≥40 kg: 500 mg tid or 875 mg bid x 10 days
Tab: 250, 500, 875 mg; *Chew tab:* 125, 250 mg (lemon-lime); 200, 400 mg (cherry-banana) (phenylalanine); *Oral susp:* 125 mg/5 ml (banana), 250 mg/5 ml (75, 100, 150 ml) (orange); 200, 400 mg/5 ml (50, 75, 100 ml) (orange) (phenylalanine)
Augmentin ES-600 <3 months: not recommended; ≥3 months, <40 kg: 90 mg/kg/day divided q 12 hours x 10 days; *see page 546 for dose by weight table;* ≥40 kg: not recommended
Oral susp: 600 mg/5 ml (50, 75, 100, 125, 150, 200 ml) (strawberry cream) (phenylalanine)
Augmentin XR <16 years: use other forms; ≥16 years: 2 tabs q 12 hours x 7-10 days
Tab: 1000*mg ext-rel
▶ *cefaclor* (B)(G) <1 month: not recommended; 1 month-12 years: 20-40 mg/kg in 2 or 3 divided doses x 10 days; *see page 549 for dose by weight table;* >12 years: 250-500 mg q 8 hours x 7-10 days; max 2 gm/day
Tab: 500 mg; *Cap:* 250, 500 mg; *Susp:* 125 mg/5 ml (75, 150 ml) (strawberry); 187 mg/5 ml (50, 100 ml) (strawberry); 250 mg/5 ml (75, 150 ml) (strawberry); 375 mg/5 ml (50, 100 ml) (strawberry)
Cefaclor Extended Release <16 years: not recommended; ≥16 years: 500 mg bid x 10 days; clinically equivalent to 250 mg immed-rel caps tid; swallow whole; take with meals
Tab: 375, 500 mg ext-rel
▶ *dicloxacillin* (B) <12 years: 12.5-25 mg/kg/day in 4 divided doses x 10 days; *see page 560 for dose by weight table;* ≥12 years: 500 mg q 6 hours x 10 days
Dynapen *Cap:* 125, 250, 500 mg; *Oral susp:* 62.5 mg/5 ml (80, 100, 200 ml)
▶ *trimethoprim/sulfamethoxazole* (C)(G)
Bactrim, Septra <12 years: not recommended; ≥12 years: 2 tabs bid x 10 days
Tab: trim 80 mg/*sulfa* 400 mg*
Bactrim DS, Septra DS <12 years: not recommended; ≥12 years: 1 tab bid x 10 days
Tab: trim 160 mg/*sulfa* 800 mg*
Bactrim Pediatric Suspension, Septra Pediatric Suspension <2 months: not recommended; ≥2 months-12 years: 40 mg/kg/day of *sulfamethoxazole* in 2 doses bid; >12 years: use tabs
Oral susp: trim 40 mg/*sulfa* 200 mg per 5 ml (100 ml) (cherry) (alcohol 0.3%)

OTITIS MEDIA: ACUTE

OTIC ANALGESIC

➤ *antipyrine/benzocaine/zinc acetate dihydrate* otic (C) fill ear canal with solution; then insert cotton plug into meatus; may repeat every 1-2 hours prn

Otozin *Otic soln:* antipyr 5.4%/benz 1%/zinc1% per ml (10 ml w. dropper)

SYSTEMIC ANTI-INFECTIVES

➤ *amoxicillin* (B)(G) <40 kg (88 lb): 80-100 mg/kg/day divided q 12 hours x 10 days; *see page 543 for dose by weight table;* ≥40 kg: 500-875 mg bid or 250-500 mg tid x 10 days

Amoxil *Cap:* 250, 500 mg; *Tab:* 875*mg; *Chew tab:* 125, 200, 250, 400 mg (cherry-banana-peppermint) (phenylalanine); *Oral susp:* 125, 250 mg/5 ml (80, 100, 150 ml) (strawberry); 200, 400 mg/5 ml (50, 75, 100 ml) (bubble gum); *Oral drops:* 50 mg/ml (30 ml) (bubble gum)

Moxatag *Tab:* 775 mg ext-rel

Trimox *Tab:* 125, 250 mg; *Cap:* 250, 500 mg; *Oral susp:* 125, 250 mg/5 ml (80, 100, 150 ml) (raspberry-strawberry)

Comment: Consider 80-90 mg/kg/day in 3 divided doses for resistant for cases

➤ *amoxicillin/clavulanate* (B)(G)

Augmentin <40 kg: 40-45 mg/kg/day divided tid x 10 days or 90 mg/kg/day divided bid x 10 days; *see page 545 for dose by weight table;* ≥40 kg: 500 mg tid or 875 mg bid x 10 days

Tab: 250, 500, 875 mg; *Chew tab:* 125, 250 mg (lemon-lime); 200, 400 mg (cherry-banana) (phenylalanine); *Oral susp:* 125 mg/5 ml (banana), 250 mg/5 ml (75, 100, 150 ml) (orange); 200, 400 mg/5 ml (50, 75, 100 ml) (orange) (phenylalanine)

Augmentin ES-600 <3 months: not recommended; ≥3 months, <40 kg: 90 mg/kg/day divided q 12 hours x 10 days; *see page 546 for dose by weight table;* ≥40 kg: not recommended

Oral susp: 600 mg/5 ml (50, 75, 100, 125, 150, 200 ml) (strawberry cream) (phenylalanine)

Augmentin XR <16 years: use other forms; ≥16 years: 2 tabs q 12 hours x 7-10 days

Tab: 1000*mg ext-rel

➤ *ampicillin* (B) <12 years: 50-100 mg/kg/day in 4 divided doses x 10 days; *see page 547 for dose by weight table;* ≥12 years: 250-500 mg qid x 10 days

Omnipen, Principen *Cap:* 250, 500 mg; *Oral susp:* 125, 250 mg/5 ml (100, 150, 200 ml) (fruit)

➤ *azithromycin* (B)(G) <12 years: 12 mg/kg/day x 5 days; *see page 548 for dose by weight table;* max 500 mg/day; ≥12 years: 500 mg x 1 dose on day 1, then 250 mg daily on days 2-5 or 500 mg daily x 3 days or **Zmax** 2 gm in a single dose

Zithromax *Tab:* 250, 500, 600 mg; *Oral susp:* 100 mg/5 ml (15 ml); 200 mg/5 ml (15, 22.5, 30 ml) (cherry); *Pkt:* 1 gm for reconstitution (cherry-banana)

Zithromax Tri-pak *Tab:* 3 x 500 mg tabs/pck

Zithromax Z-pak *Tab:* 6 x 250 mg tabs/pck

Zmax *Oral susp:* 2 gm ext-rel for reconstitution (cherry-banana) (148 mg Na$^+$)

▷ *cefaclor* (B)(G) <1 month: not recommended; 1 month-12 years: 20-40 mg/kg divided bid x 10 days; *see page 549 for dose by weight table;* max 1 gm/day; >12 years: 250-500 mg q 8 hours x 10 days; max 2 gm/day

> *Tab:* 500 mg; *Cap:* 250, 500 mg; *Susp:* 125 mg/5 ml (75, 150 ml) (strawberry); 187 mg/5 ml (50, 100 ml) (strawberry); 250 mg/5 ml (75, 150 ml) (strawberry); 375 mg/5 ml (50, 100 ml) (strawberry)

> **Cefaclor Extended Release** <16 years: not recommended; ≥16 years: 500 mg bid x 10 days (clinically equivalent to 250 mg immed-rel caps tid); swallow whole; take with meals

> *Tab:* 375, 500 mg ext-rel

▷ *cefdinir* (B) <6 months: not recommended; 6 months-12 years: 14 mg/kg/day in 1-2 divided doses x 10 days; *see page 551 for dose by weight table;* ≥12 years: 300 mg bid x 10 days or 600 mg daily x 10 days

> **Omnicef** *Cap:* 300 mg; *Oral susp:* 125 mg/5 ml (60, 100 ml) (strawberry)

▷ *cefixime* (B)(G) <6 months: not recommended; 6 months-12 years, <50 kg: 8 mg/kg/day in 1-2 divided doses x 10 days; *see page 552 for dose by weight table;* >12 years, >50 kg: 400 mg once daily x 10 days

> **Suprax** *Tab:* 400 mg; *Cap:* 400 mg; *Oral susp:* 100, 200, 500 mg/5 ml (50, 75, 100 ml) (strawberry)

▷ *cefpodoxime proxetil* (B) <2 months: not recommended; 2 months-12 years: 10 mg/kg/day (max 400 mg/dose) or 5 mg/kg/day bid (max 200 mg/dose) x 5 days; *see page 553 for dose by weight table;* >12 years: 100 mg bid x 5 days

▷ *cefprozil* (B) ≤6 months: not recommended; 6 months-12 years: 7.5 mg/kg bid x 10 days; *see page 554 for dose by weight table;* >12 years: 250-500 mg bid or 500 mg daily x 10 days

> **Cefzil** *Tab:* 250, 500 mg; *Oral susp:* 125, 250 mg/5 ml (50, 75, 100 ml) (bubble gum) (phenylalanine)

▷ *ceftibuten* (B) <12 years: 9 mg/kg daily x 10 days; max 400 mg/day; *see page 555 for dose by weight table;* ≥12 years: 400 mg daily x 10 days

> **Cedax** *Cap:* 400 mg; *Oral susp:* 90 mg/5 ml (30, 60, 90, 120 ml); 180 mg/5 ml (30, 60, 120 ml) (cherry)

▷ *ceftriaxone* (B)(G) <12 years: 50 mg/kg IM x 1 dose; ≥12 years: 1-2 gm IM x 1 dose; max 4 g

> **Rocephin** *Vial:* 250, 500 mg; 1, 2 g

▷ *cefuroxime axetil* (B)(G) <12 years: 15 mg/kg bid x 10 days; *see page 556 for dose by weight table;* ≥12 years: 250-500 mg bid x 10 days

> **Ceftin** *Tab:* 250, 500 mg; *Oral susp:* 125, 250 mg/5 ml (50, 100 ml) (tutti-frutti)

▷ *cephalexin* (B)(G) <12 years: 25-50 mg/kg/day in 4 divided doses x 10 days; *see page 557 for dose by weight table;* ≥12 years: 250 mg qid x 10 days

> **Keflex** *Cap:* 250, 333, 500, 750 mg; *Oral susp:* 125, 250 mg/5 ml (100, 200 ml) (strawberry)

▷ *clarithromycin* (C)(G) <6 months: not recommended; ≥6 months-12 years: 7.5 mg/kg divided bid x 7 days; *see page 558 for dose by weight table;* >12 years: 500 mg bid or 500 mg ext-rel daily

> **Biaxin** *Tab:* 250, 500 mg
> **Biaxin Oral Suspension** *Oral susp:* 125, 250 mg/5 ml (50, 100 ml) (fruit punch)
> **Biaxin XL** *Tab:* 500 mg ext-rel

▷ *erythromycin/sulfisoxazole* (C)(G) <2 months: not recommended; ≥2 months: 50 mg/kg/day in 3 divided doses x 10 days

> **Eryzole** *Oral susp:* eryth 200 mg/sulf 600 mg per 5 ml (100, 150, 200, 250 ml)

Pediazole *Oral susp: eryth* 200 mg/*sulf* 600 mg per 5 ml (100, 150, 200 ml) (strawberry-banana)

Comment: *erythromycin* may increase INR with concomitant **warfarin**, as well as increase serum level of **digoxin**, benzodiazepines, and statins. **Sulfamethoxazole** is not recommended in pregnancy or lactation. *CrCl 15-30 mL/min:* reduce dose by 1/2; *CrCl <15 mL/min:* not recommended.

▷ *loracarbef* (B) <12 years: 30 mg/kg/day in 2 divided doses x 10 days; *see page 570 for dose by weight table;* ≥12 years: 400 mg bid x 10 days

Lorabid *Pulvule:* 200, 400 mg; *Oral susp:* 100 mg/5 ml (50, 100 ml); 200 mg/5 ml (50, 75, 100 ml) (strawberry bubble gum)

▷ *trimethoprim/sulfamethoxazole* (C)(G)

Bactrim, Septra <12 years: not recommended; ≥12 years: 2 tabs bid x 10 days
Tab: trim 80 mg/*sulfa* 400 mg*

Bactrim DS, Septra DS <12 years: not recommended; ≥12 years: 1 tab bid x 10 days
Tab: trim 160 mg/*sulfa* 800 mg*

Bactrim Pediatric Suspension, Septra Pediatric Suspension <2 months: not recommended; ≥2 months-12 years: 40 mg/kg/day of in 2 doses bid; >12 years: use tabs
Oral susp: trim 40 mg/*sulfa* 200 mg per 5 ml (100 ml) (cherry) (alcohol 0.3%)

OTIC ANTI-INFECTIVE

▷ *ofloxacin* (C)(G) <6 months: not recommended; 6 months-12 years: 5 drops bid x 14 days; >12 years: 10 drops bid x 14 days

Floxin Otic *Otic soln:* 0.3% (5, 10 ml w. dropper)

Comment: *ofloxacin* may be used with patients with perforated tympanic membrane or tympanostomy tubes.

OTIC ANTI-INFECTIVE/CORTICOSTEROID COMBINATIONS

Comment: *neomycin* may cause ototoxicity. Do not use with known or suspected tympanic membrane rupture.

▷ *chloroxylenol/pramoxine/hydrocortisone* (C) <12 years: 3 drops tid-qid x 5-10 days; ≥12 years: 4 drops tid-qid x 5-10 days

Cortane Ear Drops, *Otic drops:* 10 ml

▷ *ciprofloxacin/hydrocortisone* (C) <1 year: not recommended; ≥1 year: 3 drops bid x 7 days

Cipro HC *Otic susp: cipro* 0.3%/*dexa* 0.1% (10 ml)

▷ *ciprofloxacin/dexamethasone* (C) <6 months: not recommended; ≥6 months: 4 drops bid x 7 days

Ciprodex *Otic susp: cipro* 0.3%/*dexa* 1% (7.5 ml)

Comment: **Ciprodex** is indicated for the treatment of otitis media in pediatric patients with tympanostomy tubes (PE tubes).

▷ *colistin/neomycin/hydrocortisone/thonzonium* (C) <12 years: 4 drops tid-qid x 5-10 days; ≥12 years: 5 drops tid-qid x 5-10 days

Coly-Mycin S *Otic susp:* 5, 10 ml

▷ *polymyxin b/neomycin/hydrocortisone* (C)(G) <12 years: 3 drops tid-qid; max 10 days; ≥12 years: 4 drops tid-qid; max 10 days

Cortisporin *Otic susp:* 10 ml w. dropper; *Otic soln:* 10 ml w. dropper

PediOtic *Otic susp:* 7.5 ml w. dropper
▷ *polymyxin B/neomycin/hydrocortisone/surfactant* (C) <12 years: 3 drops tid-qid; max 10 days; ≥12 years: 4 drops tid-qid
Cortisporin-TC *Otic susp:* 10 ml w. dropper

OTIC ANESTHETIC/ANALGESIC COMBINATIONS

▷ *antipyrine/benzocaine/glycerine* (C) fill ear canal and insert cotton plug; may repeat q 1-2 hours as needed
A/B Otic *Otic soln:* antipy 5.4%/*benzo* 1.4% 15 ml w. dropper
▷ *benzocaine* (C)(OTC)(G) <1 year: not recommended; ≥1 year: 4-5 drops q 1-2 hours
Americaine Otic *Otic soln:* 15 ml w. dropper
Benzotic *Otic soln:* 20% (15 ml w. dropper)

OTITIS MEDIA: SEROUS

Anti-infectives *see Otitis Media: Acute page* 291
Oral Prescription Drugs for the Management of Allergy, Cough, and Cold Symptoms *see page* 523
Oral Corticosteroids *see page* 498

PAGET'S DISEASE: BONE

Comment: Calcium decreases *tetracycline* absorption. calcium absorption is decreased by corticosteroids. calcium absorption is decreased by foods such as rhubarb, spinach, and bran.

BISPHOSPHONATES (CALCIUM MODIFIERS)

Comment: Bisphosphonates should be swallowed whole in the AM with 6-8 oz of plain water 30 minutes before first meal, beverage, or other medications of the day. Monitor serum alkaline phosphatase. Contraindications include abnormalities of the esophagus, which delay esophageal emptying such as stricture or achalasia, inability to stand or sit upright for at least 30 minutes post-dose, patients at risk of aspiration, and hypocalcemia. Co-administration of bisphosphonates and calcium, antacids, or oral medications containing multivalent cations will interfere with absorption of the biphosphonate. Therefore, instruct patients to wait at least half hour after taking the biphosphonate before taking any other oral medications.
▷ *alendronate (as sodium)* (C) <12 years: not recommended; ≥12 years: take once weekly, in the AM, 30 minutes before the first food, beverage, or medication of the day; do not lie down (remain upright) for at least 30 minutes and after the first food of the day; not recommended with *CrCl <35 mL/min.*
Binosto dissolve the effervescent tab in 4 oz (120 ml) of plain, room temperature, water (not mineral or flavored); wait 5 minutes after the effervescence has subsided, then stir for 10 seconds, then drink
Tab: 70 mg effervescent for buffered solution (4, 12/carton) (strawberry)
Fosamax (G) swallow tab whole; *Prevention:* 5 mg once daily or 35 mg once weekly; *Treatment:* 10 mg once daily or 70 mg once weekly

Tab: 5, 10, 35, 40, 70 mg

➤ *alendronate/cholecalciferol (vit d3)* (C)(G) 12 years: not recommended; ≥12 years: take 1 tab once weekly, in the AM, with plain water (not mineral) 30 minutes before the first food, beverage, <u>or</u> medication of the day; do not lie down (remain upright) for at least 30 minutes and after the first food of the day

Fosamax Plus D
Tab: **Fosamax Plus D 70/2800** *alen* 70 mg/*chole* 2800 IU
Fosamax Plus D 70/5600 *alen* 70 mg/*chole* 5600 IU

➤ *ibandronate (as monosodium monohydrate)* (C)(G) <12 years: not recommended; ≥12 years:

Boniva take 2.5 mg once daily <u>or</u> 150 mg once monthly on the same day; take in the AM, with plain water (not mineral) 60 minutes before the first food, beverage, <u>or</u> medication of the day; do not lie down (remain upright) for at least 30 minutes and after the first food of the day
Tab: 2.5, 150 mg
Boniva Injection administer 3 mg every 3 months by IV bolus over 15-30 seconds; if dose is missed, administer as soon as possible, then every 3 months from the date of the last dose
Prefilled syringe: 3 mg/3 ml (5 ml)
Comment: **Boniva Injection** must be administered by a qualified health care professional.

➤ *risedronate (as sodium)* (C)(G) <12 years: not recommended; ≥12 years: take in the AM; swallow whole with a full glass of plain water (not mineral) do not lie down (remain upright) for 30 minutes afterward

Actonel take at least 30 minutes before any food <u>or</u> drink; *Females:* 5 mg once daily <u>or</u> 35 mg once weekly <u>or</u> 75 mg on two consecutive days monthly <u>or</u> 150 mg once monthly; *Males:* 35 mg once weekly; *Tab:* 5, 30, 35, 75, 150 mg
Atelvia 35 mg once weekly immediately after breakfast
Tab: 35 mg del-rel

➤ *risedronate/calcium* (C) 1 x 5 mg *risedronate* tab weekly <u>and</u> 1 x 500 mg *calcium* tab on days 2-7 weekly

Actonel with Calcium *Tab:* *risedronate* 5 mg <u>and</u> *Tab:* **calcium** 500 mg (4 *risedronate* tabs + 30 *calcium* tabs/pck)

➤ *zoledronic acid* (D)(G) <12 years: not recommended; ≥12 years:

Reclast administer 5 mg via IV infusion over at least 15 minutes mg once a year (for osteoporosis) <u>or</u> once every 2 years (for osteopenia <u>or</u> prophylaxis)
Bottle: 5 mg/100 ml (single dose)
Comment: **Reclast** is indicated for the treatment of postmenopausal osteoporosis in females who are at high risk for fracture and to increase bone mass in men with primary <u>or</u> hypogonadal osteoporosis who are at high risk for fracture. Must be administered by a qualified health care professional. Contraindicated in hypocalcemia.
Zometa administer 4 mg via IV infusion over at least 15 minutes every 3-4 weeks; optimal duration of treatment not known
Bottle: 4 mg/5 ml; *Vial:* 4 mg/5 ml (single dose)
Comment: **Zometa** is indicated for the treatment of hypercalcemia of malignancy. The safety and efficacy of **Zometa** in the treatment of hypercalcemia associated with hyperparathyroidism <u>or</u> with other non-tumor-related conditions has not been established.

PAIN

Antidepressants *see Depression* page 97
Skeletal Muscle Relaxants *see Muscle Strain* page 261

ACETAMINOPHEN FOR IV INFUSION

▶ *acetaminophen* injectable (**B**) <2 years: not recommended; 2-<13 years, <50 kg: 15 mg/kg q 6 hours prn <u>or</u> 2.5 mg/kg q 4 hours prn; max 750 mg single dose; max 75 mg/kg per day; ≥13 years: administer by IV infusion over 15 minutes; 1,000 mg q 6 hours prn <u>or</u> 650 mg q 4 hours prn; max 4,000 mg/day

Ofirmev *Vial:* 10 mg/ml (100 ml) (preservative-free)

Comment: The **Ofirmev** vial is intended for single use. If any portion is withdrawn from the vial, use within 6 hours. Discard the unused portion. For pediatric patients, withdraw the intended dose and administer via syringe pump. Do not admix **Ofirmev** with any other drugs. **Ofirmev** is physically incompatible with *diazepam* and *chlorpromazine hydrochloride.*

IBUPROFEN FOR IV INFUSION

▶ *ibuprofen* (**B**) <6 months; not recommended; 6 months-<12 years: 10 mg/kg q 4-6 hours prn; max 400 mg/dose; max 40 mg/kg <u>or</u> 2,400 mg/24 hours, whichever is less; 12-<17 years: 400 mg q 4-6 hours prn; max 2,400 mg/24 hours; ≥17 years: dilute dose in 0.9% NS, D5W, <u>or</u> Lactated Ringers (LR) solution; administer by IV infusion over at least 10 minutes; do not administer via IV bolus <u>or</u> IM; 400-800 mg q 6 hours prn; maximum 3,200 mg/day

Caldolor *Vial:* 800 mg/8 ml single dose

Comment: Prepare Caldolor solution for IV administration as follows: 100 mg dose: dilute 1 ml of **Caldolor** in at least 100 ml of diluent (IVF); 200 mg dose: dilute 2 ml of **Caldolor** in at least 100 ml of diluent; 400 mg dose: dilute 4 ml of **Caldolor** in at least 100 ml of diluent; 800 mg dose: dilute 8 ml of **Caldolor** in at least 200 ml of diluent. **Caldolor** is also indicated for management of fever. For patients ≥18 years-of-age with fever, 400 mg via IV infusion, followed by 400 mg q 4-6 hours <u>or</u> 100-200 mg q 4 hours prn.

OCULAR PAIN

▶ *difluprednate* (**C**) <12 years: not recommended; ≥12 years: apply 1 drop to affected eye qid; for post-op ocular pain, begin treatment 24 hours post-op and continue x 2 weeks; then bid daily x 1 week; then taper

Durezol *Ophth emul:* 0.05% (5 ml)

Comment: **Durezol** is an ophthalmic steroid.

▶ *nepafenac* (**C**) <10 years: not recommended; ≥10 years: apply 1 drop to affected eye tid; for post-op ocular pain, begin treatment 24 hours before surgery and continue day of surgery and for two weeks post-op

Nevanac *Ophth susp:* 0.1% (3 ml) (benzalkonium chloride)

Comment: **Nevanac** is an ophthalmic NSAID.

TOPICAL/TRANSDERMAL NSAIDs

▶ *capsaicin* cream (**B**)(**G**) <2 years: not recommended; 2-12 years: apply sparingly to intact skin bid prn; >12 years: apply tid-qid prn

      Axsain *Crm:* 0.075% (1, 2 oz)
      Capsin (OTC) *Lotn:* 0.025, 0,075% (59 ml)
      Capzasin-P (OTC) *Crm:* 0.025% (1.5 oz); *Lotn:* 0.025% (2 oz)
      Capzasin-HP (OTC) *Crm:* 0.025% (1.5 oz); *Lotn:* 0.075% (2 oz)
      Dolorac *Crm:* 0.025% (28 gm)
      Double Cap (OTC) *Crm:* 0.05% (2 oz)
      R-Gel *Gel:* 0.025% (15, 30 gm)
      Zostrix (OTC) *Crm:* 0.025% (0.7, 1.5, 3 oz)
      Zostrix HP (OTC) *Emol crm:* 0.075% (1, 2 oz)
Comment: Provides some relief by 1-2 weeks; optimal benefit may take 4-6 weeks. Avoid contact with mucous membranes.

▷ *capsaicin* 8% patch **(B)** <18 years: not recommended; ≥18 years: apply sparingly tid-qid prn apply up to 4 patches for one 60-minute application to clean dry skin; may prep area with topical anesthetic; wear non-latex gloves; patches may be cut to size/shape; treatment may be repeated every 3 months; remove with cleansing gel after treatment
      Qutenza *Patch:* 8% 1640 mcg/cm (179 mg) (1 or 2 patches, each w. 1-50 gm tube cleansing gel/carton)

▷ *diclofenac epolamine transdermal patch* **(C; D ≥30 wks)** <12 years: not recommended; ≥12 years: apply one patch to affected area bid; remove during bathing; avoid non-intact skin
      Flector Patch *Patch:* 180 mg/patch (30/carton)

▷ *diclofenac epolamine transdermal patch* **(C; D ≥30 wks)** <12 years: not recommended; ≥12 years: apply sparingly tid-qid prn apply one patch to affected area bid; remove during bathing; avoid non-intact skin
      Flector Patch *Patch:* 180 mg/patch (30/carton)

▷ *diclofenac sodium* **(C; D ≥30 wks)(G)** <12 years: not recommended; ≥12 years: apply sparingly to intact skin qid prn
      Voltaren Gel *Gel:* 1% (100 gm)

▷ *diclofenac sodium* **(C; D ≥30 wks)(G)** <18 years: not established; ≥18 years:
      Pennsaid 1.5% in 10 drop increments, dispense and rub into front, side, and back of knee; usually; 40 drops (40 mg) qid
        Topical soln: 1.5% (150 ml)
      Pennsaid 2% <12 years: not recommended; ≥12 years: apply 2 pump actuations (40 mg) and rub into front, side, and back of knee bid
        Topical soln: 2% (20 mg/pump actuation, 112 gm)
Comment: **Pennsaid** is indicated for the treatment of pain associated with osteoarthritis of the knee.
      Solaraze Gel *Gel:* 3% (50 gm) (benzyl alcohol)
Comment: Contraindicated with *aspirin* allergy. As with other NSAIDs, **Solaraze Gel** should be avoided in late pregnancy (≥30 weeks) because it may cause premature closure of the ductus arteriosus.
      Voltaren Gel <12 years: not recommended; ≥12 years: apply qid; avoid non-intact skin
        Gel: 1% (100 gm)
Comment: *diclofenac* is contraindicated with *aspirin* allergy. As with other NSAIDs, **Voltaren Gel** should be avoided in late pregnancy (≥30 weeks) because it may cause premature closure of the ductus arteriosus.
Other Prescription NSAIDs *see page 490*

TOPICAL/TRANSDERMAL LIDOCAINE

▷ *lidocaine* transdermal patch (C)(G) <12 years: not recommended; ≥12 years: apply one patch to affected area for 12 hours (then off for 12 hours); remove during bathing; avoid non-intact skin; do not reuse

    Lidoderm *Patch:* 5% (10 cm x 14 cm, 30/carton)

OPIOIDS AND OTHER ORAL ANALGESICS

▷ *butalbital/acetaminophen* (C)(G) <12 years: not recommended; ≥12 years: 1 tab q 4 hours prn; max 6 tabs/day

    Tab: but 50 mg/*acet* 325 mg

    Phrenilin 1-2 tabs q 4 hours prn; max 6 tabs/day

    Tab: but 50 mg/*acet* 325 mg

    Phrenilin Forte 1 tab or cap q 4 hours prn; max 6 caps/day

    Cap: but 50 mg/*acet* 325 mg; *Tab: but* 50 mg/*acet* 325 mg

▷ *butalbital/acetaminophen/caffeine* (C)(G) <12 years: not recommended; ≥12 years:

    Fioricet 1-2 tabs q 4 hours prn; max 6/day

    Tab: but 50 mg/*acet* 325 mg/*caf* 40 mg

    Zebutal 1 cap q 4 hours prn; max 5/day

    Cap: but 50 mg/*acet* 325 mg/*caf* 40 mg

▷ *butalbital/aspirin/caffeine* (C)(III)(G)

    Fiorinal <12 years: not recommended; ≥12 years: 1-2 tabs or caps q 4 hours prn; max 6 caps/day

    Tab/Cap: but 50 mg/*asp* 325 mg/*caf* 40 mg

▷ *butalbital/aspirin/codeine/caffeine* (C)(III)(G)

    Fiorinal with Codeine <12 years: contraindicated; 12-<18 years: use extreme caution; not recommended for children and adolescents with obesity, asthma, obstructive sleep apnea, or other chronic breathing problem, or for post-tonsillectomy/ adenoidectomy pain; ≥18 years: 1-2 caps q 4 hours prn; max 6 caps/day

    Cap: but 50 mg/*asp* 325 mg/*cod* 40 mg

Comment: *Codeine* is known to be excreted in breast milk. <12 years: not recommended; 12-<18 years: use extreme caution; not recommended for children and adolescents with asthma or other chronic breathing problem. The FDA and the European Medicines Agency (EMA) are investigating the safety of using *codeine* containing medications to treat pain, cough and colds, in children 12-<18 years because of the potential for serious side effects, including slowed or difficult breathing.

▷ *codeine sulfate* (C)(III)(G) <12 years: contraindicated; 12-<18 years: use extreme caution; not recommended for children and adolescents with obesity, asthma, obstructive sleep apnea, or other chronic breathing problem, or for post-tonsillectomy/adenoidectomy pain; ≥18 years: 15-60 q 4-6 hours prn; max 60 mg/day

    Tab: 15, 30, 60 mg

Comment: *Codeine* is known to be excreted in breast milk. <12 years: not recommended; 12-<18 years: use extreme caution; not recommended for children and adolescents with asthma or other chronic breathing problem. The FDA and the European Medicines Agency (EMA) are investigating the safety of using *codeine* containing medications to treat pain, cough and colds, in children 12-<18 years because of the potential for serious side effects, including slowed or difficult breathing.

▷ *codeine/acetaminophen* (C)(III)(G) <12 years: contraindicated; 12-<18: use extreme caution; not recommended for children and adolescents with obesity, asthma, obstructive sleep apnea, or other chronic breathing problem, or for post-tonsillectomy/adenoidectomy pain; ≥18 years: 15-60 mg of *codeine* q 4 hours prn; max 360 mg of *codeine*/day

> *Tab:* Tylenol #1 *cod* 7.5 mg/*acet* 300 mg (sulfites)
> Tylenol #2 *cod* 15 mg/*acet* 300 mg (sulfites)
> Tylenol #3 *cod* 30 mg/*acet* 300 mg (sulfites)
> Tylenol #4 *cod* 60 mg/*acet* 300 mg (sulfites)

Comment: *Codeine* is known to be excreted in breast milk. <12 years: not recommended; 12-<18: use extreme caution; not recommended for children and adolescents with asthma or other chronic breathing problem. The FDA and the European Medicines Agency (EMA) are investigating the safety of using *codeine* containing medications to treat pain, cough and colds, in children 12-<18 years because of the potential for serious side effects, including slowed or difficult breathing.

> Tylenol with Codeine Elixir (C)(III) <12 years: contraindicated; 12-<18: use extreme caution; not recommended for children and adolescents with obesity, asthma, obstructive sleep apnea, or other chronic breathing problem, or for post-tonsillectomy/adenoidectomy pain; ≥18 years: 10 ml tid-qid; ≥12 year: 15-60 mg of *codeine* q 4 hours prn; max 360 mg of *codeine*/day
>
> *Elix: cod* 12 mg/*acet* 120 mg per 5 ml (cherry) (alcohol)

Comment: *Codeine* is known to be excreted in breast milk. <12 years: not recommended; 12-<18: use extreme caution; not recommended for children and adolescents with asthma or other chronic breathing problem. The FDA and the European Medicines Agency (EMA) are investigating the safety of using *codeine* containing medications to treat pain, cough and colds, in children 12-<18 years because of the potential for serious side effects, including slowed or difficult breathing.

▷ *dihydrocodeine/acetaminophen/caffeine* (C)(III)(G) <18: use extreme caution; not recommended for children and adolescents with obesity, asthma, obstructive sleep apnea, or other chronic breathing problem, or for post-tonsillectomy/adenoidectomy pain; ≥18 years:

> Panlor DC 1-2 caps q 4-6 hours prn; max 10 caps/day
> *Cap: dihydro* 16 mg/*acet* 325 mg/*caf* 30 mg
> Panlor SS 1 tab q 4 hours prn; max 5 tabs/day
> *Tab: dihydro* 32 mg/*acet* 325 mg/*caf* 60*mg

Comment: *Codeine* is known to be excreted in breast milk. <12 years: not recommended; 12-<18: use extreme caution; not recommended for children and adolescents with asthma or other chronic breathing problem. The FDA and the European Medicines Agency (EMA) are investigating the safety of using *codeine* containing medications to treat pain, cough and colds, in children 12-<18 years because of the potential for serious side effects, including slowed or difficult breathing.

▷ *dihydrocodeine/aspirin/caffeine* (D)(III)(G) <12 years: contraindicated; 12-<18: use extreme caution; not recommended for children and adolescents with obesity, asthma, obstructive sleep apnea, or other chronic breathing problem, or for post-tonsillectomy/adenoidectomy pain; ≥18 years: 1-2 caps q 4 hours prn

> Synalgos-DC *Cap: dihydro* 16 mg/*asp* 356.4 mg/*caf* 30 mg

Comment: *Codeine* is known to be excreted in breast milk. <12 years: not recommended; 12-<18: use extreme caution; not recommended for children and adolescents with asthma or other chronic breathing problem. The FDA and the European Medicines Agency (EMA) are investigating the safety of using *codeine* containing medications to treat pain, cough and colds, in children 12-<18 years because of the potential for serious side effects, including slowed or difficult breathing.

➤ *hydrocodone bitartrate* (C)(II) <18 years: not recommended; ≥18 year:

    Hysingla ER swallow whole; 1 tab once daily at the same time each day
      Tab: 20, 30, 40, 60, 80, 100, 120 mg ext-rel

    Vantrela ER swallow whole; 1 tab once daily at the same time each day
      Tab: 15, 30, 45, 60, 90 mg ext-rel

    Zohydro ER swallow whole; *Opioid naïve:* 10 mg q 12 hours; may increase by 10 mg q 12 hours every 3-7 days; when discontinuing, titrate downward every 2-4 days
      Cap: 10, 15, 20, 30, 40, 50 mg ext-rel

➤ *hydrocodone bitartrate/acetaminophen* (C)(II)(G) <12 years: not recommended; ≥12 years:

    Hycet 3 tsp (15 ml) q 4-6 hours prn; max 18 tsp/day
      Liq: hydro 7.5 mg/acet 325 mg per 15 ml

    Lorcet 1-2 caps q 4-6 hours prn; max 8 caps/day
      Cap: hydro 5 mg/acet 325 mg

    Lorcet 10/650 1 tab q 4-6 hours prn; max 6 tabs/day
      Tab: hydro 10 mg/acet 325 mg

    Lorcet-HD 1 cap q 4-6 hours prn; max 6 tabs/day
      Cap: hydro 5 mg/acet 325 mg

    Lorcet Plus 1 tab q 4-6 hours prn; max 6 tabs/day
      Tab: hydro 7.5 mg/acet 325 mg

    Lortab 2.5/500 1-2 tabs q 4-6 hours prn; max 8 tabs/day
      Tab: hydro 2.5 mg/acet 325*mg

    Lortab 5/500 1-2 tabs q 4-6 hours prn; max 8 tabs/day
      Tab: hydro 5 mg/acet 325*mg

    Lortab 7.5/500 1 tab q 4-6 hours prn; max 6 tabs/day
      Tab: hydro 7.5 mg/acet 325*mg

    Lortab 10/500 1 tab q 4-6 hours prn; max 6 tabs/day
      Tab: hydro 10 mg/acet 325*mg

    Lortab Elixir 3 tsp q 4-6 hours prn; max 18 tsp/day
      Liq: hydro 7.5 mg/acet 300 mg per 15 ml (tropical fruit punch) (alcohol)

    Maxidone 1 tab q 4-6 hours prn; max 5 tabs/day
      Tab: hydro 10 mg/acet 325*mg

    Norco 5/325 1 tab q 4-6 hours prn; max 8 tabs/day
      Tab: hydro 5 mg/acet 325*mg

    Norco 7.5/325 1 tab q 4-6 hours prn; max 6 tabs/day
      Tab: hydro 7.5 mg/acet 325*mg

    Norco 10/325 1 tab q 4-6 hours prn; max 6 tabs/day
      Tab: hydro 10 mg/acet 325*mg

    Vicodin 1-2 tabs q 4-6 hours prn; max 8 tabs/day
      Tab: hydro 5 mg/acet 300*mg

    Vicodin ES 1 tab q 4-6 hours prn; max 6 tabs/day
      Tab: hydro 7.5 mg/acet 300*mg

    Vicodin HP 1 tab q 4-6 hours prn; max 6 tabs/day
      Tab: hydro 10 mg/*acet* 300*mg
    Xodol 5/300 1-2 tabs q 4-6 hours prn; max 8 caps/day
      Tab: hydro 5 mg/*acet* 300*mg
    Xodol 7.5/300 1 tab q 4-6 hours prn; max 6 caps/day
      Tab: hydro 7.5 mg/*acet* 300*mg
    Xodol 10/300 1 tab q 4-6 hours prn; max 6 caps/day
      Tab: hydro 10 mg/*acet* 300*mg
    Zamicet 10/325 1-2 tabs q 4-6 hours prn; max 8 caps/day
      Liq: hydro 10 mg/*acet* 325 mg per 15 ml
    Zydone 5/400 1-2 tabs q 4-6 hours prn; max 8 caps/day
      Tab: hydro 5 mg/*acet* 400 mg
    Zydone 7.5/400 1 tab q 4-6 hours prn; max 6 caps/day
      Tab: hydro 7.5 mg/*acet* 400 mg
    Zydone 10/400 1 tab q 4-6 hours prn; max 6 caps/day
      Tab: hydro 10 mg/*acet* 400 mg
▶ *hydrocodone/ibuprofen* (C; not for use in 3rd)(II)(G) <12 years: not recommended;
≥12 years:
    Ibudone 5/200 1 tab q 4-6 hours prn; max 5 tabs/day
      Tab: hydro 5 mg/*ibup* 200 mg
    Ibudone 10/200 1 tab q 4-6 hours prn; max 5 tabs/day
      Tab: hydro 10 mg/*ibup* 200 mg
    Reprexain 1 tab q 4-6 hours prn; max 5 tabs/day
      Tab: hydro 5 mg/*ibup* 200 mg
    Vicoprofen 1 tab q 4-6 hours prn; max 5 tabs/day
      Tab: hydro 7.5 mg/*ibup* 200 mg
▶ *hydromorphone* (C)(II)(G) <12 years: not recommended; ≥12 years:
    Dilaudid initially 2-4 mg q 4-6 hours prn
      Tab: 2, 4, 8 mg (sulfites)
    Dilaudid Oral Liquid 2.5-10 mg q 3-6 hours prn
      Liq: 5 mg/5 ml (sulfites)
    Dilaudid Rectal Suppository 2.5-10 mg q 6-8 hours prn
      Rectal supp: 3 mg
    Dilaudid Injection initially 1-2 mg SC or IM q 4-6 hours prn
      Amp: 1, 2, 4 mg/ml (1 ml)
    Dilaudid-HP Injection initially 1-2 mg SC or IM q 4-6 hours prn
      Amp: 10 mg/ml (1 ml)
    Exalgo initially 8-64 mg once daily
      Tab: 8, 12, 16, 32 mg ext-rel (sulfites)
▶ *meperidine* (C; D in 2nd, 3rd)(II)(G) <12 years: 0.5-0.8 mg/lb q 3-4 hours prn; ≥12
years: 50-150 mg q 3-4 hours prn
    Demerol *Tab:* 50, 100 mg; *Syr:* 50 mg/5 ml (banana) (alcohol-free)
▶ *meperidine/promethazine* (C; D in 2nd, 3rd)(II)(G) <12 years: not recommended;
≥12 years:
    Mepergan 1-2 tsp q 3-4 hours prn
      Syr: mep 25 mg/*prom* 25 mg per ml
    Mepergan Fortis 1-2 tsp q 4-6 hours prn
      Tab: mep 50 mg/*prom* 25 mg
▶ *methadone* (C)(II) <12 years: not recommended; ≥12 years: 2.5-10 mg PO, SC, or
IM q 3-4 hours prn

Dolophine *Tab:* 5, 10 mg; *Dispersible tab:* 40 mg (dissolve in 120 ml orange juice
or other citrus drink); *Oral conc:* 5, 10 mg/5 ml; 10 mg/10 ml; *Inj:* 10 mg/ml
Comment: *methadone* maintenance is allowed only by approved treatment
programs with strict state and federal regulations.

➤ *morphine sulfate* (C)(II)(G) <18 years: not recommended; ≥18 years: *Tabs:* usually
15-30 mg q 4 hours prn; *Solution:* usually 10-20 mg q 4 hours prn
Tab: 15*, 30*mg; *Oral soln:* 10 mg/5 ml, 20 mg/5 ml (100, 500 ml), 100 mg/5
ml (30, 120 ml)

➤ *morphine sulfate (immed- and sust-rel)* (C)(II) <18 years: not recommended
Comment: Dosage dependent upon previous opioid dosage; see mfr pkg insert
for conversion guidelines; not for prn use; swallow whole or sprinkle contents of
caps on applesauce (do not crush, chew, or dissolve). Generic *morphine sulfate*
is available in the following forms: *Tab:* 15*, 30*mg; *Oral soln:* 10, 20 mg/5 ml
(100 ml); 100 mg/5 ml (30, 120 ml w. oral syringe)
Arymo ER swallow whole; 1 tab once daily at the same time each day
Tab: 15, 30, 60 mg ext-rel
Duramorph administer per anesthesia
IV/Intrathecal/Epidural: 0.5, 1 mg/ml
Infumorph administer per anesthesia
Intrathecal/Epidural: 10, 20 mg/ml
Kadian (G) 1 cap every 12-24 hours
Cap: 10, 20, 30, 50, 60, 80, 100, 200 mg sust-rel
MS Contin (G) 1 tab every 24 hours
Tab: 15, 30, 60, 100, 200 mg sust-rel
MSIR 5-30 mg q 4 hours prn
Tab: 15*, 30*mg; *Cap:* 15, 30 mg
MSIR Oral Solution 5-30 mg q 4 hours prn
Oral soln: 10, 20 mg/5 ml (120 ml)
MSIR Oral Solution Concentrate 5-30 mg q 4 hours prn
Oral conc: 20 mg/ml (30, 120 ml w. dropper)
Oramorph SR 1 cap every 12-24 hours
Tab: 15, 30, 60, 100 mg sust-rel
Roxanol Oral Solution 10-30 mg q 4 hours prn
Oral soln: 20 mg/ml (1, 4, 8 oz)
Roxanol Rescudose
Oral soln: 10 mg/2.5 ml (25 single dose)

➤ *morphine sulfate/naltrexone* (C)(II) <18 years: not recommended; ≥18 years:
Embeda 1 cap q 12-24 hours
Cap: **Embeda 20/0.8** *morph* 20 mg/*nal* 0.8 mg ext-rel
Embeda 30/1.2 *morph* 30 mg/*nal* 1.2 mg ext-rel
Embeda 50/2 *morph* 50 mg/*nal* 2 mg ext-rel
Embeda 60/2.4 *morph* 60 mg/*nal* 2.4 mg ext-rel
Embeda 80/3.2 *morph* 80 mg/*nal* 3.2 mg ext-rel
Embeda 100/4 *morph* 100 mg/*nal* 4 mg ext-rel
Comment: **Embeda** is not for prn use; for use in opioid-tolerant patients only;
swallow whole or sprinkle contents of caps on applesauce (do not crush, chew,
or dissolve); do not administer via NG or gastric tube (PEG tube).

➤ *oxycodone* (B)(II)(G) <18 years: not recommended; ≥18 year: 5-15 mg q 4-6 hours
prn

Comment: Concomitant use of CYP3A4 inhibitors may increase opioid effects and CYP3A4 inducers may decrease effects or possibly cause development of an abstinence syndrome (withdrawal symptoms) in patients who are physically *oxycodone* dependent/addicted.

Oxaydo *Tab:* 5, 7.5 mg

Comment: **Oxaydo** is the first and only immediate-release oral *oxycodone* that discourages intranasal abuse. **Oxaydo** is formulated with sodium lauryl sulfate, an inactive ingredient that may cause nasal burning and throat irritation when snorted and, thus potentially reducing abuse liability. There is no generic equivalent.

Oxecta *Tab:* 5, 7.5 mg

Oxycodone Oral Solution (G) *Oral soln:* 5 mg/5 ml (15, 30 ml)

OxyIR (G) *Cap:* 5 mg

Roxycodone *Tab:* 5, 15*, 30*mg; *Oral soln:* 5 mg/ml

Roxycodone Intensol *Oral soln:* 20 mg/ml

➤ *oxycodone cont-rel* (B)(II)(G) dosage dependent upon previous opioid be taking and tolerating dosages; see mfr pkg insert: <11 years: not recommended; 11-16 years: the child's pain must be severe enough to require around-the-clock, long-term treatment not managed well by other treatments; must already tolerate minimum opium dose equal to *oxycodone* 20 mg/day x 5 consecutive days; >16 years: no previous treatment with *oxycodone* required

OxyContin dose q 12 hours

  Tab: 10, 15, 20, 30, 40, 60, 80 mg cont-rel

OxyFast dose q 6 hours

  Oral conc: 20 mg/ml (30 ml w. dropper)

Xtampza ER dose q 12 hours

  Cap: 10, 15, 20, 30, 40 mg ext-rel

Comment: May open the **Xtampza ER** capsule and sprinkle in water or on soft food.

➤ *oxycodone/acetaminophen* (C)(II)(G) <12 years: not recommended; ≥12 years:

Comment: Maximum 4 grams acetaminophen per day.

Magnacet 2.5/400 1 tab q 6 hours prn; max 10 tabs/day

  Tab: oxy 2.5 mg/*acet* 325 mg

Magnacet 5/400 1 tab q 6 hours prn; max 10 tabs/day

  Tab: oxy 5 mg/*acet* 325 mg

Magnacet 7.5/400 1 tab q 6 hours prn; max 8 tabs/day

  Tab: oxy 7.5 mg/*acet* 325 mg

Magnacet 10/400 1 tab q 6 hours prn; max 6 tabs/day

  Tab: oxy 10 mg/*acet* 325 mg

Percocet 2.5/325 1 tab q 6 hours prn; max 4 gm acet/day

  Tab: oxy 2.5 mg/*acet* 325 mg

Percocet 5/325 1 tab q 6 hours prn; max 4 gm acet/day

  Tab: oxy 5 mg/*acet* 325*mg

Percocet 7.5/325 1 tab q 6 hours prn; max 4 gm acet/day

  Tab: oxy 7.5 mg/*acet* 325 mg

Percocet 7.5/500 1 tabs q 6 hours prn; max 4 gm acet/day

  Tab: oxy 7.5 mg/*acet* 325 mg

Percocet 10/325 1 tabs q 6 hours prn; max 4 gm acet/day

  Tab: oxy 10 mg/*acet* 325 mg

Percocet 10/650 1 tab q 6 hours prn; max 4 gm acet/day
  Tab: oxy 10 mg/*acet* 325 mg
Roxicet 5/325 1 tab/tsp q 6 hours prn
  Tab: oxy 5 mg/*acet* 325 mg; *Oral soln: oxy* 5 mg/*acet* 325 mg per 5 ml
Roxicet 5/500 1 caplet q 6 hours prn
  Cplt: oxy 5 mg/*acet* 325 mg
Roxicet Oral Solution 1 tsp q 6 hours prn
  Oral soln: oxy 5 mg/*acet* 325 mg per 5 ml (alcohol 0.4%)
Tylox 1 cap q 6 hours prn
  Cap: oxy 5 mg/*acet* 325 mg
Xartemis XR 2 tabs q 12 hours prn
  Tab: oxy 7.5 mg/*acet* 325 mg

➤ *oxycodone/aspirin* (D)(II)(G) <12 years: not recommended; ≥12 years:
Percodan 1 tab q 6 hours prn
  Tab: oxy 4.8355 mg/*asp* 325*mg
Percodan-Demi <6 years: not recommended: 6-12 years: 1/4 tab q 6 hours prn;
>12-18 years: 1/2 tab q 6 hours prn; >18 years: 1-2 tabs q 6 hours prn
  Tab: oxy 2.25 mg/*asp* 325 mg

➤ *oxycodone/ibuprofen* (C)(II)(G)
Combunox <12 years: not recommended; ≥12 years: 1 tab q 6 hours prn
  Tab: oxy 5 mg/*ibu* 400*mg

➤ *oxycodone/naloxone* (C)(II) <14 years: not recommended; ≥14 years: 1 tab q 3-4
hours prn
Targiniq
  Tab: Targiniq 10/5 *oxy* 10 mg/*nal* 5 mg
        Targiniq 20/10 *oxy* 20 mg/*nal* 10 mg
        Targiniq 40/20 *oxy* 40 mg/*nal* 20 mg

➤ *oxymorphone* (C)(II)(G) <18 years: not recommended; ≥18 years:
Numorphan 1 supp q 4-6 hours prn
  Rectal supp: 5 mg; *Vial:* 1 mg/ml (1 ml), *Amp:* 1.5 mg/ml (10 ml);
  Comment: Store in refrigerator in original package. 1 mg of **Numorphan** is
  approximately equivalent in analgesic activity to 10 mg of ***morphine sulfate***.
Opana 1-1 tab q 4-6 hours prn
  Tab: 5, 10 mg
Opana ER 1 tab q 12 hours prn
  Tab: 5, 7.5, 10, 15, 20, 30, 40 mg ext-rel crush-resistant
Opana Injection initially 0.5 mg IV or IM; 1 x 1 mg IM or IV q 4-6 hours prn
  Amp: 1 mg/ml (1 ml) (paraben/sodium dithionite-free)

➤ *pentazocine/aspirin* (D)(IV) <18 years: not recommended; ≥18 years: 2 cplts tid or
qid prn
Talwin Compound *Cplt: pent* 12.5 mg/*asp* 325 mg

➤ *pentazocine/naloxone* (C)(IV) <12 years: not recommended; ≥12 years: 1 tab q 3-4
hours prn
Talwin NX *Tab: pent* 50 mg/*nal* 0.5*mg

➤ *pentazocine lactate* (C)(IV) <1 year: not recommended; >1 year: 0.5 mg/kg IM 30
mg IM, SC, or IV q 3-4 hours; max 360 mg/day
Talwin Injectable *Amp:* 30 mg/ml (1, 1.5, 2 ml)

➤ *propoxyphene napsylate/acetaminophen* (C)(IV)(G)
  Comment: Max 4 gm acetaminophen per day.

Balacet 325 <12 year: not recommended; ≥12 year: 0.5 mg/kg IM 1 tab q 4 hours prn; max 6 tabs/day

Tab: prop 100 mg/*acet* 325 mg

➤ *tramadol* (C)(IV)(G)

Comment: *Tramadol* is known to be excreted in breast milk. The FDA and the European Medicines Agency (EMA) are investigating the safety of using *tramadol*-containing medications to treat pain in children 12-18 years because of the potential for serious side effects, including slowed or difficult breathing.

Rybix ODT <12 years: contraindicated; 12-<18: use extreme caution; not recommended for children and adolescents with obesity, asthma, obstructive sleep apnea, or other chronic breathing problem, or for post-tonsillectomy/adenoidectomy pain; ≥18 years: initially 100 mg once daily; may increase by 100 mg every 5 days; max 300 mg/day; *CrCl <30 mL/min* or *severe hepatic impairment:* not recommended; *Cirrhosis:* max 50 mg q 12 hours

ODT: 50 mg (mint) (phenylalanine)

Ryzolt <12 years: contraindicated; 12-<18: use extreme caution; not recommended for children and adolescents with obesity, asthma, obstructive sleep apnea, or other chronic breathing problem, or for post-tonsillectomy/adenoidectomy pain; ≥18 years: initially 100 mg once daily; may increase by 100 mg every 5 days; max 300 mg/day; *CrCl <30 mL/min* or *severe hepatic impairment:* not recommended

Tab: 100, 200, 300 mg ext-rel

Ultram <12 years: contraindicated; 12-<18: use extreme caution; not recommended for children and adolescents with obesity, asthma, obstructive sleep apnea, or other chronic breathing problem, or for post-tonsillectomy/adenoidectomy pain; ≥18 years: 50-100 mg q 4-6 hours prn; max 400 mg/day; *CrCl <30 mL/min:* max 100 mg q 12 hours; *Cirrhosis:* max 50 mg q 12 hours

Tab: 50*mg

Ultram ER <12 years: contraindicated; 12-<18: use extreme caution; not recommended for children and adolescents with obesity, asthma, obstructive sleep apnea, or other chronic breathing problem, or for post-tonsillectomy/adenoidectomy pain; ≥18 years: initially 100 mg once daily; may increase by 100 mg every 5 days; max 300 mg/day; *CrCl <30 mL/min:* or *severe hepatic impairment:* not recommended

Tab: 100, 200, 300 mg ext-rel

➤ *tramadol/acetaminophen* (C)(IV)(G) <12 years: contraindicated; 12-<18: use extreme caution; not recommended for children and adolescents with obesity, asthma, obstructive sleep apnea, or other chronic breathing problem, or for post-tonsillectomy/adenoidectomy pain; ≥18 years: 2 tabs q 4-6 hours; max 8 tabs/day; 5 days; *CrCl <30 mL/min:* max 2 tabs q 12 hours; max 4 tabs/day x 5 days

Ultracet *Tab: tram* 37.5/*acet* 325 mg

Comment: *Tramadol* is known to be excreted in breast milk. The FDA and the European Medicines Agency (EMA) are investigating the safety of using *tramadol*-containing medications to treat pain in children 12-18 years because of the potential for serious side effects, including slowed or difficult breathing.

➤ *buprenorphine* (C)(III) <16 years: not recommended; ≥16 years: change patch every 7 days; do not increase the dose until previous dose has been worn for at least 72 hours; after removal, do not reuse the site for at least 3 weeks; do not expose the patch to heat

Butrans Transdermal System *Transdermal patch:* 5, 10, 20 mcg/hour (4/pck)
▶ *fentanyl* transdermal system (C)(II) <16 years or <110 lb: not recommended; ≥16 years or ≥110 lb: apply to clean, dry, non-irritated, intact, skin; hold in place for 30 seconds; start at lowest dose and titrate upward; *Opioid-naïve:* change patch every 3 days (72 hours)

Duragesic *Transdermal patch:* 12, 25, 37.5, 50, 62.5, 75, 87.5, 100 mcg/hour (5/pck)

TRANSMUCOSAL OPIOID

Comment: For chronic severe pain. For management of breakthrough pain in patients with cancer who are already receiving and who are tolerant to opioid therapy. Opioid-tolerant patients are those taking oral *morphine* ≥60 mg/day, transdermal *fentanyl* ≥25 mcg/hr, *oxycodone* ≥30 mg/day, oral *hydromorphone* ≥8 mg/day, or an equianalgesic dose of another opioid, for ≥1 week

OPIOID PARTIAL AGONIST-ANTAGONIST

▶ *buprenorphine* (C)

Subutex <16 years: not recommended; ≥16 years: 8 mg in a single dose on day 1; then 16 mg in a single dose on day 2; target dose is 16 mg/day in a single dose; dissolve under tongue; do not chew or swallow whole

SL tab (lemon-lime) or *SL film (lime):* 2, 8 mg (30/pck)

Comment: The Transmucosal Immediate Release **Fentanyl** (TIRF) Risk Evaluation and Mitigation Strategy (REMS) program is an FDA-required program designed to ensure informed risk-benefit decisions before initiating treatment, and while patients are treated to ensure appropriate use of TIRF medicines. The purpose of the TIRF REMS Access program is to mitigate the risk of misuse, abuse, addiction, overdose and serious complications due to medication errors with the use of TIRF medicines. You must enroll in the TIRF REMS Access program to prescribe, dispense, or distribute TIRF medicines. To register, call the TIRF REMS Access program at 1-866-822-1483 or register online at https://www.tirfremsaccess.com/TirfUI/rems/home.action

▶ *fentanyl* buccal soluble film (C)(II) <18 years: not recommended; ≥18 years: dissolve 1 film on moistened area inside cheek; initially 200 mcg; no more than 4 doses/day at least 2 hours apart; max 1200 mcg/dose; do not cut film

Onsolis *Buccal film:* 200, 400, 600, 800, 1200 mcg (30 films/pck)

Comment: The Transmucosal Immediate Release **Fentanyl** (TIRF) Risk Evaluation and Mitigation Strategy (REMS) program is an FDA-required program designed to ensure informed risk-benefit decisions before initiating treatment, and while patients are treated to ensure appropriate use of TIRF medicines. The purpose of the TIRF REMS Access program is to mitigate the risk of misuse, abuse, addiction, overdose and serious complications due to medication errors with the use of TIRF medicines. You must enroll in the TIRF REMS Access program to prescribe, dispense, or distribute TIRF medicines. To register, call the TIRF REMS Access program at 1-866-822-1483 or register online at https://www.tirfremsaccess.com/TirfUI/rems/home.action

▶ *fentanyl citrate* transmucosal unit (C)(II)(G) <18 years: not recommended; ≥18 years: initially one 200 mcg unit placed between cheek and lower gum; move from side to side; suck (not chew); use 6 units before titrating; titrate dose as needed; max 4 units/day

Actiq *Unit:* 200, 400, 600, 800, 1,200, 1,600 mcg (24 units/pck)

Fentora *Unit:* 100, 200, 400, 600, 800 mcg (24 units/pck)

Comment: The Transmucosal Immediate Release **Fentanyl** (TIRF) Risk Evaluation and Mitigation Strategy (REMS) program is an FDA-required program designed to ensure informed risk-benefit decisions before initiating treatment, and while patients are treated to ensure appropriate use of TIRF medicines. The purpose of the TIRF REMS Access program is to mitigate the risk of misuse, abuse, addiction, overdose and serious complications due to medication errors with the use of TIRF medicines. You must enroll in the TIRF REMS Access program to prescribe, dispense, or distribute TIRF medicines. To register, call the TIRF REMS Access program at 1-866-822-1483 or register online at https://www.tirfremsaccess.com/TirfUI/rems/home.action

➤ *fentanyl* sublingual tab (C)(II) <18 years: not recommended; ≥18 years: initially one 100 mcg dose; if inadequate after 30 minutes, may repeat; titrate in increments of 100 mcg; max 2 doses per episode, up to 4 episodes per day; wait at least 2 hours before treating another episode; *Maintenance:* use only one tablet of appropriate strength; do not chew, suck, or swallow tablets; do not convert from other *fentanyl* products on a mcg-per-mcg basis or interchange with other *fentanyl* products

Abstral *SL tab:* 100, 200, 300, 400, 600, 800 mcg (32 tabs/pck)

Comment: The Transmucosal Immediate Release **Fentanyl** (TIRF) Risk Evaluation and Mitigation Strategy (REMS) program is an FDA-required program designed to ensure informed risk-benefit decisions before initiating treatment, and while patients are treated to ensure appropriate use of TIRF medicines. The purpose of the TIRF REMS Access program is to mitigate the risk of misuse, abuse, addiction, overdose and serious complications due to medication errors with the use of TIRF medicines. You must enroll in the TIRF REMS Access program to prescribe, dispense, or distribute TIRF medicines. To register, call the TIRF REMS Access program at 1-866-822-1483 or register online at https://www.tirfremsaccess.com/TirfUI/rems/home.action

➤ *fentanyl sublingual spray* (C)(II) <18 years: not recommended; ≥18 years:

Subsys 100, 200, 400, 600, 800 mcg/S L spray

Comment: **Subsys** is not bioequivalent with other *fentanyl* products. Do not convert patients from other *fentanyl* products to **Subsys** on a mcg-per-mcg basis. There are no conversion directions available for patients on any other *fentanyl* products other than **Actiq**. (Note: This includes oral, transdermal, or parenteral formulations of *fentanyl*.) The Transmucosal Immediate Release **Fentanyl** (TIRF) Risk Evaluation and Mitigation Strategy (REMS) program is an FDA-required program designed to ensure informed risk-benefit decisions before initiating treatment, and while patients are treated to ensure appropriate use of TIRF medicines. The purpose of the TIRF REMS Access program is to mitigate the risk of misuse, abuse, addiction, overdose and serious complications due to medication errors with the use of TIRF medicines. You must enroll in the TIRF REMS Access program to prescribe, dispense, or distribute TIRF medicines. To register, call the TIRF REMS Access program at 1-866-822-1483 or register online at https://www.tirfremsaccess.com/TirfUI/rems/home.action

PARENTERAL OPIOID AGONIST/ANTAGONIST

▷ *nalbuphine* (B)(G) <18 years: not recommended; ≥18 years: 10 mg/70 kg IM, SC, or IV q 3-6 hours prn
  Nubain *Amp:* 10, 20 mg/ml (1 ml) (sulfite-free, parabens-free)
▷ *pentazocine/naloxone* (C)(IV) <12 years: not recommended; ≥12 years: 1-2 tabs q 3-4 hours prn; max 12 tabs/day
  Talwin-NX *Tab: pent* 50 mg/*nal* 0.5*mg

INTRANASAL TRANSMUCOSAL NARCOTIC ANALGESICS

▷ *butorphanol tartrate* nasal spray(C)(IV) <18 years: not recommended; ≥18 years: initially 1 spray (1 mg) in one nostril and may repeat after 60-90 minutes in opposite nostril if needed or 1 spray in each nostril and may repeat q 3-4 hours prn
  Butorphanol Nasal Spray *Nasal spray:* 1 mg/actuation (10 mg/ml, 2.5 ml)
  Stadol Nasal Spray *Nasal spray:* 1 mg/actuation (10 mg/ml, 2.5 ml)
▷ *fentanyl* nasal spray (C)(II) <18 years: not recommended; ≥18 years: initially 1 spray (100 mcg) in one nostril and may repeat after 2 hours; when adequate analgesia is achieved, use that dose for subsequent breakthrough episodes; *Titration steps:* 100 mcg using 1 x 100 mcg spray; 200 mcg using 2 x 100 mcg spray (1 spray in each nostril); 400 mcg using 1 x 400 mcg spray; 800 mcg using 2 x 400 mcg spray (1 spray in each nostril); max 800 mcg; limit to ≤4 doses per day
  Lazanda Nasal Spray *Nasal spray:* 100, 400 mcg/100 mcl (8 sprays/bottle)
  Comment: **Lazanda Nasal Spray** is available by restricted distribution program. Call 855-841-4234 or visit https://www.fda.gov/downloads/drugs/drugsafety/ postmarketdrugsafetyinformationforpatientsandproviders/ucm261983.pdf to enroll. **Lazanda Nasal Spray** is indicated for the management of breakthrough pain in cancer patients who are already receiving and who are tolerant to opioid therapy for their underlying persistent cancer pain. Patients considered opioid tolerant are those who are taking at least 60 mg of oral morphine/day, 25 mcg of transdermal *fentanyl*/hour, 30 mg oral *oxycodone*/day, 8 mg oral *hydromorphone*/day, or 25 mg oral *oxymorphone*/day, or an equianalgesic dose of another opioid for a week or longer. Patients must remain on around-the-clock opioids when using **Lazanda Nasal Spray**. As such, it is contraindicated in the management of acute or post-op pain, including headache/migraine, or dental pain.
  Comment: The Transmucosal Immediate Release **Fentanyl** (TIRF) Risk Evaluation and Mitigation Strategy (REMS) program is an FDA-required program designed to ensure informed risk-benefit decisions before initiating treatment, and while patients are treated to ensure appropriate use of TIRF medicines. The purpose of the TIRF REMS Access program is to mitigate the risk of misuse, abuse, addiction, overdose and serious complications due to medication errors with the use of TIRF medicines. You must enroll in the TIRF REMS Access program to prescribe, dispense, or distribute TIRF medicines. To register, call the TIRF REMS Access program at 1-866-822-1483 or register online at https://www.tirfremsaccess.com/ TirfUI/rems/home.action

INTRATHECAL NARCOTIC ANALGESICS

▷ *ziconotide* intrathecal (IT) infusion (C) <12 years: not recommended; ≥12 years: initially no more than 2.4 mcg/day (0.1 mcg/hour) and titrate to upward by up to

2.4 mcg/day (0.1 mcg/day at intervals of no more than 2-3 times per week, up to a recommended maximum of 19.2 mcg/day (0.8 mcg/hr) by Day 21; dose increases in increments of less than 2.4 mcg/day (0.1 mcg/hr) and increases in dose less frequently than 2-3 times per week may be used.

Prialt *Vial:* 25 mcg/ml (20 ml), 100 mcg/ml (1, 2, 5 ml)

Comment: Patients with a pre-existing history of psychosis should not be treated with *ziconotide*. Contraindications to the use of IT analgesia include conditions such as the presence of infection at the microinfusion injection site, uncontrolled bleeding diathesis, and spinal canal obstruction that impairs circulation of CSF.

PANCREATIC ENZYME DEFICIENCY

Comment: Seen in chronic pancreatitis, post-pancreatectomy, cystic fibrosis, steatorrhea, post-GI tract bypass surgery, and ductal obstruction from neoplasia. May sprinkle cap; however, do not crush or chew cap or tab. May mix with applesauce or other acidic food; follow with water or juice. Do not let any drug remain in mouth. Take dose just prior to each meal or snack. Base dose on lipase units; adjust per diet and clinical response (i.e., steatorrhea). Pancrelipase products are interchangeable. Contraindicated with pork protein hypersensitivity.

PANCRELIPASE PRODUCTS

➤ *pancreatic enzymes* (C)

Creon <12 months: 2,000-4,000 units per 120 ml formula or per breast-feeding (do not mix directly into formula or breast milk; 12 months-4 years: 1,000 units/kg per meal; max 2,500 units/kg per meal <10,000 units/kg per day; >4 years: 500 units/kg per meal; max 2,500 units/kg per meal or <10,000 units/kg per day or <4,000 units/g fat ingested per day

Cap: **Creon 3000** *lip* 3,000 units/*pro* 9,500 units/*amyl* 15,000 units del-rel
Creon 6000 *lip* 6,000 units/*pro* 19,000 units/*amyl* 30,000 units del-rel
Creon 12000 *lip* 12,000 units/*pro* 38,000 units/amyl 60,000 units del-rel
Creon 24000 *lip* 24,000 units/*pro* 76,000 units/*amyl* 120,000 units del-rel
Creon 36000 *lip* 36,000 units/*pro* 114,000 units/*amyl* 180,000 units del-rel

Cotazym <12 years: not recommended; ≥12 years: 1-3 tabs just prior to each meal or snack

Tab: **Cotazym** *lip* 1,000 units/*pro* 12,500 units/*amyl* 12,500 units del-rel
Cotazym-S *lip* 5,000 units/*pro* 20,000 units/*amyl* 20,000 units del-rel

Donnazyme <12 years: not recommended; ≥12 years: 1-3 caps just prior to each meal or snack

Cap: **Donnazyme** *lip* 5,000 units/*pro* 20,000 units/*amyl* 20,000 units del-rel

Ku-Zyme 1-2 caps just prior to each meal or snack

Cap: **Ku-Zyme:** *lip* 12,000 units/*pro* 15,000 units/*amyl* 15,000 units del-rel

Kutrase <12 years: not recommended; ≥12 years: 1-2 caps just prior to each meal or snack

Cap: **Kutrase:** *lip* 12,000 units/*pro* 30,000 units/*amyl* 30,000 units del-rel

Pancreaze <12 months: 2,000-4,000 lipase units per 120 ml formula or per breastfeeding; ≥12 months-<4 years: 1,000 lipase units/kg per meal; 4-12 years: 500 lipase units/kg per meal; >12 years: 2,500 lipase units/kg per meal or <10,000 lipase units/kg per day or <4,000 lipase units/gram fat ingested per day

Cap: **Pancreaze 4200** *lip* 4,200 units/*pro* 10,000 units/*amyl* 17,500 units ec-microtabs

> **Pancreaze 10500** *lip* 10,500 units/*pro* 25,000 units/*amyl* 43,750 units ec microtabs
>
> **Pancreaze 16800** *lip* 16,800 units/*pro* 40,000 units/*amyl* 70,000 units ec-microtabs
>
> **Pancreaze 21000** *lip* 21,000 units/*pro* 37,000 units/*amyl* 61,000 units ec-microtabs

Pertyze 12 months-4 years and ≥8 kg: initially 1,000 lipase units/kg per meal; ≥4 years and ≥16 kg: initially 500 lipase units/kg per meal; *Both:* 2,500 lipase units/kg per meal or <10,000 units/kg per day or <4,000 lipase units/g fat ingested per day

Cap: **Pertyze 8000** *lip* 8,000 units/*pro* 28,750 units *amyl* 30,250 units del-rel
Pertyze 16000 *lip* 16,000 units/*pro* 57,500 units/*amyl* 65,000 units del-rel

Ultrase 1-3 tabs just prior to each meal or snack

Cap: **Ultrase** *lip* 4,500 units/*pro* 20,000 units/*amyl* 25,000 units del-rel
> **Ultrase MT** *lip* 12,000 units/*pro* 39,000 units/*amyl* 39,000 units del-rel
>
> **Ultrase MT 18** *lip* 18,000 units/*pro* 58,500 units/*amyl* 58,500 units del-rel
>
> **Ultrase MT 20** *lip* 20,000 units/*pro* 65,000 units/*amyl* 65,000 units del-rel

Viokace <12 years: not established; ≥12 years: initially 500 lip units/kg per meal; max 2,500 lipase units/kg per meal, or <10,000 lipase units/kg per meal, or <4,000 units/g fat ingested per day

Tab: **Viokace 8** *lip* 8,000 units/*pro* 30,000 units/*amyl* 30,000 units
> **Viokace 16** *lip* 16,000 units/*pro* 60,000 units *amyl* 60,000 units
>
> **Viokace 10440** *lip* 10,440 units/*pro* 39,150 units *amyl* 39,150 units
>
> **Viokace 20880** *lip* 20,880 units/*pro* 78,300 units *amyl* 78,300 units
>
> Comment: **Viokace 10440** and **Viokace 20880** should be taken with a daily proton pump inhibitor.
>
> **Viokace Powder** 1/4 tsp (0.7 gm) with meals
>
> **Viokace Powder** *lip* 16,800 units/*pro* 70,000 units/*amyl* 70,000 units per ¼ tsp (8 oz)

Zenpep <12 months: 2,000-4,000 units per 120 ml formula or per breast feeding (do not mix directly into formula or breast milk); 12 months-4 years: 1,000 units/kg per meal; max 2,500 units/kg per meal <10,000 units/kg per day; >4 years: 500 units/kg per meal; max 2,500 units/kg per meal or <10,000 units/kg per day or <4,000 units/g fat ingested per day

Cap: **Zenpep 5000** *lip* 5,000 units/*pro* 17,000 units/*amyl* 27,000 units del-rel
> **Zenpep 10000** *lip* 10,000 units/*pro* 34,000 units/*amyl* 55,000 units del-rel
>
> **Zenpep 15000** *lip* 15,000 units/*pro* 51,000 units/*amyl* 82,000 units del-rel
>
> **Zenpep 20000** *lip* 20,000 units/*pro* 68,000 units/*amyl* 109,000 units del-rel

Zymase <12 years: not recommended; ≥12 years: 1-3 caps just prior to each meal or snack

Cap: **Zymase** *lip* 12,000 units/*prot* 24,000 units/*amyl* 24,000 units del-rel

PANIC DISORDER

Comment: If possible when considering a benzodiazepine to treat anxiety, a short-acting benzodiazepines should be used only prn to avert intense anxiety and panic for the least time necessary while a different non-addictive antianxiety regimen (e.g., SSRI, SNRI, TCA, buspirone, beta-blocker) is established and effective treatment goals achieved. Co-administration of SSRIs with TCAs requires extreme caution. Concomitant use of MAOIs and SSRIs is absolutely contraindicated. Avoid other serotonergic drugs. A potentially fatal adverse event is *serotonin syndrome,* caused by serotonin excess. Milder symptoms require HCP intervention to avert severe symptoms that can be rapidly fatal without urgent/emergent medical care. Symptoms include restlessness, agitation, confusion, hallucinations, tachycardia, hypertension, dilated pupils, muscle twitching, muscle rigidity, loss of muscle coordination, diaphoresis, diarrhea, headache, shivering, piloerection, hyperpyrexia, cardiac arrhythmias, seizures, loss of consciousness, coma, death. Abrupt withdrawal or interruption of treatment with an antidepressant medication is sometimes associated with an *antidepressant discontinuation syndrome,* which may be mediated by gradually tapering the drug over a period of two weeks or longer, depending on the dose strength and length of treatment. Common symptoms of the *serotonin discontinuation syndrome* include flu-like symptoms (nausea, vomiting, diarrhea, headaches, sweating), sleep disturbances (insomnia, nightmares, constant sleepiness), mood disturbances (dysphoria, anxiety, agitation), cognitive disturbances (mental confusion, hyperarousal), sensory and movement disturbances (imbalance, tremors, vertigo, dizziness, electric shock-like sensations in the brain, often described by sufferers as "brain zaps").

SELECTIVE SEROTONIN REUPTAKE INHIBITORS (SSRIs)

➤ *citalopram* (C)(G) <12 years: not recommended; ≥12 years: initially 20 mg once daily; may increase after one week to 40 mg once daily; max 40 mg
  Celexa *Tab:* 10, 20, 40 mg; *Oral soln:* 10 mg/5 ml (120 ml) (pepper mint)(sugar-free, alcohol-free, parabens)

➤ *escitalopram* (C)(G) <12 years: not recommended; 12-17 years: initially 10 mg daily; may increase to 20 mg daily after 3 weeks; >17 years: initially 10 mg daily; may increase to 20 mg daily after 1 week; *Hepatic impairment:* 10 mg once daily
  Lexapro *Tab:* 5, 10*, 20*mg
  Lexapro Oral Solution *Oral soln:* 1 mg/ml (240 ml) (peppermint) (parabens)

➤ *fluoxetine* (C)(G)
  Prozac <8 years: not recommended; 8-17 years: initially 10 mg/day; may increase after 1 week to 20 mg/day; range 20-60 mg/day; range for lower weight children, 20-30 mg/day; >17 years: initially 20 mg daily; may increase after 1 week; doses >20 mg/day should be divided into AM and noon doses; max 80 mg/day
    Cap: 10, 20, 40 mg; *Tab:* 30*, 60*mg; *Oral soln:* 20 mg/5 ml (4 oz) (mint)
  Prozac Weekly <12 years: not recommended; ≥12 years: following daily *fluoxetine* therapy at 20 mg/day for 13 weeks, may initiate **Prozac Weekly** 7 days after the last 20 mg *fluoxetine* dose
    Cap: 90 mg ent-coat del-rel pellets

▶ *levomilnacipran* (C) <12 years: not recommended; ≥12 years: swallow whole; initially 20 mg once daily for 2 days; then increase to 40 mg once daily; may increase dose in 40 mg increments at intervals of ≥2 days; max 120 mg once daily; *CrCl 30-59 mL/min:* max 80 mg once daily; *CrCl 15-29 mL/min:* max 40 mg once daily
    Fetzima *Cap:* 20, 40, 80, 120 mg ext-rel

▶ *paroxetine maleate* (D)(G)
    Paxil <12 years: not recommended; ≥12 years: initially 20 mg daily in AM; may increase by 10 mg/day at weekly intervals as needed; max 60 mg/day
        Tab: 10*, 20*, 30, 40 mg
    Paxil CR <12 years: not recommended; ≥12 years: initially 25 mg daily in AM; may increase by 12.5 mg at weekly intervals as needed; max 62.5 mg/day
        Tab: 12.5, 25, 37.5 mg cont-rel ent-coat
    Paxil Suspension <12 years: not recommended; ≥12 years: initially 20 mg daily in AM; may increase by 10 mg/day at weekly intervals as needed; max 60 mg/day
        Oral susp: 10 mg/5 ml (250 ml) (orange)

▶ *sertraline* (C)(G) <6 years: not recommended; 6-<12 years: initially 25 mg daily; max 200 mg/day; 12-17 years: initially 50 mg daily; max 200 mg/day ≥17 years: initially 50 mg daily; increase at 1 week intervals if needed; max 200 mg daily; dilute oral concentrate immediately prior to administration in 4 oz water, ginger ale, lemon/lime soda, lemonade, or orange juice
    Zoloft *Tab:* 25*, 50*, 100*mg; *Oral conc:* 20 mg per ml (60 ml) (alcohol 12%)

SEROTONIN-NOREPINEPHRINE REUPTAKE INHIBITORS (SNRIs)

▶ *desvenlafaxine* (C)(G) <18 years: not recommended; ≥18 years: swallow whole; initially 50 mg once daily; max 120 mg/day
    Pristiq *Tab:* 50, 100 mg ext-rel

▶ *duloxetine* (C)(G) <12 years: not recommended; ≥12 years: swallow whole; initially 30 mg once daily x 1 week; then, increase to 60 mg once daily; max 120 mg/day
    Cymbalta *Cap:* 20, 30, 40, 60 mg del-rel

▶ *venlafaxine* (C)(G)
    Effexor initially <12 years: not recommended; ≥12 years: 75 mg/day in 2-3 divided doses; may increase at 4 day intervals in 75 mg increments to 150 mg/day; max 225 mg/day
        Tab: 37.5, 75, 150, 225 mg
    Effexor XR <18 years: not recommended; ≥18 years: initially 75 mg q AM; may start at 37.5 mg daily x 4-7 days, then increase by increments of up to 75 mg/day at intervals of at least 4 days; usual max 375 mg/day
        Tab/Cap: 37.5, 75, 150 mg ext-rel

▶ *vortioxetine* (C) <18 years: not established; ≥18 years: initially 10 mg once daily; max 30 mg/day
    Brintellix *Tab:* 5, 10, 15, 20 mg

TRICYCLIC ANTIDEPRESSANTS (TCAs)

Comment: Co-administration of SSRIs and TCAs requires extreme caution.

▶ *amitriptyline* (C)(G) <12 years: not recommended; ≥12 years: 10-20 mg q HS *Tab:* 10, 25, 50, 75, 100, 150 mg

▶ *amoxapine* (C) <12 years: not recommended; ≥12 years: initially 50 mg bid-tid; after 1 week may increase to 100 mg bid-tid; usual effective dose 200-300 mg/day; if total dose exceeds 300 mg/day, give in divided doses (max 400 mg/day); may give as a single bedtime dose (max 300 mg q HS)

Tab: 25, 50, 100, 150 mg

▷ *clomipramine* (C)(G) <10 years: not recommended; 10-<16 years: initially 25 mg daily in divided doses; gradually increase; max 3 mg/kg or 100 mg, whichever is smaller; >16 years: initially 25 mg daily in divided doses; gradually increase to 100 mg during first 2 weeks; max 250 mg/day; total maintenance dose may be given at HS

Anafranil *Cap:* 25, 50, 75 mg

▷ *desipramine* (C)(G) <12 years: not recommended; ≥12 years: 100-200 mg/day in single or divided doses; max 300 mg/day

Norpramin *Tab:* 10, 25, 50, 75, 100, 150 mg

▷ *doxepin* (C)(G) <12 years: not recommended; ≥12 years: 75 mg/day; max 150 mg/day

Cap: 10, 25, 50, 75, 100, 150 mg; Oral conc: 10 mg/ml (4 oz w. dropper)

▷ *imipramine* (C)(G) <12 years: not recommended; ≥12 years:

Tofranil initially 75 mg daily (max 200 mg); adolescents initially 30-40 mg daily (max 100 mg/day); if maintenance dose exceeds 75 mg daily, may switch to **Tofranil PM** for divided or bedtime dose

Tab: 10, 25, 50 mg

Tofranil PM initially 75 mg daily 1 hour before HS; max 200 mg

Cap: 75, 100, 125, 150 mg

▷ *nortriptyline* (D)(G) <12 years: not recommended; ≥12 years: initially 25 mg tid-qid; max 150 mg/day

Pamelor *Cap:* 10, 25, 50, 75 mg; *Oral soln:* 10 mg/5 ml (16 oz)

▷ *protriptyline* (C) <12 years: not recommended; ≥12 years: initially 5 mg tid; usual dose 15-40 mg/day in 3-4 divided doses; max 60 mg/day

Vivactil *Tab:* 5, 10 mg

▷ *trimipramine* (C) <12 years: not recommended; ≥12 years: initially 75 mg/day in divided doses; max 200 mg/day

Surmontil *Cap:* 25, 50, 100 mg

1ST GENERATION ANTIHISTAMINE

▷ *hydroxyzine* (C)(G) <6 years: 50 mg/day divided qid; 6-12 years: 50-100 mg/day divided qid; >12 years: 50-100 mg qid; max 600 mg/day

Atarax *Tab:* 10, 25, 50, 100 mg; *Syr:* 10 mg/5 ml (alcohol 0.5%)

Vistaril *Cap:* 25, 50, 100 mg; *Oral susp:* 25 mg/5 ml (4 oz) (lemon)

Comment: *hydroxyzine* is contraindicated in early pregnancy and in patients with a prolonged QT interval. It is not known whether this drug is excreted in human milk; therefore, *hydroxyzine* should not be given to nursing mothers.

AZAPIRONE

▷ *buspirone* (B) <6 years: not recommended; ≥6 years: initially 7.5 mg bid; may increase by 5 mg/day q 2-3 days; max 60 mg/day

BuSpar *Tab:* 5, 10, 15*, 30* mg

BENZODIAZEPINES

Short Acting

▷ *alprazolam* (D)(IV)(G)

Niravam <18 years: not recommended; ≥18 years: initially 0.25-0.5 mg tid; may titrate every 3-4 days; max 4 mg/day

Tab: 0.25*, 0.5*, 1*, 2*mg orally-disint

Xanax <18 years: not recommended; ≥18 years: initially 0.25-0.5 mg tid; may titrate every 3-4 days; max 4 mg/day

Tab: 0.25*, 0.5*, 1*, 2*mg

Xanax XR <18 years: not recommended; ≥18 years: initially 0.5-1 mg once daily, preferably in the AM; increase at intervals of at least 3-4 days by up to 1 mg/day; taper no faster than 0.5 mg every 3 days; max 10 mg/day; when switching from immed-rel to ext-rel *alprazolam*, once daily dose of ext-rel equals total daily dose of immed-rel

Tab: 0.5, 1, 2, 3 mg ext-rel

▷ *oxazepam* (C)(IV)(G) <12 years: not recommended; ≥12 years: 10-15 mg tid-qid for moderate symptoms; 15-30 mg tid-qid for severe symptoms

Tab: 15 mg; *Cap:* 10, 15, 30 mg

Intermediate Acting

▷ *lorazepam* (D)(IV)(G) <18 years: not recommended; ≥18 years: 1-10 mg/day in 2-3 divided doses

Ativan *Tab:* 0.5, 1*, 2*mg

Lorazepam Intensol *Oral conc:* 2 mg/ml (30 ml w. graduated dropper)

Long Acting

▷ *chlordiazepoxide* (D)(IV)(G)

Librium <6 years: not recommended; ≥6 years: 5 mg bid-qid; may increase to 10 mg bid-tid; *Moderate symptoms:* 5-10 mg tid-qid; *Severe symptoms:* 20-25 mg tid-qid

Cap: 5, 10, 25 mg

Librium Injectable <18 years: not recommended; ≥18 years: 50-100 mg IM or IV; then 25-50 mg IM tid-qid prn; max 300 mg/day

Inj: 100 mg

▷ *chlordiazepoxide/clidinium* (D)(IV) <18 years: not recommended; ≥18 years: 1-2 caps tid-qid: max 8 caps/day

Librax *Cap: chlor* 5 mg/*clid* 2.5 mg

▷ *clonazepam* (D)(IV)(G) <18 years: not recommended; ≥18 years: initially 0.25 mg bid; increase to 1 mg/day after 3 days

Klonopin *Tab:* 0.5*, 1, 2 mg

Klonopin Wafers dissolve in mouth with or without water

Wafer: 0.125, 0.25, 0.5, 1, 2 mg orally-disint

▷ *clorazepate* (D)(IV)(G) <9 years: not recommended; ≥9 years: 30 mg/day in divided doses; max 60 mg/day

Tranxene *Tab:* 3.75, 7.5, 15 mg

Tranxene SD do not use for initial therapy

Tab: 22.5 mg ext-rel

Tranxene SD Half Strength do not use for initial therapy

Tab: 11.25 mg ext-rel

Tranxene T-Tab *Tab:* 3.75*, 7.5*, 15*mg

▷ *diazepam* (D)(IV)(G) <12 years: not recommended; ≥12 years: 2-10 mg bid to qid

Diastat *Rectal gel delivery system:* 2.5 mg

Diastat AcuDial *Rectal gel delivery system:* 10, 20 mg
Valium *Tab:* 2*, 5*, 10*mg
Valium Injectable *Vial:* 5 mg/ml (10 ml); *Amp:* 5 mg/ml (2 ml); *Prefilled syringe:* 5 mg/ml (5 ml)
Valium Intensol Oral Solution *Conc oral soln:* 5 mg/ml (30 ml w. dropper) (alcohol 19%)
Valium Oral Solution *Oral soln:* 5 mg/5 ml (500 ml) (wintergreen spice)

PHENOTHIAZINES

▷ *prochlorperazine* (C)(G) **Compazine** <12 years: not recommended; ≥12 years: 5 mg tid-qid
  Tab: 5 mg; *Syr:* 5 mg/5 ml (4 oz) (fruit); *Rectal supp:* 2.5, 5, 25 mg
  Compazine Spansule <12 years: not recommended; ≥12 years: 15 mg q AM <u>or</u> 10 mg q 12 hours
  Spansule: 10, 15 mg sust-rel
▷ *trifluoperazine* (C)(G) <12 years: not recommended; ≥12 years: 1-2 mg bid; max 6 mg/day; max 12 weeks
  Stelazine *Tab:* 1, 2, 5, 10 mg

PARONYCHIA (PERIUNGUAL ABSCESS)

▷ *cephalexin* (B)(G) <12 years: 25-50 mg/kg/day in 4 divided doses x 10 days; *see page 557 for dose by weight table;* ≥12 years: mg bid x 10 days
  Keflex *Cap:* 250, 333, 500, 750 mg; *Oral susp:* 125, 250 mg/5 ml (100, 200 ml) (strawberry)
▷ *clindamycin* (B)(G) <12 years: 8-16 mg/kg/day in 3-4 divided doses x 10 days; *see page 559 for dose by weight table;* ≥12 years: 150-300 mg q 6 hours x 10 days
  Cleocin *Cap:* 75 (tartrazine), 150 (tartrazine), 300 mg
  Cleocin Pediatric Granules *Oral susp:* 75 mg/5 ml (100 ml) (cherry)
▷ *dicloxacillin* (B)(G) <12 years: 12.5-25 mg/kg/day in 4 divided doses x 10 days; *see page 560 for dose by weight table;* ≥12 years: 500 mg q 6 hours x 10 days
  Dynapen *Cap:* 125, 250, 500 mg; *Oral susp:* 62.5 mg/5 ml (80, 100, 200 ml)
▷ *erythromycin base* (B)(G) <45 kg: 30-50 mg in 2-4 doses x 10 days; ≥45 kg: 500 mg q 6 hours x 10 days
  Ery-Tab *Tab:* 250, 333, 500 mg ent-coat
  PCE *Tab:* 333, 500 mg
▷ *erythromycin ethylsuccinate* (B)(G) <12 years: 30-50 mg/kg/day in 4 divided doses q 6 hours x 10 days; may double dose with severe infection; max 100 mg/kg/day <u>or</u> 400 mg qid; *see page 563 for dose by weight table*
  EryPed *Oral susp:* 200 mg/5 ml (100, 200 ml) (fruit); 400 mg/5 ml (60, 100, 200 ml) (banana); *Oral drops:* 200, 400 mg/5 ml (50 ml) (fruit); *Chew tab:* 200 mg wafer (fruit)
  E.E.S. *Oral susp:* 200, 400 mg/5 ml (100 ml) (fruit)
  E.E.S. Granules *Oral susp:* 200 mg/5 ml (100, 200 ml) (cherry)
  E.E.S. 400 Tablets *Tab:* 400 mg

PEDICULOSIS: PEDICULOSIS HUMANUS CAPITIS (HEAD LICE)/PHTHIRUS (PUBIC LICE)

➤ *ivermectin* (C) <6 months, <33 lbs: not recommended; ≥6 months, ≥33 lbs: same thoroughly wet hair; leave on for 10 minutes; then rinse off with water; do not retreat
Sklice *Lotn:* 0.5% (4 oz, 117 g, laminate tube)

➤ *lindane* (C)(G) <2 years: not recommended; ≥2 years: apply, leave on for 4 minutes, then thoroughly wash off
Kwell Shampoo *Shampoo:* 1% (60 ml)

➤ *malathion* (B)(G) <12 years: not recommended; ≥12 years: thoroughly wet hair; allow to dry naturally; shampoo and rinse after 8-12 hours; use a fine tooth comb to remove lice and nits; if lice persist after 7-9 days, may repeat treatment
Ovide (OTC) *Lotn:* 59% (2 oz)

➤ *permethrin* (B)(G) <2 months: not recommended; ≥2 months: apply to washed and towel-dried hair; allow to remain on for 10 minutes, then rinse off; repeat after 7 days if needed
Nix (OTC) *Crm rinse:* 1% (2 oz w. comb)

➤ *pyrethrins with piperonyl butoxide* (C)(G) <2 months: not recommended; ≥2 months: apply and leave on for 10 minutes, then wash off
A-200 *Shampoo:* pyr 0.33%/pip but 3%
Rid Mousse *Shampoo:* pyr 0.33%/pip but 4%
Rid Shampoo *Shampoo:* pyr 0.33%/pip but 3%

Comment: To remove nits, soak hair in equal parts white vinegar and water for 15-20 minutes.

PELVIC INFLAMMATORY DISEASE (PID)

Comment: The following treatment regimens are published in the **2015 CDC Sexually Transmitted Diseases Treatment Guidelines.** Treatment regimens are presented by generic drug name first, followed by information about brands and dose forms. Treat all sexual partners. Because of the high risk for maternal morbidity and preterm delivery, pregnant females who have suspected PID should be hospitalized and treated with parenteral antibiotics. HIV-infected females with PID respond equally well to standard parenteral and antibiotic regimens as HIV-negative females.

OUTPATIENT REGIMENS

Regimen 1

➤ *ceftriaxone* 250 mg IM in a single dose <u>plus</u>
➤ *doxycycline* 100 mg bid x 14 days with <u>or</u> without
➤ *metronidazole* 500 mg PO bid x 14 days

Regimen 2

➤ *cefoxitin* 2 gm IM in a single dose <u>plus</u>
➤ *probenecid* 1 gm PO in a single dose administered concurrently with *doxycycline* 100 mg bid x 14 days with <u>or</u> without
➤ *metronidazole* 500 mg PO bid x 14 days

Regimen 3

▷ Other parenteral third-generation cephalosporin (e.g., **_ceftizoxime_** <u>or</u> **_cefotaxime_**) in a single dose) <u>plus</u>

▷ **_doxycycline_** 100 mg bid x 14 days with <u>or</u> without

▷ **_metronidazole_** 500 mg PO bid x 14 days

DRUG BRANDS AND DOSE FORMS

▷ **_cefoxitin_** (B)(G)
>   **Mefoxin** *Vial:* 1, 2 g

▷ **_ceftriaxone_** (B)(G)
>   **Rocephin** Vials 250, 500 mg: 1, 2 g

▷ **_doxycycline_** (D)(G)
>   **Acticlate** *Tab:* 75, 150** mg
>   **Adoxa** *Tab:* 50, 75, 100, 150 mg ent-coat
>   **Doryx** *Tab:* 50, 75, 100, 150, 200 mg del-rel
>   **Monodox** *Cap:* 50, 75, 100 mg
>   **Oracea** *Cap:* 40 mg del-rel
>   **Vibramycin** *Tab:* 100 mg; *Cap:* 50, 100 mg; *Syr:* 50 mg/5 ml (raspberry-apple) (sulfites); *Oral susp:* 25 mg/5 ml (raspberry)
>   **Vibra-Tab** *Tab:* 100 mg film-coat

Comment: **_doxycycline_** is contraindicated <8 years-of-age, in pregnancy, and lactation (discolors developing tooth enamel). A side effect may be photosensitivity (photophobia). Do not take with antacids, calcium supplements, milk <u>or</u> other dairy, <u>or</u> within 2 hours of taking another drug.

▷ **_metronidazole_** (not for use in 1st; B in 2nd, 3rd)
>   **Flagyl** *Tab:* 250*, 500* mg
>   **Flagyl 375** *Cap:* 375 mg
>   **Flagyl ER** *Tab:* 750 mg ext-rel

Comment: Alcohol is contraindicated during treatment with oral **_metronidazole_** and for 72 hours after therapy due to a possible **_disulfiram_**-like reaction (nausea, vomiting, flushing, headache).

▷ **_probenecid_** (B)(G)
>   **Benemid** *Tab:* 500* mg; *Cap:* 500 mg

PEPTIC ULCER DISEASE (PUD)

Helicobacter pylori **Eradication Regimens** *see page 173*

H2 ANTAGONISTS

▷ **_cimetidine_** (B)(G) <16 years: not recommended; ≥16 years:
>   **Tagamet** 800 mg bid <u>or</u> 400 mg qid; max 2.4 gm/day
>   *Tab:* 300, 400*, 800* mg
>   **Tagamet HB (OTC)** *Prophylaxis:* 1 tab ac; *Treatment:* 1 tab bid
>   *Tab:* 200 mg
>   **Tagamet HB Oral Suspension (OTC)** *Prophylaxis:* 1 tsp ac; *Treatment:* 1 tsp bid
>   *Oral susp:* 200 mg/20 ml (12 oz)
>   **Tagamet Liquid** *Liq:* 300 mg/5 ml (mint-peach) (alcohol 2.8%)

➤ *famotidine* (B)(G) <12 years: 0.5 mg/kg/day q HS or in 2 divided doses; max 40 mg/day; ≥12 years: 20 mg bid or 40 mg q HS; *max 6 weeks*

> **Pepcid** *Tab:* 20, 40 mg; *Oral susp:* 40 mg/5 ml (50 ml)
> **Pepcid AC (OTC)** *Tab/Rapid dissolving tab:* 10 mg
> **Pepcid Complete (OTC)** *Tab: fam* 10 mg/*CaCO$_2$* 800 mg/*Mg hydroxide* 165 mg
> **Pepcid RPD** *Tab:* 20, 40 mg rapid-dissolving

➤ *nizatidine* (B)(G) <12 years: not recommended; ≥12 years: 150 mg bid; max 12 weeks

> **Axid** *Cap:* 150, 300 mg
> **Axid AR (OTC)** 1 tab ac; max 150 mg/day
> *Tab:* 75 mg

➤ *ranitidine* (B)(G) <1 month: not recommended; 1 month-16 years: 2-4 mg/kg/day in 2 divided doses; max 300 mg/day; *Duodenal/Gastric Ulcer:* 2-4 mg/kg/day divided bid; max 300 mg/day; *Erosive Esophagitis:* 5-10 mg/kg/day divided bid; max 300 mg/day; >16 years:

> **Zantac** 150 mg bid or 300 mg q HS
> *Tab:* 150, 300 mg
> **Zantac 75 (OTC)** 1 tab ac
> *Tab:* 75 mg
> **Zantac EFFERdose** dissolve 25 mg tab in 5 ml water; dissolve 150 mg tab in 6-8 oz water
> *Efferdose:* 25, 150 mg effervescent (phenylalanine)
> **Zantac Syrup** *Syr:* 15 mg/ml (peppermint) (alcohol 7.5%)

➤ *ranitidine bismuth citrate* (C) <12 years: not recommended; ≥12 years: 400 mg bid

> **Tritec** *Tab:* 400 mg

PROTON PUMP INHIBITORS (PPIs)

Comment: If hepatic impairment, or if patient is Asian, consider reducing the PPI dosage. Research has demonstrated associations between PPI use and fractures of the hip, wrist, and spine, hypomagnesemia, kidney injuries and chronic kidney disease, possible cardiovascular drug interactions, and infections (e.g., *Clostridium difficile* and pneumonia). Reducing the acidity of the stomach allows bacteria to thrive and spread to other organs like the lungs and intestines. This risk is increased with high dose and chronic use and greatest in the elderly. The most recent class-wide FDA warning cites reports of cutaneous and systemic lupus erythematosis (CLS/SLE) associated with PPIs in patients with both new onset and exacerbation of existing autoimmune disease. PPI treatment should be discontinued and the patient should be referred to a specialist. (http://www.fda.gov/Drugs/DrugSafety/InformationbyDrugClass/ucm213259.htm)

➤ *dexlansoprazole* (B)(G) <18 years: not recommended; ≥18 years: 30-60 mg daily for up to 4 weeks

> **Dexilant** *Cap:* 30, 60 mg ent-coat del-rel granules; may open and sprinkle on applesauce; do not crush or chew granules
> **Dexilant SoluTab** *Tab:* 30 mg del-rel orally-disint

➤ *esomeprazole* (B)(OTC)(G) <1 year: not recommended; 1-11 years: <20 kg: 10 mg; ≥20 kg: 10-20 mg once daily; ≥12 years: 20-40 mg daily; max 8 weeks; take 1 hour before food; swallow whole or mix granules with food or juice and take immediately; do not crush or chew granules

> **Nexium** *Cap:* 20, 40 mg ent-coat del-rel pellets
> **Nexium for Oral Suspension** *Oral susp:* 10, 20, 40 mg ent-coat del-rel granules/pkt; mix in 2 tbsp water and drink immediately; 30 pkt/carton

➢ *lansoprazole* (B)(OTC)(G) year: not recommended; 1-11, <30 kg: 15 mg once daily; ≥12 years: 15-30 mg daily for up to 8 weeks; may repeat course; take before eating
>   **Prevacid** *Cap:* 15, 30 mg ent-coat del-rel granules; swallow whole or mix granules with food or juice and take immediately; do not crush or chew granules; follow with water
>   **Prevacid for Oral Suspension** *Oral susp:* 15, 30 mg ent-coat del-rel granules/pkt; mix in 2 tbsp water and drink immediately; 30 pkt/carton (strawberry)
>   **Prevacid SoluTab** *ODT:* 15, 30 mg (strawberry) (phenylalanine)
>   **Prevacid 24HR** 15 mg ent-coat del-rel granules; swallow whole or mix granules with food or juice and take immediately; do not crush or chew granules; follow with water

➢ *omeprazole* (C)(OTC)(G) <1 year: not recommended; 5-<10 kg: 5 mg daily; 10-<20 kg: 10 mg daily; ≥20 kg: 20-40 mg daily; take before eating; swallow whole or mix granules with applesauce and take immediately; do not crush or chew; follow with water
>   **Prilosec** *Cap:* 10, 20, 40 mg del-rel granules
>   **Prilosec OTC** *Tab:* 20 mg del-rel (regular, wild berry)

➢ *pantoprazole* (B) <12 years: not recommended; ≥12 years: 40 mg bid
>   **Protonix** (G) *Tab:* 40 mg ent-coat del-rel
>   **Protonix for Oral Suspension** *Oral susp:* 40 mg ent-coat del-rel granules/pkt; mix in 1 tsp apple juice for 5 seconds or sprinkle on 1 tsp applesauce, and swallow immediately; do not mix in water or any other liquid or food; take approximately 30 minutes prior to a meal; 30 pkt/carton

➢ *rabeprazole* (B)(OTC)(G) 12 years: not recommended; ≥12 years: initially 20 mg daily; then titrate; may take 100 mg daily in divided doses or 60 mg bid; max 8 weeks
>   **AcipHex** *Tab:* 20 mg ent-coat del-rel
>   **AcipHex Sprinkle** *Cap:* 5, 10 mg del-rel

Antacids *see GERD page* 144

OTHER

➢ *glycopyrrolate* (B)(G) <12 years: not recommended; ≥12 years: initially 1-2 mg bid-tid; *Maintenance:* 1 mg bid; max 8 mg/day
>   **Robinul** *Tab:* 1 mg (dye-free)
>   **Robinul Forte** *Tab:* 2 mg (dye-free)

Comment: *glycopyrrolate* is an anticholinergic adjunct to PUD treatment.

➢ *mepenzolate* (B)(G) 25-50 mg divided qid, with meals and at HS
>   **Cantil** *Tab:* 25 mg

➢ *sucralfate* (B)(G) Active ulcer: 1 gm qid; *Maintenance:* 1 gm bid
>   **Carafate** *Tab:* 1*g; *Oral susp:* 1 gm/10 ml (14 oz)

PROPHYLAXIS

➢ *misoprostol* (X) <12 years: not recommended; ≥12 years: 200 mg qid with food for prevention of NSAID-induced gastric ulcers
>   **Cytotec** *Tab:* 100, 200 mg

Comment: *misoprostol* is a prostaglandin E1 analog indicated for the prevention of NSAID-induced gastric ulcers. Females of childbearing potential should have a negative serum pregnancy test within 2 weeks before starting and first dose on the 2nd or 3rd day of the next menstrual period. A contraceptive method should be maintained during therapy. Risks to pregnant females include: spontaneous abortion, premature birth, fetal anomalies, and uterine rupture.

PERIPHERAL NEURITIS, DIABETIC NEUROPATHIC PAIN, PERIPHERAL NEUROPATHIC PAIN

▷ **Acetaminophen for IV Infusion** *see Pain page* 296
▷ *acetaminophen* **(B)(G)** *see Fever page* 137
▷ *aspirin* **(D)(G)** *see Fever page* 137
   Comment: *aspirin*-containing medications are contraindicated with history of allergic-type reaction to *aspirin*, children and adolescents with *Varicella* or other viral illness, and 3rd trimester pregnancy.

α₂-DELTA LIGAND

▷ *pregabalin (GABA analog)* **(C)(V)** <18 years: not recommended; ≥18 years: initially 150 mg daily divided bid-tid; may titrate within one week; max 600 mg divided bid-tid; discontinue over one week
   Lyrica *Cap:* 25, 50, 75, 100, 150, 200, 225, 300 mg; *Oral soln:* 20 mg/ml

SEROTONIN AND NOREPINEPHRINE REUPTAKE INHIBITOR (SNRI)

▷ *duloxetine* **(C)** <12 years: not recommended; ≥12 years: swallow whole; 30-60 mg once daily; may increase by 30 mg at 1 week intervals; usual target 60 mg daily; max 120 mg/day
   Cymbalta *Cap:* 20, 30, 60 mg ent-coat pellets
   Comment: **Cymbalta** is indicated for chronic pain syndromes (e.g., arthritis, fibromyalgia, low back pain).

TOPICAL/TRANSDERMAL NSAIDs

▷ *capsaicin* cream **(B)(G)** <2 years: not recommended; 2-12 years: apply sparingly to intact skin bid prn; >12 years: apply tid-qid prn
   Axsain *Crm:* 0.075% (1, 2 oz)
   Capsin (OTC) *Lotn:* 0.025, 0, 075% (59 ml)
   Capzasin-P (OTC) *Crm:* 0.025% (1.5 oz); *Lotn:* 0.025% (2 oz)
   Capzasin-HP (OTC) *Crm:* 0.075% (1.5 oz); *Lotn:* 0.075% (2 oz)
   Dolorac *Crm:* 0.025% (28 gm)
   Double Cap (OTC) *Crm:* 0.05% (2 oz)
   R-Gel *Gel:* 0.025% (15, 30 gm)
   Zostrix (OTC) *Crm:* 0.025% (0.7, 1.5, 3 oz)
   Zostrix HP (OTC) *Emol crm:* 0.075% (1, 2 oz)
   Comment: Provides some relief by 1-2 weeks; optimal benefit may take 4-6 weeks. Avoid contact with mucous membranes.
▷ *capsaicin* 8% patch **(B)** <18 years: not recommended; ≥18 years: apply up to 4 patches for one 60-minute application to clean dry skin; may prep area with topical anesthetic; wear non-latex gloves; patches may be cut to size/shape; treatment may be repeated every 3 months; remove with cleansing gel after treatment

> **Qutenza** *Patch:* 8% 1640 mcg/cm (179 mg) (1 <u>or</u> 2 patches, each w. 1-50 gm tube cleansing gel/carton)

▶ *diclofenac epolamine transdermal patch* (C) <12 years: not recommended; ≥12 years: apply one patch to affected area bid; remove during bathing; avoid non-intact skin

> **Flector Patch** *Patch:* 180 mg/patch (30/carton)

▶ *capsaicin* cream (B)(G) <2 years: not recommended; 2-12 years: apply sparingly to intact skin bid prn; >12 years: apply tid-qid prn

> **Axsain** *Crm:* 0.075% (1, 2 oz)
> **Capsin** (OTC) *Lotn:* 0.025, 0, 075% (59 ml)
> **Capzasin-P** (OTC) *Crm:* 0.025% (1.5 oz); *Lotn:* 0.025% (2 oz)
> **Capzasin-HP** (OTC) *Crm:* 0.075% (1.5 oz); *Lotn:* 0.075% (2 oz)
> **Dolorac** *Crm:* 0.025% (28 gm)
> **Double Cap** (OTC) *Crm:* 0.05% (2 oz)
> **R-Gel** *Gel:* 0.025% (15, 30 gm)
> **Zostrix** (OTC) *Crm:* 0.025% (0.7, 1.5, 3 oz)
> **Zostrix HP** (OTC) *Emol crm:* 0.075% (1, 2 oz)

Comment: Provides some relief by 1-2 weeks; optimal benefit may take 4-6 weeks. Avoid contact with mucous membranes.

▶ *capsaicin* 8% patch (B) <18 years: not recommended; ≥18 years: apply up to 4 patches for one 60-minute application to clean dry skin; may prep area with topical anesthetic; wear non-latex gloves; patches may be cut to size/shape; treatment may be repeated every 3 months; remove with cleansing gel after treatment

> **Qutenza** *Patch:* 8% 1640 mcg/cm (179 mg) (1 <u>or</u> 2 patches w. 1-50 gm tube cleansing gel/carton)

▶ *lidocaine* 5% patch (B)(G) <18 years: not recommended; ≥18 years: apply up to 3 patches at one time for up to 12 hours/24-hour period (12 hours on/12 hours off); patches may be cut into smaller sizes before removal of the release liner; do not reuse

> **Lidoderm** *Patch:* 5% (10 x 14 cm, 30/carton)

ORAL ANALGESICS

▶ *tramadol* (C)(IV)(G)

Comment: *Tramadol* is known to be excreted in breast milk. The FDA and the European Medicines Agency (EMA) are investigating the safety of using *tramadol*-containing medications to treat pain in children 12-18 years because of the potential for serious side effects, including slowed or difficult breathing.

> **Rybix ODT** <12 years: contraindicated; 12-<18: use extreme caution; not recommended for children and adolescents with obesity, asthma, obstructive sleep apnea, or other chronic breathing problem, or for post-tonsillectomy/adenoidectomy pain; ≥18 years: initially 100 mg once daily; may increase by 100 mg every 5 days; max 300 mg/day; *CrCl <30 mL/min <u>or</u> severe hepatic impairment:* not recommended; *Cirrhosis:* max 50 mg q 12 hours
>
> *ODT:* 50 mg (mint) (phenylalanine)
>
> **Ryzolt** <12 years: contraindicated; 12-<18: use extreme caution; not recommended for children and adolescents with obesity, asthma, obstructive sleep apnea, or other chronic breathing problem, or for post-tonsillectomy/adenoidectomy pain; ≥18 years: initially 100 mg once daily; may increase by 100 mg every 5 days; max 300 mg/day; *CrCl <30 mL/min <u>or</u> severe hepatic impairment:* not recommended

Tab: 100, 200, 300 mg ext-rel
Ultram <12 years: contraindicated; 12-<18: use extreme caution; not recommended for children and adolescents with obesity, asthma, obstructive sleep apnea, or other chronic breathing problem, or for post-tonsillectomy/adenoidectomy pain; ≥18 years: 50-100 mg q 4-6 hours prn; max 400 mg/day; *CrCl <30 mL/min:* max 100 mg q 12 hours; *Cirrhosis:* max 50 mg q 12 hours
Tab: 50*mg
Ultram ER <12 years: contraindicated; 12-<18: use extreme caution; not recommended for children and adolescents with obesity, asthma, obstructive sleep apnea, or other chronic breathing problem, or for post-tonsillectomy/adenoidectomy pain; ≥18 years: initially 100 mg once daily; may increase by 100 mg every 5 days; max 300 mg/day; *CrCl <30 mL/min:* or severe hepatic impairment: not recommended
Tab: 100, 200, 300 mg ext-rel
➤ *tramadol/acetaminophen* **(C)(IV)(G)** <12 years: contraindicated; 12-<18: use extreme caution; not recommended for children and adolescents with obesity, asthma, obstructive sleep apnea, or other chronic breathing problem, or for post-tonsillectomy/adenoidectomy pain; ≥18 years: 2 tabs q 4-6 hours; max 8 tabs/day; 5 days; *CrCl <30 mL/min:* max 2 tabs q 12 hours; max 4 tabs/day x 5 days
Ultracet *Tab:* tram 37.5/acet 325 mg
Comment: *Tramadol* is known to be excreted in breast milk. The FDA and the European Medicines Agency (EMA) are investigating the safety of using *tramadol*-containing medications to treat pain in children 12-18 years because of the potential for serious side effects, including slowed or difficult breathing.

MU-OPIOID AGONIST/NOREPINEPHRINE REUPTAKE INHIBITOR

➤ *tapentadol* **(C)** <18 years: not recommended; ≥18 years:
Nucynta 50-100 mg q 4-6 hours prn; max 700 mg/day on the first day; 600 mg/day on subsequent days
Tab: 50, 75, 100 mg
Nucynta ER *Opioid-naïve:* initially 50 mg q 12 hours, then titrate to optimal dose within therapeutic range; usual therapeutic range 100-250 mg q 12 hours; doses >500 mg not recommended; *Converting from Nucynta:* divide total **Nucynta** daily dose into 2 **Nucynta ER** doses and administer q 12 hours; converting from *oxycodone CR* and other opioids, see mfr recommendations
Tab: 50, 100, 150, 200, 250 mg ext-rel
Other Oral Analgesics see *Pain* page 298

PERTUSSIS (WHOOPING COUGH)

Prophylaxis see *Childhood Immunizations* page 473

POSTEXPOSURE PROPHYLAXIS AND TREATMENT

Comment: Antibiotics do not alter the course of illness, but they do prevent transmission. Infected persons should be isolated until after the fifth day of antibiotic treatment.

➤ *azithromycin* (B)(G) <12 years: 12 mg/kg/day x 5 days; *see page 548 for dose by weight table;* ≥12 years: 500 mg x 1 dose on day 1, then 250 mg daily on days 2-5 <u>or</u> 500 mg daily x 3 days <u>or</u> **Zmax** 2 gm in a single dose

    Zithromax *Tab:* 250, 500, 600 mg; *Oral susp:* 100 mg/5 ml (15 ml); 200 mg/5 ml (15, 22.5, 30 ml) (cherry); *Pkt:* 1 gm for reconstitution (cherry-banana)

    Zithromax Tri-pak *Tab:* 3 x 500 mg tabs/pck

    Zithromax Z-pak *Tab:* 6 x 250 mg tabs/pck

    Zmax *Oral susp:* 2 gm ext-rel for reconstitution (cherry-banana) (148 mg Na+)

Comment: *azithromycin* is the drug of choice for infants <1 month-of-age.

➤ *clarithromycin* (C)(G) <6 months: not recommended; ≥6 months-12 years: 7.5 mg/kg divided bid x 10 days; *see page 558 for dose by weight table;* >12 years: 250 mg bid or 500 mg ext-rel daily x 10 days

    Biaxin *Tab:* 250, 500 mg

    Biaxin Oral Suspension *Oral susp:* 125, 250 mg/5 ml (50, 100 ml) (fruit punch)

    Biaxin XL *Tab:* 500 mg ext-rel

➤ *erythromycin base* (B)(G) <12 years: 40 mg/kg/day in divided doses x 14 days; ≥12 years: 1 gm/day divided qid x 14 days

    Ery-Tab *Tab:* 250, 333, 500 mg ent-coat

    PCE *Tab:* 333, 500 mg

➤ *erythromycin ethylsuccinate* (B)(G) 40-50 mg/kg/day in 4 divided doses x 14 days; may double dose with severe infection; max 100 mg/kg/day <u>or</u> 400 mg qid; *see page 563 for dose by weight table*

    EryPed *Oral susp:* 200 mg/5 ml (100, 200 ml) (fruit); 400 mg/5 ml (60, 100, 200 ml) (banana); *Oral drops:* 200, 400 mg/5 ml (50 ml) (fruit); *Chew tab:* 200 mg wafer (fruit)

    E.E.S. *Oral susp:* 200, 400 mg/5 ml (100 ml) (fruit)

    E.E.S. Granules *Oral susp:* 200 mg/5 ml (100, 200 ml) (cherry)

    E.E.S. 400 Tablets *Tab:* 400 mg

➤ *trimethoprim/sulfamethoxazole* (C)(G)

    Bactrim, Septra <12 years: not recommended; ≥12 years: 2 tabs bid x 10 days

        Tab: trim 80 mg/*sulfa* 400 mg*

    Bactrim DS, Septra DS <12 years: not recommended; ≥12 years: 1 tab bid x 10 days

        Tab: trim 160 mg/*sulfa* 800 mg*

    Bactrim Pediatric Suspension, Septra Pediatric Suspension <2 months: not recommended; 2 months-12 years: 40 mg/kg/day of *sulfamethoxazole* in 2 doses bid; >12 years: use tabs

        Oral susp: trim 40 mg/*sulfa* 200 mg per 5 ml (100 ml) (cherry) (alcohol 0.3%)

TREATMENT

Same as Postexposure Prophylaxis

☐ PHARYNGITIS: GONOCOCCAL

Comment: Treat all sexual contacts. Empiric therapy requires concomitant treatment for *Chlamydia*. Post-treatment culture recommended with PMHx history rheumatic fever.

PRIMARY THERAPY

▶ *azithromycin* (B)(G) <12 years: 12 mg/kg/day x 5 days; *see page 548 for dose by weight table*; max 500 mg/day; ≥12 years: 500 mg x 1 dose on day 1, then 250 mg daily on days 2-5 or 500 mg daily x 3 days or **Zmax** 2 gm in a single dose
    Zithromax *Tab*: 250, 500, 600 mg; *Oral susp*: 100 mg/5 ml (15 ml); 200 mg/5 ml (15, 22.5, 30 ml) (cherry); *Pkt*: 1 gm for reconstitution (cherry-banana)
    Zithromax Tri-pak *Tab*: 3 x 500 mg tabs/pck
    Zithromax Z-pak *Tab*: 6 x 250 mg tabs/pck
    Zmax *Oral susp*: 2 gm ext-rel for reconstitution (cherry-banana) (148 mg Na+)
    Comment: Per the CDC 2015 STD Treatment Guidelines, *azithromycin* should be used with ceftriaxone 250 mg.
▶ *ceftriaxone* (B)(G) <45 kg: 125 mg IM x 1 dose; ≥45 kg: 250 mg IM x 1 dose
    Rocephin *Vial*: 250, 500 mg; 1, 2 g

PHARYNGITIS: STREPTOCOCCAL

▶ *amoxicillin* (B)(G) <40 kg (88 lb): 20-40 mg/kg/day in 3 divided doses x 10 days or 25-45 mg/kg/day in 2 divided doses x 10 days; *see page 543 for dose by weight table*; ≥40 kg: 500-875 mg bid or 250-500 mg tid x 10 days
    Amoxil *Cap*: 250, 500 mg; *Tab*: 875*mg; *Chew tab*: 125, 200, 250, 400 mg (cherry-banana-peppermint) (phenylalanine); *Oral susp*: 125, 250 mg/5 ml (80, 100, 150 ml) (strawberry); 200, 400 mg/5 ml (50, 75, 100 ml) (bubble gum); *Oral drops*: 50 mg/ml (30 ml) (bubble gum)
    Moxatag *Tab*: 775 mg ext-rel
    Trimox *Tab*: 125, 250 mg; *Cap*: 250, 500 mg; *Oral susp*: 125, 250 mg/5 ml (80, 100, 150 ml) (raspberry-strawberry)
▶ *amoxicillin/clavulanate* (B)(G)
    Augmentin <40 kg: 40-45 mg/kg/day divided tid x 10 days or 90 mg/kg/day divided bid x 10 days; *see page 545 for dose by weight table*; ≥40 kg: 500 mg tid or 875 mg bid x 10 days
        Tab: 250, 500, 875 mg; *Chew tab*: 125, 250 mg (lemon-lime); 200, 400 mg (cherry-banana) (phenylalanine); *Oral susp*: 125 mg/5 ml (banana), 250 mg/5 ml (75, 100, 150 ml) (orange); 200, 400 mg/5 ml (50, 75, 100 ml) (orange) (phenylalanine)
    Augmentin ES-600 <3 months: not recommended; ≥3 months, <40 kg: 90 mg/kg/day divided q 12 hours x 10 days; *see page 546 for dose by weight table*; ≥40 kg: not recommended
        Oral susp: 600 mg/5 ml (50, 75, 100, 125, 150, 200 ml) (strawberry cream) (phenylalanine)
    Augmentin XR <16 years: use other forms; ≥16 years: 2 tabs q 12 hours x 7-10 days
        Tab: 1000*mg ext-rel
▶ *azithromycin* (B)(G) <12 years: 12 mg/kg/day x 5 days; *see page 548 for dose by weight table*; max 500 mg/day; ≥12 years: 500 mg x 1 dose on day 1, then 250 mg daily on days 2-5 or 500 mg daily x 3 days or **Zmax** 2 gm in a single dose
    Zithromax *Tab*: 250, 500, 600 mg; *Oral susp*: 100 mg/5 ml (15 ml); 200 mg/5 ml (15, 22.5, 30 ml) (cherry); *Pkt*: 1 gm for reconstitution (cherry-banana)
    Zithromax Tri-pak *Tab*: 3 x 500 mg tabs/pck

Zithromax Z-pak *Tab:* 6 x 250 mg tabs/pck

Zmax *Oral susp:* 2 gm ext-rel for reconstitution (cherry-banana) (148 mg Na⁺)

▶ *cefaclor* (B)(G) <1 month: not recommended; 1 month-12 years: 20-40 mg/kg in 2 or 3 divided doses x 10 days; *see page 549 for dose by weight table;* max 1 gm/day; >12 years: 375 mg bid x 10 days; max 2 gm/day

 Tab: 500 mg; *Cap:* 250, 500 mg; *Susp:* 125 mg/5 ml (75, 150 ml) (strawberry); 187 mg/5 ml (50, 100 ml) (strawberry); 250 mg/5 ml (75, 150 ml) (strawberry); 375 mg/5 ml (50, 100 ml) (strawberry)

 Cefaclor Extended Release <16 years: not recommended; ≥16 years: 500 mg bid x 10 days (clinically equivalent to 250 mg immed-rel caps tid); swallow whole; take with meals

 Tab: 375, 500 mg ext-rel

▶ *cefadroxil* <12 years: 30 mg/kg/day in 2 divided doses x 10 days; *see page 550 for dose by weight table;* ≥12 years: 1-2 gm in a single or 2 divided doses x 10 days

 Duricef *Cap:* 500 mg; *Tab:* 1 g; *Oral susp:* 250 mg/5 ml (100 ml); 500 mg/5 ml (75, 100 ml) (orange-pineapple)

▶ *cefdinir* (B) <6 months: not recommended; 6 months-12 years: 14 mg/kg/day in 1-2 divided doses x 10 days; *see page 551 for dose by weight table;* ≥12 years: 300 mg bid x 10 days or 600 mg daily x 10 days

 Omnicef *Cap:* 300 mg; *Oral susp:* 125 mg/5 ml (60, 100 ml) (strawberry)

▶ *cefditoren pivoxil* (B) <12 years: not recommended; ≥12 years: 200 mg bid x 10 days

 Spectracef *Tab:* 200 mg

 Comment: **Spectracef** is contraindicated with milk protein allergy or carnitine deficiency.

▶ *cefixime* (B)(G) <6 months: not recommended; 6 months-12 years, <50 kg: 8 mg/kg/day in 1-2 divided doses x 10 days; >12 years, ≥50 kg: same as adult; *see page 552 for dose by weight table;* >12 years: 400 mg daily x 10 days

 Suprax *Tab:* 400 mg; *Cap:* 400 mg; *Oral susp:* 100, 200, 500 mg/5 ml (50, 75, 100 ml) (strawberry)

▶ *cefpodoxime proxetil* (B) <2 months: not recommended; 2 months-12 years: 10 mg/kg/day in 2 divided doses x 5-7 days; *see page 553 for dose by weight table;* >12 yours: 100 mg bid x 5-7 days

▶ *cefprozil* (B) ≤6 months: not recommended; 6 months-12 years: 7.5 mg/kg divided bid x 10 days; *see page 554 for dose by weight table;* >12 years: 500 mg daily x 10 days

 Cefzil *Tab:* 250, 500 mg; *Oral susp:* 125, 250 mg/5 ml (50, 75, 100 ml) (bubble gum) (phenylalanine)

▶ *ceftibuten* (B) <12 years: 9 mg/kg daily x 10 days; max 400 mg/day; *see page 555 for dose by weight table;* ≥12 years: 400 mg daily x 10 days

 Cedax *Cap:* 400 mg; *Oral susp:* 90 mg/5 ml (30, 60, 90, 120 ml); 180 mg/5 ml (30, 60, 120 ml) (cherry)

▶ *cefuroxime axetil* (B)(G) <3 months: not recommended; ≥3 months-12 years: 20 mg/kg/day divided bid x 10 days; *see page 556 for dose by weight table;* ≥12 years: 250-500 mg bid x 10 days

 Ceftin *Tab:* 250, 500 mg; *Oral susp:* 125, 250 mg/5 ml (50, 100 ml) (tutti-frutti)

▶ *cephalexin* (B)(G) <12 years: 25-50 mg/kg/day in 4 divided doses x 10 days; *see page 557 for dose by weight table;* ≥12 years: 500 mg bid x 10 days

 Keflex *Cap:* 250, 333, 500, 750 mg; *Oral susp:* 125, 250 mg/5 ml (100, 200 ml) (strawberry)

> *clarithromycin* (C)(G) <6 months: not recommended; ≥6 months-12 years: 7.5 mg/kg divided bid x 10 days; *see page 558 for dose by weight table;* >12 years: 250 mg bid or 500 mg ext-rel daily x 10 days
>> **Biaxin** *Tab:* 250, 500 mg
>> **Biaxin Oral Suspension** *Oral susp:* 125, 250 mg/5 ml (50, 100 ml) (fruit punch)
>> **Biaxin XL** *Tab:* 500 mg ext-rel

> *dirithromycin* (C)(G) <12 years: not recommended; ≥12 years: 500 mg daily x 10 days
>> **Dynabac** *Tab:* 250 mg

> *erythromycin base* (B)(G) <45 kg: 30-50 mg divided bid-qid x 10 days; ≥45 kg: 500 mg qid x 10 days
>> **Ery-Tab** *Tab:* 250, 333, 500 mg ent-coat
>> **PCE** *Tab:* 333, 500 mg

> *erythromycin estolate* (B)(G) <12 years: 20-50 mg/kg divided q 6 hours x 10 days; *see page 562 for dose by weight table;* ≥12 years: 250-500 mg qid x 10 days
>> **Ilosone** *Pulvule:* 250 mg; *Tab:* 500 mg; *Liq:* 125, 250 mg/5 ml (100 ml)

> *erythromycin ethylsuccinate* (B)(G) 30-50 mg/kg/day in 4 divided doses x 7 days; may double dose with severe infection; max 100 mg/kg/day or 400 mg qid; *see page 563 for dose by weight table*
>> **EryPed** *Oral susp:* 200 mg/5 ml (100, 200 ml) (fruit); 400 mg/5 ml (60, 100, 200 ml) (banana); *Oral drops:* 200, 400 mg/5 ml (50 ml) (fruit); *Chew tab:* 200 mg wafer (fruit)
>> **E.E.S.** *Oral susp:* 200, 400 mg/5 ml (100 ml) (fruit)
>> **E.E.S. Granules** *Oral susp:* 200 mg/5 ml (100, 200 ml) (cherry)
>> **E.E.S. 400 Tablets** *Tab:* 400 mg

> *loracarbef* (B) <12 years: 15 mg/kg/day in 2 divided doses x 5 days; *see page 570 for dose by weight table;* ≥12 years: 200 mg bid x 5 days
>> **Lorabid** *Pulvule:* 200, 400 mg; *Oral susp:* 100 mg/5 ml (50, 100 ml); 200 mg/5 ml (50, 75, 100 ml) (strawberry bubble gum)

> *penicillin g (benzathine)* (B)(G) <60 lb: 300,000-600,000 units IM x 1 dose; ≥60 lb, ≥12-18 years: 900,000 units x 1 dose; ≥18 years: 1.2 million units IM x 1 dose
>> **Bicillin L-A** *Cartridge-needle unit:* 600,000 units (1 ml); 1.2 million units (2 ml)

> *penicillin g (benzathine and procaine)* (B)(G) <30 lb: 600,000 units IM x 1 dose; 30-<60 lb: 900,000-1.2 million units IM x 1 dose; ≥60 mg, >12 years: 2.4 million units IM x 1 dose
>> **Bicillin C-R** *Cartridge-needle unit:* 600,000 units (1 ml); 1.2 million units; (2 ml); 2.4 million units (4 ml)

> *penicillin v potassium* (B)(G) <12 years: 25-75 mg/kg day divided q 6-8 hours x 10 days; *see page 572 for dose by weight table;* ≥12 years: 500 mg bid or 250 mg qid x 10 days
>> **Pen-Vk** *Tab:* 250, 500 mg; *Oral soln:* 125 mg/5 ml (100, 200 ml); 250 mg/5 ml (100, 150, 200 ml)
>> **Veetids** *Tab:* 250, 500 mg; *Oral soln:* 125, 250 mg/5 ml (100, 200 ml)

PINWORM (*ENTEROBIUS VERMICULARIS*)

ANTHELMINTICS

Comment: Oral bioavailability of anthelmintics is enhanced when administered with a fatty meal (estimated fat content 40 g). Treatment of all family members is recommended. Some clinicians recommend all household contacts of infected patients receive treatment, especially when multiple or repeated symptomatic infections occur, since such contacts commonly also are infected; retreatment after 14 to 21 days may be needed.

▶ *albendazole* (C) take with a meal; chew or crush and mix with food; may repeat in 2-3 weeks; <20 kg: 200 mg as a single dose; ≥20 kg: 400 mg as a single dose

    Albenza *Tab:* 200 mg

▶ *mebendazole* (C) take with a meal; chew or crush and mix with food; may repeat in 3 weeks if needed <2 years: not recommended; ≥2 years: 100 mg as a single dose;

    Emverm *Chew tab:* 100 mg

    Vermox (G) *Chew tab:* 100 mg

▶ *pyrantel pamoate* (C) take with a meal; may open capsule and sprinkle or mix with food; may repeat in 2-3 weeks if needed; 11 mg/kg x 1 dose; max 1 gm/dose; 25-37 lb: 1/2 tsp x 1 dose; 38-62 lb: 1 tsp x 1 dose; 63-87 lb: 1 tsp x 1 dose; 88-112 lb: 2 tsp x 1 dose; 113-137 lb: 2 tsp x 1 dose; 138-162 lb: 3 tsp x 1 dose; 163-187 lb: 3 tsp x 1 dose; >187 lb: 4 tsp x 1 dose

    Antiminth (OTC) *Cap:* 180 mg; *Liq:* 50 mg/ml (30 ml); 144 mg/ml (30 ml); *Oral susp:* 50 mg/ml (60 ml)

    Pin-X (OTC); *Cap:* 180 mg; *Liq:* 50 mg/ml (30 ml); 144 mg/ml (30 ml); *Oral susp:* 50 mg/ml (30 ml)

▶ *thiabendazole* (C) take with a meal; chew or crush and mix with food; <30 lb: consult mfr pkg insert; ≥30 lb: 25 mg/kg x 1 dose; 30-50 lb: 250 mg x 1 dose; >50 lb: 10 mg/lb x 1 dose; take with a meal; max 1.5 gm/dose

    Mintezol *Chew tab:* 500*mg (orange); *Oral susp:* 500 mg/5 ml (120 ml) (orange)

Comment: *thiabendazole* is not for prophylaxis and should not be used as first-line therapy for pinworms. May impair mental alertness. May not be available in the US.

PITYRIASIS ALBA

Comment: Pityriasis alba is a chronic skin disorder seen in children with a genetic predisposition to atopic disease. Treatment is directed toward controlling roughness and pruritus. There is no known treatment for the associated skin pigment changes. Pityriasis alba resolves spontaneously and permanently in the 2nd or 3rd decade of life.

Topical Corticosteroids *see page 494*

COAL TAR PREPARATIONS

▶ *coal tar* (C)

    Scytera (OTC) apply qd-qid; use lowest effective dose

    Foam: 2%

    T/Gel Shampoo Extra Strength (OTC) use every other day; max 4 x/week; massage into affected area for 5 minutes; rinse; repeat

    Shampoo: 1%

    T/Gel Shampoo Original Formula (OTC) use every other day; max 7 x/week; massage into affected area for 5 minutes; rinse; repeat

    Shampoo: 0.5%

    T/Gel Shampoo Stubborn Itch Control (OTC) use every other day; max 7 x/ week; massage into affected area for 5 minutes; rinse; repeat

    Shampoo: 0.5%

EMOLLIENTS AND OTHER MOISTURIZING AGENTS

See **Dermatitis: Atopic** *page* 102

PITYRIASIS ROSEA

Topical Corticosteroids *see page* 494
Oral Prescription Drugs for the Management of Allergy, Cough, and Cold Symptoms
see page 523

PLAGUE (*YERSINIA PESTIS*)

Comment: *Yersinia pestis* is transmitted via the bite of a flea from an infected rodent or the bite, lick, or scratch of an infected cat. Untreated bubonic plague may progress to secondary pneumonic plague, which may be transmitted via contaminated respiratory droplet spread.

➤ *streptomycin* (C)(G) 15 mg/kg IM bid x 10 days
  Amp: 1 gm/2.5 ml or 400 mg/ml (2.5 ml)
  Comment: For patients with renal impairment, reduce dose of *streptomycin* to 20 mg/kg/day if mild and 8 mg/kg/day q 3 days if advanced. For patients who are pregnant or who have hearing impairment, shorten the course of treatment to 3 days after fever has resolved.

➤ *moxifloxacin* (C)(G) <18 years: not recommended; ≥18 years: 400 mg daily x 10 days
  Avelox *Tab:* 400 mg; IV soln: 400 mg/250 mg (latex-free, preservative-free)
  Comment: *moxifloxacin* is for prophylaxis as well as treatment for pneumonia and septic plague. *moxifloxacin* is contraindicated <18 years-of-age and during pregnancy and lactation. Risk of tendonitis or tendon rupture.

➤ *tetracycline* (D)(G) <8 years: not recommended; ≥8 years, ≤100 lb: 25-50 mg/kg/day in 4 divided doses x 10 days; *see page 572 for dose by weight table*; ≥8 years, >100 lb: 500 mg qid x 10 days
  Achromycin V *Cap:* 250, 500 mg
  Sumycin *Tab:* 250, 500 mg; *Cap:* 250, 500 mg; *Oral susp:* 125 mg/5 ml (100, 200 ml) (fruit) (sulfites)
  Comment: *tetracycline* is contraindicated <8 years-of-age, in pregnancy, and lactation (discolors developing tooth enamel). A side effect may be photosensitivity (photophobia). Do not give with antacids, calcium supplements, milk or other dairy, or within two hours of taking another drug.

PNEUMOCYSTIS JIROVECII PNEUMONIA

➤ *atovaquone* (C) <12 years: see mfr pkg insert for weight-based dosing table; ≥12 years: take as a single dose with food or a milky drink at the same time each day; repeat dose if vomited within 1 hour; *Prophylaxis:* 1,500 mg once daily; *Treatment:* 750 mg bid x 21 days
  Mepron *Susp:* 750 mg/5 ml (citrus)

▷ *trimethoprim/sulfamethoxazole* (C)(G) <2 months: not recommended; ≥2 months-12 years: 40 mg/kg/day of *sulfamethoxazole* in 2 doses bid x 10 days; >12 years: *Prophylaxis:* 1 tab 3 x/week; *Treatment:* 1 tab daily x 3 weeks; *Septra* can be given if intolerable to *Bactrim*

    Bactrim, Septra <12 years: not recommended; ≥12 years: 2 tabs bid x 10 days
        Tab: trim 80 mg/*sulfa* 400 mg*
    Bactrim DS, Septra DS <12 years: not recommended; ≥12 years: 1 tab bid x 10 days
        Tab: trim 160 mg/*sulfa* 800 mg*
    Bactrim Pediatric Suspension, Septra Pediatric Suspension <2 months: not recommended; ≥2 months-12 years: 40 mg/kg/day of *sulfamethoxazole* in 2 doses bid; >12 years: use tabs
        Oral susp: trim 40 mg/*sulfa* 200 mg per 5 ml (100 ml) (cherry) (alcohol 0.3%)

PNEUMONIA: CHLAMYDIAL

RECOMMENDED REGIMEN

▷ *erythromycin base* (B)(G) <45 kg: 50 mg in 4 divided doses x 10-14 days; ≥45 kg: 500 mg qid hours x 10-14 days
    Ery-Tab *Tab:* 250, 333, 500 mg ent-coat
    PCE *Tab:* 333, 500 mg
▷ *erythromycin ethylsuccinate* (B)(G) <45 kg: 50 mg/kg/day in 4 divided doses x 10-14 days; ≥45 kg: same as adult; *see page 563 for dose by weight table*
    EryPed *Oral susp:* 200 mg/5 ml (100, 200 ml) (fruit); 400 mg/5 ml (60, 100, 200 ml) (banana); *Oral drops:* 200, 400 mg/5 ml (50 ml) (fruit); *Chew tab:* 200 mg wafer (fruit)
    E.E.S. *Oral susp:* 200, 400 mg/5 ml (100 ml) (fruit)
    E.E.S. Granules *Oral susp:* 200 mg/5 ml (100, 200 ml) (cherry)
    E.E.S. 400 Tablets *Tab:* 400 mg

ALTERNATE REGIMENS

▷ *azithromycin* (B)(G) <12 years: 20 mg/kg per dose once daily x 10 days; *see page 548 for dose by weight table;* max 500 mg/day; ≥12 years: 500 mg once daily x 10 days
    Zithromax *Tab:* 250, 500, 600 mg; Oral susp: 100 mg/5 ml (15 ml); 200 mg/5 ml (15, 22.5, 30 ml) (cherry); Pkt: 1 gm for reconstitution (cherry-banana)
    Zithromax Tri-pak *Tab:* 3 x 500 mg tabs/pck
    Zithromax Z-pak *Tab:* 6 x 250 mg tabs/pck
    Zmax *Oral susp:* 2 gm ext-rel for reconstitution (cherry-banana) (148 mg Na⁺)
▷ *levofloxacin* (C) <18 years: not recommended; ≥18 years: *Uncomplicated:* 500 mg daily x 7 days; *Complicated:* 750 mg daily x 7 days
    Levaquin *Tab:* 250, 500, 750 mg; *Oral soln:* 25 mg/ml (480 ml) (benzyl alcohol); *Inj conc:* 25 mg/ml for IV infusion after dilution (20, 30 ml single-use vial) (preservative-free); *Premix soln:* 5 mg/ml for IV infusion (50, 100, 150 ml) (preservative-free)
Comment: *levofloxacin* is contraindicated <18 years-of-age, and during pregnancy and lactation. Risk of tendonitis or tendon rupture.

PNEUMONIA: COMMUNITY ACQUIRED (CAP)/COMMUNITY ACQUIRED BACTERIAL PNEUMONIA (CABP)

ANTI-INFECTIVES

Age 3 Months-5 Years

▷ *amoxicillin* (B)(G) <40 kg (88 lb): 80-100 mg/kg/day divided q 12 hours x 10 days; *see page 543 for dose by weight table;* ≥40 kg: 500-875 mg bid <u>or</u> 250-500 mg tid x 10 days

    Amoxil *Cap:* 250, 500 mg; *Tab:* 875 mg; *Chew tab:* 125, 200, 250, 400 mg (cherry-banana-peppermint) (phenylalanine); *Oral susp:* 125, 250 mg/5 ml (80, 100, 150 ml) (strawberry); 200, 400 mg/5 ml (50, 75, 100 ml) (bubble gum); *Oral drops:* 50 mg/ml (30 ml) (bubble gum)

    Moxatag *Tab:* 775 mg ext-rel

    Trimox *Tab:* 125, 250 mg; *Cap:* 250, 500 mg; *Oral susp:* 125, 250 mg/5 ml (80, 100, 150 ml) (raspberry-strawberry)

▷ *amoxicillin/clavulanate* (B)(G)

    Augmentin <40 kg: 45-90 mg/kg/day divided q 12 hours x 10 days; *see page 545 for dose by weight table;* ≥40 kg: 500 mg tid <u>or</u> 875 mg bid x 10 days

        Tab: 250, 500, 875 mg; *Chew tab:* 125, 250 mg (lemon-lime); 200, 400 mg (cherry-banana) (phenylalanine); *Oral susp:* 125 mg/5 ml (banana), 250 mg/5 ml (75, 100, 150 ml) (orange); 200, 400 mg/5 ml (50, 75, 100 ml) (orange) (phenylalanine)

    Augmentin ES-600 <3 months: not recommended; ≥3 months, <40 kg: 90 mg/kg/day divided q 12 hours x 10 days; *see page 546 for dose by weight table;* ≥40 kg: not recommended

        Oral susp: 600 mg/5 ml (50, 75, 100, 125, 150, 200 ml) (strawberry cream) (phenylalanine)

    Augmentin XR <16 years: use other forms; ≥16 years: 2 tabs q 12 hours x 7-10 days

        Tab: 1000*mg ext-rel

▷ *azithromycin* (B)(G) <12 years: 12 mg/kg/day x 5 days; *see page 548 for dose by weight table;* max 500 mg/day; ≥12 years: 500 mg x 1 dose on day 1, then 250 mg once daily on days 2-5 <u>or</u> 500 mg once daily x 7-10 days

    Zithromax *Tab:* 250, 500, 600 mg; *Oral susp:* 100 mg/5 ml (15 ml); 200 mg/5 ml (15, 22.5, 30 ml) (cherry); *Pkt:* 1 gm for reconstitution (cherry-banana)

    Zithromax Tri-pak *Tab:* 3 x 500 mg tabs/pck

    Zithromax Z-pak *Tab:* 6 x 250 mg tabs/pck

    Zmax *Oral susp:* 2 gm ext-rel for reconstitution (cherry-banana) (148 mg Na$^+$)

▷ *cefaclor* (B)(G) <1 month: not recommended; 1 month-12 years: 20-40 mg/kg divided bid x 10 days; *see page 549 for dose by weight table;* max 1 gm/day; >12 years: 250 mg tid <u>or</u> 375 mg bid x 10 days; max 2 gm/day

        Tab: 500 mg; *Cap:* 250, 500 mg; *Susp:* 125 mg/5 ml (75, 150 ml) (strawberry); 187 mg/5 ml (50, 100 ml) (strawberry); 250 mg/5 ml (75, 150 ml) (strawberry); 375 mg/5 ml (50, 100 ml) (strawberry)

    Cefaclor Extended Release <16 years: not recommended; ≥16 years: 500 mg bid x 10 days (clinically equivalent to 250 mg immed-rel caps tid); swallow whole; take with meals

    Tab: 375, 500 mg ext-rel

▷ *ceftriaxone* (B)(G)50-75 mg/kg IM in 2 divided doses; max 2 gm/day
    Rocephin *Vial:* 250, 500 mg; 1, 2 g

▷ *clarithromycin* (C) <6 months: not recommended; ≥6 months-12 years: 7.5 mg/kg divided bid x 7-14 days; *see page 558 for dose by weight table;* >12 years: 500 mg q 12 hours or 500 mg ext-rel daily x 10 days
    Biaxin *Tab:* 250, 500 mg
    Biaxin Oral Suspension *Oral susp:* 125, 250 mg/5 ml (50, 100 ml) (fruit punch)
    Biaxin XL *Tab:* 500 mg ext-rel

▷ *erythromycin base* (B)(G) <45 kg: 30-50 mg in 2-4 divided doses x 7-10 days; ≥45 kg: 500 mg qid hours x 7-10 days
    Ery-Tab *Tab:* 250, 333, 500 mg ent-coat
    PCE *Tab:* 333, 500 mg

▷ *erythromycin estolate* (B)(G)30-50 mg/kg/day in divided doses x 10 days; *see page 562 for dose by weight table*
    Ilosone *Pulvule:* 250 mg; *Tab:* 500 mg; *Liq:* 125, 250 mg/5 ml (100 ml)

Age 5-18 Years

▷ *amoxicillin* (B)(G) <40 kg (88 lb): 20-40 mg/kg/day in 3 divided doses x 10 days or 25-45 mg/kg/day in 2 divided doses x 10 days; *see page 543 for dose by weight table;* ≥40 kg: 500-875 mg bid or 250-500 mg tid x 10 days
    Amoxil *Cap:* 250, 500 mg; *Tab:* 875*mg; *Chew tab:* 125, 200, 250, 400 mg (cherry-banana-peppermint) (phenylalanine); *Oral susp:* 125, 250 mg/5 ml (80, 100, 150 ml) (strawberry); 200, 400 mg/5 ml (50, 75, 100 ml) (bubble gum); *Oral drops:* 50 mg/ml (30 ml) (bubble gum)
    Trimox *Tab:* 125, 250 mg; *Cap:* 250, 500 mg; *Oral susp:* 125, 250 mg/5 ml (80, 100, 150 ml) (raspberry-strawberry)

▷ *amoxicillin/clavulanate* (B)(G)
    Augmentin <40 kg: 40-45 mg/kg/day divided tid x 10 days or 90 mg/kg/day divided bid x 10 days; *see page 545 for dose by weight table;* ≥40 kg: 500 mg tid or 875 mg bid x 10 days
    Tab: 250, 500, 875 mg; *Chew tab:* 125, 250 mg (lemon-lime); 200, 400 mg (cherry-banana) (phenylalanine); *Oral susp:* 125 mg/5 ml (banana), 250 mg/5 ml (75, 100, 150 ml) (orange); 200, 400 mg/5 ml (50, 75, 100 ml) (orange) (phenylalanine)
    Augmentin ES-600 <3 months: not recommended; ≥3 months, <40 kg: 90 mg/kg/day divided q 12 hours x 10 days; *see page 546 for dose by weight table;* ≥40 kg: not recommended
    Oral susp: 600 mg/5 ml (50, 75, 100, 125, 150, 200 ml) (strawberry cream) (phenylalanine)
    Augmentin XR <16 years: use other forms; ≥16 years: 2 tabs q 12 hours x 7-10 days
    Tab: 1000*mg ext-rel

▷ *azithromycin* (B)(G) <12 years: 10 mg/kg x 1 dose on day 1, then 5 mg/kg/day on days 2-5; *see page 548 for dose by weight table*; max 500 mg/day; ≥12 years: 500 mg x 1 dose on day 1, then 250 mg daily on days 2-5 or 500 mg daily x 3 days or **Zmax** 2 gm in a single dose
    Zithromax *Tab:* 250, 500, 600 mg; *Oral susp:* 100 mg/5 ml (15 ml); 200 mg/5 ml (15, 22.5, 30 ml) (cherry); *Pkt:* 1 gm for reconstitution (cherry-banana)
    Zithromax Tri-pak *Tab:* 3 x 500 mg tabs/pck

       Zithromax Z-pak *Tab:* 6 x 250 mg tabs/pck

▷ *cefaclor* (B)(G) <1 month: not recommended; 1 month-12 years: 20-40 mg/kg divided bid x 10 days; *see page 549 for dose by weight table;* max 1 gm/day; >12 years: 250 mg tid or 375 mg bid x 10 days; max 2 gm/day
       Tab: 500 mg; *Cap:* 250, 500 mg; *Susp:* 125 mg/5 ml (75, 150 ml) (strawberry); 187 mg/5 ml (50, 100 ml) (strawberry); 250 mg/5 ml (75, 150 ml) (strawberry); 375 mg/5 ml (50, 100 ml) (strawberry)
       Cefaclor Extended Release <16 years: not recommended; ≥16 years: 500 mg bid x 10 days (clinically equivalent to 250 mg immed-rel caps tid); swallow whole; take with meals
       Tab: 375, 500 mg ext-rel

▷ *cefdinir* (B) <6 months: not recommended; 6 months-12 years: 14 mg/kg/day in 1-2 divided doses x 10 days; *see page 551 for dose by weight table;* ≥12 years: 300 mg bid x 10 days or 600 mg daily x 10 days
       Omnicef *Cap:* 300 mg; *Oral susp:* 125 mg/5 ml (60, 100 ml) (strawberry)

▷ *cefpodoxime proxetil* (B) <2 months: nor recommended; 2 months-12 years: 10 mg/kg/day in 2 doses x 14 days; *see page 553 for dose by weight table;* >12 years: 200 mg bid x 14 days

▷ *ceftriaxone* (B) 50-75 mg/kg IM in 2 divided doses; max 2 gm/day
       Rocephin *Vial:* 250, 500 mg; 1, 2 g

▷ *clarithromycin* (C) <6 months: not recommended; ≥6 months: 7.5 mg/kg bid x 7-14 days
       Biaxin *Tab:* 250, 500 mg
       Biaxin Oral Suspension *Oral susp:* 125, 250 mg/5 ml (50, 100 ml) (fruit punch)
       Biaxin XL *Tab:* 500 mg ext-rel

▷ *dirithromycin* (C)(G) <12 years: not recommended; ≥12 years: 500 mg daily x 7-14 days
       Dynabac *Tab:* 250 mg

▷ *erythromycin base* (B)(G) <45 kg: 30-50 mg in 2-4 divided doses x 10 days; ≥45 kg: 500 mg q 6 hours x 10 days
       Ery-Tab *Tab:* 250, 333, 500 mg ent-coat
       PCE *Tab:* 333, 500 mg

▷ *erythromycin estolate* (B) <12 years: 30-50 mg/kg/day in divided doses x 10 days; *see page 562 for dose by weight table;* ≥12 years: 250 mg q 6 hours or 500 mg bid x 10 days
       Ilosone *Pulvule:* 250 mg; *Tab:* 500 mg; *Liq:* 125, 250 mg/5 ml (100 ml)

Age ≥18 Years Without Comorbidity

▷ *amoxicillin* (B)(G) 500-875 mg bid or 250-500 mg tid x 10 days
       Amoxil *Cap:* 250, 500 mg; *Tab:* 875*mg; *Chew tab:* 125, 200, 250, 400 mg (cherry-banana-peppermint) (phenylalanine); *Oral susp:* 125, 250 mg/5 ml (80, 100, 150 ml) (strawberry); 200, 400 mg/5 ml (50, 75, 100 ml) (bubble gum); *Oral drops:* 50 mg/ml (30 ml) (bubble gum)
       Moxatag *Tab:* 775 mg ext-rel
       Trimox *Tab:* 125, 250 mg; *Cap:* 250, 500 mg; *Oral susp:* 125, 250 mg/5 ml (80, 100, 150 ml) (raspberry-strawberry)

▷ *amoxicillin/clavulanate* (B)(G)
       Augmentin <40 kg: 40-45 mg/kg/day divided tid x 10 days or 90 mg/kg/day divided bid x 10 days; *see page 545 for dose by weight table;* ≥40 kg: 500 mg tid or bid x 10 days

Tab: 250, 500, 875 mg; *Chew tab:* 125, 250 mg (lemon-lime); 200, 400 mg (cherry-banana) (phenylalanine); *Oral susp:* 125 mg/5 ml (banana), 250 mg/5 ml (75, 100, 150 ml) (orange); 200, 400 mg/5 ml (50, 75, 100 ml) (orange) (phenylalanine)

Augmentin ES-600 <3 months: not recommended; ≥3 months, <40 kg: 90 mg/kg/day divided q 12 hours x 10 days; *see page 546 for dose by weight table;* ≥40 kg: not recommended

Oral susp: 600 mg/5 ml (50, 75, 100, 125, 150, 200 ml) (strawberry cream) (phenylalanine)

Augmentin XR <16 years: use other forms; ≥16 years: 2 tabs q 12 hours x 7-10 days

Tab: 1000*mg ext-rel

➤ *azithromycin* (B)(G) 500 mg x 1 dose on day 1, then 250 mg daily on days 2-5 or 500 mg daily x 3 days or **Zmax** 2 gm in a single dose

Zithromax *Tab:* 250, 500, 600 mg; *Oral susp:* 100 mg/5 ml (15 ml); 200 mg/5 ml (15, 22.5, 30 ml) (cherry); *Pkt:* 1 gm for reconstitution (cherry-banana)

Zithromax Tri-pak *Tab:* 3 x 500 mg tabs/pck

Zithromax Z-pak *Tab:* 6 x 250 mg tabs/pck

Zmax *Oral susp:* 2 gm ext-rel for reconstitution (cherry-banana) (148 mg Na⁺)

➤ *cefaclor* (B)(G) 250 mg tid or 375 mg bid x 10 days

Tab: 500 mg; *Cap:* 250, 500 mg; *Susp:* 125 mg/5 ml (75, 150 ml) (strawberry); 187 mg/5 ml (50, 100 ml) (strawberry); 250 mg/5 ml (75, 150 ml) (strawberry); 375 mg/5 ml (50, 100 ml) (strawberry)

Cefaclor Extended Release <16 years: not recommended; ≥16 years: 500 mg bid x 10 days (clinically equivalent to 250 mg immed-rel caps tid); swallow whole; take with food

Tab: 375, 500 mg ext-rel

➤ *cefdinir* (B) <6 months: not recommended; 6 months-12 years: 14 mg/kg/day in 1-2 divided doses x 10 days; *see page 551 for dose by weight table;* ≥12 years: 300 mg bid x 10 days or 600 mg daily x 10 days

Omnicef *Cap:* 300 mg; *Oral susp:* 125 mg/5 ml (60, 100 ml) (strawberry)

➤ *cefpodoxime proxetil* (B) 200 mg bid x 14 days

➤ *ceftaroline fosamil* (B) administer by IV infusion after reconstitution every 12 hours x 5-7 days; *CrCl ≥50 mL/min:* 600 mg; *CrCl >30-<50 mL/min:* 400 mg; *CrCl: >15-<30 mL/min:* 300 mg; ES RD: 200 mg

Teflaro *Vial:* 400, 600 mg

➤ *ceftriaxone* (B)(G) 50-75 mg/kg IM in 2 divided doses; max 2 gm/day

Rocephin *Vial:* 250, 500 mg; 1, 2 g

➤ *clarithromycin* (C)(G) 500 mg bid or 500 mg ext-rel daily x 7-14 days

Biaxin *Tab:* 250, 500 mg

Biaxin Oral Suspension *Oral susp:* 125, 250 mg/5 ml (50, 100 ml) (fruit punch)

Biaxin XL *Tab:* 500 mg ext-rel

➤ *dirithromycin* (C)(G) 500 mg daily x 14 days

Dynabac *Tab:* 250 mg

➤ *doxycycline* (D)(G)

Acticlate *Tab:* 75, 150** mg

Adoxa *Tab:* 50, 75, 100, 150 mg ent-coat

Doryx *Tab:* 50, 75, 100, 150, 200 mg del-rel

Monodox *Cap:* 50, 75, 100 mg

Oracea *Cap:* 40 mg del-rel

Vibramycin *Tab:* 100 mg; *Cap:* 50, 100 mg; *Syr:* 50 mg/5 ml (raspberry-apple) (sulfites); *Oral susp:* 25 mg/5 ml (raspberry)
Vibra-Tab *Tab:* 100 mg film-coat

▷ *ertapenem* (B) 1 gm daily; *CrCl <30 mL/min:* 500 mg daily x 3-10 days; may switch to an oral antibiotic after 3 days if warranted; *IV infusion:* administer over 30 minutes; *IM injection:* reconstitute with lidocaine only
Invanz *Vial:* 1 gm pwdr for reconstitution

▷ *erythromycin base* (B)(G) 500 mg q 6 hours x 14-21 days
Ery-Tab *Tab:* 250, 333, 500 mg ent-coat
PCE *Tab:* 333, 500 mg

▷ *erythromycin estolate* (B) 500 mg q 6 hours x 14-21 days
Ilosone *Pulvule:* 250 mg; *Tab:* 500 mg; *Liq:* 125, 250 mg/5 ml (100 ml)

▷ *gemifloxacin* (C)(G) <18 years: not recommended; ≥18 years: 320 mg daily x 5-7 days
Factive *Tab:* 320* mg
Comment: *gemifloxacin* is contraindicated <18 years-of-age and during pregnancy and lactation. Risk of tendonitis or tendon rupture.

▷ *levofloxacin* (C) *Uncomplicated:* 500 mg once daily x 7-14 days; *Complicated:* 750 mg once daily x 7-14 days
Levaquin *Tab:* 250, 500, 750 mg; *Oral soln:* 25 mg/ml (480 ml) (benzyl alcohol); *Inj conc:* 25 mg/ml for IV infusion after dilution (20, 30 ml single-use vial) (preservative-free); *Premix soln:* 5 mg/ml for IV infusion (50, 100, 150 ml) (preservative-free)
Comment: *levofloxacin* is contraindicated <18 years-of-age and during pregnancy and lactation. Risk of tendonitis or tendon rupture.

▷ *linezolid* (C)(G) <5 years: 10 mg/kg q 8 hours x 10-14 days; 5-11 years: 10 mg/kg q 12 hours x 10-14 days; >11 years: 400-600 mg q 12 hours x 10-14 days
Zyvox *Tab:* 400, 600 mg; *Oral susp:* 100 mg/5 ml (150 ml) (orange) (phenylalanine)
Comment: *linezolid* is indicated to treat susceptible vancomycin-resistant *E. faecium* infections.

▷ *loracarbef* (B) <12 years: 15 mg/kg/day in 2 divided doses x 10 days; *see page* 570 *for dose by weight table;* ≥12 years: 200 mg bid x 10 days
Lorabid *Pulvule:* 200, 400 mg; *Oral susp:* 100 mg/5 ml (50, 100 ml); 200 mg/5 ml (50, 75, 100 ml) (strawberry bubble gum)

▷ *moxifloxacin* (C)(G) <18 years: not recommended; ≥18 years: 400 mg daily x 5 days
Avelox *Tab:* 400 mg; IV soln: 400 mg/250 ml (latex-free, preservative-free)
Comment: *moxifloxacin* is contraindicated during pregnancy and lactation. Risk of tendonitis or tendon rupture.

▷ *ofloxacin* (C)(G) <18 years: not recommended; ≥18 years: 400 mg bid x 10 days
Floxin *Tab:* 200, 300, 400 mg
Comment: *ofloxacin* is contraindicated <18 years-of-age and during pregnancy and lactation. Risk of tendonitis or tendon rupture.

▷ *tedizolid phosphate* (B) administer 200 mg once daily x 6 days, via PO or IV infusion over 1 hour
Sivextro *Tab:* 200 mg (6/blister pck)
Comment: **Sivextro** is indicated for the treatment of community acquired bacterial pneumonia (CABP)

▷ *telithromycin* (C) 2 x 400 mg tabs in a single dose daily x 7-10 days
Ketek *Tab:* 300, 400 mg

Comment: *telithromycin* is contraindicated with PMHx hepatitis or jaundice associated with macrolide use.
➤ *tigecycline* (D)(G) 100 mg once; then 50 mg q 12 hours x 7-14 days; *Severe hepatic impairment (Child Pugh C):* 100 mg once; then 25 mg q 12 hours

    Tygacil *Vial:* 50 mg pwdr for reconstitution and IV infusion (preservative-free)

    Comment: **Tygacil** is contraindicated in pregnancy, and lactation (discolors developing tooth enamel). A side effect may be photo-sensitivity (photophobia). Do not give with antacids, calcium supplements, milk or other dairy, or within two hours of taking another drug.

PNEUMONIA: LEGIONELLA

➤ *ciprofloxacin* (C) <18 years: 20-40 mg/kg/day divided q 12 hours x 14-21 days; ≥18 years: 500 mg bid x 14-21 days; max 1.5 gm/day

    Cipro (G) *Tab:* 250, 500, 750 mg; *Oral susp:* 250, 500 mg/5 ml (100 ml) (strawberry)

    Cipro XR *Tab:* 500, 1,000 mg ext-rel

    ProQuin XR *Tab:* 500 mg ext-rel
➤ *clarithromycin* (C)(G) 500 mg bid or 500 mg ext-rel daily x 14-21 days

    Biaxin *Tab:* 250, 500 mg

    Biaxin Oral Suspension *Oral susp:* 125, 250 mg/5 ml (50, 100 ml) (fruit punch)

    Biaxin XL *Tab:* 500 mg ext-rel
➤ *dirithromycin* (C)(G) 500 mg once daily x 14-21 days

    Dynabac *Tab:* 250 mg
➤ *erythromycin base* (B)(G) <45 kg: 30-50 mg in 2-4 divided doses x 14-21 days; ≥45 kg: 500 mg qid x 14-21 days

    Ery-Tab *Tab:* 250, 333, 500 mg ent-coat

    PCE *Tab:* 333, 500 mg
➤ *erythromycin estolate* (B)(G) <12 years: 30-50 mg/kg/day in divided doses x 14-21 days; *see page 562 for dose by weight table;* ≥12 years: 1-2 gm daily in divided doses x 14-21 days

    Ilosone *Pulvule:* 250 mg; *Tab:* 500 mg; *Liq:* 125, 250 mg/5 ml (100 ml)
➤ *trimethoprim/sulfamethoxazole* (C)(G)

    Bactrim, Septra <12 years: not recommended; ≥12 years: 2 tabs bid x 10 days

        Tab: trim 80 mg/*sulfa* 400 mg*

    Bactrim DS, Septra DS <12 years: not recommended; ≥12 years: 1 tab bid x 10 days

        Tab: trim 160 mg/*sulfa* 800 mg*

    Bactrim Pediatric Suspension, Septra Pediatric Suspension <2 months: not recommended; ≥2 months-12 years: 40 mg/kg/day of *sulfamethoxazole* in 2 doses bid x 10 days; >12 years: use tabs

        Oral susp: trim 40 mg/*sulfa* 200 mg per 5 ml (100 ml) (cherry) (alcohol 0.3%)

PNEUMONIA: MYCOPLASMA

ANTI-INFECTIVES

➤ *azithromycin* (B)(G) <12 years: 12 mg/kg/day x 5 days; *see page 548 for dose by weight table;* max 500 mg/day; ≥12 years: 500 mg x 1 dose on day 1, then 250 mg daily on days 2-5 or 500 mg daily x 3 days or **Zmax** 2 gm in a single dose

Zithromax *Tab:* 250, 500, 600 mg; *Oral susp:* 100 mg/5 ml (15 ml); 200 mg/5 ml (15, 22.5, 30 ml) (cherry); *Pkt:* 1 gm for reconstitution (cherry-banana)
Zithromax Tri-pak *Tab:* 3 x 500 mg tabs/pck
Zithromax Z-pak *Tab:* 6 x 250 mg tabs/pck
Zmax *Oral susp:* 2 gm ext-rel for reconstitution (cherry-banana) (148 mg Na⁺)

▶ *clarithromycin* (C)(G) <6 months: not recommended; ≥6 months-12 years: 7.5 mg/kg bid x 14-21 days; *see page 558 for dose by weight table*; >12 years: 500 mg bid or 500 mg ext-rel daily x 14-21 days
Biaxin *Tab:* 250, 500 mg
Biaxin Oral Suspension *Oral susp:* 125, 250 mg/5 ml (50, 100 ml) (fruit punch)
Biaxin XL *Tab:* 500 mg ext-rel

▶ *erythromycin base* (B)(G) <45 kg: 30-50 mg in 2-4 doses x 14-21 days; ≥45 kg: 500 mg q 6 hours x 14-21 days
Ery-Tab *Tab:* 250, 333, 500 mg ent-coat
PCE *Tab:* 333, 500 mg

▶ *erythromycin ethylsuccinate* (B)(G) 30-50 mg/kg/day in 4 divided doses x 14-21 days; may double dose with severe infection; max 100 mg/kg/day or 400 mg qid; *see page 563 for dose by weight table*
EryPed *Oral susp:* 200 mg/5 ml (100, 200 ml) (fruit); 400 mg/5 ml (60, 100, 200 ml) (banana); *Oral drops:* 200, 400 mg/5 ml (50 ml) (fruit); *Chew tab:* 200 mg wafer (fruit)
E.E.S. *Oral susp:* 200, 400 mg/5 ml (100 ml) (fruit)
E.E.S. Granules *Oral susp:* 200 mg/5 ml (100, 200 ml) (cherry)
E.E.S. 400 Tablets *Tab:* 400 mg

▶ *tetracycline* (D)(G) <8 years: not recommended; ≥8 years, ≤100 lb: 25-50 mg/kg/day in 4 divided doses x 14-21 days; *see page 574 for dose by weight table*; ≥8 years, >100 lb: 500 mg qid x 14-21 days
Achromycin V *Cap:* 250, 500 mg
Sumycin *Tab:* 250, 500 mg; *Cap:* 250, 500 mg; *Oral susp:* 125 mg/5 ml (100, 200 ml) (fruit) (sulfites)

Comment: *tetracycline* is contraindicated <8 years-of-age, in pregnancy, and lactation (discolors developing tooth enamel). A side effect may be photo-sensitivity (photophobia). Do not give with antacids, calcium supplements, milk or other dairy, or within two hours of taking another drug.

▮ PNEUMONIA: PNEUMOCOCCAL

PROPHYLAXIS

▶ *pneumococcal* vaccine (C) <2 years: not recommended; ≥2 years: 0.5 ml IM or SC in deltoid x 1 dose
Pneumovax *Vial:* 25 mcg/0.5 ml (0.5 ml single dose, 10/pck; 2.5 ml)
Pnu-Imune 23 *Vial:* 25 mcg/0.5 ml (0.5 ml single dose, 5/pck; 2.5 ml)

Comment: Pneumococcal vaccine contains 23 polysaccharide isolates representing approximately 85-90% of common U.S. isolates. Administer the pneumococcal vaccine in the anterolateral aspect of the thigh for infants and the deltoid for toddlers and children.

TREATMENT

see **CAP/CABP** *page* 330

POLIOMYELITIS

PROPHYLAXIS

▷ *trivalent poliovirus vaccine, inactivated (type 1, 2, and 3)* **(C)** <6 weeks: not recommended; ≥6 weeks: one dose at 2, 4, 6-18 months and 4-6 years-of-age
   Ipol 0.5 ml SC <u>or</u> IM in deltoid area

POLYCYSTIC OVARIAN SYNDROME (PCOS, STEIN-LEVENTHAL DISEASE)

See **Contraceptives** *page* 475
See **Type 2 Diabetes Mellitus** *page* 422

POLYMYALGIA RHEUMATICA

Comment: Initial treatment is low-dose prednisone at 12-25 mg/day. May attempt a very slow tapering regimen after 2-4 weeks. If relapse occurs, increase the daily dose of corticosteroid to the previous effective dose. Most people with polymyalgia rheumatica need to continue corticosteroid treatment for at least a year. Approximately 30-60% of people will have at least one relapse during corticosteroid tapering. Joint guidelines from the American Academy of Rheumatology (AAR) and the European League Against Rheumatism (ELAR) suggest using concomitant methotrexate (MTX) along with corticosteroids in some patients. It may be useful early in the course of treatment <u>or</u> later, if the patient relapses <u>or</u> does not respond to corticosteroids. The American Academy of Rheumatology (AAR) recommends the following daily doses for anyone on a chronic oral corticosteroid regimen: Calcium 1,200-1,500 mg/day and vitamin D 800-1,000 IU/day.

Oral Corticosteroids *see page* 498

For calcium and vitamin D supplementation, see **Hypocalcemia** *page* 219

▷ *methotrexate* **(X)** <2 years: not recommended; 2-12 years: 10 mg/m² once weekly; max 20 mg/m²; >12 years: 7.5 mg x 1 dose per week <u>or</u> 2.5 mg x 3 at 12 hour intervals once a week; max 20 mg/week; therapeutic response begins in 3-6 weeks; administer *methotrexate* injection SC only into the abdomen <u>or</u> thigh
   Rasuvo *Autoinjector:* 7.5 mg/0.15 ml, 10 mg/0.20 ml, 12.5 mg/0.25 ml, 15 mg/0.30 ml, 17.5 mg/0.35 ml, 20 mg/0.40 ml, 22.5 mg/0.45 ml, 25 mg/0.50 ml, 27.5 mg/0.55 ml, 30 mg/0.60 ml (solution concentration for SC injection is 50 mg/ml)
   Rheumatrex *Tab:* 2.5*mg (5, 7.5, 10, 12.5, 15 mg/week, 4/card unit dose pack)
   Trexall R *Tab:* 5*, 7.5*, 10*, 15*mg (5, 7.5, 10, 12.5, 15 mg/week, 4/card unit dose pack)

Comment: *methotrexate* (MTX) is contraindicated with immunodeficiency, blood dyscrasias, alcoholism, and chronic liver disease.

POSTHERPETIC NEURALGIA

GAMMA AMINOBUTYRIC ACID ANALOG

▶ *gabapentin* (C) <3 years: not recommended; 3-12 years: initially 10-15 mg/kg/day in 3 divided doses; max 12 hours between doses; titrate over 3 days; 3-4 years: titrate to 40 mg/kg/day; 5-12 years: titrate to 25-35 mg/kg/day; max 50 mg/kg/day; >12 years: initially 300 mg on Day 1; then 600 mg on Day 2; then 900 mg on Days 3-6; then 1200 mg on Days 7-10; then 1500 mg on Days 11-14; titrate up to 1800 mg on Day 15; take entire dose once daily with the evening meal; do not crush, split, or chew

    Gralise (C) *Tab:* 300, 600 mg

    Neurontin (G) *Tab:* 600*, 800* mg; *Cap:* 100, 300, 400 mg; *Oral soln:* 250 mg/5 ml (480 ml) (strawberry-anise)

      Tab: 600·, 800· mg; *Cap:* 100, 300, 400 mg; *Oral soln:* 250 mg/5 ml (480 ml) (strawberry-anise)

Comment: Avoid abrupt cessation of *gabapentin*. To discontinue, withdraw gradually over 1 week or longer.

▶ *gabapentin enacarbil* (C) <18 years: not recommended; ≥18 years: 600 mg once daily at about 5: 00 PM; if dose not taken at recommended time, next dose should be taken the following day; swallow whole; take with food; *CrCl 30-59 mL/min:* 600 mg on Day 1, Day 3, and every day thereafter; *CrCl <30 mL/min:* or on hemodialysis: not recommended

    Horizant *Tab:* 600 ext-rel

Comment: Avoid abrupt cessation of *gabapentin enacarbil*. To discontinue, withdraw gradually over 1 week or longer.

TRICYCLIC ANTIDEPRESSANTS (TCAs)

Comment: Co-administration of SSRIs and TCAs requires extreme caution.

▶ *amitriptyline* (C)(G) <12 years: not recommended; ≥12 years: 10-20 mg q HS *Tab:* 10, 25, 50, 75, 100, 150 mg

▶ *amoxapine* (C) <12 years: not recommended; ≥12 years: initially 50 mg bid-tid; after 1 week may increase to 100 mg bid-tid; usual effective dose 200-300 mg/day; if total dose exceeds 300 mg/day, give in divided doses (max 400 mg/day); may give as a single bedtime dose (max 300 mg q HS)

    Tab: 25, 50, 100, 150 mg

▶ *clomipramine* (C)(G) <10 years: not recommended; 10-<16 years: initially 25 mg daily in divided doses; gradually increase; max 3 mg/kg or 100 mg, whichever is smaller; >16 years: initially 25 mg daily in divided doses; gradually increase to 100 mg during first 2 weeks; max 250 mg/day; total maintenance dose may be given at HS

    Anafranil *Cap:* 25, 50, 75 mg

▶ *desipramine* (C)(G) <12 years: not recommended; ≥12 years: 100-200 mg/day in single or divided doses; max 300 mg/day

    Norpramin *Tab:* 10, 25, 50, 75, 100, 150 mg

▶ *doxepin* (C)(G) <12 years: not recommended; ≥12 years: 75 mg/day; max 150 mg/day

    Cap: 10, 25, 50, 75, 100, 150 mg; *Oral conc:* 10 mg/ml (4 oz w. dropper)

▶ *imipramine* (C)(G) <12 years: not recommended; ≥12 years:

    Tofranil initially 75 mg daily (max 200 mg); adolescents initially 30-40 mg daily (max 100 mg/day); if maintenance dose exceeds 75 mg daily, may switch to **Tofranil PM** for divided or bedtime dose

Tab: 10, 25, 50 mg

Tofranil PM initially 75 mg daily 1 hour before HS; max 200 mg
Cap: 75, 100, 125, 150 mg

➤ *nortriptyline* **(D)(G)** <12 years: not recommended; ≥12 years: initially 25 mg tid-qid; max 150 mg/day

Pamelor *Cap:* 10, 25, 50, 75 mg; *Oral soln:* 10 mg/5 ml (16 oz)

➤ *protriptyline* **(C)** <12 years: not recommended; ≥12 years: initially 5 mg tid; usual dose 15-40 mg/day in 3-4 divided doses; max 60 mg/day

Vivactil *Tab:* 5, 10 mg

➤ *trimipramine* **(C)** <12 years: not recommended; ≥12 years: initially 75 mg/day in divided doses; max 200 mg/day

Surmontil *Cap:* 25, 50, 100 mg

α₂-DELTA LIGAND

➤ *pregabalin (GABA analog)* **(C)(V)** <18 years: not recommended; ≥18 years: initially 150 mg daily divided bid-tid and may titrate within one week; max 600 mg divided bid-tid; discontinue over one week

Lyrica *Cap:* 25, 50, 75, 100, 150, 200, 225, 300 mg; *Oral soln:* 20 mg/ml

TOPICAL/TRANSDERMAL ANALGESICS

➤ *capsaicin* cream **(B)(G)** <2 years: not recommended; 2-12 years: apply sparingly to intact skin bid prn; >12 years: apply tid-qid prn

Axsain *Crm:* 0.075% (1, 2 oz)
Capsin (OTC) *Lotn:* 0.025, 0, 075% (59 ml)
Capzasin-P (OTC) *Crm:* 0.025% (1.5 oz); *Lotn:* 0.025% (2 oz)
Capzasin-HP (OTC) *Crm:* 0.075% (1.5 oz); *Lotn:* 0.075% (2 oz)
Dolorac *Crm:* 0.025% (28 gm)
Double Cap (OTC) *Crm:* 0.05% (2 oz)
R-Gel *Gel:* 0.025% (15, 30 gm)
Zostrix (OTC) *Crm:* 0.025% (0.7, 1.5, 3 oz)
Zostrix HP (OTC) *Emol crm:* 0.075% (1, 2 oz)

Comment: Provides some relief by 1-2 weeks; optimal benefit may take 4-6 weeks. Avoid contact with mucous membranes.

➤ *diclofenac epolamine* **(C)** <12 years: not recommended; ≥12 years: apply one patch to affected area bid; remove during bathing; avoid non-intact skin; do not reuse

Flector Patch *Patch:* 180 mg/patch (30/carton)

Comment: *diclofenac* is contraindicated with *aspirin* allergy and late pregnancy.

➤ *doxepin* cream **(B)** <12 years: not recommended; ≥12 years: apply to affected area qid at intervals of at least 3-4 hours; max 8 days

Prudoxin *Crm:* 5% (45 gm)
Zonalon *Crm:* 5% (30, 45 gm)

➤ *pimecrolimus* 1% cream **(C)** <2 years: not recommended; ≥2 years: apply to affected area bid; do not occlude

Elidel *Crm:* 1% (30, 60, 100 gm)

Comment: *pimecrolimus* is indicated for short-term and intermittent long-term use. Discontinue use when resolution occurs. Contraindicated if the patient is immunosuppressed. Change to the 0.1% preparation _or_ if secondary bacterial infection is present.

▷ *tacrolimus* (C) <2 years: not recommended; 2-15 years: use 0.03% strength; apply to affected area bid; continue for 1 week after clearing; >15 years: apply to affected area bid; do not occlude or apply to wet skin; continue for 1 week after clearing
  Protopic *Oint:* 0.03, 0.1% (30, 60, 100 gm)

▷ *trolamine salicylate* (NE) <2 years: not recommended; ≥2 years: apply tid-qid prn to intact skin
  Mobisyl *Crm:* 10%
  Comment: Provides some relief by 1-2 weeks; optimal benefit

TOPICAL/TRANSDERMAL ANESTHETICS

▷ *lidocaine* cream (B) <12 years: not recommended; ≥12 years:
  LidaMantle *Crm:* 3% (1, 2 oz)
  Lidoderm *Crm:* 3% (85 gm)

▷ *lidocaine* lotion (B) <12 years: not recommended; ≥12 years:
  LidaMantle *Lotn:* 3% (177 ml)

▷ *lidocaine* 5% patch (B)(G) <12 years: not recommended; ≥12 years: apply up to 3 patches at one time for up to 12 hours/24-hour period (12 hours on/12 hours off); patches may be cut into smaller sizes before removal of the release liner; do not reuse
  Lidoderm *Patch:* 5% (10 x 14 cm; 30/carton)

▷ *lidocaine/dexamethasone* (B) <12 years: not recommended; ≥12 years:
  Decadron Phosphate with Xylocaine *dexa* 4 mg/*lido* 10 mg per ml (5 ml)

▷ *lidocaine/hydrocortisone* (B)(G) <12 years: not recommended; ≥12 years:
  LidaMantle HC *Crm:* lido 3%/hydro 0.5% (1, 3 oz); *Lotn:* (177 ml)

ORAL ANALGESICS

▷ *acetaminophen* (B)(G) *see Fever page* 137

▷ *aspirin* (D)(G) *see Fever page* 137
  Comment: *aspirin*-containing medications are contraindicated with history of allergic-type reaction to *aspirin*, children and adolescents with *Varicella* or other viral illness, and 3rd trimester pregnancy.

▷ *tramadol* (C)(IV)(G)
  Comment: *Tramadol* is known to be excreted in breast milk. The FDA and the European Medicines Agency (EMA) are investigating the safety of using *tramadol*-containing medications to treat pain in children 12-18 years because of the potential for serious side effects, including slowed or difficult breathing.
  Rybix ODT <12 years: contraindicated; 12-<18: use extreme caution; not recommended for children and adolescents with obesity, asthma, obstructive sleep apnea, or other chronic breathing problem, or for post-tonsillectomy/adenoidectomy pain; ≥18 years: initially 100 mg once daily; may increase by 100 mg every 5 days; max 300 mg/day; *CrCl <30 mL/min or severe hepatic impairment:* not recommended; *Cirrhosis:* max 50 mg q 12 hours
    ODT: 50 mg (mint) (phenylalanine)
  Ryzolt <12 years: contraindicated; 12-<18: use extreme caution; not recommended for children and adolescents with obesity, asthma, obstructive sleep apnea, or other chronic breathing problem, or for post-tonsillectomy/adenoidectomy pain; ≥18 years: initially 100 mg once daily; may increase by 100 mg every 5 days; max 300 mg/day; *CrCl <30 mL/min or severe hepatic impairment:* not recommended

Tab: 100, 200, 300 mg ext-rel

Ultram <12 years: contraindicated; 12-<18: use extreme caution; not recommended for children and adolescents with obesity, asthma, obstructive sleep apnea, or other chronic breathing problem, or for post-tonsillectomy/adenoidectomy pain; ≥18 years: 50-100 mg q 4-6 hours prn; max 400 mg/day; *CrCl <30 mL/min:* max 100 mg q 12 hours; *Cirrhosis:* max 50 mg q 12 hours

Tab: 50*mg

Ultram ER <12 years: contraindicated; 12-<18: use extreme caution; not recommended for children and adolescents with obesity, asthma, obstructive sleep apnea, or other chronic breathing problem, or for post-tonsillectomy/adenoidectomy pain; ≥18 years: initially 100 mg once daily; may increase by 100 mg every 5 days; max 300 mg/day; *CrCl <30 mL/min:* or *severe hepatic impairment:* not recommended

Tab: 100, 200, 300 mg ext-rel

➤ *tramadol/acetaminophen* (C)(IV)(G) <12 years: contraindicated; 12-<18: use extreme caution; not recommended for children and adolescents with obesity, asthma, obstructive sleep apnea, or other chronic breathing problem, or for post-tonsillectomy/adenoidectomy pain; ≥18 years: 2 tabs q 4-6 hours; max 8 tabs/day; 5 days; *CrCl <30 mL/min:* max 2 tabs q 12 hours; max 4 tabs/day x 5 days

Ultracet *Tab:* tram 37.5/acet 325 mg

Comment: *Tramadol* is known to be excreted in breast milk. The FDA and the European Medicines Agency (EMA) are investigating the safety of using *tramadol*-containing medications to treat pain in children 12-18 years because of the potential for serious side effects, including slowed or difficult breathing.

Other Oral Analgesics *see Pain page 298*

TRICYCLIC ANTIDEPRESSANTS (TCAs)

Comment: Co-administration of SSRIs and TCAs requires extreme caution.

➤ *amitriptyline* (C)(G) <12 years: not recommended; ≥12 years: 10-20 mg q HS *Tab:* 10, 25, 50, 75, 100, 150 mg

➤ *amoxapine* (C) <12 years: not recommended; ≥12 years: initially 50 mg bid-tid; after 1 week may increase to 100 mg bid-tid; usual effective dose 200-300 mg/day; if total dose exceeds 300 mg/day, give in divided doses (max 400 mg/day); may give as a single bedtime dose (max 300 mg q HS)

Tab: 25, 50, 100, 150 mg

➤ *clomipramine* (C)(G) <10 years: not recommended; 10-<16 years: initially 25 mg daily in divided doses; gradually increase; max 3 mg/kg or 100 mg, whichever is smaller; >16 years: initially 25 mg daily in divided doses; gradually increase to 100 mg during first 2 weeks; max 250 mg/day; total maintenance dose may be given at HS

Anafranil *Cap:* 25, 50, 75 mg

➤ *desipramine* (C)(G) <12 years: not recommended; ≥12 years: 100-200 mg/day in single or divided doses; max 300 mg/day

Norpramin *Tab:* 10, 25, 50, 75, 100, 150 mg

➤ *doxepin* (C)(G) <12 years: not recommended; ≥12 years: 75 mg/day; max 150 mg/day

Cap: 10, 25, 50, 75, 100, 150 mg; Oral conc: 10 mg/ml (4 oz w. dropper)

➤ *imipramine* (C)(G) <12 years: not recommended; ≥12 years:

Tofranil initially 75 mg daily (max 200 mg); adolescents initially 30-40 mg daily (max 100 mg/day); if maintenance dose exceeds 75 mg daily, may switch to **Tofranil PM** for divided <u>or</u> bedtime dose

    Tab: 10, 25, 50 mg

Tofranil PM initially 75 mg daily 1 hour before HS; max 200 mg

    Cap: 75, 100, 125, 150 mg

➤ *nortriptyline* (D)(G) <12 years: not recommended; ≥12 years: initially 25 mg tid-qid; max 150 mg/day

    Pamelor *Cap:* 10, 25, 50, 75 mg; *Oral soln:* 10 mg/5 ml (16 oz)

➤ *protriptyline* (C) <12 years: not recommended; ≥12 years: initially 5 mg tid; usual dose 15-40 mg/day in 3-4 divided doses; max 60 mg/day

    Vivactil *Tab:* 5, 10 mg

➤ *trimipramine* (C) <12 years: not recommended; ≥12 years: initially 75 mg/day in divided doses; max 200 mg/day

    Surmontil *Cap:* 25, 50, 100 mg

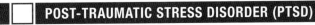

POST-TRAUMATIC STRESS DISORDER (PTSD)

Comment: No one pharmacological agent has emerged as the best treatment for PTSD. A combination of pharmacological agents (e.g., antidepressants, non-adrenergic agents, antipsychosis drugs) may comprise an individualized treatment plan to successfully manage core symptoms of PTSD as well as associated anxiety, depression, sleep disturbances, and co-occurring psychiatric disorders.

SELECTIVE SEROTONIN REUPTAKE INHIBITORS (SSRIs)

Comment: The FDA has approved two SSRIs for the treatment of PTSD: *paroxetine* and *sertraline*. However, the safety and efficacy of other SSRIs (*fluoxetine, citalopram, escitalopram, fluvoxamine*) have been tested in clinical practice. Co-administration of SSRIs with TCAs requires extreme caution. Concomitant use of MAOIs and SSRIs is absolutely contraindicated. Avoid St. John's wort and other serotonergic agents. A potentially fatal adverse event is *serotonin syndrome*, caused by serotonin excess. Milder symptoms require HCP intervention to avert severe symptoms that can be rapidly fatal without urgent/emergent medical care. Symptoms include restlessness, agitation, confusion, hallucinations, tachycardia, hypertension, dilated pupils, muscle twitching, muscle rigidity, loss of muscle coordination, diaphoresis, diarrhea, headache, shivering, piloerection, hyperpyrexia, cardiac arrhythmias, seizures, loss of consciousness, coma, and death. Abrupt withdrawal or interruption of treatment with an antidepressant medication is sometimes associated with an *antidepressant discontinuation syndrome*, which may be mediated by gradually tapering the drug over a period of two weeks or longer, depending on the dose strength and length of treatment. Common symptoms of the *serotonin discontinuation syndrome* include flu-like symptoms (nausea, vomiting, diarrhea, headaches, sweating), sleep disturbances (insomnia, nightmares, constant sleepiness), mood disturbances (dysphoria, anxiety, agitation), cognitive disturbances (mental confusion, hyperarousal), sensory and movement disturbances (imbalance, tremors, vertigo, dizziness, electric-shock-like sensations in the brain, often described by sufferers as "brain zaps").

▷ *citalopram* (C)(G) <12 years: not recommended; ≥12 years: initially 20 mg once daily; may increase after one week to 40 mg once daily; max 40 mg
    Celexa *Tab:* 10, 20, 40 mg; *Oral soln:* 10 mg/5 ml (120 ml) (pepper mint)(sugar-free, alcohol-free, parabens)

▷ *escitalopram* (C)(G) <12 years: not recommended; 12-17 years: initially 10 mg daily; may increase to 20 mg daily after 3 weeks; ≥17 years: initially 10 mg daily; may increase to 20 mg daily after 1 week; *Hepatic impairment:* 10 mg once daily
    Lexapro *Tab:* 5, 10*, 20*mg
    Lexapro Oral Solution *Oral soln:* 1 mg/ml (240 ml) (peppermint) (parabens)

▷ *fluoxetine* (C)(G)
    Prozac <8 years: not recommended; 8-17 years: initially 10 mg/day; may increase after 1 week to 20 mg/day; range 20-60 mg/day; range for lower weight children, 20-30 mg/day; ≥17 years: initially 20 mg daily; may increase after 1 week; doses >20 mg/day should be divided into AM and noon doses; max 80 mg/day
        Cap: 10, 20, 40 mg; *Tab:* 30*, 60*mg; *Oral soln:* 20 mg/5 ml (4 oz) (mint)
    Prozac Weekly <12 years: not recommended; ≥12 years: following daily *fluoxetine* therapy at 20 mg/day for 13 weeks, may initiate **Prozac Weekly** 7 days after the last 20 mg *fluoxetine* dose
        Cap: 90 mg ent-coat del-rel pellets

▷ *levomilnacipran* (C) <12 years: not recommended; ≥12 years: swallow whole; initially 20 mg once daily for 2 days; then increase to 40 mg once daily; may increase dose in 40 mg increments at intervals of ≥2 days; max 120 mg once daily; *CrCl 30-59 mL/min:* max 80 mg once daily; *CrCl 15-29 mL/min:* max 40 mg once daily
    Fetzima *Cap:* 20, 40, 80, 120 mg ext-rel

▷ *paroxetine maleate* (D)(G)
    Paxil <12 years: not recommended; ≥12 years: initially 20 mg daily in AM; may increase by 10 mg/day at weekly intervals as needed; max 60 mg/day
        Tab: 10*, 20*, 30, 40 mg
    Paxil CR <12 years: not recommended; ≥12 years: initially 25 mg daily in AM; may increase by 12.5 mg at weekly intervals as needed; max 62.5 mg/day
        Tab: 12.5, 25, 37.5 mg cont-rel ent-coat
    Paxil Suspension <12 years: not recommended; ≥12 years: initially 20 mg daily in AM; may increase by 10 mg/day at weekly intervals as needed; max 60 mg/day
        Oral susp: 10 mg/5 ml (250 ml) (orange)

▷ *sertraline* (C)(G) <6 years: not recommended; 6-<12 years: initially 25 mg daily; max 200 mg/day; 12-17 years: initially 50 mg daily; max 200 mg/day ≥17 years: initially 50 mg daily; increase at 1 week intervals if needed; max 200 mg daily; dilute oral concentrate immediately prior to administration in 4 oz water, ginger ale, lemon/lime soda, lemonade, or orange juice
    Zoloft *Tab:* 25*, 50*, 100*mg; *Oral conc:* 20 mg per ml (60 ml) (alcohol 12%)

ATYPICAL ANTIPSYCHOSIS DRUGS

▷ *olanzapine* (C)(G) <13 years: not recommended; 13-17 years: initially 2.5-5 mg once daily at HS; >17 years: initially 5-10 mg once daily at HS; titrate weekly, max 20 mg at HS; usual maintenance 10-20 mg/day
    Zyprexa *Tab:* 2.5, 5, 7.5, 10, 15, 20 mg
    Zyprexa Zydis *ODT:* 5, 10, 15, 20 mg (phenylalanine)

▷ *quetiapine* (C)(G)

    SeroQUEL <10 years: not recommended; 10-17 years: initially 25 mg bid, titrate q 2nd <u>or</u> 3rd day in increments of 25-50 mg bid-tid; max 600 mg/day in 2-3 divided doses; >17 years: initially 25 mg bid, titrate q 2nd <u>or</u> 3rd day in increments of 25-50 mg bid-tid; usual maintenance 400-600 mg/day in 2-3 divided doses

      Tab: 25, 50, 100, 200, 300, 400 mg

    SeroQUEL XR <18 years: not recommended; ≥18 years: swallow whole; administer once daily in the PM; *Day 1:* 50 mg; *Day 2:* 100 mg; *Day 3:* 200 mg; *Day 4:* 300 mg; usual range 400-600 mg/day

      Tab: 50, 150, 200, 300, 400 mg ext-rel

▷ *risperidone* (C)

Comment: **Risperdal** tabs, oral solution, and M-tabs are indicated for the short-term monotherapy of acute mania <u>or</u> mixed episodes associated with bipolar I disorder, <u>or</u> in combination with *lithium* <u>or</u> *valproic acid* in patients >12 years-of-age. **Risperdol Consta** is indicated as monotherapy <u>or</u> adjunctive therapy to *lithium* <u>or</u> *valproic acid* for the maintenance treatment mania and mixed episodes in bipolar I disorder.

    Risperdal <5 years: not established; 5-10 years: initially 0.5 mg once daily at the same time each day adjust at 24 hour intervals by 0.5-1 mg to target dose 2.5 mg/day; usual range 1-6 mg/day; max 6 mg/day; >10 years: *Tab:* initially 2-3 mg once daily; may adjust at 24 hour intervals by 1 mg/day; usual range 1-6 mg/day; max 6 mg/day; *Oral soln:* do not take with cola <u>or</u> tea

      Tab: 0.25, 0.5, 1, 2, 3, 4 mg; *Oral soln:* 1 mg/ml (100 ml)

    Risperdal Consta <18 years: not established; ≥18 years: administer deep IM in the deltoid <u>or</u> gluteal; give with oral *respiridone* <u>or</u> other antipsychotic x 3 weeks; then stop oral form; 25 mg IM every 2 weeks; max 50 mg every 2 weeks

      Vial: 12.5, 25, 37.5, 50 mg pwdr for long-acting IM inj after reconstitution, single use w. diluent and supplies

    Risperdal M-Tab <10 years: not established; ≥10 years: dissolve on tongue with <u>or</u> without fluid

      M-Tab: 0.5, 1, 2, 3, 4 mg orally-disint (phenylalanine)

NON-ADRENERGIC AGENTS

ALPHA-1 ANTAGONISTS

▷ *prazosin* (C)(G) <12 years: not recommended: ≥12 years: first dose at HS, 1 mg bid-tid; increase dose slowly; usual range 6-15 mg/day in divided doses; max 20-40 mg/day

    Minipress *Cap:* 1, 2, 5 mg

Comment: *prazosin* is useful in reducing nightmares and other sleep disturbances.

CENTRAL ALPHA2A-AGONISTS

▷ *clonidine* (C)

Comment: *clonidine* is useful to reduce nightmares, hypervigilance, startle reactions, and outbursts of rage.

    Catapres <12 years: not recommended; ≥12 years: initially 0.1 mg bid; usual range 0.2-0.6 mg/day in divided doses; max 2.4 mg/day

      Tab: 0.1*, 0.2*, 0.3*mg

Catapres-TTS <12 years: not recommended; ≥12 years: initially 0.1 mg patch weekly; increase after 1-2 weeks if needed; max 0.6 mg/day
Patch: 0.1, 0.2 mg/day (12/carton); 0.3 mg/day (4/carton)
Kapvay (G) <12 years: not recommended; ≥12 years: initially 0.1 mg bid; usual range 0.2-0.6 mg/day in divided doses; max 2.4 mg/day
Tab: 0.1, 0.2 mg
Nexiclon XR <12 years: not recommended; ≥12 years: initially 0.18 mg (2 ml) suspension or 0.17 mg tab once daily; usual max 0.52 mg (6 ml suspension) once daily
Tab: 0.17, 0.26 mg ext-rel; *Oral susp:* 0.09 mg/ml ext-rel (4 oz)

BETA-ADRENERGIC BLOCKER (NON-CARDIOSELECTIVE)

▷ *propranolol* (C)(G)
Comment: *propranolol* is useful to mediate hyperarousal. For other non-cardioselective beta-adrenergic blockers, *see* **Hypertension** *page* 200
Inderal <12 years: not recommended; ≥12 years: initially 10 mg bid; usual range 160-320 mg/day in divided doses
Tab: 10*, 20*, 40*, 60*, 80*mg
Inderal LA <12 years: not recommended; ≥12 years: initially 80 mg daily in a single dose; increase q 3-7 days; usual range 120-160 mg/day; max 320 mg/day in a single dose
Cap: 60, 80, 120, 160 mg sust-rel
InnoPran XL <12 years: not recommended; ≥12 years: initially 80 mg q HS; max 120 mg/day
Cap: 80, 120 mg ext-rel

SEROTONIN AND NOREPINEPHRINE REUPTAKE INHIBITORS (SNRIs)

▷ *desvenlafaxine* (C)(G) <18 years: not recommended; ≥18 years: swallow whole; initially 50 mg once daily; max 120 mg/day
Pristiq *Tab:* 50, 100 mg ext-rel
▷ *duloxetine* (C)(G) <12 years: not recommended; ≥12 years: swallow whole; initially 30 mg once daily x 1 week; then, increase to 60 mg once daily; max 120 mg/day
Cymbalta *Cap:* 20, 30, 40, 60 mg del-rel
▷ *venlafaxine* (C)(G)
Effexor <12 years: not recommended; ≥12 years: initially 75 mg/day in 2-3 divided doses; may increase at 4 day intervals in 75 mg increments to 150 mg/day; max 225 mg/day
Tab: 37.5, 75, 150, 225 mg
Effexor XR <18 years: not recommended; ≥18 years: initially 75 mg q AM; may start at 37.5 mg daily x 4-7 days, then increase by increments of up to 75 mg/day at intervals of at least 4 days; usual ax 375 mg/day
Tab/Cap: 37.5, 75, 150 mg ext-rel
▷ *vortioxetine* (C) <18 years: not established; ≥18 years: initially 10 mg once daily; max 30 mg/day
Brintellix *Tab:* 5, 10, 15, 20 mg

5HT2/3 RECEPTOR BLOCKERS

▷ *mirtazapine* (C) <12 years: not established; ≥12 years: initially 15 mg q HS; increase at intervals of 1-2 weeks; 1-2 weeks; usual range 15-60 mg/day; max 60 mg/day

Remeron *Tab:* 15*, 30*, 45*mg
Remeron SolTab *ODT:* 15, 30, 45 mg (orange) (phenylalanine)

SEROTONIN/ACETYLCHOLINE/NOREPINEPHRINE/DOPAMINE BLOCKER

▷ *trazodone* (C)(G) <18 years: not recommended; ≥18 years: initially 150 mg/day in divided doses with food; increase by 50 mg/day q 3-4 days; max 400 mg/day in divided doses or 50-400 mg at HS
    Oleptro *Tab:* 50, 100*, 150*, 200, 250, 300 mg

TRICYCLIC ANTIDEPRESSANTS (TCAs)

Comment: Co-administration of SSRIs and TCAs requires extreme caution.
▷ *amitriptyline* (C)(G) <12 years: not recommended; ≥12 years: 10-20 mg q HS *Tab:* 10, 25, 50, 75, 100, 150 mg
▷ *amoxapine* (C) <12 years: not recommended; ≥12 years: initially 50 mg bid-tid; after 1 week may increase to 100 mg bid-tid; usual effective dose 200-300 mg/day; if total dose exceeds 300 mg/day, give in divided doses (max 400 mg/day); may give as a single bedtime dose (max 300 mg q HS)
    Tab: 25, 50, 100, 150 mg
▷ *clomipramine* (C)(G) <10 years: not recommended; 10-<16 years: initially 25 mg daily in divided doses; gradually increase; max 3 mg/kg or 100 mg, whichever is smaller; >16 years: initially 25 mg daily in divided doses; gradually increase to 100 mg during first 2 weeks; max 250 mg/day; total maintenance dose may be given at HS
    Anafranil *Cap:* 25, 50, 75 mg
▷ *desipramine* (C)(G) <12 years: not recommended; ≥12 years: 100-200 mg/day in single or divided doses; max 300 mg/day
    Norpramin *Tab:* 10, 25, 50, 75, 100, 150 mg
▷ *doxepin* (C)(G) <12 years: not recommended; ≥12 years: 75 mg/day; max 150 mg/day
    Cap: 10, 25, 50, 75, 100, 150 mg; Oral conc: 10 mg/ml (4 oz w. dropper)
▷ *imipramine* (C)(G) <12 years: not recommended; ≥12 years:
    Tofranil initially 75 mg daily (max 200 mg); adolescents initially 30-40 mg daily (max 100 mg/day); if maintenance dose exceeds 75 mg daily, may switch to Tofranil PM for divided or bedtime dose
        Tab: 10, 25, 50 mg
    Tofranil PM initially 75 mg daily 1 hour before HS; max 200 mg
        Cap: 75, 100, 125, 150 mg
▷ *nortriptyline* (D)(G) <12 years: not recommended; ≥12 years: initially 25 mg tid-qid; max 150 mg/day
    Pamelor *Cap:* 10, 25, 50, 75 mg; *Oral soln:* 10 mg/5 ml (16 oz)
▷ *protriptyline* (C) <12 years: not recommended; ≥12 years: initially 5 mg tid; usual dose 15-40 mg/day in 3-4 divided doses; max 60 mg/day
    Vivactil *Tab:* 5, 10 mg
▷ *trimipramine* (C) <12 years: not recommended; ≥12 years: initially 75 mg/day in divided doses; max 200 mg/day
    Surmontil *Cap:* 25, 50, 100 mg

MONOAMINE OXIDASE INHIBITORS (MAOIS)

Comment: Many drug and food interactions with this class of drugs; use cautiously. MAOIs should be reserved for refractory depression that has not responded to other classes of antidepressants. Concomitant use of MAOIs and SSRIs is contraindicated. See mfr pkg insert for drug and food interactions. MAOIs have been used to reduce recurrent recollections of the trauma, nightmares, flashbacks, numbing, sleep disturbances, and social withdrawal in PTSD.

▶ *phenelzine* (C)(G) <16 years: not recommended; ≥16 years: initially 15 mg tid; max 90 mg/day

Nardil *Tab:* 15 mg

▶ *selegiline* (C) <12 years: not recommended; ≥12 years: initially 10 mg tid; max 60 mg/day

Emsam *Transdermal patch:* 6 mg/24 hrs, 9 mg/24 hrs, 12 mg/24 hrs

Comment: At the **Emsam** transdermal patch 6 mg/24 hrs dose, the dietary restrictions commonly required when using non-selective MAOIs are not necessary.

PREGNANCY

see **Appendix Z: Prescription Prenatal Vitamins** *page 520*

Comment: Prenatal vitamins should have at least 400 mcg of folic acid content. Take one dose once daily. It is recommended that prenatal vitamins be started at least 3 months prior to conception to improve preconception nutritional status, and continued throughout pregnancy and the postnatal period, in lactating and non-lactating females, and throughout the childbearing years.

NAUSEA/VOMITING

▶ *doxylamine succinate/pyridoxine* (A)(G) do not crush or chew; take on an empty stomach with water; initially 2 tabs at HS on day 1; may increase to 1 tab AM and 2 tabs at HS day 2; may increase to 1 tab AM, 1 tab mid-afternoon, 2 tabs at HS; max 4 tabs/day

Diclegis *Tab: doxyl* 10 mg/*pyri* 10 mg del-rel

Comment: **Diclegis** is the only FDA-approved drug for the treatment of morning sickness. It has not been studied in females with hyperemesis gravidarum.

▶ *promethazine* (C) <2 years: not recommended; 2-12 years: 0.5 mg/lb or 6.25-25 mg q 4-6 hours PO or rectally; >12 years: 12.5-25 q 4-6 hours PO or rectally

Phenergan *Tab:* 12.5*, 25*, 50 mg; *Plain syr:* 6.25 mg/5 ml; *Fortis syr:* 25 mg/5 ml; *Rectal supp:* 12.5, 25, 50 mg; *Amp:* 25, 50 mg/ml (1 ml)

Comment: *promethazine* is contraindicated in children with uncomplicated nausea, dehydration, Reye's syndrome, history of sleep apnea, asthma, and lower respiratory disorders in children. *Promethazine* lowers the seizure threshold in children, may cause cholestatic jaundice, anticholinergic effects, extrapyramidal effects, and potentially fatal respiratory depression.

▶ *ondansetron* (C)(G) <4 years: not recommended; 4-11 years: 4-8 mg bid prn; >11 hours: 8 mg q 8 hours prn

Zofran *Tab:* 4, 8, 24 mg

Zofran Injection *Vial:* 2 mg/ml (2 ml single dose); 2 mg/ml (20 ml multidose) for IV or IM administration

Zofran ODT *ODT:* 4, 8 mg (strawberry) (phenylalanine)

Zofran Oral Solution *Oral soln:* 4 mg/5 ml (50 ml) (strawberry)
Zuplenz Oral Soluble Film: 4, 8 mg orally-disint (10/carton) (peppermint)

▢ PREMENSTRUAL DYSPHORIC DISORDER (PMDD)

Oral Prescription NSAIDs *see page* 490
Other Oral Analgesics *see* **Pain** *page* 298
Other Oral Contraceptives *see page* 475

ORAL ESTROGEN/PROGESTERONE COMBINATIONS

Comment: **Rajani** (a generic form of **Beyaz**) and **Yaz,** also available in generic forms (**Gianvi, Ocella, Syeda, Vestura, Yasmin, Zarah**), have an FDA indication for treatment of PMDD in post-menarchal females who choose to use an OCP. Contraindicated with renal and adrenal insufficiency. Monitor K⁺ level during the first cycle if the patient is at risk for hyperkalemia for any reason. If the patient is taking a drug that increases serum potassium (e.g., ACEIs, ARBS, NSAIDs, K⁺ sparing diuretics), the patient is at risk for hyperkalemia.

▷ *ethinyl estradiol/drospirenone* (X)(G) Pre-menarchal: not indicated; Post-menarchal: 1 tab once daily x 28 days; repeat cycle; start on first Sunday after menses begins or on first day of next menses
   Yaz *Tab: ethin estra* 20 mcg/*drospir* 3 mg
▷ *ethinyl/estradiol/drospirenone/levomefolate calcium* (X)(G) Pre-menarchal: not indicated; Post-menarchal: 1 tab once daily x 28 days; repeat cycle; start on first Sunday after menses begins or on first day of next menses preceded by a negative pregnancy test
   Beyaz *Tab: ethin estra* 20 mcg/*drospir* 3 mg/*levo* 0.451 mg
   Rajani *Tab: ethin estra* 20 mcg/*drospir* 3 mg/*levo* 0.451 mg

DIURETICS

▷ *spironolactone* (D)(G) <12 years: not recommended; ≥12 years: initially 50-100 mg once daily or in divided doses; titrate at 2-week intervals
   Aldactone *Tab:* 25, 50*, 100*mg

ANTIDEPRESSANTS

▷ *fluoxetine* (C)(G)
   Prozac <8 years: not recommended; 8-17 years: initially 10 or 20 mg/day; start lower weight children at 10 mg/day; if starting at 10 mg/day, may increase after 1 week to 20 mg/day; ≥17 years: initially 20 mg daily; may increase after 1 week; doses >20 mg/day should be divided into AM and noon doses; max 80 mg/day
   Tab: 10*mg; *Cap:* 10, 20, 40 mg; *Oral soln:* 20 mg/5 ml (4 oz) (mint)
   Prozac Weekly <8 years: not recommended; ≥8 years: following daily *fluoxetine* therapy at 20 mg/day for 13 weeks, may initiate **Prozac Weekly** 7 days after the last 20 mg *fluoxetine* dose
   Cap: 90 mg ent-coat del-rel pellets
   Sarafem <8 years: not recommended; ≥8 years: administer daily or 14 days before expected menses and through first full day of menses; initially 20 mg/day; max 80 mg/day
   Tab: 10, 15, 20 mg; *Cap:* 20 mg

▷ *paroxetine maleate* (D)(G)
  Paxil <12 years: not recommended; ≥12 years: initially 20 mg daily in AM; may increase by 10 mg/day at weekly intervals as needed; max 60 mg/day
    Tab: 10*, 20*, 30, 40 mg
  Paxil CR <12 years: not recommended; ≥12 years: initially 25 mg daily in AM; may increase by 12.5 mg at weekly intervals as needed; max 62.5 mg/day; may start 14 days before and continue through day one of menses
    Tab: 12.5, 25, 37.5 mg cont-rel ent-coat
  Paxil Suspension <12 years: not recommended; ≥12 years: initially 20 mg daily in AM; may increase by 10 mg/day at weekly intervals as needed; max 60 mg/day
    Oral susp: 10 mg/5 ml (250 ml) (orange)
▷ *sertraline* (C) <12 years: not recommended; ≥12 years: *For 2 weeks prior to onset of menses:* initially 50 mg daily x 3; then increase to 100 mg daily for remainder of the cycle; *For full cycle:* initially 50 mg daily; then may increase by 50 mg/day each cycle to max 150 mg/day
  Zoloft *Tab:* 25*, 50*, 100*mg; *Oral conc:* 20 mg per ml (60 ml) (alcohol 12%); dilute just before administering in 4 oz water, ginger ale, lemon-lime soda, lemonade, or orange juice
▷ *nortriptyline* (D)(G) <12 years: not recommended; ≥12 years: initially 25 mg tid-qid; max 150 mg/day
  Pamelor *Cap:* 10, 25, 50, 75 mg; *Oral soln:* 10 mg/5 ml

CALCIUM SUPPLEMENTS

▷ *calcium* (C) 1200 mg/day
See *Osteoporosis page 282*

PROCTITIS: ACUTE (PROCTOCOLITIS/ENTERITIS)

Comment: The following regimen for the treatment of proctitis, proctocolitis, and enteritis is published in the **2015 CDC Sexually Transmitted Diseases Treatment Guidelines**.

RECOMMENDED REGIMEN

▷ *ceftriaxone* (B)(G) 250 mg IM in a single dose
  Rocephin *Vial:* 250, 500 mg; 1, 2 g
    plus
▷ *doxycycline* (D)(G) <8 years: not recommended; ≥8 years, ≤100 lb: 2 mg/lb on first day in 2 divided doses, followed by 1 mg/lb/day in 1-2 divided doses x 7 days; ≥8 years, >100 lb: 100 mg bid x 7 days; *see page 561 for dose by weight table*
  Acticlate *Tab:* 75, 150** mg
  Adoxa *Tab:* 50, 75, 100, 150 mg ent-coat
  Doryx *Tab:* 50, 75, 100, 150, 200 mg del-rel
  Monodox *Cap:* 50, 75, 100 mg
  Oracea *Cap:* 40 mg del-rel
  Vibramycin *Tab:* 100 mg; *Cap:* 50, 100 mg; *Syr:* 50 mg/5 ml (raspberry-apple) (sulfites); *Oral susp:* 25 mg/5 ml (raspberry)
  Vibra-Tab *Tab:* 100 mg film-coat

Comment: *doxycycline* is contraindicated <8 years-of-age, in pregnancy, and lactation (discolors developing tooth enamel). A side effect may be photo-sensitivity (photophobia). Do not take with antacids, calcium supplements, milk or other dairy, or within 2 hours of taking another drug.

PROSTATITIS: ACUTE

ANTI-INFECTIVES

▶ *ciprofloxacin* (C) <18 years: not recommended; ≥18 years: 500 mg bid x 4-6 weeks; max 1.5 gm/day
   Cipro (G) *Tab:* 250, 500, 750 mg; *Oral susp:* 250, 500 mg/5 ml (100 ml) (strawberry)
   Cipro XR *Tab:* 500, 1,000 mg ext-rel
   ProQuin XR *Tab:* 500 mg ext-rel
Comment: *ciprofloxacin* is contraindicated <18 years-of-age, and during pregnancy and lactation. Risk of tendonitis or tendon rupture.
▶ *norfloxacin* (C) <18 years: not recommended; ≥18 years: 400 mg bid x 28 days
   Noroxin *Tab:* 400 mg
Comment: *norfloxacin* is contraindicated <18 years-of-age, and during pregnancy and lactation. Risk of tendonitis or tendon rupture.
▶ *ofloxacin* (C)(G) <18 years: not recommended; ≥18 years: 300 mg x bid x 6 weeks
   Floxin *Tab:* 200, 300, 400 mg
Comment: *ofloxacin* is contraindicated <18 years-of-age, and during pregnancy and lactation. Risk of tendonitis or tendon rupture.
▶ *trimethoprim/sulfamethoxazole* (C)(G)
   Bactrim, Septra <12 years: not recommended; ≥12 years: 2 tabs bid x 10 days
      Tab: trim 80 mg/*sulfa* 400 mg*
   Bactrim DS, Septra DS <12 years: not recommended; ≥12 years: 1 tab bid x 10 days
      Tab: trim 160 mg/*sulfa* 800 mg*
   Bactrim Pediatric Suspension, Septra Pediatric Suspension <2 months: not recommended; ≥2 months-12 years: 40 mg/kg/day of *sulfamethoxazole* in 2 doses bid x 10 days
      Oral susp: trim 40 mg/*sulfa* 200 mg per 5 ml (100 ml) (cherry) (alcohol 0.3%)
Comment: *CrCl 15-30 mL/min:* reduce dose by 1/2; *CrCl <15 mL/min:* not recommended.

PROSTATITIS: CHRONIC

ANTI-INFECTIVES

▶ *carbenicillin* (B) <12 years: not recommended; ≥12 years: 1-2 tabs qid x 7-14 days
   Geocillin *Tab:* 382 mg
▶ *ciprofloxacin* (C) <18 years: not recommended; ≥18 years: 500 mg bid x 3 or more months; max 1.5 gm/day
   Cipro (G) *Tab:* 250, 500, 750 mg; *Oral susp:* 250, 500 mg/5 ml (100 ml) (strawberry)
   Cipro XR *Tab:* 500, 1000 mg ext-rel

ProQuin XR *Tab:* 500 mg ext-rel

Comment: *ciprofloxacin* is contraindicated <18 years-of-age, and during pregnancy and lactation. Risk of tendonitis or tendon rupture.

▶ *ofloxacin* (C)(G) <18 years: not recommended; ≥18 years: 300 mg bid x 4-12 weeks
Floxin *Tab:* 200, 300, 400 mg

Comment: *ofloxacin* is contraindicated <18 years-of-age, and during pregnancy and lactation. Risk of tendonitis or tendon rupture.

▶ *norfloxacin* (C) <18 years: not recommended; ≥18 years: 400 mg bid x 4-12 weeks
Noroxin *Tab:* 400 mg

Comment: *norfloxacin* contraindicated <18 years-of-age, and during pregnancy and lactation. Risk of tendonitis or tendon rupture.

▶ *trimethoprim/sulfamethoxazole* (C)(G)
Bactrim, Septra <12 years: not recommended; ≥12 years: 2 tabs bid x 10 days
Tab: trim 80 mg/*sulfa* 400 mg*
Bactrim DS, Septra DS <12 years: not recommended; ≥12 years: 1 tab bid x 10 days
Tab: trim 160 mg/*sulfa* 800 mg*
Bactrim Pediatric Suspension, Septra Pediatric Suspension <2 months: not recommended; ≥2 months-12 years: 40 mg/kg/day of *sulfamethoxazole* in 2 doses bid x 10 days
Oral susp: trim 40 mg/*sulfa* 200 mg per 5 ml (100 ml) (cherry) (alcohol 0.3%)
Comment: *CrCl 15-30 mL/min: reduce dose by 1/2; CrCl <15 mL/min: not recommended.*

SUPPRESSION THERAPY

▶ *trimethoprim/sulfamethoxazole* (C)(G)
Bactrim, Septra <12 years: not recommended; ≥12 years: 2 tabs bid x 10 days
Tab: trim 80 mg/*sulfa* 400 mg*
Bactrim DS, Septra DS <12 years: not recommended; ≥12 years: 1 tab bid x 10 days
Tab: trim 160 mg/*sulfa* 800 mg*
Bactrim Pediatric Suspension, Septra Pediatric Suspension <2 months: not recommended; ≥2 months-12 years: 40 mg/kg/day of *sulfamethoxazole* in 2 doses bid; >12 years: use tabs
Oral susp: trim 40 mg/*sulfa* 200 mg per 5 ml (100 ml) (cherry) (alcohol 0.3%)
Comment: *CrCl 15-30 mL/min: reduce dose by 1/2; CrCl <15 mL/min: not recommended.*

PRURITUS

Oral Prescription Drugs for the Management of Allergy, Cough, and Cold Symptoms *see page* 523
Topical Corticosteroids *see page* 494
Parenteral Corticosteroids *see page* 499
Oral Corticosteroids *see page* 498
Eucerin Products (OTC)
Lac-Hydrin Products (OTC)
Lubriderm Products (OTC)

Aveeno Products (OTC)

TOPICAL OIL

▶ *fluocinolone acetamide* 0.01% topical oil (C) <6 years: not recommended; ≥6 years: apply sparingly bid for up to 4 weeks
> **Derma-Smoothe/FS Topical Oil** apply sparingly tid
> *Topical oil:* 0.01% (4 oz) (peanut oil)

TOPICAL ANALGESICS

▶ *capsaicin* cream (B)(G) <2 years: not recommended; 2-12 years: apply sparingly to intact skin bid prn; >12 years: apply tid-qid prn
> **Axsain** *Crm:* 0.075% (1, 2 oz)
> **Capsin** (OTC) *Lotn:* 0.025, 0, 075% (59 ml)
> **Capzasin-P** (OTC) *Crm:* 0.025% (1.5 oz); *Lotn:* 0.025% (2 oz)
> **Capzasin-HP** (OTC) *Crm:* 0.075% (1.5 oz); *Lotn:* 0.075% (2 oz)
> **Dolorac** *Crm:* 0.025% (28 gm)
> **Double Cap** (OTC) *Crm:* 0.05% (2 oz)
> **R-Gel** *Gel:* 0.025% (15, 30 gm)
> **Zostrix** (OTC) *Crm:* 0.025% (0.7, 1.5, 3 oz)
> **Zostrix HP** (OTC) *Emol crm:* 0.075% (1, 2 oz)

Comment: Provides some relief by 1-2 weeks; optimal benefit may take 4-6 weeks. Avoid contact with mucous membranes.

▶ *doxepin* cream (B) <12 years: not recommended; ≥12 years: apply to affected area qid at intervals of at least 3-4 hours; max 8 days
> **Prudoxin** *Crm:* 5% (45 gm)
> **Zonalon** *Crm:* 5% (30, 45 gm)

▶ *pimecrolimus* 1% cream (C) <2 years: not recommended; ≥2 years: apply to affected area bid; do not occlude
> **Elidel** *Crm:* 1% (30, 60, 100 gm)

Comment: *pimecrolimus* is indicated for short-term and intermittent long-term use. Discontinue use when resolution occurs. Contraindicated if the patient is immunosuppressed. Change to the 0.1% preparation or if secondary bacterial infection is present.

▶ *tacrolimus* (C) <2 years: not recommended; 2-15 years: use 0.03% strength; apply to affected area bid; continue for 1 week after clearing; >15 years: apply to affected area bid; do not occlude or apply to wet skin; continue for 1 week after clearing
> **Protopic** *Oint:* 0.03, 0.1% (30, 60, 100 gm)

▶ *trolamine salicylate* (NE) <2 years: not recommended; ≥2 years: apply tid-qid prn to intact skin
> **Mobisyl** *Crm:* 10%

Comment: Provides some relief by 1-2 weeks; optimal benefit

▢ PSEUDOGOUT

Oral Prescription NSAIDs *see page* 490
Other Oral Analgesics *see **Pain** page* 298
Topical/Transdermal NSAIDs *see **Pain** page* 298

Parenteral Corticosteroids *see page* 499
Oral Corticosteroids *see page* 498
Topical Analgesic and Anesthetic Agents *see page* 488

PSEUDOMEMBRANOUS COLITIS

Comment: Staphylococcal enterocolitis and antibiotic-associated pseudomembranous colitis caused by *C. difficile*.

ANTI-INFECTIVES

▷ *vancomycin* (B, caps; C, susp)(G)40 mg/kg/day in 3-4 doses x 7-10 days; max 2 gm/day; ≥40 kg: 500 mg to 2 gm in 3-4 doses x 7-10 days; max 2 gm/day
▷ *metronidazole* (not for use in 1st; B in 2nd, 3rd)(G) 500 mg tid x 14 days
    Flagyl *Tab:* 250*, 500*mg
    Flagyl 375 *Cap:* 375 mg
    Flagyl ER *Tab:* 750 mg ext-rel
    Comment: Alcohol is contraindicated during treatment with oral *metronidazole* and for 72 hours after therapy due to a possible *disulfiram*-like reaction (nausea, vomiting, flushing, headache).

PSITTACOSIS

ANTI-INFECTIVES

▷ *tetracycline* (D)(G) <8 years: not recommended; ≥8 years, ≤100 lb: 25-50 mg/kg/day in 4 divided doses x 7-14 days; *see page 574 for dose by weight table*; ≥8 years, >100 lb: 250 mg qid or 500 mg tid x 7-14 days
    Achromycin V *Cap:* 250, 500 mg
    Sumycin *Tab:* 250, 500 mg; *Cap:* 250, 500 mg; *Oral susp:* 125 mg/5 ml (100, 200 ml) (fruit) (sulfites)
    Comment: *tetracycline* is contraindicated <8 years-of-age, in pregnancy, and lactation (discolors developing tooth enamel). A side effect may be photo-sensitivity (photophobia). Do not give with antacids or calcium supplements or within two hours of another drug.

PSORIASIS

Emollients *see Dermatitis: Atopic page* 102
Topical Corticosteroids *see page* 494

VITAMIN D-3 DERIVATIVES

▷ *calcipotriene* (C) <12 years: not recommended; ≥12 years: apply bid to lesions and gently rub in completely
    Dovonex *Crm:* 0.005% (30, 120 gm)

VITAMIN D-3 DERIVATIVE/CORTICOSTEROID COMBINATIONS

▷ *calcipotriene/betamethasone dipropionate* (C)(G)

Enstilar <18 years: not recommended; ≥18 years: apply to affected area and gently rub in once daily x up to 4 weeks; limit treatment area to 30% of body surface area; do not occlude; do not use on face, axillae, groin, <u>or</u> atrophic skin; max 100 gm/week

Foam: calci 0.005%/*beta* 0.064% (60 gm spray can)

Taclonex <18 years: not recommended; ≥18 years: apply to affected area and gently rub in once daily as needed, up to 4 weeks

Taclonex Ointment <18 years: not recommended; ≥18 years: apply bid to lesions and gently rub in completely; limit treatment area to 30% of body surface area; do not occlude; do not use on face, axillae, groin, <u>or</u> atrophic skin; max 100 gm/week

Oint: calci 0.005%/*beta* 0.064% (60, 100 gm)

Taclonex Scalp Topical Suspension <18 years: not recommended; ≥18 years: apply to affected area and gently rub in once daily x 2 weeks <u>or</u> until cleared; max 8 weeks; limit treatment area to 30% of body surface area; do not occlude; do not use on face, axillae, groin, <u>or</u> atrophic skin; max 100 gm/week

Bottle: (30, 60 g; 120 gm [2 x 60 g])

▷ *Calcitriol* (C) <18 years: not recommended; ≥18 years: apply bid to lesions and gently rub in completely; max weekly dose should not exceed 200 g

Vectical *Oint:* 3 mcg/g (100 gm)

IMMUNOSUPPRESSANTS

▷ *alefacept* (B) <12 years: not recommended; ≥12 years: 7.5 mg IV bolus <u>or</u> 15 mg IM once weekly x 12 weeks; may retreat x 12 weeks

Amevive *IV dose pack:* 7.5 mg single use (w. 10 ml sterile water diluents [use 0.6 ml]; 1, 4/pck); *IM dose pack:* 15 mg single use (w. 10 ml sterile water diluent [use 0.6 ml]; 1, 4/pck)

Comment: CD4+ and T-lymphocyte count should be checked prior to initiating treatment with *alefacept* and then monitored. Treatment should be withheld if CD4+ T-lymphocyte counts are below 250 cells/mcl.

▷ *cyclosporine* (C) <18 years: not recommended; ≥18 years: 1.25 mg/kg bid; may increase after 4 weeks by 0.5 mg/kg/day; then adjust at 2-week intervals; max 4 mg/kg/day; administer with meals

Neoral *Cap:* 25, 100 mg (alcohol)

Neoral Oral Solution *Oral soln:* 100 mg/ml (50 ml) may dilute in room temperature apple juice <u>or</u> orange juice (alcohol)

ANTIMITOTICS

▷ *anthralin* (C) <12 years: not recommended; ≥12 years: apply once daily

Zithranol-RR *Crm:* 1.2% (15, 45 gm)

RETINOIDS

▷ *acitretin* (X)(G) <12 years: not recommended; ≥12 years: 25-50 mg once daily with main meal

Soriatane *Cap:* 10, 25 mg

▷ *tazarotene* (X)(G) <12 years: not recommended; ≥12 years: apply once daily at HS
    Avage Cream *Crm:* 0.1% (30 gm)
    Tazorac Cream *Crm:* 0.05, 0.1% (15, 30, 60 gm)
    Tazorac Gel *Gel:* 0.05, 0.1% (30, 100 gm)

COAL TAR PREPARATIONS

▷ *coal tar* (C)(G)
    Scytera (OTC) apply qd-qid; use lowest effective dose
        Foam: 2%
    T/Gel Shampoo Extra Strength (OTC) use every other day; max 4 x/week;
    massage into affected areas for 5 minutes; rinse; repeat
        Shampoo: 1%
    T/Gel Shampoo Original Formula (OTC) use every other day; max 7 x/week;
    massage into affected areas for 5 minutes; rinse; repeat
        Shampoo: 0.5%
    T/Gel Shampoo Stubborn Itch Control (OTC) use every other day; max 7 x/
    week; massage into affected areas for 5 minutes; rinse; repeat
        Shampoo: 0.5%

INTERLEUKIN-17A ANTAGONIST

▷ *secukinumab* (B) <18 years: not recommended; ≥18 years: inject SC into the upper
    arm, abdomen, or thigh; rotate sites; administer 300 mg SC (as two separate 150
    mg SC injections) at weeks 0, 1, 2, 3, and 4; then 300 mg every 4 weeks; for some
    patients, 150 mg/dose may be sufficient
    Cosentyx *Vial:* 150 mg/ml pwdr for SC inj after reconstitution single use
    (preservative-free)
    Comment: **Cosentyx** may be used as monotherapy or in combination with
    methotrexate (MTX).

INTERLEUKIN-12/INTERLEUKIN-23 ANTAGONIST

▷ *ustekinumab* (B) <18 years: not recommended; ≥18 years: inject SC; rotate sites;
    <100 kg: 45 mg once; then 4 weeks later; then every 12 weeks; ≥100 kg: 90 mg once;
    then 4 weeks later; then every 12 weeks
    Stelara *Vial:* 45 mg/0.5 ml single use (preservative-free)
    Comment: **Stelara** may be used as monotherapy or in combination with
    methotrexate (MTX).

TUMOR NECROSIS FACTOR (TNF) BLOCKERS

▷ *etanercept* (B) <18 years: not recommended; ≥18 years: inject SC into thigh, abdo-
    men, or upper arm; rotate sites; initially 50 mg twice weekly (3-4 days apart) for 3
    months; then 50 mg/week maintenance or 25 mg or 50 mg per week for 3 months;
    then 50 mg/week maintenance
    Enbrel *Vial:* 25 mg pwdr for SC injection after reconstitution (4/carton w. sup-
    plies) (preservative-free, diluent contains benzyl alcohol); *Prefilled syringe:* 50
    mg/ml (preservative-free); *SureClick Autoinjector:* 25 mg/ml (preservative-free)
▷ *adalimumab* (B) <18 years: not recommended; ≥18 years: initially 80 mg SC once
    followed by 40 mg once every other week starting one week after initial dose; inject
    into thigh or abdomen; rotate sites

Humira *Prefilled syringe:* 20 mg/0.4 ml; 40 mg/0.8 ml single dose (2/pck; 2, 6/ starter pck) (preservative-free)

▷ *golimumab* (B) <18 years: not established; ≥18 years: administer SC or IV infusion (in combination with *methotrexate [MTX]*)

Simponi 50 mg SC once monthly; rotate sites
Prefilled syringe, SmartJect Autoinjector: 50 mg/0.5 ml, single use (preservative-free)

Simponi Aria 2 mg/kg IV infusion week 0 and week 4; then every 8 weeks thereafter
Vial: 50 mg/4 ml, single-use, soln for IV infusion after dilution (latex-free, preservative-free)

▷ *infliximab* (B) <6 years: not recommended; ≥6 years: administer by IV infusion over 2 hours; 5 mg/kg weeks 0, 2, 6; then once every 8 weeks

Remicade *Vial:* 100 mg pwdr for reconstitution for IV infusion (preservative-free)

MOISTURIZING AGENTS

Aquaphor Healing Ointment (OTC) *Oint:* (1.75, 3.5, 14 oz) (alcohol)
Eucerin Daily Sun Defense (OTC) *Lotn:* 6 oz (fragrance-free)
Comment: **Eucerin Daily Sun Defense** is a moisturizer with SPF 15.
Eucerin Facial Lotion (OTC) *Lotn:* 4 oz
Eucerin Light Lotion (OTC) *Lotn:* 8 oz
Eucerin Lotion (OTC) *Lotn:* 8, 16 oz
Eucerin Original Creme (OTC) *Crm:* 2, 4, 16 oz (alcohol)
Eucerin Plus Creme *Crm:* 4 oz
Eucerin Plus Lotion (OTC) *Lotn:* 6, 12 oz
Eucerin Protective Lotion (OTC) *Lotn:* 4 oz (alcohol)
Comment: **Eucerin Protective Lotion** is a moisturizer with SPF 25.
Lac-Hydrin Cream (OTC) *Crm:* 280, 385 g
Lac-Hydrin Lotion (OTC) *Lotn:* 225, 400 g
Lubriderm Dry Skin Scented (OTC) *Lotn:* 6, 10, 16, 32 oz
Lubriderm Dry Skin Unscented (OTC) *Lotn:* 3.3, 6, 10, 16 oz (fragrance-free)
Lubriderm Sensitive Skin Lotion (OTC) *Lotn:* 3.3, 6, 10, 16 oz (lanolin-free)
Lubriderm Dry Skin (OTC) *Lotn (scented):* 2.5, 6, 10, 16 oz; *Lotn (fragrance-free):* 1, 2.5, 6, 10, 16 oz
Lubriderm Bath 1-2 capfuls in bath or rub onto wet skin as needed; then rinse *Oil:* 8 oz

PSORIATIC ARTHRITIS

Oral Prescription NSAIDs *see page* 490
Other Oral Analgesics *see Pain page* 298
Topical/Transdermal NSAIDs *see Pain page* 298
Parenteral Corticosteroids *see page* 499
Oral Corticosteroids *see page* 498
Topical Analgesic and Anesthetic Agents *see page* 488

TOPICAL ANALGESICS

▷ *capsaicin* cream (B)(G) <2 years: not recommended; 2-12 years: apply sparingly to intact skin bid prn; >12 years: apply tid-qid prn

> **Axsain** *Crm:* 0.075% (1, 2 oz)
> **Capsin (OTC)** *Lotn:* 0.025, 0, 075% (59 ml)
> **Capzasin-P (OTC)** *Crm:* 0.025% (1.5 oz); *Lotn:* 0.025% (2 oz)
> **Capzasin-HP (OTC)** *Crm:* 0.075% (1.5 oz); *Lotn:* 0.075% (2 oz)
> **Dolorac** *Crm:* 0.025% (28 gm)
> **Double Cap (OTC)** *Crm:* 0.05% (2 oz)
> **R-Gel** *Gel:* 0.025% (15, 30 gm)
> **Zostrix (OTC)** *Crm:* 0.025% (0.7, 1.5, 3 oz)
> **Zostrix HP (OTC)** *Emol crm:* 0.075% (1, 2 oz)

Comment: Provides some relief by 1-2 weeks; optimal benefit may take 4-6 weeks. Avoid contact with mucous membranes.

▷ *diclofenac sodium* (C; D ≥30 wks)

> **Pennsaid 1.5%** <12 years: not established; ≥12 years: in 10 drop increments, dispense and rub into front, side, and back of knee: usually; 40 drops (40 mg) qid
> *Topical soln:* 1.5% (150 ml)
> **Pennsaid 2%** <12 years: not established; ≥12 years: apply 2 pump actuations (40 mg) and rub into front, side, and back of knee bid
> *Topical soln:* 2% (20 mg/pump actuation, 112 gm)

Comment: **Pennsaid** is indicated for the treatment of pain associated with osteoarthritis of the knee.

> **Solaraze Gel** *Gel:* 3% (50 gm) (benzyl alcohol)

Comment: Contraindicated with *aspirin* allergy. As with other NSAIDs, **Solaraze Gel** should be avoided in late pregnancy (≥30 weeks) because it may cause premature closure of the ductus arteriosus.

> **Voltaren Gel (G)** <12 years: not established; ≥12 years: apply sparingly and rub in
> *Gel:* 1% (100 gm)

Comment: Contraindicated with *aspirin* allergy. As with other NSAIDs, **Voltaren Gel** should be avoided in late pregnancy (≥30 weeks) because it may cause premature closure of the ductus arteriosus.

▷ *trolamine salicylate* (NE) <2 years: not recommended; ≥2 years: apply tid-qid

> **Mobisyl** *Crm:* 10%

Comment: Provides some relief by 1-2 weeks; optimal benefit may take 4-6 weeks.

ORAL SALICYLATE

▷ *indomethacin* (C) <14 years: usually not recommended; >2 years, if risk warranted: 1-2 mg/kg/day in divided doses; max 3-4 mg/kg/day or 150-200 mg/day, whichever is less; <14 years, ER cap not recommended; ≥14 years: initially 25 mg bid-tid, increase as needed at weekly intervals by 25-50 mg/day; max 200 mg/day

> *Cap:* 25, 50 mg; *Susp:* 25 mg/5 ml (pineapple-coconut, mint; alcohol 1%); *Supp:* 50 mg; *ER Cap:* 75 mg ext-rel

Comment: *indomethacin* is indicated only for acute painful flares. Administer with food and/or antacids. Use lowest effective dose for shortest duration.

ORAL NSAIDs

See more **Oral NSAIDs** page 490
➤ *diclofenac sodium* (C)
> **Voltaren** <12 years: not established; ≥12 years: 50 mg bid-qid <u>or</u> 75 mg bid <u>or</u> 25 mg qid with an additional 25 mg at HS if necessary
> *Tab:* 25, 50, 75 mg ent-coat
> **Voltaren XR** <18 years: not established; ≥18 years: 100 mg once daily; rarely, 100 mg bid may be used
> *Tab:* 100 mg ext-rel

NSAID PLUS PPI

➤ *esomeprazole/naproxen* (C; not for use in 3rd)(G) <18 years: not recommended; ≥18 years: 1 tab bid; use lowest effective dose for the shortest duration; swallow whole; take at least 30 minutes before a meal
> **Vimovo** *Tab: nap* 375 mg/*eso* 20 mg ext-rel; *nap* 500 mg/*eso* 20 mg ext-rel
> Comment: **Vimovo** is indicated to improve signs/symptoms, and risk of gastric ulcer in patients at risk of developing NSAID-associated gastric ulcer.

COX-2 INHIBITORS

Comment: Cox-2 inhibitors are contraindicated with history of asthma, urticaria, and allergic-type reactions to **aspirin**, other NSAIDs, and sulfonamides, 3rd trimester of pregnancy, and coronary artery bypass graft (CABG) surgery.
➤ *celecoxib* (C)(G) <18 years: not recommended; ≥18 years: 50-400 mg qd-bid; max 800 mg/day
> **Celebrex** *Cap:* 50, 100, 200, 400 mg
➤ *meloxicam* (C)(G)
> **Mobic** <2 years, <60 kg: not recommended; ≥2, >60 kg: 0.125 mg/kg; max 7.5 mg once daily; ≥18 years: initially 7.5 mg once daily; max 15 mg once daily; *Hemodialysis:* max 7.5 mg/day
> *Tab:* 7.5, 15 mg; *Oral susp:* 7.5 mg/5 ml (100 ml) (raspberry)
> **Vivlodex** <18 years: not established; ≥18 years: initially 5 mg qd; may increase to max 10 mg/day; *Hemodialysis:* max 5 mg/day
> *Cap:* 5, 10 mg

PHOSPHODIESTERASE 4 (PDE4) INHIBITOR

➤ *apremilast* (C) <18 years: not established; ≥18 years: swallow whole; initial titration over 5 days; maintenance 30 mg bid; *Day 1:* 10 mg in AM; *Day 2:* 10 mg AM and 10 mg PM; *Day 3:* 10 mg AM and 20 mg PM; *Day 4:* 20 mg AM and 20 mg PM; *Day 5:* 20 mg AM and 30 mg PM; *Day 6 and ongoing:* 30 mg AM and 30 mg PM
> **Otezla** *Tab:* 10, 20, 30 mg; *2-Week Starter Pack*
Comment: Register pregnant patients exposed to by calling 877-311-8972.

INTERLEUKIN-12/INTERLEUKIN-23 ANTAGONIST

➤ *ustekinumab* (B) <18 years: not established; ≥18 years: inject SC; rotate sites; <100 kg: 45 mg once; then 4 weeks later; then every 12 weeks; ≥100 kg: 90 mg once; then 4 weeks later; then every 12 weeks
> **Stelara** *Vial:* 45 mg/0.5 ml single use (preservative-free)

Comment: **Stelara** may be used as monotherapy <u>or</u> in combination with *methotrexate* (MTX).

TUMOR NECROSIS FACTOR (TNF) BLOCKERS

▷ *adalimumab* (B) <2 years, <10 kg: not recommended; 10-<15 kg: 10 mg every other week; 15-<30 kg: 20 mg every other week; ≥30-40 kg: 40 mg every other week; >40 kg 40 mg SC once every other week; may increase to once weekly without *methotrexate* (MTX); administer in abdomen <u>or</u> thigh; rotate sites; 2-17 years, supervise first dose

> **Humira** *Prefilled syringe:* 20 mg/0.4 ml; 40 mg/0.8 ml single dose (2/pck; 2, 6/ starter pck) (preservative-free)
>
> Comment: **Humira** may use with *methotrexate* (MTX), DMARDs, corticoids, salicylates, NSAIDs, <u>or</u> analgesics.

▷ *etanercept* (B) <4 years: not recommended; 4-17 years: 0.4 mg/kg SC twice weekly, 72-96 hours apart <u>or</u> 0.8 mg/kg SC weekly (max 50 mg/dose); >17 years: 25 mg SC twice weekly, 72-96 hours apart <u>or</u> 50 mg SC weekly; rotate sites

> **Enbrel** *Vial:* 25 mg pwdr for SC injection after reconstitution (4/carton w. supplies) (preservative-free; diluent contains benzyl alcohol); *Prefilled syringe:* 50 mg/ml (preservative-free); *SureClick Autoinjector:* 25 mg/ml (preservative-free)

Comment: *etanercept* reduces pain, morning stiffness, and swelling. May be administered in combination with *methotrexate*. Live vaccines should not be administered concurrently. Do not administer with active infection.

▷ *golimumab* (B) <18 years: not established; ≥18 years: administer SC <u>or</u> IV infusion (in combination with *methotrexate* [MTX])

> **Simponi** 50 mg SC once monthly; rotate sites
> *Prefilled syringe, SmartJect Autoinjector:* 50 mg/0.5 ml, single use (preservative-free)
> **Simponi Aria** 2 mg/kg IV infusion week 0 and week 4; then every 8 weeks thereafter
> *Vial:* 50 mg/4 ml, single-use, soln for IV infusion after dilution (latex-free, preservative-free)

Comment: Corticosteroids, non-biologic DMARDs, <u>and/or</u> NSAIDs may be continued during treatment with *golimumab*.

▷ *infliximab* (B) <18 years: not established; ≥18 years: administer SC <u>or</u> IV infusion (in combination with *methotrexate* [MTX]) administer by IV infusion over at least 2 hours; 5 mg/kg once weekly at weeks 0, 2, 6, and then every 8 weeks

> **Remicade** *Vial:* 100 mg pwdr for reconstitution and dilution; (preservative-free)

PULMONARY ARTERIAL HYPERTENSION (PAH; WHO GROUP I)

PROSTACYCLIN RECEPTOR AGONIST

▷ *selexipag* (X) <12 years: not established; ≥12 years: initially 200 mcg bid; increase by 200 mcg bid to highest tolerated dose up to 1600 mcg bid; *Moderate hepatic impairment (Child-Pugh B):* initially 200 mcg once daily; increase by 200 mcg once daily at weekly intervals as tolerated; swallow whole; may take with food to improve tolerability

Uptravi
>   *Tab:* 200, 400, 600, 800, 1000, 1200, 1400, 1600 mcg; *Titration pck:* 140 x 200
>   mcg + 60 x 800 mcg)
>   Comment: Discontinue **Uptravi** if pulmonary veno-occlusive disease is
>   confirmed or severe hepatic impairment (Child-Pugh C). May be potentiated by
>   concomitant strong CYP2C8 inhibitors (e.g., gemfibrozil); *Nursing mothers:* not
>   recommended. Discontinue breastfeeding or discontinue the drug.

GUANYLATE CYCLASE STIMULATOR

▷ *riociguat* (X) <12 years: not established; ≥12 years: initially 0.5-1 mg tid; titrate
   every 2 weeks as tolerated (SBP ≥95 and absence of hypotensive symptoms) to
   highest tolerated dose; max 2.5 mg tid
   Adempas *Tab:* 0.5, 1, 1.5, 2, 2.5 mg
   Comment: If **Adempas** is interrupted for ≥3 days, retitrate. Consider titrating
   to dosage higher than 2.5 mg tid, if tolerated, in patients who smoke. Consider
   a starting dose of 0.5 mg tid when initiating **Adempas** in patients receiving
   strong cytochrome P450 (CYP) and P-glycoprotein/breast cancer resistance
   protein (P-gp/BCRP) inhibitors such as azole antimycotics (e.g., *ketoconazole,
   itraconazole*) or HIV protease inhibitors (e.g., *ritonavir*). Monitor for signs and
   symptoms of hypotension with strong CYP and P-gp/BCRP inhibitors. Obtain
   pregnancy tests prior to initiation and monthly during treatment. **Adempas** has
   consistently shown to have teratogenic effects when administered to animals.
   Females can only receive **Adempas** through the Adempas Risk Evaluation and
   Mitigation Strategy (REMS) Program, a restricted distribution program: www.
   AdempasREMS.com or 855-4 ADEMPAS. It is not known if **Adempas** is present
   in human milk; however, *riociguat* or its metabolites were present in the milk
   of rats. Because of the potential for serious adverse reactions in nursing infants
   from *riociguat*, discontinue nursing or **Adempas**. In placebo-controlled clinical
   trials, serious bleeding has occurred (including hemoptysis, hematemesis,
   vaginal hemorrhage, catheter site hemorrhage, subdural hematoma, and intra-
   abdominal hemorrhage. Safety and efficacy have not been demonstrated in
   patients with creatinine clearance <15 mL/min or on dialysis or severe hepatic
   impairment (Child-Pugh C).
      Endothelin Receptor Antagonist, Selective for the Endothelin Type-A (ETA)
      Receptor
▷ *ambrisentan* (X) <12 years: not established; ≥12 years: 20 mg once daily; at 4-week
   intervals, either the dose of **Letairis** initially 5 mg once daily, with or without or
   tadalafil can be increased, as needed and tolerated, to **Letairis** 10 mg or *tadalafil* 40
   mg; do not split, crush, or chew.
   Letairis *Tab:* 5, 10 mg *film-coat*
   Comment: In patients with PAH, plasma ET-1 concentrations are increased as
   much as 10-fold and correlate with increased mean right atrial pressure and
   disease severity. ET-1 and ET-1 mRNA concentrations are increased as much as
   9-fold in the lung tissue of patients with PAH, primarily in the endothelium of
   pulmonary arteries. These findings suggest that ET-1 may play a critical role in
   the pathogenesis and progression of PAH. When taken with *tadalafil*, **Letairis** is
   indicated to reduce the risk of disease progression and hospitalization, to reduce
   the risk of hospitalization due to worsening PAH, and to improve exercise
   tolerance. **Letairis** is contraindicated in idiopathic pulmonary fibrosis (IPF).

Exclude pregnancy before the initiation of treatment with **Letairis**. Females of reproductive potential must use acceptable methods of contraception during treatment with **Letairis** and for one month after treatment. Obtain monthly pregnancy tests during treatment and 1 month after discontinuation of treatment. Females can only receive **Letairis** through the **Letairis** Risk Evaluation and Mitigation Strategy (REMS) Program, a restricted distribution program, because of the risk of embryo-fetal toxicity: **www. Letairisrems.com** or **1-866-664-5327.**

PHOSPHODIESTERASE TYPE 5 (PDE5) INHIBITORS, CGMP-SPECIFIC DRUGS

▷ *sildenafil citrate* (B)(G) <12 years: not established; ≥12 years: *Orally:* initially 5 or 20 mg tid, 4-6 hours apart; max 20 mg tid; *IV bolus:* 2.5 mg or 10 mg bolus injection tid, 4-6 hours apart; max 10 mg tid; the dose does not need to be adjusted for body weight.

Revatio *Tab:* 20 mg film-coat; *Oral susp:* 10 mg/ml pwdr for reconstitution (1.12 g, 112 ml) (grape) (sorbitol); *Vial:* 10 mg/12.5 ml (0.8 mg/ml)

Comment: A 10 mg IV dose is predicted to provide pharmacological effect equivalent to the 20 mg oral dose. **Revatio** is contraindicated with concomitant nitrate drugs including **nitroglycerin, isosorbide dinitrate,** isosorbide mononitrate, and some recreational drugs such as "poppers." Taking **Revatio** with a nitrate can cause a sudden and serious decrease in blood pressure. **Revatio** is contraindicated with concomitant guanylate cyclase stimulator drugs such as **riociguat (Adempas).** Avoid the use of grapefruit products while taking **Revatio.** Stop **Revatio** and get emergency medical help if sudden vision loss. **Revatio** is contraindicated with other phosphodiesterase type 5 (PDE5) Inhibitors, cGMP-specific drugs such as **avanafil (Stendra), tadalafil (Cialis),** or **vardenafil (Levitra).** Caution with history of recent MI, stroke, life-threatening arrhythmia, hypotension, hypertension, cardiac failure, unstable angina, retinitis pigmentosa, CYP3A4 inhibitors (e.g., **cimetidine,** the azoles, **erythromycin,** protease inhibitors (e.g., **ritonavir**), CYP3A4 inducers (e.g., **rifampin, carbamazepine, phenytoin, phenobarbital**), alcohol, and antihypertensive agents. Side effects include headache, flushing, nasal congestion, rhinitis, dyspepsia, and diarrhea. Use **Revatio** with caution in patients with anatomical deformation of the penis (e.g., angulation, cavernosal fibrosis, or Peyronie's disease) or in patients who have conditions, which may predispose them to priapism (e.g., sickle cell anemia, multiple myeloma, or leukemia). In the event of an erection that persists longer than 4 hours, the patient should seek immediate medical assistance. If priapism (painful erection greater than 6 hours in duration) is not treated immediately, penile tissue damage and permanent loss of potency could result.

▷ *tadalafil* (B)(G) <12 years: not established; ≥12 years: 40 mg once daily; *CrCl 31-80 mL/min:* initially 20 mg once daily; increase to 40 mg once daily if tolerated; *CrCl <30 mL/min:* not recommended; *Mild or moderate hepatic cirrhosis (Child Pugh Class A or B):* initially 20 mg once daily; *Severe hepatic cirrhosis (Child Pugh Class C):* not recommended; *use with ritonavir; Receiving ritonavir for at least 1 week:* initiate *tadalafil* at 20 mg once daily; may increase to 40 mg once daily if tolerated; *Already on tadalafil:* stop *tadalafil* at least 24 hours prior to initiating *ritonavir;* resume *tadalafil* at 20 mg once daily after at least 1 week; may increase to 40 mg once daily if tolerated

Adcirca *Tab:* 20 mg

Comment: Contraindicated with concomitant organic nitrates and guanylate cyclase stimulators (e.g., *riociguat*).

▶ *treprostinil* (B) <12 years: not established; ≥12 years: swallow whole; take with food

Orenitram *Tab:* 0.125, 0.25, 1, 2.5 mg ext-rel

Comment: **Orenitram** is indicated to improve exercise capacity. It is contraindicated with severe hepatic impairment (Child-Pugh C). **Orenitram** inhibits platelet aggregation and increases the risk of bleeding. Concomitant administration of **Orenitram** with diuretics, antihypertensive agents, or other vasodilators increases the risk of symptomatic hypotension.

PYELONEPHRITIS: ACUTE

URINARY TRACT ANALGESIA

▶ *phenazopyridine* (B)(G) <12 years: not recommended; ≥12 years: 95-200 mg q 6 hours prn; max 2 days

AZO Standard, Prodium, Uristat (OTC) *Tab:* 95 mg

AZO Standard Maximum Strength (OTC) *Tab:* 97.5 mg

Pyridium, Urogesic *Tab:* 100, 200 mg

OUTPATIENT ANTI-INFECTIVE TREATMENT

Comment: Acute pyelonephritis can be treated with a single IM antibiotic administration followed by a PO antibiotic regimen and close follow up. Example: **Rocephin** 1 gm IM followed by **Bactrim DS**, *cephalexin, ciprofloxacin, levofloxacin,* or *loracarbef.*

▶ *cephalexin* (B)(G) 25-50 mg/kg/day in 4 divided doses x 10-14 days; *see page 557 for dose by weight table;* 1-4 gm/day in 4 divided doses x 10-14 days

Keflex *Cap:* 250, 333, 500, 750 mg; *Oral susp:* 125, 250 mg/5 ml (100, 200 ml) (strawberry)

▶ *ciprofloxacin* (C) <18 years: not recommended; ≥18 years: 500 mg bid or 1000 mg XR once daily x 3-14 days; max 1.5 gm/day

Cipro (G) *Tab:* 250, 500, 750 mg; *Oral susp:* 250, 500 mg/5 ml (100 ml) (strawberry)

Cipro XR *Tab:* 500, 1000 mg ext-rel

ProQuin XR *Tab:* 500 mg ext-rel

Comment: *ciprofloxacin* is contraindicated <18 years-of-age, and during pregnancy and lactation. Risk of tendonitis or tendon rupture.

▶ *levofloxacin* (C) <18 years: not recommended; ≥18 years: *Uncomplicated:* 500 mg once daily x 10 days; *Complicated:* 750 mg once daily x 10 days

Levaquin *Tab:* 250, 500, 750 mg; *Oral soln:* 25 mg/ml (480 ml) (benzyl alcohol); *Inj conc:* 25 mg/ml for IV infusion after dilution for IV infusion (50, 100, 150 ml) (preservative-free)

Comment: *levofloxacin* is contraindicated <18 years-of-age, and during pregnancy and lactation. Risk of tendonitis or tendon rupture.

▶ *loracarbef* (B) <12 years: 15 mg/kg/day in 2 divided doses x 10 days; *see page 570 for dose by weight table;* ≥12 years: 200 mg bid x 10 days

Lorabid *Pulvule:* 200, 400 mg; *Oral susp:* 100 mg/5 ml (50, 100 ml); 200 mg/5 ml (50, 75, 100 ml) (strawberry bubble gum)

▷ *trimethoprim/sulfamethoxazole* (D)(G)

Bactrim, Septra <12 years: not recommended; ≥12 years: 2 tabs bid x 10 days
Tab: trim 80 mg/*sulfa* 400 mg*

Bactrim DS, Septra DS <12 years: not recommended; ≥12 years: 1 tab bid x 10 days
Tab: trim 160 mg/*sulfa* 800 mg*

Bactrim Pediatric Suspension, Septra Pediatric Suspension <2 months: not recommended; ≥2 months-12 years: 40 mg/kg/day of *sulfamethoxazole* in 2 doses bid; >12 years: use tabs
Oral susp: trim 40 mg/*sulfa* 200 mg per 5 ml (100 ml) (cherry) (alcohol 0.3%)

RABIES

PRE-EXPOSURE PROPHYLAXIS

Comment: Postpone pre-exposure prophylaxis during acute febrile illness <u>or</u> infection. Have *epinephrine* 1:1000 readily available.

▷ *rabies immune globulin, human (HRIG)* (C) 3 injections of 1 ml IM each on day 0, 7, and either day 21 <u>or</u> 28; booster doses 1 ml IM every 2 years; for infants, administer in the vastus lateralis muscle
Imovax *Vial:* 2.5 u/ml (1 ml, single dose)

POSTEXPOSURE PROPHYLAXIS

Comment: Have *epinephrine* 1:1000 readily available.

▷ *rabies immune globulin, human (HRIG)* (C) 20 IU/kg infiltrated into wound area as much as feasible, then remaining dose administered IM at site remote from vaccine administration
BayRab, Imogam Rabies *Vial:* 150 IU/ml (2, 10 ml)

▷ *rabies vaccine, human diploid cell* (C) *Not previously immunized:* administer first dose 1 ml in the deltoid as soon as possible after exposure; then repeat on days 3, 7, 14, 28 <u>or</u> 30, and 90; administer 1st dose with rabies immune globulin; *Previously immunized:* only 2 doses are administered, immediately after exposure and again 3 days later; no rabies immune globulin is needed; for infants, administer in the vastus lateralis muscle
Imovax, RabAvert *Vial:* 2.5 IU/ml (2.5 IU of freeze-dried vaccine w. diluent)

TETANUS PROPHYLAXIS

See Tetanus page 398 for patients not previously immunized

RESPIRATORY SYNCYTIAL VIRUS (RSV)

PROPHYLAXIS

▷ *palivizumab* 15 mg/kg IM administered monthly throughout the RSV season
Synagis *Vial:* 100 mg/ml
Treatment *see Bronchiolitis page 54*

RETINITIS: CYTOMEGALOVIRUS (CMV)

Comment: *cidofovir* and *valganciclovir* are nucleoside analogs and prodrugs of *ganciclovir* indicated for the treatment of AIDS-related *cytomegalovirus* (CMV) retinitis and prevention of CMV disease in patients ≥18 years with kidney, heart, and kidney-pancreas transplant patients at high risk, and for prevention of CMV disease in pediatric kidney and heart transplant patients at high risk.

▶ *cidofovir* (C) <12 years: not recommended; ≥12 years: administer via IV infusion over 1 hour; pretreat with oral *probenecid* (2 g, 3 hours prior to starting the *cidofovir* infusion and 1 g, 2 and 8 hours after the infusion is ended) and 1 liter of IV NaCl should be infused immediately before each dose of *cidofovir* (a 2nd liter of NaCl should also be infused either during or after each dose of *cidofovir* if a fluid load is tolerable); *Induction:* 5 mg/kg once weekly for 2 consecutive weeks; *Maintenance:* 5 mg/kg once every 2 weeks; reduce to 3 mg/kg if serum Cr increases 0.3-0.4 mg/dL above baseline; discontinue if serum Cr increases to >0.5 mg/dL above baseline or if >3+ proteinuria develops

Vistide *Vial:* 75 mg/ml (5 ml) (preservative-free)

Comment: *cidofovir* is a nucleoside analog indicated for treatment of AIDS-related *cytomegalovirus* (CMV) retinitis.

▶ *valganciclovir* (C)(G) take with food; <4 months: not recommended; 4 months-16 years: see mfr pkg insert for dosing calculation equation; >16 years: *Induction:* 900 mg bid x 21 days; *Maintenance:* 900 mg daily; *CrCl <60 mL/min:* reduce dose (see mfr pkg insert; hemodialysis or CrCl <10 mL/min not recommended (use *ganciclovir*)

Valcyte *Tab:* 450 mg (preservative-free); *Oral pwdr for reconstitution:* 50 mg/ml (tutti-frutti)

RHEUMATOID ARTHRITIS (RA)

Oral Prescription NSAIDs *see page* 490
Other Oral Analgesics *see Pain page* 298
Topical/Transdermal NSAIDs *see Pain page* 298
Parenteral Corticosteroids *see page* 499
Oral Corticosteroids *see page* 498
Topical Analgesic and Anesthetic Agents *see page* 488

TOPICAL ANALGESICS

▶ *capsaicin* cream (B)(G) <2 years: not recommended; 2-12 years: apply sparingly to intact skin bid prn; >12 years: apply tid-qid prn

Axsain *Crm:* 0.075% (1, 2 oz)
Capsin (OTC) *Lotn:* 0.025, 0, 075% (59 ml)
Capzasin-P (OTC) *Crm:* 0.025% (1.5 oz); *Lotn:* 0.025% (2 oz)
Capzasin-HP (OTC) *Crm:* 0.075% (1.5 oz); *Lotn:* 0.075% (2 oz)
Dolorac *Crm:* 0.025% (28 gm)
Double Cap (OTC) *Crm:* 0.05% (2 oz)
R-Gel *Gel:* 0.025% (15, 30 gm)
Zostrix (OTC) *Crm:* 0.025% (0.7, 1.5, 3 oz)

    Zostrix HP (OTC) *Emol crm:* 0.075% (1, 2 oz)
Comment: Provides some relief by 1-2 weeks; optimal benefit may take 4-6 weeks. Avoid contact with mucous membranes.
▷ *trolamine salicylate* **(NE)** <2 years: not recommended; ≥2 years: apply tid-qid prn to intact skin
    Mobisyl *Crm:* 10%
Comment: Provides some relief by 1-2 weeks; optimal benefit may take 4-6 weeks.

ORAL SALICYLATE

▷ *indomethacin* **(C)** <14 years: usually not recommended; >2 years, if risk warranted: 1-2 mg/kg/day in divided doses; max 3-4 mg/kg/day (or 150-200 mg/day, whichever is less); <14 years, ER cap not recommended; ≥14 years: initially 25 mg bid-tid, increase as needed at weekly intervals by 25-50 mg/day; max 200 mg/day
    Cap: 25, 50 mg; *Susp;* 25 mg/5 ml (pineapple-coconut, mint; alcohol 1%); *Supp:* 50 mg; *ER Cap:* 75 mg ext-rel
Comment: *indomethacin* is indicated only for acute painful flares. Administer with food and/or antacids. Use lowest effective dose for shortest duration.

NSAID

See more Oral NSAIDs *page* 490
▷ *diclofenac sodium* **(C)(G)**
    Voltaren <12 years: not recommended; ≥12 years: 50 mg bid-qid <u>or</u> 75 mg bid <u>or</u> 25 mg qid with an additional 25 mg at HS if necessary
    Tab: 25, 50, 75 mg ent-coat
    Voltaren XR <18: not recommended; ≥18 years: 100 mg once daily; rarely, 100 mg bid may be used
    Tab: 100 mg ext-rel

NSAID PLUS PPI

▷ *esomeprazole/naproxen* **(C; not for use in 3rd)(G)** <18 years: not recommended; ≥18 years: 1 tab bid; use lowest effective dose for the shortest duration; swallow whole; take at least 30 minutes before a meal
    Vimovo *Tab: nap* 375 mg/*eso* 20 mg ext-rel; *nap* 500 mg/*eso* 20 mg ext-rel
    Comment: **Vimovo** is indicated to improve signs/symptoms, and risk of gastric ulcer in patients at risk of developing NSAID-associated gastric ulcer.

COX-2 INHIBITORS

Comment: Cox-2 inhibitors are contraindicated with history of asthma, urticaria, and allergic-type reactions to *aspirin*, other NSAIDs, and sulfonamides, 3rd trimester of pregnancy, and coronary artery bypass graft (CABG) surgery.
▷ *celecoxib* **(C)(G)** <18 years: not recommended; ≥18 years: 100-400 mg bid; max 800 mg/day
    Celebrex *Cap:* 50, 100, 200, 400 mg
▷ *meloxicam* **(C)(G)**
    Mobic <2 years, <60 kg: not recommended; ≥2, >60 kg: 0.125 mg/kg; max 7.5 mg once daily; ≥18 years: initially 7.5 mg once daily; max 15 mg once daily; *Hemodialysis:* max 7.5 mg/day

Tab: 7.5, 15 mg; *Oral susp:* 7.5 mg/5 ml (100 ml) (raspberry)

Vivlodex <18 years: not established; ≥18 years: initially 5 mg qd; may increase to max 10 mg/day; *Hemodialysis:* max 5 mg/day

Cap: 5, 10 mg

JANUS KINASE (JAK) INHIBITOR

▷ *tofacitinib* (C) <12 years: not established; ≥12 years: 5 mg twice daily; reduce to 5 mg once daily for moderate-to-severe renal impairment or moderate hepatic impairment, concomitant potent CYP3A4 inhibitors, or drugs that result in both CYP3A4 and potent CYP2C19 inhibition

Xeljanz *Tab:* 5 mg

Xeljanz XR *Tab:* 11 mg ext-rel

Comment: **Xeljanz** is indicated for moderate-to-severe RA as monotherapy in patients who have inadequate response or intolerance to *methotrexate* (MTX) and/or in combination with other non-biologic DMARDs.

DISEASE MODIFYING ANTIRHEUMATIC DRUGS (DMARDs)

Comment: DMARDs are first-line treatment options for RA. DMARDs include penicillamine, gold salts (*auranofin*, *aurothio-glucose*), immunosuppressants, and *hydroxychloroquine*. The DMARDs reduce ESR, reduce RF, and favorably affect the outcome of RA. Immunosuppressants may require 6 weeks to affect benefits and 6 months for full improvement.

▷ *auranofin (gold salt)* (C) <12 years: not recommended; ≥12 years: 3 mg bid or 6 mg once daily; if inadequate response after 6 months, increase to 3 mg tid

Ridaura *Vial:* 100 mg/20 ml

▷ *azathioprine* (D) <12 years: not established; ≥12 years: 1 mg/kg/day in a single or divided doses; may increase by 0.5 mg/kg/day q 4 weeks; max 2.5 mg/kg/day; minimum trial to ascertain effectiveness is 12 weeks

Azasan *Tab* 75*, 100*mg

Imuran *Tab* 50*mg

▷ *cyclosporine (immunosuppressant)* (C) <12 years: not recommended; ≥12 years: 1.25 mg/kg bid; may increase after 4 weeks by 0.5 mg/kg/day; then adjust at 2 week intervals; max 4 mg/kg/day; administer with meals

Neoral *Cap:* 25, 100 mg (alcohol)

Neoral Oral Solution *Oral soln:* 100 mg/ml (50 ml) may dilute in room temperature apple juice or orange juice (alcohol)

Comment: **Neoral** is indicated for RA unresponsive to *methotrexate* (MTX).

▷ *hydroxychloroquine* (C) <12 years: not recommended; ≥12 years: 400-600 mg/day

Plaquenil *Tab:* 200 mg

Comment: May require several weeks to achieve beneficial effects. If no improvement in 6 months, discontinue.

▷ *leflunomide* (X)(G) <18 years: not recommended; ≥18 years: initially 100 mg once daily x 3 days; maintenance dose 20 mg once daily; max 20 mg daily

Arava *Tab:* 10, 20, 100 mg

Comment: **Arava** is contraindicated with breastfeeding.

▷ *methotrexate* (X) <2 years: not recommended; ≥2 years-12 years: 10 mg/m² once weekly; max 20 mg/m²; >12 years: 7.5 mg x 1 dose per week or 2.5 mg x 3 at 12 hour intervals once a week; max 20 mg/week; therapeutic response begins in 3-6 weeks; administer *methotrexate* injection SC only into the abdomen or thigh

Rasuvo *Autoinjector:* 7.5 mg/0.15 ml, 10 mg/0.20 ml, 12.5 mg/0.25 ml, 15 mg/0.30 ml, 17.5 mg/0.35 ml, 20 mg/0.40 ml, 22.5 mg/0.45 ml, 25 mg/0.50 ml, 27.5 mg/0.55 ml, 30 mg/0.60 ml (solution concentration for SC injection is 50 mg/ml)

Rheumatrex *Tab:* 2.5*mg (5, 7.5, 10, 12.5, 15 mg/week, 4/card unit-of-use dose pack)

Trexall *Tab:* 5*, 7.5*, 10*, 15*mg (5, 7.5, 10, 12.5, 15 mg/week, 4/card unit-of-use dose pack)

Comment: ***methotrexate*** (MTX) is contraindicated with immunodeficiency, blood dyscrasias, alcoholism, and chronic liver disease.

➤ ***penicillamine*** (D) <12 years: not recommended; ≥12 years: 125-250 mg once daily initially; may increase by 125-250 mg/day q 1-3 months; max 1.5 gm/day

Cuprimine *Cap:* 125, 250 mg

Depen *Tab:* 250 mg

➤ ***sulfasalazine*** (C; D in 2nd, 3rd)(G) <6 years: not recommended; 6-16 years: initially 1/4 to 1/3 of maintenance dose; increase weekly; maintenance 30-50 mg/kg/day in 2 divided doses at regular intervals; max 2 gm/day; >16 years: initially 0.5 gm once daily bid; gradually increase every 4 days; usual maintenance 2-3 gm/day in equally divided doses at regular intervals; max 4 gm/day

Azulfidine *Tab:* 500 mg

Azulfidine EN *Tab:* 500 mg ent-coat

TUMOR NECROSIS FACTOR (TNF) BLOCKERS

➤ ***adalimumab*** (B) <2 years, <10 kg: not recommended; ≥2 years: 10-<15 kg: 10 mg every other week; 15-<30 kg: 20 mg every other week; ≥30 kg: 40 mg SC every other week; ≥17 years: may increase to once weekly without ***methotrexate*** (MTX); administer in abdomen or thigh; rotate sites; 2-17 years, supervise first dose

Humira *Prefilled syringe:* 20 mg/0.4 ml; 40 mg/0.8 ml single dose (2/pck; 2, 6/starter pck) (preservative-free)

Comment: **Humira** may use with ***methotrexate*** (MTX), DMARDs, corticosteroids, salicylates, NSAIDs, or analgesics.

➤ ***certolizumab pegol*** (B) <12 years: not recommended; ≥12 years: 400 mg SC on Day 1, at week 2, and at week 4; then 200 give for other week; rotate sites

Cimzia *Vial:* 200 mg single dose w. supplies (2/pck, 2, 6/starter pck); *Prefilled syringe:* 200 mg single dose w. supplies (2/pck, 2, 6/starter pck) (preservative-free)

➤ ***etanercept*** (B) <4 years: not recommended; 4-<17 years: 0.4 mg/kg SC twice weekly, 72-96 hours apart (max 25 mg/dose) or 0.8 mg/kg SC weekly (max 50 mg/dose); ≥17 years: 25 mg SC twice weekly, 72-96 hours apart or 50 mg SC weekly; rotate sites

Enbrel *Vial:* 25 mg pwdr for SC injection after reconstitution (4/carton w. supplies) (preservative-free; diluent contains benzyl alcohol); *Prefilled syringe:* 50 mg/ml (preservative-free); *SureClick Autoinjector:* 50 mg/ml (preservative-free)

Comment: ***etanercept*** reduces pain, morning stiffness, and swelling. May be administered in combination with ***methotrexate***. Live vaccines should not be administered concurrently. Do not administer with active infection.

➤ ***golimumab*** (B) <18 years: not recommended; ≥18 years: administer SC or IV infusion (in combination with ***methotrexate*** [MTX])

Simponi 50 mg SC once monthly; rotate sites

Prefilled syringe, SmartJect Autoinjector: 50 mg/0.5 ml, single use (preservative-free)

Simponi Aria 2 mg/kg IV infusion week 0 and week 4; then every 8 weeks thereafter

Vial: 50 mg/4 ml, single-use, soln for IV infusion after dilution (latex-free, preservative-free)

Comment: corticosteroids, non-biologic DMARDs, <u>and/or</u> NSAIDs may be continued during treatment with *golimumab.*

➤ *infliximab* (B) <18 years: not recommended; ≥18 years: administer SC <u>or</u> IV infusion (in combination with *methotrexate* [MTX]) administer by IV infusion over at least 2 hours; 3 mg/kg once weekly at weeks 0, 2, 6, and then every 8 weeks; may increase to 10 mg/kg <u>or</u> *administer* every 4 weeks

Remicade *Vial:* 100 mg pwdr for reconstitution and dilution; (preservative-free)

Comment: Use *infliximab* concomitantly with *methotrexate* when there has been insufficient response to *methotrexate* alone.

Interleukin-1 Receptor Antagonist

➤ *anakinra (interleukin-1 receptor antagonist)* (B) <12 years: not recommended; ≥12 years: 100 mg SC once daily; discard any unused portion

Kineret *Prefilled syringe:* 100 mg/single-dose syringe (7, 28/pk) (preservative-free)

Interleukin-6 Receptor Antagonist

➤ *sarilumab* <18 years: not recommended; ≥18 years: 200 mg SC every 2 weeks on the same day; if necessary, the dosage can be reduced 150 mg every 2 weeks to manage potential laboratory abnormalities, such as neutropenia, thrombocytopenia, and liver enzyme elevations; SC injections may be self-administered

Kevzara *Prefilled syringe:* 150, 200 mg (1.4 ml, single-use)

Comment: *sarilumab* is a human monoclonal antibody that binds to the interleukin-6 receptor (IL-6R), and has been shown to inhibit IL-6R mediated signaling. IL-6 is a cytokine in the body that, in excess and over time, can contribute to the inflammation associated with RA. **Kevzara** received FDA approval in May, 2017 for use in patients with active moderate-to-severe rheumatoid arthritis (RA) in adults who have had an inadequate response <u>or</u> intolerance to one <u>or</u> more disease modifying antirheumatic drugs (DMARDs). **Kevzara** may be used as monotherapy <u>or</u> in combination with *methotrexate* <u>or</u> other conventional DMARDs. Monitor patient for dose related laboratory changes including elevated LFTs, neutropenia, and thrombocytopenia. **Kevzara** should not be initiated in patients with an absolute neutrophil count (ANC) <2000/mm3, platelet count <150,000/mm3, <u>or</u> liver transaminases above 1.5 times the upper limit of normal (ULN). Registration in the Pregnancy Exposure Registry (1-877-311-8972) is encouraged for monitoring pregnancy outcomes in women exposed to **Kevzara** during pregnancy. Negative side effects of **Kevzara** should be reported to the FDA at www.fda.gov/medwatch <u>or</u> call 1-800-FDA-1088 <u>or</u> call Sanofi-Aventis at 1-800-633-1610. The limited available data with **Kevzara** in pregnant women are not sufficient to determine whether there is a drug-associated risk for major birth defects and miscarriage. Monoclonal antibodies, such as *sarilumab*, are actively transported across the placenta during the third trimester of pregnancy and may affect immune response in the infant exposed *in utero*. It is not known whether *sarilumab* passes into breast milk; therefore, breastfeeding is not recommended while using **Kevzara**.

▶ *tocilizumab* (B) <2 years: not recommended; ≥2 years: weight-based dosing according to diagnosis: *PJIA: ≥30 kg:* 8 mg/kg SC every 4 weeks; *<30 kg:* 10 mg/kg SC every 4 weeks; *SJIA: ≥30 kg:* 8 mg/kg SC every 2 weeks; *<30 kg:* 12 mg/kg SC every 2 weeks; *IV Infusion:* administer over 1 hour; do not administer as bolus or IV push; *PJIA, and SJIA, ≥30 kg:* dilute to 100 mL in 0.9% or 0.45% NaCl. *PJIA and SJIA, <30 kg:* dilute to 50 mL in 0.9% or 0.45% NaCl; ≥18 years: whether used in combination with DMARDs or as monotherapy, the recommended IV infusion starting dose is 4 mg/kg IV every 4 weeks followed by an increase to 8 mg/kg IV every 4 weeks based on clinical response; Max 800 mg per infusion in RA patients; *SC Administration:* ≥100 kg: 162 mg SC once weekly on the same day; SC injections may be self-administered

    Actemra *Vial:* 80 mg/4 ml, 200 mg/10 ml, 400 mg/20 ml, single-use, for IV infusion after dilution; *Prefilled syringe:* 162 mg (0.9 ml, single-dose)

Comment: *tocilizumab* is an interleukin-6 receptor-α inhibitor indicated for use in moderate-to-severe rheumatoid arthritis (RA) that has not responded to conventional therapy, and also for some subtypes of juvenile idiopathic arthritis (JIA). **Actemra** may be used alone or in combination with *methotrexate* and in RA, other DMARDs may be used. Monitor patient for dose related laboratory changes including elevated LFTs, neutropenia, and thrombocytopenia. **Actemra** should not be initiated in patients with an absolute neutrophil count (ANC) <2000/mm3, platelet count <100,000/mm3, or who have ALT or AST above 1.5 times the upper limit of normal (ULN). Registration in the Pregnancy Exposure Registry (1-877-311-8972) is encouraged for monitoring pregnancy outcomes in women exposed to **Actemra** during pregnancy. The limited available data with **Actemra** in pregnant women are not sufficient to determine whether there is a drug-associated risk for major birth defects and miscarriage. Monoclonal antibodies, such as *tocilizumab*, are actively transported across the placenta during the third trimester of pregnancy and may affect immune response in the infant exposed *in utero*. It is not known whether *tocilizumab* passes into breast milk; therefore, breastfeeding is not recommended while using **Actemra**.

Selective Costimulation Modulator

▶ *abatacept* (C) <6 years: not recommended; 6-17 years: administer as an IV infusion over 30 minutes at weeks 0, 2, and 4; then every 4 weeks thereafter; <75 kg, administer 10 mg/kg; max 1 g; ≥17 years: administer as an IV infusion over 30 minutes at weeks 0, 2, and 4; then every 4 weeks thereafter; <60 kg, administer 500 mg/dose; 60-100 kg, administer 750 mg/dose; >100 kg, administer 1 gm/dose

    Orencia *Vial:* 250 mg pwdr for IV infusion after reconstitution (silicone-free) (preservative-free); *Prefilled syringe:* 125 mg/ml soln for SC injection (preservative-free); *ClickJect Autoinjector:* 125 mg/ml soln for SC injection

CD20 ANTIBODY

▶ *rituximab* (C) <6 years: not recommended; ≥6 years: administer corticosteroid 30 minutes prior to each infusion; concomitant *methotrexate* therapy, administer a 1,000 mg IV infusion at 0 and 2 weeks; then every 24 weeks or based on response, but not sooner than every 16 weeks.

    Rituxan *Vial:* 10 mg/ml (10, 50 ml) (preservative-free)

INTRA-ARTICULAR INJECTION

▷ *sodium hyaluronate* <*12 years*: not recommended; ≥12 years: 20 mg as intra-articular injection weekly x 5 weeks

　　Hyalgan *Prefilled syringe:* 20 mg/2 ml

　　Comment: Remove joint effusion and inject with *lidocaine* if possible before injecting **Hyalgan**.

 RHINITIS/SINUSITIS: ALLERGIC

Oral Prescription Drugs for the Management of Allergy, Cough, and Cold Symptoms *see page 523*
Parenteral Corticosteroids *see page 499*
Oral Corticosteroids *see page 498*

SECOND GENERATION ANTIHISTAMINES

Comment: Second generation antihistamines are sedating, but much less so than the first generation antihistamines. All antihistamines are excreted into breast milk.

▷ *cetirizine* (C)(OTC)(G) <6 years: not recommended; ≥6-<65 years: initially 5-10 mg once daily; ≥65 years: 5 mg once daily

　　Children's Zyrtec Chewable *Chew tab:* 5, 10 mg (grape)
　　Children's Zyrtec Allergy Syrup *Syr:* 1 mg/ml (4 oz) (grape, bubble gum) (sugar-free, dye-free)
　　Zyrtec *Tab:* 10 mg
　　Zyrtec Hives Relief *Tab:* 10 mg
　　Zyrtec Liquid Gels *Liq gel:* 10 mg

▷ *desloratadine* (C)

　　Clarinex <6 years: not recommended; ≥6 years: 1/2-1 tab once daily
　　　Tab: 5 mg
　　Clarinex RediTabs <6 years: not recommended; 6-12 years: 2.5 mg once daily; ≥12 years: 5 mg once daily
　　　ODT: 2.5, 5 mg (tutti-frutti) (phenylalanine)
　　Clarinex Syrup <6 months: not recommended; 6-11 months: 1 mg (2 ml) once daily; 1-5 years: 1.25 mg (2.5 ml) once daily; 6-11 years: 2.5 mg (5 ml) once daily; ≥12 years: 5 mg (10 ml) once daily
　　　Tab: 0.5 mg per ml (4 oz) (tutti-frutti) (phenylalanine)
　　Desloratadine ODT

▷ *fexofenadine* (C)(OTC)(G) 6 months-2 years: 15 mg bid; *CrCl ≤90 mL/min:* 15 mg once daily; 2-11 years: 30 mg bid; *CrCl ≤90 mL/min:* 30 mg once daily ≥12 years and older: ≥ 12 years: 60 mg once daily-bid *or* 180 mg once daily; *CrCl <90 mL/ min:* 60 mg once daily **Allegra** *Tab:* 30, 60, 180 mg film-coat

　　Allegra Allergy *Tab:* 60, 180 mg film-coat
　　Allegra ODT *ODT:* 30 mg (phenylalanine)
　　Allegra Oral Suspension *Oral susp:* 30 mg/5 ml (6 mg/ml) (4 oz)

▷ *loratadine* (C)(OTC)(G) <2 years: not recommended; 2-5 years: 5 mg once daily; ≥6 years: 5 mg bid or 10 mg once daily; *Hepatic or Renal Insufficiency:* (see mfr pkg insert)

　　Children's Claritin Chewables *Chew tab:* 5 mg (grape) (phenylalanine)

Children's Claritin Syrup 1 mg/ml (4 oz) (fruit) (sugar-free, alcohol-free, dye-free; sodium 6 mg/5 ml)
Claritin *Tab:* 10 mg
Claritin Hives Relief *Tab:* 10 mg
Claritin Liqui-Gels *Liq gel:* 10 mg
Claritin RediTabs 12 Hours *ODT:* 5 mg (mint)
Claritin RediTabs 24 Hours *ODT:* 10 mg (mint)

▷ *levocetirizine* (B)(OTC) administer dose in the PM; *Seasonal Allergic Rhinitis:* <2 years: not recommended; may start at ≥2 years; *Chronic Idiopathic Urticaria (CIU), Perennial Allergic Rhinitis:* <6 months: not recommended; may start at ≥ 6 months; *Dosing by Age:* 6 months-5 years: max 1.25 mg once daily; 6-11 years: max 2.5 mg once daily; ≥12 years: 2.5-5 mg once daily; *Renal Dysfunction <12 years:* contraindicated; *Renal Dysfunction ≥12 years:* CrCl 50-80 ml/min: 2.5 mg once daily; CrCl 30-50 mL/min: 2.5 mg every other day; CrCl: 10-30 mL/min: 2.5 mg twice weekly (every 3-4 days); *CrCl <10 mL/min,* ESRD or hemodialysis: contraindicated;
Xyzal *Tab:* 5*mg
Xyzal Oral Solution *Oral soln:* 0.5 mg/ml (150 ml)

FIRST GENERATION ANTIHISTAMINES

▷ *hydroxyzine* (C)(G) <6 years: 50 mg/day divided qid prn; ≥6 years: 50-100 mg/day divided qid prn; max 600 mg/day; 25 mg tid prn; max 600 mg/day
Atarax *Tab:* 10, 25, 50, 100 mg; *Syr:* 10 mg/5 ml (alcohol 0.5%)
Vistaril *Cap:* 25, 50, 100 mg; *Oral susp:* 25 mg/5 ml (4 oz) (lemon)

ALLERGEN EXTRACTS

Comment: Allergen extracts (**Grastek, Oralair, Ragwitek**) are not for immediate relief of allergic symptoms. Contraindicated with severe, unstable, and uncontrolled asthma, history of eosinophilic esophagitis, and severe local or systemic reaction. First dose under supervision HCP and observe ≥30 minutes. Subsequent doses may be taken at home.

▷ *short ragweed pollen allergen extract* (C) <18 years: not recommended; ≥18 years: one SL tab once daily
Ragwitek *SL tab: ambrosia artemisiifolia 12 amb a 1-unit* (30, 90/blister pck)
Comment: Initiate **Ragwitek** at least 12 weeks before onset of ragweed pollen season and continue throughout season.

▷ *sweet vernal, orchard, perennial rye, timothy, Kentucky blue grass mixed pollen allergen extract* (C) <10 years: not established; 10-17 years: Day 1: 100 IR; Day 2: 200 IR; Day 3 and thereafter: 300 IR once daily; >17 years: 300 IR once daily
Oralair *SL tab:* 100, 300 IR (index of reactivity) (30/blister pck)
Comment: **Oralair** is indicated for grass pollen-induced allergic rhinitis with or without conjunctivitis confirmed by positive skin test. Initiate **Oralair** at least 4 months before onset of grass pollen season and continue throughout season.

▷ *Timothy grass pollen allergen extract* (C) <5 years: not established; ≥5 years: one SL tab once daily
Grastek *SL tab:* 2800 bioequivalent allergy units (BAUS) (30/blister pck)
Comment: **Grastek** is indicated for grass pollen-induced allergic rhinitis with or without conjunctivitis confirmed by positive skin test. Initiate **Grastek** at least 12 weeks before onset of grass pollen season and continue throughout season.

NASAL DECONGESTANT

▷ *tetrahydrozoline* (C)
>   **Tyzine**
>   *Nasal spray:* 0.1% (15 ml); *Nasal drops:* 0.1% (30 ml)
>   **Tyzine Pediatric Nasal Drops** 2-3 sprays or drops in each nostril q 3-6 hours prn
>   *Nasal drops:* 0.05% (15 ml)

LEUKOTRIENE RECEPTOR ANTAGONISTS (LRAs)

Comment: The LRAs are indicated for prophylaxis and chronic treatment, only. Not for primary (rescue) treatment of acute asthma attack.

▷ *montelukast* (B)(G) <12 months: not recommended; 12-23 months: one 4 mg granule pkt daily; 2-5 years: one 4 mg chew tab or granule pkt daily; >5-14 years: one 5 mg chew tab daily; >14 years: 10 mg once daily in the PM; for EIB, take at least 2 hours before exercise; max 1 dose/day
>   **Singulair** *Tab:* 10 mg
>   **Singulair Chewable** *Chew tab:* 4, 5 mg (cherry) (phenylalanine)
>   **Singulair Oral Granules** *Granules:* 4 mg/pkt; take within 15 minutes of opening pkt; may mix with applesauce, carrots, rice, or ice cream

▷ *zafirlukast* (B) <7 years: not recommended; 7-11 years: 10 mg bid 1 hour ac or 2 hours pc; >11 years: 20 mg bid, 1 hour ac or 2 hours pc
>   **Accolate** *Tab:* 10, 20 mg

▷ *zileuton* (C)
>   **Zyflo** <12 years: not recommended; ≥12 years: 1 tab qid; max 2400 mg/day
>   *Tab:* 600 mg
>   **Zyflo CR** <12 years: not recommended; ≥12 years: 2 tabs bid; max 1200 mg/day
>   *Tab:* 600 mg ext-rel

NASAL CORTICOSTEROIDS

▷ *beclomethasone dipropionate* (C)
>   **Beconase** <6 years: not recommended; 6-12 years: 1 spray in each nostril tid; >12 years: 1 spray in each nostril bid-qid
>   *Nasal spray:* 42 mcg/actuation (6.7 g, 80 sprays; 16.8 g, 200 sprays)
>   **Beconase AQ** <6 years: not recommended; ≥6 years: 1-2 sprays in each nostril bid
>   *Nasal spray:* 42 mcg/actuation (25 g, 180 sprays)
>   **Beconase Inhalation Aerosol** <6 years: not recommended; 6-12 years: 1 spray in each nostril tid; >12 years: 1-2 sprays in each nostril bid to qid
>   *Nasal spray:* 42 mcg/actuation (6.7 g, 80 sprays; 16.8 g, 200 sprays)
>   **Vancenase AQ** <6 years: not recommended; ≥6 years: 1-2 sprays in each nostril bid
>   *Nasal spray:* 84 mcg/actuation (25 g, 200 sprays)
>   **Vancenase AQ DS** <6 years: not recommended; ≥6 years: 1-2 sprays in each nostril once daily
>   *Nasal spray:* 84, 168 mcg/actuation (19 g, 120 sprays)
>   **Vancenase Pockethaler** <6 years: not recommended; ≥6 years: 1 spray in each nostril bid or tid
>   *Pockethaler:* 42 mcg/actuation (7 g, 200 sprays)

QNASL Nasal Aerosol <12 years: 2 sprays, 40 mcg/spray, in each nostril once daily; ≥12 years: 2 sprays, 80 mcg/spray, in each nostril once daily
Nasal spray: 40 mcg/actuation (4.9 g, 60 sprays); 80 mcg/actuation (8.7 g, 120 sprays)

► *budesonide* (C)

Rhinocort <6 years: not recommended; >6 years: initially 2 sprays in each nostril bid in the AM and PM, <u>or</u> 4 sprays in each nostril in the AM; max 4 sprays each nostril/day; use lowest effective dose
Nasal spray: 32 mcg/actuation (7 g, 200 sprays)

Rhinocort Aqua Nasal Spray <6 years: not recommended; ≥6-12 years: initially 1 spray in each nostril once daily; max 2 sprays in each nostril daily; >12 years: initially 1 spray in each nostril once daily; max 4 sprays in each nostril once daily
Nasal spray: 32 mcg/actuation (10 ml, 60 sprays)

► *ciclesonide* (C)

Omnaris <6 years: not recommended; ≥6 years: 2 sprays in each nostril once daily
Nasal spray: 50 mcg/actuation (12.5 g, 120 sprays)

Zetonna <6 years: not recommended; ≥6 years: 1-2 sprays in each nostril once daily
Nasal spray: 37 mcg/actuation (6.1 g, 60 sprays) (HFA)

► *dexamethasone* (C) <6 years: not recommended; ≥6-12 years: 1-2 sprays in each nostril bid; max 8 sprays/day; maintain at lowest effective dose; >12 years: 2 sprays in each nostril bid-tid; max 12 sprays/day; maintain at lowest effective dose

Dexacort Turbinaire *Nasal spray:* 84 mcg/actuation (12.6 g, 170 sprays)

► *fluticasone furoate* (C) <2 years: not recommended; ≥2-11 years: 1 spray in each nostril once daily; ≥12 years: 2 sprays in each nostril once daily; may reduce to 1 spray each nostril once daily

Veramyst *Nasal spray:* 27.5 mcg/actuation (10 g, 120 sprays) (alcohol-free)

► *fluticasone propionate* (C)(OTC)(G) <4 years: not recommended; >4-12 years: initially 1 spray in each nostril once daily; may increase to 2 sprays in each nostril once daily; maintenance 1 spray in each nostril once daily; max 2 sprays in each nostril/day; >12 years: initially 2 sprays in each nostril once daily <u>or</u> 1 spray bid; maintenance 1 spray once daily

Flonase *Nasal spray:* 50 mcg/actuation (16 g, 120 sprays)

► *flunisolide* (C) <6 years: not recommended; 6-14 years: initially 1 spray in each nostril tid <u>or</u> 2 sprays in each nostril bid; max 4 sprays/nostril/day; >14 years: 2 sprays in each nostril bid; may increase to 2 sprays in each nostril tid; max 8 sprays/nostril/day

Nasalide *Nasal spray:* 25 mcg/actuation (25 ml, 200 sprays)
Nasarel *Nasal spray:* 25 mcg/actuation (25 ml, 200 sprays)

► *mometasone furoate* (C)(G) <2 years: not recommended; 2-11 years: 1 spray in each nostril once daily; max 2 sprays in each nostril once daily; >11 years: 2 sprays in each nostril once daily

Nasonex *Nasal spray:* 50 mcg/actuation (17 g, 120 sprays)

► *olopatadine* (C) <6 years: not recommended; 6-11 years: 1 spray each nostril bid; >11 years: 2 sprays in each nostril bid

Patanase *Nasal spray:* 0.6%; 665 mcg/actuation (30.5 g, 240 sprays) (benzalkonium chloride)

▷ *triamcinolone acetonide* (C)(G) <6 years: not recommended; ≥6 years-12 years: 1 spray in each nostril once daily; max 2 sprays in each nostril once daily; >12 years: initially 2 sprays in each nostril once daily; max 4 sprays in each nostril once daily or 2 sprays in each nostril bid or 1 spray in each nostril qid; maintain at lowest effective dose
   Nasacort Allergy 24HR (OTC) *Nasal spray:* 55 mcg/actuation (10 g, 120 sprays)
   Tri-Nasal *Nasal spray:* 50 mcg/actuation (15 ml, 120 sprays)

NASAL MAST CELL STABILIZERS

▷ *cromolyn sodium* (B)(OTC) <2 years: not recommended; ≥2 years: 1 spray in each nostril tid-qid; max 6 sprays in each nostril/day
   Children's NasalCrom, NasalCrom *Nasal spray:* 5.2 mg/spray (13 ml, 100 sprays; 26 ml, 200 sprays)
   Comment: Begin use 1-2 weeks before exposure to known allergen. May take 2-4 weeks to achieve maximum effect.

NASAL ANTIHISTAMINES

▷ *azelastine* (C)
   Astelin Ready Spray <5 years: not recommended; ≥5-12 years: 1 spray in each nostril qd-bid; >12 years: 2 sprays in each nostril bid
      Nasal spray: 137 mcg/actuation (30 ml, 200 sprays) (benzalkonium chloride)
   Astepro 0.15% Nasal Spray <2 years: not recommended; ≥2 years: 1 or 2 sprays each nostril once daily bid
      Nasal spray: 205.5 mcg/actuation (17 ml, 106 sprays; 30 ml, 200 sprays) (benzalkonium chloride)

NASAL ANTIHISTAMINE/CORTICOSTEROID COMBINATION

▷ *azelastine/fluticasone* (C) <6 years: not recommended; ≥6 years: 1 spray in each nostril bid
   Dymista *Nasal spray:* azel 137 mcg/*flutic* 50 mcg per actuation (23 g, 120 sprays) (benzalkonium chloride)

NASAL ANTICHOLINERGICS

▷ *ipratropium bromide* (B)(G)
   Atrovent Nasal Spray 0.03% <6 years: not recommended; ≥6 years: 2 sprays in each nostril bid-tid
      Nasal spray: 21 mcg/actuation (30 ml, 345 sprays)
   Atrovent Nasal Spray 0.06% 2 <5 years: not recommended; 5-11 years: 2 sprays in each nostril tid; >11 years: sprays in each nostril tid-qid; max 5-7 days
      Nasal spray: 42 mcg/actuation (15 ml, 165 sprays)
   Comment: Avoid use with narrow-angle glaucoma, prostate hyperplasia, and bladder neck obstruction.

RHINITIS MEDICAMENTOSA

Comment: The nasal/oral regimen selected should be instituted with concurrent weaning from the nasal decongestant.

Oral Prescription Drugs for the Management of Allergy, Cough, and Cold Symptoms
see page 523
Nasal Corticosteroids *see Rhinitis/Sinusitis: Allergic page* 370
Oral Corticosteroids *see page* 498
Parenteral Corticosteroids *see page* 499

NASAL ANTICHOLINERGICS

➢ *ipratropium bromide* (B)(G)
>   **Atrovent Nasal Spray 0.03%** <6 years: not recommended; ≥6 years: stop nasal
>   decongestant; 2 sprays in each nostril bid-tid with progressive weaning as
>   tolerated
>   *Nasal spray:* 21 mcg/actuation (30 ml, 345 sprays)
>   **Atrovent Nasal Spray 0.06%** <5 years: not recommended; ≥5-11 years: 2 sprays
>   in each nostril tid; ≥11 years: 2 sprays in each nostril tid-qid with progressive
>   weaning as tolerated
>   *Nasal spray:* 42 mcg/actuation (15 ml, 165 sprays)

Comment: Avoid use with narrow-angle glaucoma, prostate hyperplasia, and
bladder neck obstruction

NASAL ANTIHISTAMINE

➢ *azelastine* (C) <5 years: not recommended; ≥5-12 years: 1 spray in each nostril bid
>12 years: 2 sprays in each nostril bid
>   **Astelin Ready Spray** *Nasal spray:* 137 mcg/actuation (30 ml, 200 sprays)

SECOND GENERATION ANTIHISTAMINES

Comment: Second generation antihistamines are sedating, but much less so than the
first generation antihistamines. All antihistamines are excreted into breast milk.
➢ *cetirizine* (C)(OTC)(G) <6 years: not recommended; ≥6-<65 years: initially 5-10
mg once daily; ≥65 years: 5 mg once daily
>   **Children's Zyrtec Chewable** *Chew tab:* 5, 10 mg (grape)
>   **Children's Zyrtec Allergy Syrup** *Syr:* 1 mg/ml (4 oz) (grape, bubble gum)
>   (sugar-free, dye-free)
>   **Zyrtec** *Tab:* 10 mg
>   **Zyrtec Hives Relief** *Tab:* 10 mg
>   **Zyrtec Liquid Gels** *Liq gel:* 10 mg
➢ *desloratadine* (C)
>   **Clarinex** <6 years: not recommended; ≥6 years: 1/2-1 tab once daily
>   *Tab:* 5 mg
>   **Clarinex RediTabs** <6 years: not recommended; 6-12 years: 2.5 mg once daily;
>   ≥12 years: 5 mg once daily
>   *ODT:* 2.5, 5 mg (tutti-frutti) (phenylalanine)
>   **Clarinex Syrup** <6 months: not recommended; 6-11 months: 1 mg (2 ml) once
>   daily; 1-5 years: 1.25 mg (2.5 ml) once daily; 6-11 years: 2.5 mg (5 ml) once
>   daily; ≥12 years: 5 mg (10 ml) once daily
>   *Tab:* 0.5 mg per ml (4 oz) (tutti-frutti) (phenylalanine)
>   **Desloratadine ODT**
➢ *fexofenadine* (C)(OTC)(G) 6 months-2 years: 15 mg bid; *CrCl ≤90 mL/min:* 15 mg
once daily; 2-11 years: 30 mg bid; *CrCl ≤90 mL/min:* 30 mg once daily ≥12 years

and older: ≥12 years: 60 mg once daily-bid or 180 mg once daily; *CrCl <90 mL/min:* 60 mg once daily **Allegra** *Tab:* 30, 60, 180 mg film-coat

    Allegra Allergy *Tab:* 60, 180 mg film-coat

    Allegra ODT *ODT:* 30 mg (phenylalanine)

    Allegra Oral Suspension *Oral susp:* 30 mg/5 ml (6 mg/ml) (4 oz)

▷ *loratadine* (C)(OTC)(G) <2 years: not recommended; 2-5 years: 5 mg once daily; ≥6 years: 5 mg bid or 10 mg once daily; *Hepatic or Renal Insufficiency:* (see mfr pkg insert)

    Children's Claritin Chewables *Chew tab:* 5 mg (grape) (phenylalanine)

    Children's Claritin Syrup 1 mg/ml (4 oz) (fruit) (sugar-free, alcohol-free, dye-free; sodium 6 mg/5 ml)

    Claritin *Tab:* 10 mg

    Claritin Hives Relief *Tab:* 10 mg

    Claritin Liqui-Gels *Liq gel:* 10 mg

    Claritin RediTabs 12 Hours *ODT:* 5 mg (mint)

    Claritin RediTabs 24 Hours *ODT:* 10 mg (mint)

▷ *levocetirizine* (B)(OTC) administer dose in the PM; *Seasonal Allergic Rhinitis:* <2 years: not recommended; may start at ≥2 years; *Chronic Idiopathic Urticaria (CIU), Perennial Allergic Rhinitis:* <6 months: not recommended; may start at ≥ 6 months; *Dosing by Age:* 6 months-5 years: max 1.25 mg once daily; 6-11 years: max 2.5 mg once daily; ≥12 years: 2.5-5 mg once daily; *Renal Dysfunction <12 years:* contraindicated; *Renal Dysfunction ≥12 years:* CrCl 50-80 ml/min: 2.5 mg once daily; CrCl 30-50 mL/min: 2.5 mg every other day; CrCl: 10-30 mL/min: 2.5 mg twice weekly (every 3-4 days); *CrCl <10 mL/min,* ESRD or hemodialysis: contraindicated;

    Xyzal *Tab:* 5*mg

    Xyzal Oral Solution *Oral soln:* 0.5 mg/ml (150 ml)

FIRST GENERATION ANTIHISTAMINES

▷ *hydroxyzine* (C)(G) <6 years: 50 mg/day divided qid prn; ≥6 years: 50-100 mg/day divided qid prn; max 600 mg/day; 25 mg tid prn; max 600 mg/day

    Atarax *Tab:* 10, 25, 50, 100 mg; *Syr:* 10 mg/5 ml (alcohol 0.5%)

    Vistaril *Cap:* 25, 50, 100 mg; *Oral susp:* 25 mg/5 ml (4 oz) (lemon)

☐ RHINITIS: VASOMOTOR

NASAL ANTICHOLINERGICS

▷ *ipratropium bromide* (B)(G)

    Atrovent Nasal Spray 0.03% <6 years: not recommended; ≥6 years: stop nasal decongestant; 2 sprays in each nostril bid-tid with progressive weaning as tolerated

    Nasal spray: 21 mcg/actuation (30 ml, 345 sprays)

    Atrovent Nasal Spray 0.06% <5 years: not recommended; ≥5-11 years: 2 sprays in each nostril tid; >11 years: stop nasal decongestant; 2 sprays in each nostril tid-qid with progressive weaning as tolerated

    Nasal spray: 42 mcg/actuation (15 ml, 165 sprays)

Comment: Avoid use with narrow-angle glaucoma, prostate hyperplasia, and bladder neck obstruction

ROSEOLA (EXANTHEM SUBITUM)

Antipyretics *see Fever* page 136

 ROCKY MOUNTAIN SPOTTED FEVER (*RICKETTSIA RICKETTSII*)

ANTI-INFECTIVES

▶ *doxycycline* (D)(G) <8 years: not recommended; ≥8 years, ≤100 lb: 2-2.5 mg/kg q 12 hours x 7-10 days; ≥8 years, >100 lb: 200 mg on first day; then 100 mg bid x 7-10 days

  Acticlate *Tab:* 75, 150**mg
  Adoxa *Tab:* 50, 75, 100, 150 mg ent-coat
  Doryx *Tab:* 50, 75, 100, 150, 200 mg del-rel
  Monodox *Cap:* 50, 75, 100 mg
  Oracea *Cap:* 40 mg del-rel
  Vibramycin *Tab:* 100 mg; *Cap:* 50, 100 mg; *Syr:* 50 mg/5 ml (raspberry-apple) (sulfites); *Oral susp:* 25 mg/5 ml (raspberry)
  Vibra-Tab *Tab:* 100 mg film-coat

Comment: *doxycycline* contraindicated <8 years-of-age, in pregnancy, and lactation (discolors developing tooth enamel). A side effect may be photo-sensitivity (photophobia). Do not take with antacids, calcium supplements, milk or other dairy, or within 2 hours of taking another drug.

▶ *tetracycline* (D)(G) <8 years: not recommended; ≥8 years, ≤100 lb: 10 mg/kg/day divided q 6 hours x 7-10 days; *see page 574 for dose by weight table*; ≥8 years, >100 lb: 500 mg q 6 hours x 7-10 days

  Achromycin V *Cap:* 250, 500 mg
  Sumycin *Tab:* 250, 500 mg; *Cap:* 250, 500 mg; *Oral susp:* 125 mg/5 ml (100, 200 ml) (fruit) (sulfites)

Comment: *tetracycline* is contraindicated <8 years-of-age, in pregnancy, and lactation (discolors developing tooth enamel). A side effect may be photo-sensitivity (photophobia). Do not give with antacids, calcium supplements, milk or other dairy, or within two hours of taking another drug.

 ROTAVIRUS GASTROENTERITIS

PROPHYLAXIS

Comment: RotaTeq targets the most common strains of rotavirus (G1, G2, G3, G4), which are responsible for more than 90% of rotavirus disease in the United States.

▶ *rotavirus vaccine, live* <6 weeks or >32 weeks: not recommended; >6 weeks and <32 weeks: administer 1st dose at 6-12 weeks of age; administer 2nd and 3rd doses at 4-10-week intervals for a total of 3 doses; if an incomplete dose is administered, do not administer a replacement dose, but continue with the remaining doses in the recommended series

RotaTeq *Oral susp:* 2 ml single-use tube (fetal bovine serum [trace], preservative-free, thimerosal-free)

ROUNDWORM (ASCARIASIS)

ANTHELMINTICS

Comment: Oral bioavailability of anthelmintics is enhanced when administered with a fatty meal (estimated fat content 40 g).

▸ *albendazole* (C) take with a meal; may crush and mix with food; may repeat in 3 weeks if needed; <2 years: 200 mg as a single dose; >2 years: 400 mg as a single dose;

   Albenza Tab: 200 mg

▸ *mebendazole* (C) take with a meal; may crush and mix with food; may repeat in 3 weeks if needed; <2 years: not recommended; >2 years: 100 mg bid x 3 days;

   Emverm *Chew tab:* 100 mg
   Vermox (G) *Chew tab:* 100 mg

▸ *pyrantel pamoate* (C) take with a meal; may open capsule and sprinkle or mix with food; treat x 3 days; may repeat in 2-3 weeks if needed; 11 mg/kg/dose; max 1 gm/dose; <25 lb: not recommended; 25-37 lb: 1/2 tsp/dose; 38-62 lb: 1 tsp/dose; 63-87 lb: 1 tsp/dose; 88-112 lb: 2 tsp/dose; 113-137 lb: 2 tsp/dose; 138-162 lb: 3 tsp/dose; 163-187 lb: 3 tsp/dose; >187 lb: 4 tsp/dose

   Antiminth (OTC) *Cap:* 180 mg; *Liq:* 50 mg/ml (30 ml); 144 mg/ml (30 ml); *Oral susp:* 50 mg/ml (60 ml)
   Pin-X (OTC) *Cap:* 180 mg; *Liq:* 50 mg/ml (30 ml); 144 mg/ml (30 ml); *Oral susp:* 50 mg/ml (30 ml)

▸ *thiabendazole* (C) take with a meal; may crush and mix with food; treat x 7 days; max 1.5 gm/dose; max 3 g/day <30 lb: consult mfr pkg insert; ≥30 lb: 25 mg/kg/dose bid; 30-50 lb: 250 mg bid; >50 lb: 10 mg/lb/dose bid

   Mintezol *Chew tab:* 500*mg (orange); *Oral susp:* 500 mg/5 ml (120 ml) (orange)

   Comment: *thiabendazole* is not for prophylaxis. May impair mental alertness. May not be available in the US.

RUBELLA (GERMAN MEASLES)

PROPHYLAXIS

See Childhood Immunizations page 473

▸ *rubella virus, live, attenuated/neomycin* vaccine (C) <12 months: not recommended; ≥12 months: 25 mcg SC; if vaccinated <12 months, revaccinate at 12 months;

   Meruvax II 25 mcg SC

▸ *measles, mumps, rubella, live, attenuated, neomycin vaccine* (C)

   MMR II 25 mcg SC (preservative-free)

Comment: Contraindications: hypersensitivity to *neomycin* or eggs, primary or acquired immune deficiency, immunosuppressant therapy, bone marrow or lymphatic malignancy, and pregnancy (within 3 months following vaccination).

TREATMENT

➤ *immune globulin* (Ig) 0.25 ml/kg IM (0.5 mg/kg in immunocompromised children)

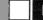 **RUBEOLA (RED MEASLES)**

PROPHYLAXIS

➤ *measles, mumps, rubella, live, attenuated, neomycin vaccine* (C)
  MMR II 25 mcg SC (preservative-free)
  Comment: Contraindications: hypersensitivity to *neomycin* or eggs, primary or acquired immune deficiency, immunosuppressant therapy, bone marrow or lymphatic malignancy, and pregnancy (within 3 months following vaccination). *See Childhood Immunizations page* 473

TREATMENT

➤ *immune globulin* (Ig) 0.25 ml/kg IM (0.5 mg/kg in immunocompromised children)

SALMONELLOSIS

➤ *ciprofloxacin* (C) <18 years: not recommended; ≥18 years: 500 mg bid x 3-5 days; max 1.5 gm/day
  Cipro (G) *Tab:* 250, 500, 750 mg; *Oral susp:* 250, 500 mg/5 ml (100 ml) (strawberry)
  Cipro XR *Tab:* 500, 1000 mg ext-rel
  ProQuin XR *Tab:* 500 mg ext-rel
  Comment: *ciprofloxacin* is contraindicated <18 years-of-age, and during pregnancy and lactation. Risk of tendonitis or tendon rupture.
➤ *trimethoprim/sulfamethoxazole* (D)(G)
  Bactrim, Septra <12 years: not recommended; ≥12 years: 2 tabs bid x 10 days
    Tab: trim 80 mg/*sulfa* 400 mg*
  Bactrim DS, Septra DS <12 years: not recommended; ≥12 years: 1 tab bid x 10 days
    Tab: trim 160 mg/*sulfa* 800 mg*
  Bactrim Pediatric Suspension, Septra Pediatric Suspension <2 months: not recommended; ≥2 months-12 years: 40 mg/kg/day of *sulfamethoxazole* in 2 doses bid; >12 years: use tabs
    Oral susp: trim 40 mg/*sulfa* 200 mg per 5 ml (100 ml) (cherry) (alcohol 0.3%)

 SCABIES (*SARCOPTES SCABIEI*)

Comment: This section presents treatment regimens for scabies infestation published in the **2015 CDC Sexually Transmitted Diseases Treatment Guidelines**, as well as other available treatments.

RECOMMENDED REGIMEN

➤ *permethrin* (B)(G) <2 months: not recommended; ≥2 months: massage into skin from head to soles of feet; leave on x 8-14 hours, then rinse off
   Acticin, Elimite *Crm:* 5% (60 gm)

ALTERNATIVE REGIMEN

➤ *lindane* (B)(G) <2 months: not recommended; ≥2 months: 1 oz of lotion or 30 gm of cream apply to all skin surfaces from neck down to the soles of the feet; leave on x 8 hours, then wash off thoroughly; may repeat if needed in 14 days
   Kwell *Lotn:* 1% (60, 473 ml); *Crm:* 1% (60 gm); *Shampoo:* 1% (60, 473 ml)

OTHER TOPICAL TREATMENTS

➤ *crotamiton* (C) <12 years: not recommended; ≥12 years: massage into skin from chin down; repeat in 24 hours
   Eurax *Lotn:* 10% (60 gm); *Crm:* 10% (60 gm)

SCARLET FEVER (SCARLATINA)

Comment: Microorganism responsible for scarlet fever is Group A beta-hemolytic *Streptococcus* (GABHS). Strep cultures and screens will be positive.

➤ *azithromycin* (B)(G) <12 years: 12 mg/kg/day x 5 days; *see page 548 for dose by weight table;* max 500 mg/day; ≥12 years: 500 mg x 1 dose on day 1, then 250 mg once daily on days 2-5 or 500 mg once daily x 5 days
   Zithromax *Tab:* 250, 500, 600 mg; *Oral susp:* 100 mg/5 ml (15 ml); 200 mg/5 ml (15, 22.5, 30 ml) (cherry); *Pkt:* 1 gm for reconstitution (cherry-banana)
   Zithromax Tri-pak *Tab:* 3 x 500 mg tabs/pck
   Zithromax Z-pak *Tab:* 6 x 250 mg tabs/pck
   Zmax *Oral susp:* 2 gm ext-rel for reconstitution (cherry-banana) (148 mg Na⁺)

➤ *cefadroxil* <12 years: 30 mg/kg/day in 2 divided doses x 10 days; *see page 550 for dose by weight table;* ≥12 years: 1-2 gm in a single or 2 divided doses x 10 days
   Duricef *Cap:* 500 mg; *Tab:* 1 g; *Oral susp:* 250 mg/5 ml (100 ml); 500 mg/5 ml (75, 100 ml) (orange-pineapple)

➤ *cephalexin* (B)(G) 25-50 mg/kg/day in 2 divided doses x 10 days; *see page 557 for dose by weight table*
   Keflex *Cap:* 250, 333, 500, 750 mg; *Oral susp:* 125, 250 mg/5 ml (100, 200 ml) (strawberry)

➤ *clarithromycin* (C)(G) <6 months: not recommended; ≥6 months-12 years: 7.5 mg/kg bid x 14-21 days; *see page 558 for dose by weight table;* >12 years: 500 mg bid or 500 mg ext-rel daily x 14-21 days
   Biaxin *Tab:* 250, 500 mg
   Biaxin Oral Suspension *Oral susp:* 125, 250 mg/5 ml (50, 100 ml) (fruit punch)
   Biaxin XL *Tab:* 500 mg ext-rel

➤ *clindamycin* (B)(G) <12 years: 8-16 mg/kg/day in 3-4 divided doses x 10 days; *see page 559 for dose by weight table;* ≥12 years: 150-300 mg q 6 hours x 10 days
   Cleocin *Cap:* 75 (tartrazine), 150 (tartrazine), 300 mg
   Cleocin Pediatric Granules *Oral susp:* 75 mg/5 ml (100 ml) (cherry)

➤ *erythromycin estolate* (B)(G) <12 years: 20-50 mg/kg q 6 hours x 10 days; *see page 562 for dose by weight table;* ≥12 years: 250 mg q 6 hours x 10 days
    Ilosone *Pulvule:* 250 mg; *Tab:* 500 mg; *Liq:* 125, 250 mg/5 ml (100 ml)

➤ *erythromycin ethylsuccinate* (B)(G) 30-50 mg/kg/day in 4 divided doses x 10 days; may double dose with severe infection; max 100 mg/kg/day <u>or</u> 400 mg qid; *see page 563 for dose by weight table*
    EryPed *Oral susp:* 200 mg/5 ml (100, 200 ml) (fruit); 400 mg/5 ml (60, 100, 200 ml) (banana); *Oral drops:* 200, 400 mg/5 ml (50 ml) (fruit); *Chew tab:* 200 mg wafer (fruit)
    E.E.S. *Oral susp:* 200, 400 mg/5 ml (100 ml) (fruit)
    E.E.S. Granules *Oral susp:* 200 mg/5 ml (100, 200 ml) (cherry)
    E.E.S. 400 Tablets *Tab:* 400 mg

➤ *penicillin g (benzathine and procaine)* (B)(G) <30 lb: 600,000 IM x 1 dose; 30-60 lb: 900,000-1.2 million units IM x 1 dose; >60 lbs: 2.4 million units IM x 1 dose
    Bicillin C-R Cartridge-needle unit: 600,000 units (1 ml); 1.2 million units; (2 ml); 2.4 million units (4 ml)

➤ *penicillin v potassium* (B) <12 years: 25-75 mg/kg day divided q 6-8 hours x 10 days; *see page 572 for dose by weight table;* ≥12 years: 250 mg tid x 10 days
    Pen-VK *Tab:* 250, 500 mg; *Oral soln:* 125 mg/5 ml (100, 200 ml); 250 mg/5 ml (100, 150, 200 ml)

◻ SEIZURE DISORDER

Status Epilepticus *see* ***Status Epilepticus*** *page 392*
Anticonvulsant Drugs *see page 509*

◻ SEXUAL ASSAULT (STD/STI/VD EXPOSURE)

Comment: The following treatment regimens for victims of sexual assault are published in the **2015 CDC Sexually Transmitted Diseases Treatment Guidelines**.

RECOMMENDED PROPHYLAXIS REGIMEN

➤ *ceftriaxone* 250 mg IM in a single dose <u>plus</u> *metronidazole* 2 gm in a single dose <u>plus</u> *azithromycin* 1 gm in a single dose

ALTERNATE PROPHYLAXIS REGIMENS

Regimen 1

➤ *ceftriaxone* 250 mg IM in a single dose <u>plus</u> *metronidazole* 2 gm in a single dose <u>plus</u> *doxycycline* 100 mg bid x 7 days

Regimen 2

➤ *cefixime* 400 mg in a single dose <u>plus</u> *metronidazole* 2 gm in a single dose <u>plus</u> *azithromycin* 1 gm in a single dose

Regimen 3

▶ *cefixime* 400 mg in a single dose <u>plus</u> *metronidazole* 2 gm in a single dose <u>plus</u> *doxycycline* 100 mg bid x 7 days

Regimen 4

▶ *azithromycin* (B)(G) 1 gm as a single dose <u>plus</u> *metronidazole* 2 gm in a single dose

DRUG BRANDS AND DOSE FORMS

▶ *azithromycin* (B)(G)
   Zithromax *Tab:* 250, 500, 600 mg; *Oral susp:* 100 mg/5 ml (15 ml); 200 mg/5 ml (15, 22.5, 30 ml) (cherry); *Pkt:* 1 gm for reconstitution (cherry-banana)
   Zithromax Tri-pak *Tab:* 3 x 500 mg tabs/pck
   Zithromax Z-pak *Tab:* 6 x 250 mg tabs/pck
   Zmax *Oral susp:* 2 gm ext-rel for reconstitution (cherry-banana) (148 mg Na$^+$)
▶ *cefixime* (B)(G)
   Suprax *Tab:* 400 mg; *Cap:* 400 mg; *Oral susp:* 100, 200, 500 mg/5 ml (50, 75, 100 ml) (strawberry)
▶ *ceftriaxone* (B)(G)
   Rocephin *Vial:* 250, 500 mg; 1, 2 g
▶ *doxycycline* (D)(G)
   Acticlate *Tab:* 75, 150**mg
   Adoxa *Tab:* 50, 75, 100, 150 mg ent-coat
   Doryx *Tab:* 50, 75, 100, 150, 200 mg del-rel
   Monodox *Cap:* 50, 75, 100 mg
   Oracea *Cap:* 40 mg del-rel
   Vibramycin *Tab:* 100 mg; *Cap:* 50, 100 mg; *Syr:* 50 mg/5 ml (raspberry-apple) (sulfites); *Oral susp:* 25 mg/5 ml (raspberry)
   Vibra-Tab *Tab:* 100 mg film-coat
   Comment: *doxycycline* is contraindicated <8 years-of-age, in pregnancy, and lactation (discolors developing tooth enamel). A side effect may be photo-sensitivity (photophobia). Do not take with antacids, calcium supplements, milk <u>or</u> other dairy, <u>or</u> within 2 hours of taking another drug.
▶ *metronidazole* (not for use in 1st; B in 2nd, 3rd)(G) **Flagyl** *Tab:* 250*, 500*mg
   Flagyl 375 *Cap:* 375 mg
   Flagyl ER *Tab:* 750 mg ext-rel
   Comment: Alcohol is contraindicated during treatment with oral *metronidazole* and for 72 hours after therapy due to a possible *disulfiram*-like reaction (nausea, vomiting, flushing, headache).

SHIGELLOSIS

ANTI-INFECTIVES

▶ *azithromycin* (B) <6 months: not recommended; ≥6 months-12 years: 10 mg/kg x 1 dose on day 1; then 5 mg/kg/day on days 2-5; *see page 548 for dose by weight table*; max 500 mg/day; >12 years: 500 mg x 1 dose on day 1, then 250 mg once daily on days 2-5 <u>or</u> 500 mg once daily x 3 days <u>or</u> **Zmax** 2 gm in a single dose

Zithromax *Tab:* 250, 500, 600 mg; *Oral susp:* 100 mg/5 ml (15 ml); 200 mg/5 ml (15, 22.5, 30 ml) (cherry); *Pkt:* 1 gm for reconstitution (cherry-banana)

Zithromax Tri-pak *Tab:* 3 x 500 mg tabs/pck

Zithromax Z-pak *Tab:* 6 x 250 mg tabs/pck

Zmax *Oral susp:* 2 gm ext-rel for reconstitution (cherry-banana) (148 mg Na⁺)

➤ *ciprofloxacin* (C) <18 years: not recommended; ≥18 years: 500 mg bid x 3 days; max 1.5 gm/day

Cipro (G) *Tab:* 250, 500, 750 mg; *Oral susp:* 250, 500 mg/5 ml (100 ml) (strawberry)

Cipro XR *Tab:* 500, 1000 mg ext-rel

ProQuin XR *Tab:* 500 mg ext-rel

Comment: *ciprofloxacin* is contraindicated <18 years-of-age, and during pregnancy and lactation. Risk of tendonitis <u>or</u> tendon rupture.

➤ *ofloxacin* (C)(G) <18 years: not recommended; ≥18 years: 400 mg bid x 3 days

Floxin *Tab:* 200, 300, 400 mg

Comment: *ofloxacin* is contraindicated <18 years-of-age, and during pregnancy and lactation. Risk of tendonitis <u>or</u> tendon rupture.

➤ *tetracycline* (D)(G) <8 years: not recommended; ≥8 years, ≤100 lb: 25-50 mg/kg/day in 4 divided doses x 5 days; *see page 574 for dose by weight table;* ≥8 years, >100 lb: 250-500 mg qid x 5 days

Achromycin V *Cap:* 250, 500 mg

Sumycin *Tab:* 250, 500 mg; *Cap:* 250, 500 mg; *Oral susp:* 125 mg/5 ml (100, 200 ml) (fruit) (sulfites)

Comment: *tetracycline* is contraindicated <8 years-of-age, in pregnancy, and lactation (discolors developing tooth enamel). A side effect may be photo-sensitivity (photophobia). Do not give with antacids, calcium supplements, milk <u>or</u> other dairy, <u>or</u> within two hours of taking another drug.

➤ *trimethoprim/sulfamethoxazole* (D)(G)

Bactrim, Septra <12 years: not recommended; ≥12 years: 2 tabs bid x 10 days
Tab: trim 80 mg/*sulfa* 400 mg*

Bactrim DS, Septra DS <12 years: not recommended; ≥12 years: 1 tab bid x 10 days
Tab: trim 160 mg/*sulfa* 800 mg*

Bactrim Pediatric Suspension, Septra Pediatric Suspension <2 months: not recommended; ≥2 months-12 years: 40 mg/kg/day of *sulfamethoxazole* in 2 doses bid; >12 years: use tabs
Oral susp: trim 40 mg/*sulfa* 200 mg per 5 ml (100 ml) (cherry) (alcohol 0.3%)

SINUSITIS/RHINOSINUSITIS: ACUTE BACTERIAL (ABRS)

ANTI-INFECTIVES

➤ *amoxicillin* (B)(G) <40 kg (88 lb): 20-40 mg/kg/day in 3 divided doses x 10 days <u>or</u> 25-45 mg/kg/day in 2 divided doses x 10 days; *see page 543 for dose by weight table;* ≥40 kg: 500-875 mg bid <u>or</u> 250-500 mg tid x 10 days

Amoxil *Cap:* 250, 500 mg; *Tab:* 875*mg; *Chew tab:* 125, 200, 250, 400 mg (cherry-banana-peppermint) (phenylalanine); *Oral susp:* 125, 250 mg/5 ml (80, 100, 150 ml) (strawberry); 200, 400 mg/5 ml (50, 75, 100 ml) (bubble gum); *Oral drops:* 50 mg/ml (30 ml) (bubble gum)

Moxatag *Tab:* 775 mg ext-rel
Trimox *Tab:* 125, 250 mg; *Cap:* 250, 500 mg; *Oral susp:* 125, 250 mg/5 ml (80, 100, 150 ml) (raspberry-strawberry)

➤ *amoxicillin/clavulanate* (B)(G)
    Augmentin <40 kg: 40-45 mg/kg/day divided tid x 10 days or 90 mg/kg/day divided bid x 10 days; *see page 545 for dose by weight table;* ≥40 kg: 500 mg tid or 875 mg bid x 10 days
        Tab: 250, 500, 875 mg; *Chew tab:* 125, 250 mg (lemon-lime); 200, 400 mg (cherry-banana) (phenylalanine); *Oral susp:* 125 mg/5 ml (banana), 250 mg/5 ml (75, 100, 150 ml) (orange); 200, 400 mg/5 ml (50, 75, 100 ml) (orange) (phenylalanine)
    Augmentin ES-600 <3 months: not recommended; ≥3 months, <40 kg: 90 mg/kg/day divided q 12 hours x 10 days; *see page 546 for dose by weight table;* ≥40 kg: use tab
        Oral susp: 600 mg/5 ml (50, 75, 100, 125, 150, 200 ml) (strawberry cream) (phenylalanine)
    Augmentin XR <16 years: use other forms; ≥16 years: 2 tabs q 12 hours x 7-10 days
        Tab: 1000*mg ext-rel

➤ *cefaclor* (B)(G) <1 month: not recommended; 1 month-12 years: 20-40 mg/kg divided bid x 10 days; *see page 549 for dose by weight table;* max 1 gm/day; >12 years: 250-500 mg q 8 hours x 10 days; max 2 gm/day
        Tab: 500 mg; *Cap:* 250, 500 mg; *Susp:* 125 mg/5 ml (75, 150 ml) (strawberry); 187 mg/5 ml (50, 100 ml) (strawberry); 250 mg/5 ml (75, 150 ml) (strawberry); 375 mg/5 ml (50, 100 ml) (strawberry)
    Cefaclor Extended Release <16 years: not recommended; ≥16 years: 500 mg bid x 10 days (clinically equivalent to 250 mg immed-rel caps tid); swallow whole; take with food
        Tab: 375, 500 mg ext-rel

➤ *cefdinir* (B) <6 months: not recommended; 6 months-12 years: 14 mg/kg/day in a single or 2 divided doses x 10 days; *see page 551 for dose by weight table;* >12 years: 300 mg bid or 600 mg once daily x 10 days
    Omnicef *Cap:* 300 mg; *Oral susp:* 125 mg/5 ml (60, 100 ml) (strawberry)

➤ *cefixime* (B)(G) <6 months: not recommended; 6 months-12 years, <50 kg: 8 mg/kg/day in 1-2 divided doses x 10 days; *see page 552 for dose by weight table;* >12 years, >50 kg: 400 mg once daily x 10 days
    Suprax *Tab:* 400 mg; *Cap:* 400 mg; *Oral susp:* 100, 200, 500 mg/5 ml (50, 75, 100 ml) (strawberry)

➤ *cefpodoxime proxetil* <2 months: not recommended; 2 months-12 years: 10 mg/kg/day (max 400 mg/dose) or 5 mg/kg/day bid (max 200 mg/dose) x 10 days; *see page 553 for dose by weight table;* >12 years: 200 mg bid x 10 days

➤ *cefprozil* (B) <6 months: not recommended; 6 months-12 years: *Mild:* 7.5 mg/kg bid x 10 days; *Moderate/Severe:* 15 mg/kg q 12 hours x 10 days; *see page 554 for dose by weight table;* >12 years: 250-500 mg bid x 10 days
    Cefzil *Tab:* 250, 500 mg; *Oral susp:* 125, 250 mg/5 ml (50, 75, 100 ml) (bubble gum) (phenylalanine)

➤ *ceftibuten* (B) <12 years: 9 mg/kg once daily x 10 days; max 400 mg/day; *see page 555 for dose by weight table;* ≥12 years: 400 mg once daily x 10 days
    Cedax *Cap:* 400 mg; *Oral susp:* 90 mg/5 ml (30, 60, 90, 120 ml); 180 mg/5 ml (30, 60, 120 ml) (cherry)

▷ *cefuroxime axetil* (B)(G) <3 months: not recommended; 3 months-12 years: 20-30 mg/kg/day in 2 divided doses x 10 days; *see page 556 for dose by weight table*; ≥12 years: 250-500 mg bid x 10 days

    Ceftin *Tab:* 250, 500 mg; *Oral susp:* 125, 250 mg/5 ml (50, 100 ml) (tutti-frutti)

▷ *ciprofloxacin* (C) <18 years: not recommended; ≥18 years: 500 mg bid x 10 days; max 1.5 gm/day

    Cipro (G) *Tab:* 250, 500, 750 mg; *Oral susp:* 250, 500 mg/5 ml (100 ml) (strawberry)

    Cipro XR *Tab:* 500, 1000 mg ext-rel

    ProQuin XR *Tab:* 500 mg ext-rel

Comment: *ciprofloxacin* is contraindicated <18 years-of-age, and during pregnancy and lactation. Risk of tendonitis or tendon rupture.

▷ *clarithromycin* (C)(G) <6 months: not recommended; ≥6 months-12 years: 7.5 mg/kg bid x 10 days; *see page 558 for dose by weight table;* >12 years: 500 mg bid or 500 mg ext-rel daily x 10 days

    Biaxin *Tab:* 250, 500 mg

    Biaxin Oral Suspension *Oral susp:* 125, 250 mg/5 ml (50, 100 ml) (fruit punch)

    Biaxin XL *Tab:* 500 mg ext-rel

▷ *levofloxacin* (C) <18 years: not recommended; ≥18 years: *Uncomplicated:* 500 mg once daily x 10-14 days; *Complicated:* 750 mg once daily x 10-14 days

    Levaquin *Tab:* 250, 500, 750 mg; *Oral soln:* 25 mg/ml (480 ml) (benzyl alcohol); *Inj conc:* 25 mg/ml for IV infusion after dilution (20, 30 ml single-use vial) (preservative-free); *Premix soln:* 5 mg/ml for IV infusion (50, 100, 150 ml) (preservative-free)

Comment: *levofloxacin* is contraindicated <18 years-of-age, and during pregnancy and lactation. Risk of tendonitis or tendon rupture.

▷ *loracarbef* (B) <12 years: 15 mg/kg/day in 2 divided doses x 10 days; *see page 570 for dose by weight table*; ≥12 years: 200 mg bid x 10 days

    Lorabid *Pulvule:* 200, 400 mg; *Oral susp:* 100 mg/5 ml (50, 100 ml); 200 mg/5 ml (50, 75, 100 ml) (strawberry bubble gum)

▷ *moxifloxacin* (C)(G) <18 years: not recommended; ≥18 years: 400 mg daily x 10 days

    Avelox *Tab:* 400 mg

Comment: *moxifloxacin* is contraindicated <18 years-of-age, and during pregnancy and lactation. Risk of tendonitis or tendon rupture.

▷ *trimethoprim/sulfamethoxazole* (D)(G)

    Bactrim, Septra <12 years: not recommended; ≥12 years: 2 tabs bid x 10 days
        Tab: trim 80 mg/*sulfa* 400 mg*

    Bactrim DS, Septra DS <12 years: not recommended; ≥12 years: 1 tab bid x 10 days
        Tab: trim 160 mg/*sulfa* 800 mg*

    Bactrim Pediatric Suspension, Septra Pediatric Suspension <2 months: not recommended; ≥2 months-12 years: 40 mg/kg/day of *sulfamethoxazole* in 2 doses bid; >12 years: use tabs
        Oral susp: trim 40 mg/*sulfa* 200 mg per 5 ml (100 ml) (cherry) (alcohol 0.3%)

SJOGREN'S SYNDROME (CHRONIC DRY MOUTH)

CHOLINERGIC/MUSCARINIC AGONIST COMBINATION

▷ *cevimeline* (C)(G) 30 mg tid

    Evoxac *Cap:* 30 mg

Comment: *cevimeline* is contraindicated in acute iritis, narrow-angle glaucoma, and uncontrolled asthma.
➤ *pilocarpine* (C)(G) 5 mg qid <u>or</u> 7.5 mg tid
   Salagen *Tab*: 5, 7.5 mg

ORAL ENZYME RINSE

➤ *xylitol/solazyme/selectobac* (NE) swish 5 ml for 30 seconds bid-tid
   Orazyme Dry Mouth Rinse *Oral soln*: 1.5, 16 oz

SKIN: CALLOUSED

KERATOLYTICS

➤ *salicylic acid* (C)(OTC) <12 years: not recommended; ≥12 years: apply lotion, cream <u>or</u> gel to affected area qd-bid; apply patch to affected area and leave on x 48 hours with max 5 applications/14 days
➤ *urea* (C)
   Carmol 40 <12 years: not recommended; ≥12 years: apply to affected area with applicator stick provided once daily-tid; smooth over until cream is absorbed; protect surrounding tissue; may cover with adhesive bandage <u>or</u> gauze secured with adhesive tape
      Crm/Gel: 40% (30 gm)
   Keratol 40 <12 years: not recommended; ≥ 12 years: apply to affected area with applicator stick provided once daily-tid; smooth over until cream is absorbed; protect surrounding tissue; may cover with adhesive bandage <u>or</u> gauze secured with adhesive tape
      Crm: 40% (1, 3, 7 oz); *Gel*: 40% (15 ml); *Lotn*: 40% (8 oz)
Comment: The moisturizing effect of **Carmol 40** and **Keratol 40** is enhanced by applying while the skin is still moist (after washing <u>or</u> bathing).

SKIN INFECTION: BACTERIAL (CARBUNCLE, FOLLICULITIS, FURUNCLE)

Comment: Abscesses usually require surgical incision and drainage.
➤ *hexachlorophene* (C) dispense 5 ml into wet hand, work up into lather; then apply to area to be cleansed; rinse thoroughly
   pHisoHex *Liq clnsr*: 5, 16 oz

TOPICAL ANTI-INFECTIVES

➤ *mupirocin* (B)(G) apply to lesions bid
   Bactroban *Oint*: 2% (22 gm); *Crm*: 2% (15, 30 gm)
   Centany *Oint*: 2% (15, 30 gm)
➤ *polymyxin B/neomycin* (C) *oint*: apply once daily-tid
   Neosporin (OTC) *Oint*: 15 g

ORAL ANTI-INFECTIVES

▷ *amoxicillin* (B)(G) <40 kg (88 lb): 20-40 mg/kg/day in 3 divided doses x 10 days or 25-45 mg/kg/day in 2 divided doses x 10 days; *see page 543 for dose by weight table;* ≥40 kg: 500-875 mg bid or 250-500 mg tid x 10 days

> **Amoxil** *Cap:* 250, 500 mg; *Tab:* 875*mg; *Chew tab:* 125, 200, 250, 400 mg (cherry-banana-peppermint) (phenylalanine); *Oral susp:* 125, 250 mg/5 ml (80, 100, 150 ml) (strawberry); 200, 400 mg/5 ml (50, 75, 100 ml) (bubble gum); *Oral drops:* 50 mg/ml (30 ml) (bubble gum)

> **Moxatag** *Tab:* 775 mg ext-rel

> **Trimox** *Tab:* 125, 250 mg; *Cap:* 250, 500 mg; *Oral susp:* 125, 250 mg/5 ml (80, 100, 150 ml) (raspberry-strawberry)

▷ *azithromycin* (B) <6 months: not recommended; ≥6 months-12 years: 10 mg/kg x 1 dose on day 1; then 5 mg/kg/day on days 2-5; *see page 548 for dose by weight table;* max 500 mg/day; >12 years: 500 mg x 1 dose on day 1, then 250 mg once daily on days 2-5 or 500 mg once daily x 3 days or **Zmax** 2 gm in a single dose

> **Zithromax** *Tab:* 250, 500, 600 mg; *Oral susp:* 100 mg/5 ml (15 ml); 200 mg/5 ml (15, 22.5, 30 ml) (cherry); *Pkt:* 1 gm for reconstitution (cherry-banana)

> **Zithromax Tri-pak** *Tab:* 3 x 500 mg tabs/pck

> **Zithromax Z-pak** *Tab:* 6 x 250 mg tabs/pck

> **Zmax** *Oral susp:* 2 gm ext-rel for reconstitution (cherry-banana) (148 mg Na$^+$)

▷ *cefaclor* (B)(G) <1 month: not recommended; 1 month-12 years: 20-40 mg/kg divided bid or tid x 10 days; *see page 549 for dose by weight table;* max 1 gm/day; >12 years: 375 mg bid x 10 days; max 2 gm/day

> *Tab:* 500 mg; *Cap:* 250, 500 mg; *Susp:* 125 mg/5 ml (75, 150 ml) (strawberry); 187 mg/5 ml (50, 100 ml) (strawberry); 250 mg/5 ml (75, 150 ml) (strawberry); 375 mg/5 ml (50, 100 ml) (strawberry)

> **Cefaclor Extended Release** <16 years: not recommended; ≥16 years: 500 mg bid x 10 days (clinically equivalent to 250 mg immed-rel caps tid); swallow whole; take with food

> > *Tab:* 375, 500 mg ext-rel

▷ *cefadroxil* <12 years: 30 mg/kg/day in 2 divided doses x 10 days; *see page 550 for dose by weight table;* ≥12 years: 1-2 gm in a single or 2 divided doses x 10 days

> **Duricef** *Cap:* 500 mg; *Tab:* 1 g; *Oral susp:* 250 mg/5 ml (100 ml); 500 mg/5 ml (75, 100 ml) (orange-pineapple)

▷ *cefdinir* (B) <6 months: not recommended; 6 months-12 years: 14 mg/kg/day in 1-2 divided doses x 10 days; *see page 551 for dose by weight table;* ≥12 years: 300 mg bid x 10 days or 600 mg daily x 10 days

> **Omnicef** *Cap:* 300 mg; *Oral susp:* 125 mg/5 ml (60, 100 ml) (strawberry)

▷ *cefditoren pivoxil* (B) <12 years: not recommended; ≥12 years: 200 mg bid x 10 days

> **Spectracef** *Tab:* 200 mg

Comment: Contraindicated with milk protein allergy or carnitine deficiency.

▷ *cefpodoxime proxetil* (B) <2 months: not recommended; 2 months-12 years: 10 mg/kg/day (max 400 mg/dose) or 5 mg/kg/day bid (max 200 mg/dose) x 7-14 days; *see page 553 for dose by weight table;* >12 years: 400 mg bid x 7-14 days

▷ *cefprozil* (B) <2 years: not recommended; 2-12 years: 7.5 mg/kg bid x 10 days; *see page 554 for dose by weight table;* >12 years: 250-500 mg bid or 500 mg once daily x 10 days

> **Cefzil** *Tab:* 250, 500 mg; *Oral susp:* 125, 250 mg/5 ml (50, 75, 100 ml) (bubble gum) (phenylalanine)

➤ *ceftriaxone* (B)(G) <12 years: 50-75 mg/kg IM in 1-2 divided doses; max 2 gm/day; ≥12 years: 1-2 gm IM once daily; max 4 gm/day
  Rocephin *Vial:* 250, 500 mg; 1, 2 g
➤ *cefuroxime axetil* (B)(G) <3 months: not recommended; 3 months-12 years: 20-30 mg/kg/day in 2 divided doses x 10 days; *see page* 556 *for dose by weight table;* ≥12 years: 250-500 mg bid x 10 days
  Ceftin *Tab:* 250, 500 mg; *Oral susp:* 125, 250 mg/5 ml (50, 100 ml) (tutti-frutti)
➤ *cephalexin* (B)(G) <12 years: 25-50 mg/kg/day in 4 divided doses x 10 days; *see page* 557 *for dose by weight table;* ≥12 years: 500 mg bid x 10 days
  Keflex *Cap:* 250, 333, 500, 750 mg; *Oral susp:* 125, 250 mg/5 ml (100, 200 ml) (strawberry)
➤ *clarithromycin* (C)(G) <6 months: not recommended; ≥6 months-12 years: 7.5 mg/kg bid x 10 days; *see page* 558 *for dose by weight table;* >12 years: 250-500 mg bid or 500-1000 mg ext-rel once daily x 10 days
  Biaxin *Tab:* 250, 500 mg
  Biaxin Oral Suspension *Oral susp:* 125, 250 mg/5 ml (50, 100 ml) (fruit punch)
  Biaxin XL *Tab:* 500 mg ext-rel
➤ *dicloxacillin* (B) <12 years: 12.5-25 mg/kg/day in 4 divided doses x 10 days; *see page* 560 *for dose by weight table;* >12 years: 500 mg qid x 10 days
  Dynapen *Cap:* 125, 250, 500 mg; *Oral susp:* 62.5 mg/5 ml (80, 100, 200 ml)
➤ *dirithromycin* (C)(G) <12 years: not recommended; ≥12 years: 500 mg once daily x 10 days
  Dynabac *Tab:* 250 mg
➤ *doxycycline* (D)(G) <8 years: not recommended; ≥8 years, ≤100 lb: 1 mg/lb in a single dose once daily x 9 days; ≥8 years, >100 lb: 100 mg bid x 9 days; *see page* 561 *for dose by weight table*
  Acticlate *Tab:* 75, 150**mg
  Adoxa *Tab:* 50, 75, 100, 150 mg ent-coat
  Doryx *Tab:* 50, 75, 100, 150, 200 mg del-rel
  Monodox *Cap:* 50, 75, 100 mg
  Oracea *Cap:* 40 mg del-rel
  Vibramycin *Tab:* 100 mg; *Cap:* 50, 100 mg; *Syr:* 50 mg/5 ml (raspberry-apple) (sulfites); *Oral susp:* 25 mg/5 ml (raspberry)
  Vibra-Tab *Tab:* 100 mg film-coat
  Comment: *doxycycline* is contraindicated <8 years-of-age, in pregnancy, and lactation (discolors developing tooth enamel). A side effect may be photosensitivity (photophobia). Do not take with antacids, calcium supplements, milk or other dairy, or within 2 hours of taking another drug.
➤ *erythromycin base* (B)(G) <45 kg: 30-50 mg in 2-4 divided doses x 10 days; ≥45 kg: 500 mg q 6 hours x 10 days
  Ery-Tab *Tab:* 250, 333, 500 mg ent-coat
  PCE *Tab:* 333, 500 mg
➤ *erythromycin estolate* (B)(G) <12 years: 20-50 mg/kg q 6 hours x 10 days; *see page* 562 *for dose by weight table;* ≥12 years: 250-500 mg q 6 hours x 10 days
  Ilosone *Pulvule:* 250 mg; *Tab:* 500 mg; *Liq:* 125, 250 mg/5 ml (100 ml)
➤ *erythromycin ethylsuccinate* (B)(G) 30-50 mg/kg/day in 4 divided doses x 10 days; may double dose with severe infection; max 100 mg/kg/day or 400 mg qid; *see page* 563 *for dose by weight table*

EryPed *Oral susp:* 200 mg/5 ml (100, 200 ml) (fruit); 400 mg/5 ml (60, 100, 200 ml) (banana); *Oral drops:* 200, 400 mg/5 ml (50 ml) (fruit); *Chew tab:* 200 mg wafer (fruit)

E.E.S. *Oral susp:* 200, 400 mg/5 ml (100 ml) (fruit)

E.E.S. Granules *Oral susp:* 200 mg/5 ml (100, 200 ml) (cherry)

E.E.S. 400 Tablets *Tab:* 400 mg

➤ *gemifloxacin* (C)(G) <18 years: not recommended; ≥18 years: 320 mg once daily x 5-7 days

Factive *Tab:* 320*mg

Comment: *gemifloxacin* is contraindicated <18 years-of-age, and during pregnancy and lactation. Risk of tendonitis o̲r tendon rupture.

➤ *levofloxacin* (C) <18 years: not recommended; ≥18 years: *Uncomplicated:* 500 mg once daily x 7-10 days; *Complicated:* 750 mg once daily x 7-10 days

Levaquin *Tab:* 250, 500, 750 mg; *Oral soln:* 25 mg/ml (480 ml) (benzyl alcohol); *Inj conc:* 25 mg/ml for IV infusion after dilution (20, 30 ml single-use vial) (preservative-free); *Premix soln:* 5 mg/ml for IV infusion (50, 100, 150 ml) (preservative-free)

Comment: *levofloxacin* is contraindicated <18 years-of-age, and during pregnancy and lactation. Risk of tendonitis o̲r tendon rupture.

➤ *linezolid* (C)(G) <5 years: 10 mg/kg q 8 hours x 10-14 days; 5-11 years: 10 mg/kg q 12 hours x 10-14 days; >11 years: 400-600 mg q 12 hours x 10-14 days

Zyvox *Tab:* 400, 600 mg; *Oral susp:* 100 mg/5 ml (150 ml) (orange) (phenylalanine)

Comment: *linezolid* is indicated to treat susceptible vancomycin-resistant *E. faecium* infections.

➤ *loracarbef* (B) <12 years: 15 mg/kg/day in 2 divided doses x 7 days; *see page 570 for dose by weight table;* ≥12 years: 200 mg bid x 7 days

Lorabid *Pulvule:* 200, 400 mg; *Oral susp:* 100 mg/5 ml (50, 100 ml); 200 mg/5 ml (50, 75, 100 ml) (strawberry bubble gum)

➤ *minocycline* (D)(G) <8 years: not recommended; ≥8 years, ≤100 lb: 2 mg/lb on first day in 2 divided doses, followed by 1 mg/lb q 12 hours x 9 more days; ≥8 years, >100 lb: 200 mg on first day; then 100 mg q 12 hours x 9 more days

Dynacin *Cap:* 50, 100 mg

Minocin *Cap:* 50, 75, 100 mg; *Oral susp:* 50 mg/5 ml (60 ml) (custard) (sulfites, alcohol 5%)

Comment: *minocycline* is contraindicated <8 years-of-age, in pregnancy, and lactation (discolors developing tooth enamel). A side effect may be photo-sensitivity (photophobia). Do not give with antacids, calcium supplements, milk o̲r other dairy, o̲r within two hours of taking another drug.

➤ *moxifloxacin* (C)(G) <18 years: not recommended; ≥18 years: 400 mg daily x 10 days

Avelox *Tab:* 400 mg

Comment: *moxifloxacin* is contraindicated <18 years-of-age, and during pregnancy and lactation. Risk of tendonitis o̲r tendon rupture.

➤ *ofloxacin* (C)(G) <18 years: not recommended; ≥18 years: 400 mg bid x 10 days

Floxin *Tab:* 200, 300, 400 mg

Comment: *ofloxacin* is contraindicated <18 years-of-age, and during pregnancy and lactation. Risk of tendonitis o̲r tendon rupture.

▶ *tetracycline* (D)(G) <8 years: not recommended; ≥8 years, ≤100 lb: 25-50 mg/kg/day in 4 divided doses x 10 days; *see page 574 for dose by weight table;* ≥8 years, >100 lb: 500 mg qid x 10 days

    Achromycin V *Cap:* 250, 500 mg

    Sumycin *Tab:* 250, 500 mg; *Cap:* 250, 500 mg; *Oral susp:* 125 mg/5 ml (100, 200 ml) (fruit) (sulfites)

Comment: *tetracycline* is contraindicated <8 years-of-age, in pregnancy, and lactation (discolors developing tooth enamel). A side effect may be photo-sensitivity (photophobia). Do not give with antacids, calcium supplements, milk <u>or</u> other dairy, <u>or</u> within two hours of taking another drug.

SLEEP APNEA (HYPOPNEA SYNDROME)

ANTINARCOLEPTIC AGENTS

▶ *armodafinil* (C)(IV)(G) <17 years: not recommended; ≥17 years: *OSAHS:* 150-250 mg once daily in the AM; *SWSD:* 150 mg 1 hour before starting shift; reduce dose with severe hepatic impairment

    Nuvigil *Tab:* 50, 150, 200, 250 mg

▶ *modafinil* (C)(IV) <16 years: not recommended; ≥16 years: 100-200 mg q AM; max 400 mg/day

    Provigil *Tab:* 100, 200*mg

Comment: *modafinil* promotes wakefulness in patients with excessive sleepiness due to obstructive sleep apnea/hypopnea syndrome.

SLEEPINESS: EXCESSIVE/SHIFT WORK SLEEP DISORDER (SWSD)

ANTINARCOLEPTIC AGENT

▶ *armodafinil* (C)(IV)(G) <17 years: not recommended; ≥17 years: *OSAHS:* 150-250 mg once daily in the AM; *SWSD:* 150 mg 1 hour before starting shift; reduce dose with severe hepatic impairment

    Nuvigil *Tab:* 50, 150, 200, 250 mg

▶ *modafinil* (C)(IV) <16 years: not recommended; ≥16 years: 100-200 mg q AM; max 400 mg/day

    Provigil *Tab:* 100, 200*mg

Comment: **Provigil** promotes wakefulness in patients with narcolepsy, shift work sleep disorder, and excessive sleepiness due to obstructive sleep apnea/hypopnea syndrome.

SMALLPOX (VARIOLA MAJOR)

PROPHYLAXIS

▶ *vaccinia virus* vaccine *(dried, calf lymph type)* (C) <12 months: not recommended; 12 months-18 years, non-emergency: not recommended

    DRYvax

Kit: vial dried smallpox vaccine (1), 0.25 ml diluent in syringe (1), vented needle (1), 100 individually wrapped bifurcated needles (5 needles/strip, 20 strips) (polymyxin B sulfate, dihydrostreptomycin sulfate, chlortetracycline HCL, neomycin sulfate, glycerin, phenol)

Comment: DRYvax is a dried live vaccine with approximately 100 million *Infectious vaccinia* viruses (pock-forming units [pfu] per ml). Contact with immunosuppressed individuals should be avoided until the scab has separated from the skin (2 to 3 weeks) <u>and/or</u> a protective occlusive dressing covers the inoculation site. Scarification only. Do not inject IV, IM, <u>or</u> SC. Revaccination is recommended every 10 years.

☐ SPRAIN

Comment: RICE: Rest; Ice; Compression; Elevation.
Oral Prescription NSAIDs *see page* 490
Other Oral Analgesics *see Pain page* 298
Topical/Transdermal NSAIDs *see Pain page* 298
Parenteral Corticosteroids *see page* 499
Oral Corticosteroids *see page* 498
Topical Analgesic and Anesthetic Agents *see page* 488

☐ STATUS ASTHMATICUS

Inhaled Beta2-Agonists (Bronchodilators) *see Asthma page* 391
Oral Beta2-Agonists (Bronchodilators) *see Asthma page* 33
Inhaled Anticholinergics *see Asthma page* 27
Inhaled Anticholinergic/Beta2-Agonist Combination *see Asthma page* 31
Methylxanthines *see Asthma page* 33
Parenteral Corticosteroids *see page* 499
Oral Corticosteroids *see page* 498

EPINEPHRINE

▷ *epinephrine* (C)(G) Use 1:1000 solution; may repeat q 20-30 minutes as needed up to 3 doses; <2 years: 0.05-0.1 ml SC; 2-<6 years: 0.1 ml SC; 6-<12 years: 0.2 ml ≥12 years: 0.3-0.5 mg SC

ANAPHYLAXIS EMERGENCY TREATMENT KITS

▷ *epinephrine* (C) 0.01 mg/kg SC <u>or</u> IM in thigh; may repeat if needed; <15 kg: not recommended; 15-30 kg: 0.15 mg; ≥30 kg: 0.3 ml IM <u>or</u> SC in thigh; may repeat if needed

AdrenaClick *Autoinjector:* 0.15, 0.3 mg (1 mg/ml; 2/carton) (sulfites)
Auvi-Q *Autoinjector:* 0.15, 0.3 mg (1 mg/ml; 2/carton w. 1 non-active training device) (sulfites)
EpiPen *Autoinjector:* 0.3 mg (*epi* 1:1000, 0.3 ml (2/carton) (sulfites)
Epi-E-Zpen *Autoinjector:* 0.15 mg (*epi* 1:2000, 0.3 ml (2/carton) (sulfites)

Twinject *Autoinjector:* 0.15, 0.3 mg (*epi* 1:1000, 2/carton) (sulfites)
▶ *epinephrine/chlorpheniramine* (C) infants-2 years: 0.05-0.1 ml SC <u>or</u> IM; 2-<6 years: 0.15 ml SC <u>or</u> IM <u>plus</u> 1 PO tab *chlorpheniramine*; 6-<12 years: 0.2 ml SC <u>or</u> IM <u>plus</u> 2 chewable *chlorpheniramine* tabs; ≥12 years: *epinephrine* 0.3 ml SC <u>or</u> IM <u>plus</u> 4 chewable *chlorpheniramine* tabs
   Ana-Kit: 0.3 ml syringes of *epi* 1:1000 (2/carton) for self-injection <u>plus</u> 4 *chlor* 2 mg chew tabs

STATUS EPILEPTICUS

Anticonvulsant Drugs *see page* 113
▶ *diazepam* injectable **(D)(IV)** <1 months: see mfr pkg insert; 1 month-5 years: 0.2-0.5 mg IV q 2-5 minutes; max 5 mg; >5-<12 years: 1 mg IV q 2-5 minutes; max 10 mg; may repeat in 2-4 hours if needed; ≥12 years: initially 5-10 mg IV in large vein; may repeat q 10-15 minutes; max 30 mg; may repeat in 2-4 hours if needed; do not dilute; may administer IM if IV not accessible
   Diastat *Rectal gel delivery system:* 2.5 mg
   Diastat AcuDial *Rectal gel delivery system:* 10, 20 mg
   Valium Injectable *Vial:* 5 mg/ml (10 ml); *Amp:* 5 mg/ml (2 ml); *Prefilled syringe:* 5 mg/ml (5 ml)
   Valium Intensol Oral Solution *Conc oral soln:* 5 mg/ml (30 ml w. dropper) (alcohol 19%)
   Valium Oral Solution *Oral soln:* 5 mg/5 ml (500 ml) (wintergreen spice)
▶ *lorazepam* injectable **(D)(IV)** <18 years: not recommended; ≥18 years: administer 4 mg IV over 2 minutes (dilute first); may repeat in 10-15 minutes; may give IM if needed (undiluted)
   Ativan Injectable *Vial:* 2 mg/ml (1, 10 ml); *Tubex:* 2 mg/ml (0.5 ml); *Cartridge:* 2, 4 mg/ml (1 ml)
▶ *phenytoin (injectable)* **(D)(G)** <12 years: 15-20 mg/kg IV, not to exceed 1-2 mg/kg/minute; ≥12 years: 10-15 mg/kg IV, not to exceed 50 mg/minute; follow with 100 mg orally <u>or</u> IV q 6-8 hours; do not dilute in IV fluid
   Dilantin *Vial:* 50 mg/ml (2, 5 ml); *Amp:* 50 mg/ml (2 ml)
Comment: Monitor *phenytoin* serum levels. Therapeutic serum level: 10-20 gm/ml. Side effects include gingival hyperplasia.

STYE (HORDEOLUM)

OPHTHALMIC ANTI-INFECTIVES

▶ *erythromycin* **ophthalmic ointment (B)** 1 cm up to 6 times/day
   Ilotycin Ophthalmic Ointment *Ophth oint:* 5 mg/g (1/8 oz)
▶ *erythromycin* ophthalmic solution **(B)** initially 1-2 drops q 1-2 hours; may then increase dose interval
   Isopto Cetamide Ophthalmic Solution *Ophth soln:* 15% (15 ml)
▶ *gentamicin* ophthalmic solution **(C)** 1 cm bid-tid
   Garamycin Ophthalmic Ointment *Ophth oint:* 3 mg/g (3.5 gm)
   Genoptic Ophthalmic Ointment *Ophth oint:* 3 mg/g (3.5 gm)
   Gentacidin Ophthalmic Ointment *Ophth oint:* 3 mg/g (3.5 gm)

➤ *polymyxin B/bacitracin* ophthalmic ointment (C) apply 1/2 inch q 3-4 hours
  Polysporin *Ophth oint: poly* 10,000 U/*bac* 500 units per gm (3.75 gm)
➤ *polymyxin B/bacitracin/neomycin* ophthalmic ointment (C)(G) apply 1/2 inch q
  3-4 hours
  Neosporin Ophthalmic Ointment *Ophth oint: poly* B 10,000 U/*bac* 400 U/*neo*
  3.5 mg/g (3.75 gm)
➤ *polymyxin B/neomycin/gramicidin* ophthalmic solution (C) 1-2 drops 2-3 times q
  1 hour; then 1-2 drops bid-qid x 7-10 days
  Neosporin Ophthalmic Solution
  Ophth soln: poly 10,000 U/*neo* 1.75 mg/*gram* 0.025 mg/ml (10 ml)
➤ *sodium sulfacetamide* ophthalmic solution and ointment (C)
  Bleph-10 Ophthalmic Solution <2 years: not recommended; ≥2-<12 years: 1-2
  drops q 2-3 hours during the day; ≥12 years: 2 drops q 4 hour x 7-14 days
  Ophth soln: 10% (2.5, 5, 15 ml) (benzalkonium chloride)
  Bleph-10 Ophthalmic Ointment <2 years: not recommended; ≥2-<12 years:
  apply 1/4-1/3 inch qid and HS; ≥12 years: apply 1/2 inch qid and HS
  Ophth oint: 10% (3.5 gm) (phenylmercuric acetate)

SUNBURN

➤ *prednisone* (C)(G) 10 mg qid x 4-6 days if severe and extensive
➤ *silver sulfadiazine* (B)(G) <12 years: not established; ≥12 years: apply bid
  Silvadene *Crm:* 1% (20 gm tube; 20, 50, 85, 400, 1,000 gm jar)
  Comment: *silver sulfadiazine* is contradicted in sulfa allergy, late pregnancy,
  within the first 2 months after birth, premature infants.

SYPHILIS (*TREPONEMA PALLIDUM*)

Comment: The following treatment regimens for *T. pallidum* are published in the **2015
CDC Sexually Transmitted Diseases Treatment Guidelines**. Treat all sexual contacts.
Consider testing for other STDs. *Penicillin G*, administered parenterally, is the
preferred drug for treating all stages of syphilis. The preparation used (i.e., benzathine,
aqueous procaine, or aqueous crystalline), the dosage, and the length of treatment
depend on the stage and clinical manifestations of the disease. Combinations of
benzathine penicillin, procaine penicillin, and oral penicillin preparations are not
appropriate (e.g., **Bicillin C-R**). Screen serologically for syphilis early in pregnancy.
There are no proven alternatives to penicillin for the treatment of syphilis during
pregnancy. Pregnant patients who are allergic to penicillin should be desensitized
and treated with *penicillin*. Sexual transmission of *T. pallidum* is thought to occur
only when mucocutaneous syphilis at any stage should be evaluated clinically and
serologically and treated with a recommended regimen according to CDC guidelines.

PRIMARY, SECONDARY, AND EARLY LATENT SYPHILIS, <1 YEAR DURATION, ≥12 YEARS-OF-AGE

Regimen 1

➤ *penicillin g (benzathine)* 2.4 million units IM in a single dose

LATE LATENT, LATENT SYPHILIS OF UNKNOWN DURATION, AND TERTIARY SYPHILIS, ≥12 YEARS-OF-AGE

Regimen 1

▷ *penicillin g (benzathine)* 2.4 million units IM in a single dose; 7.2 million units total administered in 3 divided doses of 2.4 million units each IM at 1 week intervals

REGIMEN: NEUROSYPHILIS, ≥12 YEARS-OF-AGE

Regimen 1

▷ *aqueous crystalline penicillin g* 2.4 million units IM in a single dose 18-24 million units per day, administered as 3-4 million units IV every 4 hours <u>or</u> continuous IV infusion, for 10-14 days

ALTERNATIVE REGIMEN: NEUROSYPHILIS, ≥12 YEARS-OF-AGE

Regimen 1

▷ *penicillin g (procaine)* 2.4 million units IM once daily x 10-14 days <u>plus</u> *probenecid* 500 mg qid x 10-14 days

PRIMARY AND SECONDARY SYPHILIS IN HIV-INFECTED PERSONS

Regimen 1

▷ *penicillin g (benzathine)* 2.4 million units IM in a single dose

LATENT SYPHILIS AMONG HIV-INFECTED PERSONS ≥12 YEARS-OF-AGE

Comment: Treatment is the same as for HIV-negative persons.

CONGENITAL SYPHILIS, ≥12 YEARS-OF-AGE

Regimen 1

▷ *aqueous crystalline penicillin g* 100,000-150,000 units/kg/day, administered as 50,000 units IV every 12 hours during the first 7 days of life and every 8 hours thereafter for a total of 10 days

ALTERNATE REGIMENS, ≥12 YEARS-OF-AGE

Regimen 1

▷ *penicillin g (benzathine)* 50,000 units/kg IM in a single dose

Regimen 2

▷ *penicillin g (procaine)* 50,000 units/kg/dose IM, administered in a single daily dose x 10 days

INFANTS AND CHILDREN <12 YEARS-OF-AGE

Regimen 1

▷ *aqueous crystalline penicillin g* 200,000-300,000 units/kg/day, administered as 50,000 units IV every 12 hours during the first 7 days of life and every 4-6 hours thereafter for a total of 10 days

DRUG BRANDS AND DOSE FORMS

➢ *aqueous crystalline penicillin g* (B)(G)
➢ *penicillin g (benzathine)* (B)(G)
  Bicillin L-A *Cartridge-needle unit:* 600,000 million units (1 ml); 1.2 million units (2 ml); 2.4 million units (4 ml)
➢ *penicillin g (procaine)* (B)(G)
  Bicillin C-R Cartridge-needle unit: 600,000 units (1 ml); 1.2 million units; (2 ml); 2.4 million units (4 ml)
➢ *probenecid* (B)(G)
  Benemid *Tab:* 500*mg; *Cap:* 500 mg

TAPEWORM (CESTODE)

ANTHELMINTICS

Comment: Oral bioavailability of anthelmintics is enhanced when administered with a fatty meal (estimated fat content 40 g).
➢ *albendazole* (C) take with a meal; may crush and mix with food; may repeat in 3 weeks if needed; <2 years: 200 mg bid x 7 days; 2-12 years: 400 mg once daily x 7 days; >12 years: 400 mg bid x 7 days;
  Albenza *Tab:* 200 mg
  Comment: *albendazole* is a broad-spectrum benzimidazole carbamate anthelmintic.
➢ *praziquantel* (B) take with a meal; may crush and mix with food; <4 years: not established; ≥4 years: 5-10 mg/kg as a single dose
  Biltricide *Tab:* 600**mg film-coat (cross-scored for half or quarter dose)
  Comment: Therapeutically effective levels of Biltricide may not be achieved when administered concomitantly with strong P450 inducers, such as rifampin. Females should not breastfeed on the day of Biltricide treatment and during the subsequent 72 hours. Use caution with hepatosplenic patients who have moderate to severe liver impairment (Child-Pugh class B and C).
➢ *nitazoxanide* (B) take with a meal; may crush and mix with food; <12 months: not recommended; ≥12 months: treat q 12 hours x 3 days; <11 years: [use suspension]; 12-47 months: 5 ml; 4-11 years: 10 ml; >11 years: [use tab or suspension] 500 mg
  Alinia *Tab:* 500 mg; *Oral susp:* 100 mg/5 ml (60 ml)

TARDIVE DYSKINESIA

Comment: Tardive dyskinesia is a treatable, albeit irreversible, neurological disorder characterized by repetitive involuntary movements, usually of the jaw, lips and tongue, such as grimacing, sticking out the tongue and smacking the lips. Some affected people also experience involuntary movement of the extremities or difficulty breathing. This condition is most often an adverse side effect associated with the older "typical" antipsychotic drugs. Risk is decreased with the newer "atypical" antipsychotic drugs.

VESICULAR MONOAMINE TRANSPORTER 2 (VMAT2) INHIBITOR

➢ *valbenazine* (NE) <18 years: not established; ≥18 years: initially 40 mg once daily; after one week, increase to the recommended 80 mg once daily; take with or without food; recommended dose for patients with moderate or severe hepatic impairment is 40 mg once daily; consider dose reduction based on tolerability in known CYP2D6 poor metabolizers; concomitant use of strong CYP3A4 inducers is not recommended; avoid concomitant use of MAOIs

    Ingrezza *Cap:* 40 mg

Comment: Safety and effectiveness of **Ingrezza** have not been established in pediatric patients. No dose adjustment is required for elderly patients. The limited available data on **Ingrezza** use in pregnant women are insufficient to inform a drug-associated risk. There is no information regarding the presence of **Ingrezza** or its metabolites in human milk, the effects on the breastfed infant, or the effects on milk production. However, women are advised not to breastfeed during treatment and for 5 days after the final dose. To report suspected adverse reactions, contact Neurocrine Biosciences, Inc. at 877-641-3461 or FDA at 1-800-FDA-1088 or www.fda.gov/medwatch.

TEMPOROMANDIBULAR JOINT (TMJ) DISORDER

Oral Prescription NSAIDs *see page* 490
Other Oral Analgesics see *Pain page* 298
Topical/Transdermal NSAIDs *see Pain page* 298
Parenteral Corticosteroids *see page* 499
Oral Corticosteroids *see page* 498
Topical Analgesic and Anesthetic Agents *see page* 488

TESTOSTERONE DEFICIENCY, HYPOTESTOSTERONEMIA, HYPOGONADISM

Comment: *testosterone* is contraindicated in male breast cancer and prostate cancer. *Testosterone* replacement therapy is indicated in males with primary hypogonadism (congenital or acquired due to cryptorchidism, bilateral torsion, orchitis, vanishing testis syndrome, or orchidectomy), or hypogonadotropic hypogonadism (congenital or acquired), and delayed puberty not secondary to a pathological disorder (x-ray of the hand and wrist to determine bone age should be obtained every 6 months to assess the effect of treatment on the epiphyseal centers).

ORAL ANDROGENS

▷ *fluoxymesterone* (X)(III) *Hypogonadism:* <12 years: use by specialist only; *Puberty:* 5-20 mg once daily; *Delayed puberty:* use low dose and limit duration to 4-6 months

    Halotestin *Tab:* 2*, 5*, 10*mg (tartrazine)

▷ *methyltestosterone* (X)(III) *Hypogonadism:* <12 years: use by specialist only; *Puberty:* usually 10-50 mg once daily; *Delayed puberty:* use low dose and limit duration to 4-6 months

    Android *Cap:* 10 mg
    Methitest *Tab:* 10*mg
    Testred *Cap:* 10 mg

➢ **testosterone (X)(III)** <18 years: not recommended; ≥18 years: 30 mg q 12 hours to gum region, just above the incisor tooth on either side of the mouth; hold system in place for 30 seconds; rotate sites with each application

    Striant *Buccal tab:* 30 mg (6 blister pcks; 10 buccal systems/blister pck)

    Comment: Serum total ***testosterone*** concentrations may be checked 4 to 12 weeks after initiating treatment with **Striant**. To capture the maximum serum concentration, an early morning sample (just prior to applying the AM dose) is recommended.

TOPICAL ANDROGENS

Comment: Topical androgens are not recommended under 18 years-of-age. Wash hands after application. Allow solution to dry before it touches clothing. Do not wash site for at least 2 hours after application. Pregnant and nursing females, and children, must avoid skin contact with application sites. If there is contact, wash the area as soon as possible with soap and water.

➢ **testosterone (X)(III)**

    AndroGel 1% <18 years: not recommended; ≥18 years: initially apply 5 gm once daily in the AM to clean, dry, intact skin of the shoulders, upper arms, <u>and/or</u> abdomen; do not apply to scrotum; may increase to 7.5 gm/day and then to 10 gm/day if needed

    Gel: 2.5, 5 gm (30 pkts); 75 gm (60 metered 1.25 gm doses)

    AndroGel 1.62% <18 years: not recommended; ≥18 years: initially apply 2.5 gm (2 pump actuations) once daily in the AM to clean, dry, skin of the shoulders and upper arms intact skin of the upper arms; do not apply to abdomen <u>or</u> genitals; may adjust dose between 1 and 4 pump actuations based on the predose morning serum testosterone concentration at approximately 14 and 28 days after starting treatment <u>or</u> adjusting dose

    Gel: 2.25 mg pump actuation (75 g, 60 metered 1.25 gm doses)

    Axiron <18 years: not recommended; ≥18 years: apply to clean dry intact skin of the axillae; do not apply to the scrotum, penis, abdomen, shoulders, <u>or</u> upper arms; initially apply 60 mg (30 mg/axilla) once daily in the AM; adjust dose based on serum testosterone concentration 2 to 8 hours after applying and at least 14 days after starting therapy <u>or</u> following dose adjustment; may increase dose in 30 mg increments if serum testosterone <300 ng/dL up to 120 mg; reduce dose to 30 mg if levels >1050 ng/dL; discontinue if serum testosterone remains at >1050 ng/dL

    Soln: 30 mg/1.5 ml pump actuation (90 ml; 60 metered actuations) (alcohol, latex-free)

    Fortesta (G) <18 years: not recommended; ≥18 years: initially 40 mg of testosterone (4 pump actuations) applied to the thighs once daily in the AM; may adjust between 10 mg minimum and 70 mg maximum.

    Gel: 10 mg/0.5 gm pump actuation (120 actuations)

    Comment: The **Fortesta** dose should be based on the serum ***testosterone*** concentration 2 hours after applying **Fortesta** and at approximately 14 days and 35 days after starting treatment <u>or</u> following dose adjustment. Dose adjustment criteria: ≤500 ng/dL, increase daily dose by 10 mg; 500-≤1250 ng/dL, no change; 1250-≤2500 ng/dL, decrease daily dose by 10 mg; ≥2500 ng/dL, decrease daily dose by 20 mg.

Gel: 10 mg (0.5 gm)/pump actuation (60 g; 120 metered dose actuations) (ethanol)

Testim (G) <18 years: not recommended; ≥18 years: initially apply 5 gm once daily in the AM to clean, dry, intact skin of the shoulders <u>and/or</u> upper arms; do not apply to the genitals <u>or</u> abdomen; may increase to 10 gm after 2 weeks

Gel: 1%, clear, hydroalcoholic (5 mg/5 g, 5 gm single-use tube)

Vogelxo Gel (G) <18 years: not recommended; ≥18 years: 1% initially apply 5 gm once daily in the AM to clean, dry, intact skin of the shoulders, upper arms, <u>and/or</u> abdomen; do not apply to scrotum; may increase to 7.5 gm/day and then to 10 gm/day if needed

Gel: 5 gm/pkt (30 pkts); 5 gm/tube (30 tubes); metered dose actuations (2 x 75 g, 1.25 gm actuation)

INTRANASAL ANDROGENS

➤ *testosterone (nasal gel)* **(X)(III)** <18 years: not established; ≥18 years: initially one pump actuation each nostril (33 mg) 3 x/day, at least 6-8 hours apart, at the same times each day max: 6 pump actuations/day

NatSteel: 5.5 mg/actuation, metered dose pump (11 g, 60 actuations)

TRANSDERMAL ANDROGEN

➤ *testosterone* **(X)(III)**

Androderm <15 years: not recommended; ≥15 years: initially apply 4 mg nightly at approximately 10 PM to clean, dry area of the arm, back, <u>or</u> upper buttocks; leave on x 24 hours; may increase to 7.5 mg <u>or</u> decrease to 2.5 mg based on confirmed AM serum testosterone concentrations

Transdermal patch: 2, 4 mg/24 hr

TETANUS (*CLOSTRIDIUM TETANI*)

PROPHYLAXIS

See **Childhood Immunizations** page 473

POSTEXPOSURE PROPHYLAXIS IN PREVIOUSLY NON-IMMUNIZED PERSONS

➤ *tetanus immune globulin, human* **(C)** <7 years: not recommended; ≥7 years: 250 mg deep IM in a single dose

BayTET, HyperTET *Vial:* 250 unit single dose; *Prefilled syringe:* 250 units

➤ *tetanus toxoid* **vaccine (C)** 0.5 ml IM x 3 dose series

Vial: 5 Lf units/0.5 ml (0.5, 5 ml); *Prefilled syringe:* 5 Lf units/0.5 ml (0.5 ml)

Comment: Dose of **BayTET/HyperTET** S/D is calculated as 4 units/kg. However, it may be advisable to administer the entire contents of the syringe of **BayTET/HyperTET** S/D (250 units) regardless of the child's size, since theoretically the same amount of toxin will be produced in the child's body by the infecting tetanus organism as it will in an adult's body. At the same time but in a different extremity and with a different syringe, administer Diphtheria and Tetanus Toxoids and Pertussis Vaccine Adsorbed (DTP) or Diphtheria and Tetanus Toxoids Adsorbed (For Pediatric Use) (DT), if pertussis vaccine is contraindicated, should be administered per mfr pkg insert. Tetanus immune globulin may interact with live viral vaccines such as measles, mumps, rubella, and polio. It is also unknown if **BayTET/HyperTET** can cause fetal harm when administered to a pregnant female <u>or</u> can affect reproduction capacity. The single injection of tetanus toxoid only initiates the series for producing active immunity in the recipient. The patient will need further toxoid injections in 1 month and 1 year; otherwise the active immunization series is incomplete. If a contraindication to using tetanus toxoid-containing preparations exists for a person who has not completed a primary series of tetanus toxoid immunization, and that person has a wound that is neither clean nor minor, only passive immunization should be administered using tetanus immune globulin.

THREADWORM (*STRONGYLOIDIDES STERCORALIS*)

ANTHELMINTICS

Comment: Oral bioavailability of anthelmintics is enhanced when administered with a fatty meal (estimated fat content 40 g).

➤ *albendazole* (C) take with a meal; chew or crush and mix with food; may repeat in 3 weeks if needed; <2 years: 200 mg bid x 7 days; >2 years: 400 mg bid x 7 days
   Albenza *Tab:* 200 mg

➤ *ivermectin* (C) take with water; chew <u>or</u> crush and mix with food; may repeat in 3 months if needed; <15 kg: not recommended; ≥15 kg: 200 mcg/kg as a single dose
   Stromectol *Tab:* 3, 6*mg

➤ *mebendazole* (C) take with a meal; chew <u>or</u> crush and mix with food; may repeat in 3 weeks if needed; <2 years: not recommended; ≥2 years: 100 mg bid x 3 days
   Emverm *Chew tab:* 100 mg
   Vermox (G) *Chew tab:* 100 mg

➤ *pyrantel pamoate* (C) take with a meal; may open capsule and sprinkle <u>or</u> mix with food; treat x 3 days; may repeat in 2-3 weeks if needed; treat x 3 days; 11 mg/kg/dose; max 1 gm/dose; <25 lb: not recommended; 25-37 lb: 1/2 tsp/dose; 38-62 lb: 1 tsp/dose; 63-87 lb: 1 tsp/dose; 88-112 lb: 2 tsp/dose; 113-137 lb: 2 tsp/dose; 138-162 lb: 3 tsp/dose; 163-187 lb: 3 tsp/dose; >187 lb: 4 tsp/dose
   Antiminth *Cap:* 180 mg; *Liq:* 50 mg/ml (30 ml); 144 mg/ml (30 ml); *Oral susp:* 50 mg/ml (60 ml)
   Pin-X *Cap:* 180 mg; *Liq:* 50 mg/ml (30 ml); 144 mg/ml (30 ml); *Oral susp:* 50 mg/ml (30 ml)

➤ *thiabendazole* (C) take with a meal; may crush and mix with food; treat x 7 days; <30 lb: consult mfr pkg insert; ≥30 lb: 25 mg/kg/dose bid with meals; 30-50 lb: 250 mg bid with meals; >50 lb: 10 mg/lb/dose bid with meals; max 1.5 gm/dose; max 3 g/day
   Mintezol *Chew tab:* 500*mg (orange); *Oral susp:* 500 mg/5 ml (120 ml) (orange)

Comment: *thiabendazole* is not for prophylaxis. May impair mental alertness. May not be available in the US.

TINEA CAPITIS

Comment: Tinea capitis must be treated with an oral antifungal.

FOR SEVERE KERION PRURITUS

➤ *prednisone* (C) 1 mg/kg/day for 7-14 days
   See **Oral Corticosteroids** page 498

SYSTEMIC ANTIFUNGALS

➤ *griseofulvin, microsize* (C)(G) <12 years: <30 lb: 5 mg/lb/day; 30-50 lb: 125-250 mg/day; >50 lb: 250-500 mg/day; 5 mg/lb/day x 4-6 weeks <u>or</u> longer; *see page 568 for dose by weight table*; >12 years: 500 mg once daily x 4-6 weeks <u>or</u> longer; max 1 gm/day

    Grifulvin V *Tab:* 250, 500 mg; *Oral susp:* 125 mg/5 ml (120 ml; alcohol 0.02%)

➤ *griseofulvin, ultramicrosize* (C)(G) <2 years: not recommended; 2-12 years: 3.3 mg/lb/day in a single <u>or</u> divided doses x 4-6 weeks <u>or</u> longer; >12 years: 375 mg/day in a single <u>or</u> divided doses x 4-6 weeks <u>or</u> longer

    Gris-PEG *Tab:* 125, 250 mg

    Comment: *griseofulvin* should be taken with fatty foods (e.g., milk, ice cream). Liver enzymes should be monitored.

➤ *ketoconazole* (C)(G) <2 years: not recommended; ≥2 years-12 years: 3.3-6.6 mg/kg once daily x 4 weeks; >12 years: initially 200 mg once daily; max 400 mg/day x 4 weeks

    Nizoral *Tab:* 200 mg

    Comment: Caution with *ketoconazole* due to potential for hepatotoxicity.

TINEA CORPORIS (RINGWORM)

TOPICAL ANTI-FUNGALS

➤ *butenafine* (C)(G) <12 years: not recommended; ≥12 years: apply bid x 1 week <u>or</u> once daily x 4 weeks

    Lotrimin Ultra (OTC) *Crm:* 1% (12, 24 gm)

    Mentax *Crm:* 1% (15, 30 gm)

    Comment: *butenafine* is a benzylamine, not an azole. Fungicidal activity continues for at least 5 weeks after last application.

➤ *ciclopirox* (B)

    Loprox Cream <10 years: not recommended; ≥10 years: apply bid; max 4 weeks
        Crm: 0.77% (15, 30, 90 gm)

    Loprox Lotion <10 years: not recommended; ≥10 years: apply bid; max 4 weeks
        Lotn: 0.77% (30, 60 ml)

    Loprox Gel <16 years: not recommended; ≥16 years: apply bid; max 4 weeks
        Gel: 0.77% (30, 45 gm)

➤ *clotrimazole* (B)(G) apply to affected area bid x 14 days

    Lotrimin *Crm:* 1% (15, 30, 45 gm)

    Lotrimin AF (OTC) *Crm:* 1% (12 gm); *Lotn:* 1% (10 ml); *Soln:* 1% (10 ml)

➤ *econazole* (C) apply once daily x 14 days

    Spectazole *Crm:* 1% (15, 30, 85 gm)

➤ *ketoconazole* (C) apply to affected area bid x 14 days

    Nizoral Cream *Crm:* 2% (15, 30, 60 gm)

➤ *luliconazole* (C) <18 years: not recommended; ≥18 years: apply to affected area and 1 inch into the immediate surrounding area(s) once daily

    Luzu Cream 1% *Crm:* 1% (30, 60 gm)

➤ *miconazole 2%* (C) <12 years: not recommended; ≥12 years: apply qd-bid x 2 weeks

    Lotrimin AF Spray Liquid (OTC) *Spray liq:* 2% (113 gm) (alcohol 17%)

    Lotrimin AF Spray Powder (OTC) *Spray pwdr:* 2% (90 gm) (alcohol 10%)

    Monistat-Derm *Crm:* 2% (1, 3 oz); *Spray liq:* 2% (3.5 oz); *Spray pwdr:* 2% (3 oz)

▷ *naftifine* (B)(G)
  Naftin Cream <12 years: not recommended; ≥12 years: apply once daily x 14 days
    Crm: 1% (15, 30, 60 gm)
  Naftin Gel apply <12 years: not recommended; ≥12 years: bid x 14 days
    Gel: 1% (20, 40, 60 gm)
▷ *oxiconazole nitrate* (B)(G) <12 years: not recommended; ≥12 years: apply qd-bid x
  2 weeks
  Oxistat *Crm:* 1% (15, 30, 60 gm); *Lotn:* 1% (30 ml)
▷ *sulconazole* (C) <12 years: not recommended; ≥12 years: apply qd-bid x 3 weeks
  Exelderm *Crm:* 1% (15, 30, 60 gm); *Lotn:* 1% (30 mg)
▷ *terbinafine* (B)(G)
  Lamisil Cream (OTC) <12 years: not recommended; ≥12 years: apply to
  affected and surrounding area qd-bid x 1-4 weeks until significantly improved
    Crm: 1% (15, 30 gm)
  Lamisil AT Cream (OTC) apply to affected and surrounding area qd-bid x 1-4
  weeks until significantly improved
    Crm: **1% (15, 30 gm)**
  Lamisil Solution (OTC) <12 years: not recommended; ≥12 years: apply to
  affected and surrounding area once daily x 1 week
    Soln: 1% (30 ml spray bottle)

TOPICAL ANTIFUNGAL/STEROID COMBINATION

▷ *clotrimazole/betamethasone* (C)(G) <12 years: not recommended; ≥12 years: apply
  bid x 2 weeks; max 4 weeks
  Lotrisone *Crm:* *clotrim* 1 mg/*beta* 0.5 mg (15, 45 gm); *Lotn:* *clotrim* 1 mg/*beta*
  0.5 mg (30 ml)

SYSTEMIC ANTIFUNGALS

▷ *griseofulvin, microsize* (C)(G) <12 years: <30 lb: 5 mg/lb/day; 30-50 lb: 125-250 mg/
  day; >50 lb: 250-500 mg/day; 5 mg/lb/day x 4-6 weeks or longer; *see page 568 for dose
  by weight table;* ≥12 years: 500 mg once daily x 4-6 weeks or longer; max 1 gm/day
    Grifulvin V *Tab:* 250, 500 mg; *Oral susp:* 125 mg/5 ml (120 ml; alcohol 0.02%)
▷ *griseofulvin, ultramicrosize* (C)(G) <2 years: not recommended; 2-12 years: 3.3 mg/
  lb/day in a single or divided doses x 4-6 weeks or longer; >12 years: 375 mg/day in a
  single or divided doses x 4-6 weeks or longer
    Gris-PEG *Tab:* 125, 250 mg
  Comment: *griseofulvin* should be taken with fatty foods (e.g., milk, ice cream).
  Liver enzymes should be monitored.
▷ *ketoconazole* (C)(G) <2 years: not recommended; ≥2 years-12 years: 3.3-6.6 mg/kg
  once daily x 4 weeks; >12 years: initially 200 mg once daily; max 400 mg/day x 4 weeks
    Nizoral *Tab:* 200 mg
  Comment: Caution with *ketoconazole* due to potential for hepatotoxicity.

TINEA CRURIS (JOCK ITCH)

TOPICAL ANTIFUNGALS

▷ *butenafine* (B)(G) <12 years: not recommended; ≥12 years: apply bid x 1 week or
  once daily x 4 weeks

>> **Lotrimin Ultra (C)(OTC)** *Crm:* 1% (12, 24 gm)
>> **Mentax** *Crm:* 1% (15, 30 gm)
>
> **Comment:** *butenafine* is a benzylamine, not an azole. Fungicidal activity continues for at least 5 weeks after last application.

▷ *ciclopirox* (B)
>> **Loprox Cream** <10 years: not recommended; ≥10 years: apply bid; max 4 weeks
>>> *Crm:* 0.77% (15, 30, 90 gm)
>> **Loprox Lotion** <10 years: not recommended; ≥10 years: apply bid; max 4 weeks
>>> *Lotn:* 0.77% (30, 60 ml)
>> **Loprox Gel** <16 years: not recommended; ≥16 years: apply bid; max 4 weeks
>>> *Gel:* 0.77% (30, 45 gm)

▷ *clotrimazole* (B)(G) apply to affected area bid x 7 days
>> **Lotrimin** *Crm:* 1% (15, 30, 45 gm)
>> **Lotrimin AF (OTC)** *Crm:* 1% (12 gm); *Lotn:* 1% (10 ml); *Soln:* 1% (10 ml)

▷ *econazole* (C) apply once daily x 2 weeks
>> **Spectazole** *Crm:* 1% (15, 30, 85 gm)

▷ *ketoconazole* (C) apply to affected area bid x 2 weeks
>> **Nizoral Cream** *Crm:* 2% (15, 30, 60 gm)

▷ *luliconazole* (C) <18 years: not recommended; ≥18 years: apply to affected area and 1 inch into the immediate surrounding area(s) once daily
>> **Luzu Cream** 1% *Crm:* 1% (30, 60 gm)

▷ *miconazole 2%* (C)(G) apply qd-bid x 2 weeks
>> **Lotrimin AF Spray Liquid (OTC)** *Spray liq:* 2% (113 gm) (alcohol 17%)
>> **Lotrimin AF Spray Powder (OTC)** *Spray pwdr:* 2% (90 gm) (alcohol 10%)
>> **Monistat-Derm** *Crm:* 2% (1, 3 oz); *Spray liq:* 2% (3.5 oz); *Spray pwdr:* 2% (3 oz)

▷ *naftifine* (B)(G)
>> **Naftin Cream** <12 years: not recommended; ≥12 years: apply once daily x 2 weeks
>>> *Crm:* 1% (15, 30, 60 gm)
>> **Naftin Gel** <12 years: not recommended; ≥12 years: apply bid x 2 weeks
>>> *Gel:* 1% (20, 40, 60 gm)

▷ *oxiconazole nitrate* (B)(G) apply qd-bid x 2 weeks
>> **Oxistat** *Crm:* 1% (15, 30, 60 gm); *Lotn:* 1% (30 ml)

▷ *sulconazole* (C) <12 years: not recommended; ≥12 years: apply qd-bid x 3 weeks
>> **Exelderm** *Crm:* 1% (15, 30, 60 gm); *Lotn:* 1% (30 mg)

▷ *terbinafine* (B)(G)
>> **Lamisil Cream (OTC)** <12 years: not recommended; ≥12 years: apply bid x 1-4 weeks
>>> *Crm:* 1% (15, 30 gm)
>> **Lamisil AT Cream (OTC)** <12 years: not recommended; ≥12 years: apply to affected and surrounding area qd-bid x 1-4 weeks until significantly improved
>>> *Crm:* 1% (15, 30 gm)
>> **Lamisil Solution (OTC)** <12 years: not recommended; ≥12 years: apply to affected and surrounding area once daily x 1 week
>>> *Soln:* 1% (30 ml spray bottle)

▷ *tolnaftate* (C)(OTC)(G) <2 years: not recommended; ≥2 years: apply sparingly bid x 2-4 weeks
>> **Tinactin** *Crm:* 1% (15, 30 gm); *Pwdr:* 1% (45, 90 gm); *Soln:* 1% (10 ml); *Aerosol liq:* 1% (4 oz); *Aerosol pwdr:* 1% (3.5, 5 oz)

➤ *undecylenate acid* (NE) apply bid x 4 weeks
  Desenex (OTC) *Pwdr:* 25% (1.5, 3 oz); *Spray pwdr:* 25% (2.7 oz); *Oint:* 25% (0.5, 1 oz)

TOPICAL ANTIFUNGAL/ANTI-INFLAMMATORY AGENTS

➤ *clotrimazole/betamethasone* (C)(G) <12 years: not recommended; ≥12 years: apply bid x 4 weeks; max 4 weeks
  Crm: clotrim 10 mg/*beta* 0.5 mg (15, 45 gm); *Lotn: clotrim* 10 mg/*beta* 0.5 mg (30 ml)

SYSTEMIC ANTIFUNGALS

➤ *griseofulvin, microsize* (C)(G) <12 years: <30 lb: 5 mg/lb/day; 30-50 lb: 125-250 mg/day; >50 lb: 250-500 mg/day; 5 mg/lb/day x 4-6 weeks or longer; *see page* 568 *for dose by weight table;* ≥12 years: 500 mg once daily x 4-6 weeks or longer; max 1 gm/day
  Grifulvin V *Tab:* 250, 500 mg; *Oral susp:* 125 mg/5 ml (120 ml; alcohol 0.02%)
➤ *griseofulvin, ultramicrosize* (C)(G) <2 years: not recommended; 2-12 years: 3.3 mg/lb/day in a single or divided doses x 4-6 weeks or longer; >12 years: 375 mg/day in a single or divided doses x 4-6 weeks or longer
  Gris-PEG *Tab:* 125, 250 mg
  Comment: *griseofulvin* should be taken with fatty foods (e.g., milk, ice cream). Liver enzymes should be monitored.
➤ *ketoconazole* (C)(G) <2 years: not recommended; ≥2 years-12 years: 3.3-6.6 mg/kg once daily x 4 weeks; >12 years: initially 200 mg once daily; max 400 mg/day x 4 weeks
  Nizoral *Tab:* 200 mg
Comment: Caution with *ketoconazole* due to potential for hepatotoxicity.

TINEA PEDIS (ATHLETE'S FOOT)

TOPICAL ANTIFUNGALS

➤ *butenafine* (B)(G) <12 years: not recommended; ≥12 years: apply bid x 1 week or once daily x 4 weeks
  Lotrimin Ultra (C)(OTC) *Crm:* 1% (12, 24 gm)
  Mentax *Crm:* 1% (15, 30 gm)
  Comment: *butenafine* is a benzylamine, not an azole. Fungicidal activity continues for at least 5 weeks after last application.
➤ *Burrows solution* (NE) wet dressings
➤ *ciclopirox* (B)
  Loprox Cream <10 years: not recommended; ≥10 years: apply bid; max 4 weeks
    Crm: 0.77% (15, 30, 90 gm)
  Loprox Lotion <10 years: not recommended; ≥10 years: apply bid; max 4 weeks
    Lotn: 0.77% (30, 60 ml)
  Loprox Gel <16 years: not recommended; ≥16 years: apply bid; max 4 weeks
    Gel: 0.77% (30, 45 gm)
➤ *clotrimazole* (C)(G) <12 years: not recommended; ≥12 years: apply bid to affected area x 4 weeks

Desenex *Crm:* 1% (0.5 oz)
Lotrimin *Crm:* 1% (15, 30, 45, 90 gm); *Lotn:* 1% (30 ml); *Soln:* 1% (10, 30 ml)
Lotrimin AF (OTC) *Crm:* 1% (15, 30, 45, 90 gm); *Lotn:* 1% (20 ml); *Soln:* 1% (20 ml)

▷ *econazole* (C) apply once daily x 4 weeks
Spectazole *Crm:* 1% (15, 30, 85 gm)

▷ *ketoconazole* (C) apply to affected area bid x 4 weeks
Nizoral Cream *Crm:* 2% (15, 30, 60 gm)

▷ *luliconazole* (C) <18 years: not recommended; ≥18 years: apply to affected area and 1 inch into the immediate surrounding area(s) once daily
Luzu Cream 1% *Crm:* 1% (30, 60 gm)

▷ *miconazole* 2% (C)(G) apply bid x 4 weeks
Lotrimin AF Spray Liquid (OTC) *Spray liq:* 2% (113 gm) (alcohol 17%)
Lotrimin AF Spray Powder (OTC) *Spray pwdr:* 2% (90 g; alcohol 10%)
Monistat-Derm *Crm:* 2% (1, 3 oz); *Spray liq:* 2% (3.5 oz); *Spray pwdr:* 2% (3 oz)

▷ *naftifine* (B)(G)
Naftin Cream <12 years: not recommended; ≥12 years: apply once daily x 4 weeks
Crm: 1% (15, 30, 60 gm)
Naftin Gel <12 years: not recommended; ≥12 years: apply bid x 4 weeks
Gel: 1% (20, 40, 60 gm)

▷ *oxiconazole nitrate* (B)(G)apply qd-bid x 4 weeks
Oxistat *Crm:* 1% (15, 30, 60 gm); *Lotn:* 1% (30 ml)

▷ *sertaconazole* (C) <12 years: not recommended; ≥12 years: apply qd-bid x 4 weeks
Ertaczo *Crm:* 2% (15, 30 gm)

▷ *sulconazole* (C) <12 years: not recommended; ≥12 years: apply qd-bid x 4 weeks
Exelderm *Crm:* 1% (15, 30, 60 gm); *Lotn:* 1% (30 mg)

▷ *terbinafine* (B)(G)
Lamisil Cream (OTC) <12 years: not recommended; ≥12 years: apply bid x 1-4 weeks
Crm: 1% (15, 30 gm)
Lamisil AT Cream (OTC) <12 years: not recommended; ≥12 years: apply to affected and surrounding area qd-bid x 1-4 weeks until significantly improved
Crm: 1% (15, 30 gm)
Lamisil Solution (OTC) <12 years: not recommended; ≥12 years: apply to affected and surrounding area bid x 1 week
Soln: 1% (30 ml spray bottle)

▷ *tolnaftate* (C)(OTC)(G) <2 years: not recommended; ≥2 years: apply sparingly bid x 2-4 weeks
Tinactin *Crm:* 1% (15, 30 gm); *Pwdr:* 1% (45, 90 gm); *Soln:* 1% (10 ml); *Aerosol liq:* 1% (4 oz); *Aerosol pwdr:* 1% (3.5, 5 oz)

TOPICAL ANTIFUNGAL/ANTI-INFLAMMATORY COMBINATION

▷ *clotrimazole/betamethasone* (C)(G) 12 years: not recommended; ≥12 years: apply bid x 4 weeks; max 4 weeks
Lotrisone *Crm: clotrim* 1 mg/*beta* 0.5 mg (15, 45 gm); *Lotn: clotrim* 1 mg/*beta* 0.5 mg (30 ml)

SYSTEMIC ANTIFUNGALS

▶ *griseofulvin, microsize* (C)(G) <12 years: <30 lb: 5 mg/lb/day; 30-50 lb: 125-250 mg/day; >50 lb: 250-500 mg/day; 5 mg/lb/day x 4-6 weeks <u>or</u> longer; *see page 568 for dose by weight table;* ≥12 years: 500 mg once daily x 4-6 weeks <u>or</u> longer; max 1 gm/day

    Grifulvin V *Tab:* 250, 500 mg; *Oral susp:* 125 mg/5 ml (120 ml) (alcohol 0.02%)

▶ *griseofulvin, ultramicrosize* (C)(G) <2 years: not recommended; 2-12 years: 3.3 mg/lb/day in a single <u>or</u> divided doses x 4-6 weeks <u>or</u> longer; >12 years: 375 mg/day in a single <u>or</u> divided doses x 4-6 weeks <u>or</u> longer

    Gris-PEG *Tab:* 125, 250 mg

Comment: *griseofulvin* should be taken with fatty foods (e.g., milk, ice cream). Liver enzymes should be monitored.

▶ *ketoconazole* (C)(G) <2 years: not recommended; ≥2 years-12 years: 3.3-6.6 mg/kg once daily x 4 weeks; >12 years: initially 200 mg once daily; max 400 mg/day x 4 weeks

    Nizoral *Tab:* 200 mg

Comment: Caution with *ketoconazole* due to potential for hepatotoxicity.

TINEA VERSICOLOR

Comment: Resolution may take 3-6 months.

TOPICAL ANTIFUNGALS

▶ *butenafine* (G) <12 years: not recommended; ≥12 years: apply once daily x 2 weeks

    Lotrimin Ultra (C)(OTC) *Crm:* 1% (12, 24 gm)
    Mentax (B) *Crm:* 1% (15, 30 gm)

Comment: *butenafine* is a benzylamine, not an azole. Fungicidal activity continues for at least 5 weeks after last application.

▶ *ciclopirox* (B)

    Loprox Cream <10 years: not recommended; ≥10 years: apply bid; max 4 weeks
      Crm: 0.77% (15, 30, 90 gm)
    Loprox Lotion <10 years: not recommended; ≥10 years: apply bid; max 4 weeks
      Lotn: 0.77% (30, 60 ml)
    Loprox Gel <16 years: not recommended; ≥16 years: apply bid; max 4 weeks
      Gel: 0.77% (30, 45 gm)

▶ *clotrimazole* (B)(G) apply bid x 7 days

    Lotrimin *Crm:* 1% (15, 30, 45 gm)
    Lotrimin AF (OTC) *Crm:* 1% (12 gm); *Lotn:* 1% (10 ml); *Soln:* 1% (10 ml)

▶ *econazole* (C) apply once daily x 2 weeks

    Spectazole *Crm:* 1% (15, 30, 85 gm)

▶ *miconazole 2%* (C)(G) apply once daily x 2 weeks

    Lotrimin AF Spray Liquid (OTC) *Spray liq:* 2% (113 gm) (alcohol 17%)
    Lotrimin AF Spray Powder (OTC) *Spray pwdr:* 2% (90 gm) alcohol 10%)
    Monistat-Derm *Crm:* 2% (1, 3 oz); *Spray liq:* 2% (3.5 oz); *Spray pwdr: 2% (3 oz)*

▶ *ketoconazole* (C) apply to affected area once daily x 2 weeks

    Nizoral Cream *Crm:* 2% (15, 30, 60 gm)
    Nizoral Shampoo lather into area and leave on 5 minutes x 1 application
      Shampoo: 2% (4 oz)

▷ *oxiconazole nitrate* (B)(G) apply once daily x 2 weeks
　　Oxistat *Crm:* 1% (15, 30, 60 gm); *Lotn:* 1% (30 ml)
▷ *selenium sulfide* shampoo (C)(G) apply after shower, allow to dry, leave on over-
　night; then scrub off vigorously in AM; repeat in 1 week and again q 3 months until
　resolution occurs
　　Selsun Blue *Shampoo:* 1% (120, 210, 240, 330 ml); 2.5% (120 ml)
▷ *sulconazole* (C) <12 years: not recommended; ≥12 years: apply qd-bid x 3 weeks
　　Exelderm *Crm:* 1% (15, 30, 60 gm); *Lotn:* 1% (30 mg)
▷ *terbinafine* (B) <12 years: not recommended; ≥12 years: apply bid to affected and
　surrounding area x 1 week
　　Lamisil Solution (OTC) *Soln:* 1% (30 ml spray bottle)

ORAL ANTIFUNGALS

▷ *ketoconazole* (C)(G) <2 years: not recommended; ≥2 years-12 years: 3.3-6.6 mg/
　kg once daily x 4 weeks; >12 years: initially 200 mg once daily; max 400 mg/day x 4
　weeks
　　Nizoral *Tab:* 200 mg
Comment: Caution with **ketoconazole** due to potential for hepatotoxicity.

TOBACCO DEPENDENCE/NICOTINE WITHDRAWAL SYNDROME

NON-NICOTINE PRODUCTS

Alpha$_4$-Beta$_2$ Nicotinic Acetylcholine Receptor Partial Agonist

▷ *varenicline* (C)
　　Chantix <18 years: not recommended; ≥18 years: set target quit date; begin
　　therapy 1 week prior to target quit date; take after eating with a full glass of
　　water; initially 0.5 mg once daily for 3 days; then 0.5 mg bid x 4 days; then 1 mg
　　bid; treat x 12 weeks; may continue treatment for 12 more weeks
　　　Tab: 0.5, 1 mg; *Starting Month Pak:* 0.5 mg x 11 tabs + 1 mg x 42 tabs;
　　　Continuing Month Pak: 1 mg x 56 tabs
Comment: Caution with **Chantix** due to potential risk for anxiety or suicidal ideation.

AMINOKETONES

▷ *bupropion HBr* (C)(G)
　　Aplenzin <18 years: not recommended; ≥18 years: initially 100 mg bid for at
　　least 3 days; may increase to 375 or 400 mg/day after several weeks; then after
　　at least 3 more days, 450 mg in 4 divided doses; max 450 mg/day, 174 mg/single
　　dose
　　　Tab: 174, 348, 522 mg
▷ *bupropion HCl* (B)(G)
　　Forfivo XL do not use for initial treatment; use immediate-release bupropion
　　forms for initial titration; switch to **Forfivo XL** 450 mg once daily when total
　　dose/day reaches 450 mg; may switch to **Forfivo XL** when total dose/day
　　reaches 300 mg for 2 weeks and patient needs 450 mg/day to reach therapeutic
　　target; swallow whole, do not crush or chew

Tab: 450 mg ext-rel

Wellbutrin <18 years: not recommended; ≥18 years: initially 100 mg bid for at least 3 days; may increase to 375 or 400 mg/day after several weeks; then after at least 3 more days, 450 mg in 4 divided doses; max 450 mg/day, 150 mg/single dose

Tab: 75, 100 mg

Wellbutrin SR <18 years: not recommended; ≥18 years: initially 150 mg in AM for at least 3 days; may increase to 150 mg bid if well tolerated; usual dose 300 mg/day; max 400 mg/day

Tab: 100, 150 mg sust-rel

Wellbutrin XL <18 years: not recommended; ≥18 years: initially 150 mg in AM for at least 3 days; increase to 150 mg bid if well tolerated; usual dose 300 mg/day; max 400 mg/day

Tab: 150, 300 mg sust-rel

Zyban <18 years: not recommended; ≥18 years: 150 mg once daily x 3 days; then 150 mg bid x 7-12 weeks; max 300 mg/day

Tab: 150 mg sust-rel

Comment: Contraindications to *bupropion* include seizure disorder, disorder, concurrent MAOI and alcohol use. Smoking should be discontinued after the 7th day of therapy with *bupropion*. Avoid bedtime dose.

TRANSDERMAL NICOTINE SYSTEMS (D)

Habitrol (OTC) <12 years: not recommended; ≥12 years: initially one 21 mg/24 hour patch/day x 4-6 weeks; then one 14 mg/24 hour patch/day x 2-4 weeks; then one 7 mg/24 hour patch/day x 2-4 weeks; then discontinue

Transdermal patch: 7, 14, 21 mg/24 hour

Nicoderm CQ (OTC) <12 years: not recommended; ≥12 years: initially one 21 mg/24 hour patch/day x 6 weeks, then one 14 mg/24 hour patch/day x 2 weeks; then one 7 mg/24 hour patch/day x 2 weeks

Transdermal patch: 7, 14, 21 mg/24 hour

Comment: Nicoderm CQ is available as a clear patch.

Nicotrol Step-down Patch (OTC) <12 years: not recommended; ≥12 years: 1 patch/day x 6 weeks

Transdermal patch: 5, 10, 15 mg/16 hour (7/pck)

Nicotrol Transdermal (OTC) <12 years: not recommended; ≥12 years: 1 patch/day x 6 weeks

Transdermal patch: 15 mg/16 hour (7/pck)

Prostep <12 years: not recommended; ≥12 years: initially one 22 mg/24 hour patch/day x 4-8 weeks; then discontinue or one 11 mg/24 hour patch/day x 2-4 additional weeks

Transdermal patch: 11, 22 mg/24 hour (7/pck)

NICOTINE GUM

➤ *nicotine polacrilex* (D) <12 years: not recommended; ≥12 years: chew one piece of gum slowly and intermittently over 30 minutes q 1-2 hours x 6 weeks; then q 2-4 hours x 3 weeks; then q 4-8 hours x 3 weeks; max 24 pieces/day; 2 mg if smoked <25 cigarettes/day; 4 mg if smoked >24 cigarettes/day

Nicorette (OTC) *Gum squares:* 2, 4 mg (108 piece starter kit and 48 piece refill) (orange, mint, or original, sugar-free)

NICOTINE LOZENGE

▶ *nicotine polacrilex* (X)(OTC)(G) <18 years: not recommended; ≥18 years: dissolve over 20-30 minutes; minimize swallowing; do not eat or drink for 15 min before and during use; use 2 mg lozenge if first cigarette smoked >30 minutes after waking; use 4 mg lozenge if first cigarette smoked within 30 min of waking; 1 lozenge q 1-2 hours (at least 9/day) x 6 weeks; then q 2-4 hours x 3 weeks; then q 4-8 hours x 3 weeks; then stop; max 5 lozenges/6 hours and 20 lozenges/day

Commit Lozenge *Loz:* 2, 4 mg (72/pck) (phenylalanine)
Nicorette Mini Lozenge (G) *Loz:* 2, 4 mg (72/pck) (mint) (phenylalanine)

NICOTINE INHALATION PRODUCTS

▶ *nicotine* 0.5 mg aqueous nasal spray (D)
Nicotrol NS 12 years: not recommended; ≥12 years: 1-2 doses/hour nasally; max 5 doses/hour or 40 doses/day; usual max 3 months
Nasal spray: 0.5 mg/spray; 10 mg/ml (10 ml, 200 doses)
▶ *nicotine* <12 years: not recommended; ≥12 years: 10 mg inhalation system (D)
Nicotrol Inhaler individualize therapy; at least 6 cartridges/day x 3-6 weeks; max 16 cartridges/day x first 12 weeks; then reduce gradually over 12 more weeks
Inhaler: 10 mg/cartridge, 4 mg delivered (42 cartridge/pck) (menthol)

Comment: Nicotrol Inhaler is a smoking replacement; to be used with decreasing frequency. Smoking should be discontinued before starting therapy. Side effects include cough, nausea, mouth, or throat irritation. This system delivers nicotine, but no tars or carcinogens. Each cartridge lasts about 20 minutes with frequent continuous puffing and provides nicotine equivalent to 2 cigarettes.

TONSILLITIS: ACUTE

▶ *amoxicillin* (B)(G) <40 kg (88 lb): 20-40 mg/kg/day in 3 divided doses x 10 days or 25-45 mg/kg/day in 2 divided doses x 10 days; *see page 543 for dose by weight table;* ≥40 kg: 500-875 mg bid or 250-500 mg tid x 10 days
Amoxil *Cap:* 250, 500 mg; *Tab:* 875*mg; *Chew tab:* 125, 200, 250, 400 mg (cherry-banana-peppermint) (phenylalanine); *Oral susp:* 125, 250 mg/5 ml (80, 100, 150 ml) (strawberry); 200, 400 mg/5 ml (50, 75, 100 ml) (bubble gum); *Oral drops:* 50 mg/ml (30 ml) (bubble gum)
Moxatag *Tab:* 775 mg ext-rel
Trimox *Tab:* 125, 250 mg; *Cap:* 250, 500 mg; *Oral susp:* 125, 250 mg/5 ml (80, 100, 150 ml) (raspberry-strawberry)
▶ *azithromycin* (B) <12 years: 12 mg/kg/day x 5 days; *see page 548 for dose by weight table;* max 500 mg/day; ≥12 years: 500 mg x 1 dose on day 1, then 250 mg once daily on days 2-5 or 500 mg once daily x 3 days or **Zmax** 2 gm in a single dose
Zithromax *Tab:* 250, 500, 600 mg; *Oral susp:* 100 mg/5 ml (15 ml); 200 mg/5 ml (15, 22.5, 30 ml) (cherry); *Pkt:* 1 gm for reconstitution (cherry-banana)
Zithromax Tri-pak *Tab:* 3 x 500 mg tabs/pck
Zithromax Z-pak *Tab:* 6 x 250 mg tabs/pck
Zmax *Oral susp:* 2 gm ext-rel for reconstitution (cherry-banana) (148 mg Na⁺)
▶ *cefaclor* (B)(G) <1 month: not recommended; 1 month-12 years: 20-40 mg/kg divided bid x 10 days; *see page 549 for dose by weight table;* max 1 gm/day; >12 years: 250-500 mg q 8 hours x 10 days; max 2 gm/day

>> *Tab:* 500 mg; *Cap:* 250, 500 mg; *Susp:* 125 mg/5 ml (75, 150 ml) (strawberry); 187 mg/5 ml (50, 100 ml) (strawberry); 250 mg/5 ml (75, 150 ml) (strawberry); 375 mg/5 ml (50, 100 ml) (strawberry)

Cefaclor Extended Release <16 years: not recommended; ≥16 years: 500 mg bid x 10 days (clinically equivalent to 250 mg immed-rel caps tid); swallow whole; take with meals

Tab: 375, 500 mg ext-rel

▷ *cefadroxil* <12 years: 30 mg/kg/day in 2 divided doses x 10 days; *see page 550 for dose by weight table;* ≥12 years: 1-2 gm in a single or 2 divided doses x 10 days

Duricef *Cap:* 500 mg; *Tab:* 1 g; *Oral susp:* 250 mg/5 ml (100 ml); 500 mg/5 ml (75, 100 ml) (orange-pineapple)

▷ *cefdinir* (B) <6 months: not recommended; 6 months-12 years: 14 mg/kg/day in 1-2 divided doses x 10 days; *see page 551 for dose by weight table;* ≥12 years: 300 mg bid x 10 days or 600 mg daily x 10 days

Omnicef *Cap:* 300 mg; *Oral susp:* 125 mg/5 ml (60, 100 ml) (strawberry)

▷ *cefditoren pivoxil* (B) <12 years: not recommended; ≥12 years: 200 mg bid x 10 days

Spectracef *Tab:* 200 mg

Comment: Contraindicated with milk protein allergy or carnitine deficiency.

▷ *ceftibuten* (B) <12 years: 9 mg/kg daily x 10 days; max 400 mg/day; *see page 555 for dose by weight table;* ≥12 years: 400 mg daily x 10 days

Cedax *Cap:* 400 mg; *Oral susp:* 90 mg/5 ml (30, 60, 90, 120 ml); 180 mg/5 ml (30, 60, 120 ml) (cherry)

▷ *cefixime* (B)(G) <6 months: not recommended; 6 months-12 years, <50 kg: 8 mg/kg/day in 1-2 divided doses x 10 days; *see page 552 for dose by weight table;* >12 years, >50 kg: 400 mg once daily x 10 days

Suprax *Tab:* 400 mg; *Cap:* 400 mg; *Oral susp:* 100, 200, 500 mg/5 ml (50, 75, 100 ml) (strawberry)

▷ *cefpodoxime proxetil* (B) <2 months: not recommended; 2 months-12 years: 10 mg/kg/day (max 400 mg/dose) or 5 mg/kg/day bid (max 200 mg/dose) x 5-7 days; *see page 553 for dose by weight table;* >12 years: 200 mg bid x 5-7 days

▷ *cefprozil* (B) <2 years: not recommended; 2-12 years: 7.5 mg/kg bid x 10 days; *see page 554 for dose by weight table;* >12 years: 500 mg once daily x 10 days

Cefzil *Tab:* 250, 500 mg; *Oral susp:* 125, 250 mg/5 ml (50, 75, 100 ml) (bubble gum) (phenylalanine)

▷ *cephalexin* (B)(G) <12 years: 25-50 mg/kg/day in 4 divided doses x 10 days; *see page 557 for dose by weight table;* ≥12 years: 250 mg tid x 10 days

Keflex *Cap:* 250, 333, 500, 750 mg; *Oral susp:* 125, 250 mg/5 ml (100, 200 ml) (strawberry)

▷ *clarithromycin* (C)(G) <6 months: not recommended; ≥6 months-12 years: 7.5 mg/kg bid x 10 days; *see page 558 for dose by weight table;* >12 years: 250 mg bid or 500 mg ext-rel once daily 10 days

Biaxin *Tab:* 250, 500 mg

Biaxin Oral Suspension *Oral susp:* 125, 250 mg/5 ml (50, 100 ml) (fruit punch)

Biaxin XL *Tab:* 500 mg ext-rel

▷ *dirithromycin* (C)(G) <12 years: not recommended; ≥12 years: 500 mg once daily x 10 days

Dynabac *Tab:* 250 mg

▷ *erythromycin base* (B)(G) <45 kg: 30-50 mg in 2-4 divided doses x 10 days; ≥45 kg: 500 mg q 6 hours x 10 days

     Ery-Tab *Tab:* 250, 333, 500 mg ent-coat
     PCE *Tab:* 333, 500 mg
➤ *erythromycin ethylsuccinate* **(B)(G)** 30-50 mg/kg/day in 4 divided doses x 7 days; may double dose with severe infection; max 100 mg/kg/day <u>or</u> 400 mg qid; *see page 563 for dose by weight table*
     EryPed *Oral susp:* 200 mg/5 ml (100, 200 ml) (fruit); 400 mg/5 ml (60, 100, 200 ml) (banana); *Oral drops:* 200, 400 mg/5 ml (50 ml) (fruit); *Chew tab:* 200 mg wafer (fruit)
     E.E.S. *Oral susp:* 200, 400 mg/5 ml (100 ml) (fruit)
     E.E.S. Granules *Oral susp:* 200 mg/5 ml (100, 200 ml) (cherry)
     E.E.S. 400 Tablets *Tab:* 400 mg
➤ *loracarbef* **(B)** <12 years: 15 mg/kg/day in 2 divided doses x 10 days; *see page 570 for dose by weight table;* ≥12 years: 200 mg bid x 10 days
     Lorabid *Pulvule:* 200, 400 mg; *Oral susp:* 100 mg/5 ml (50, 100 ml); 200 mg/5 ml (50, 75, 100 ml) (strawberry bubble gum)
➤ *penicillin V potassium* **(B)(G)** <12 years: 25-75 mg/kg day divided q 6-8 hours x 10 days; *see page 572 for dose by weight table;* ≥12 years: 250 mg tid x 10 days
     Pen-VK *Tab:* 250, 500 mg; *Oral soln:* 125 mg/5 ml (100, 200 ml); 250 mg/5 ml (100, 150, 200 ml)

TRICHINOSIS (*TRICHINELLA SPIRALIS*)

Comment: Trichinosis is caused by eating raw or undercooked pork or wild game infected with the larvae of a parasitic worm, *Trichinella spiralis*. The initial symptoms are abdominal discomfort, nausea, vomiting, diarrhea, fatigue, and fever beginning one to two days following ingestion. These parasites then invade other organs (e.g., muscles) causing muscle aches, itching, fever, chills, and joint pains that begins about two to eight weeks after ingestion. The treatment is oral anthelmintics, which may cause abdominal pain, diarrhea, and (rarely) hypersensitivity reactions, convulsions, neutropenia, agranulocytosis, and hepatitis.

ANTHELMINTICS

Comment: Oral bioavailability of anthelmintics is enhanced when administered with a fatty meal (estimated fat content 40 g).
➤ *albendazole* **(C)** take with a meal; may crush and mix with food; may repeat in 3 weeks if needed; <2 years: 200 mg once daily x 3 days; 2-12 years: 400 mg once daily x 3 days; >12 years: 400 mg as bid x 3 days;
     Albenza *Tab:* 200 mg
➤ *mebendazole* **(C)** <2 years: not recommended; ≥2 years: chew, swallow, <u>or</u> mix with food; 200-400 mg tid x 3 days; then 400-500 mg tid
     Emverm *Chew tab:* 100 mg
     Vermox **(G)** *Chew tab:* 100 mg
➤ *pyrantel pamoate* **(C)** take with a meal; may open capsule and sprinkle or mix with food; treat x 3 days; may repeat in 2-3 weeks if needed; 11 mg/kg/dose; max 1 gm/dose; <25 lb: not recommended; 25-37 lb: 1/2 tsp/dose; 38-62 lb: 1 tsp/dose; 63-87 lb: 1 tsp/dose; 88-112 lb: 2 tsp/dose; 113-137 lb: 2 tsp/dose; 138-162 lb: 3 tsp/dose; 163-187 lb: 3 tsp/dose; >187 lb: 4 tsp/dose
     Antiminth *Cap:* 180 mg; *Liq:* 50 mg/ml (30 ml); 144 mg/ml (30 ml); *Oral susp:* 50 mg/ml (60 ml)

Pin-X (OTC) *Cap:* 180 mg; *Liq:* 50 mg/ml (30 ml); 144 mg/ml (30 ml); *Oral susp:* 50 mg/ml (30 ml)

▷ *thiabendazole* (C) take with a meal; may crush and mix with food; treat x 7 days; may repeat in 3 weeks if needed; <30 lb: consult mfr pkg insert; ≥30 lb: 25 mg/kg/dose bid; 30-50 lb: 250 mg bid; >50 lb: 10 mg/lb/dose bid; max 1.5 gm/dose; max 3 g/day

Mintezol *Chew tab:* 500*mg (orange); *Oral susp:* 500 mg/5 ml (120 ml) (orange)

Comment: *thiabendazole* is not for prophylaxis. May impair mental alertness. May not be available in the US.

TRICHOMONIASIS (*TRICHOMONAS VAGINALIS*)

Comment: The following treatment regimens for *Trichomoniasis* are published in the **2015 CDC Sexually Transmitted Diseases Treatment Guidelines**. Treat all sexual contacts. A multidose treatment regimen should be considered in HIV-positive females.

RECOMMENDED REGIMENS (NON-PREGNANT)

Regimen 1

▷ *metronidazole* 2 gm once in a single dose

Regimen 2

▷ *tinidazole* 2 gm once in a single dose

RECOMMENDED ALTERNATE REGIMEN

Regimen 1

▷ *metronidazole* 500 mg bid x 7 days

DRUG BRANDS AND DOSE FORMS

▷ *metronidazole* (not for use in 1st; B in 2nd, 3rd)(G)
Flagyl *Tab:* 250*, 500*mg
Flagyl 375 *Cap:* 375 mg
Flagyl ER *Tab:* 750 mg ext-rel

Comment: Alcohol is contraindicated during treatment with oral *metronidazole* and for 72 hours after therapy due to a possible *disulfiram*-like reaction (nausea, vomiting, flushing, headache).

▷ *tinidazole* (not for use in 1st; B in 2nd, 3rd)
Tindamax *Tab:* 250*, 500*mg

RECOMMENDED REGIMENS: PREGNANCY/LACTATION

Comment: All pregnant females should be considered for treatment. They can be treated with 2 gm *metronidazole* in a single dose at any stage of pregnancy. Lactating females who are administered *metronidazole* should be instructed to interrupt breastfeeding for 12-24 hours after receiving the 2 gm dose of *metronidazole*.

TRIGEMINAL NEURALGIA (TIC DOULOUREUX)

▷ *baclofen* (C)(G) <12 years: not recommended; ≥12 years: initially 5-10 mg tid with food; usual dose 10-80 mg/day

Lioresal *Tab:* 10*, 20*mg

Comment: Potential for seizures <u>or</u> hallucinations on abrupt withdrawal of *baclofen*.

▷ *carbamazepine* (C)

Carbatrol <12 years: max <35 mg/kg/day; use ext-rel form above 400 mg/day; 12-15 years: max 1 gm/day in 2 divided doses; >15-18 years: usual maintenance 1.2 gm/day in 2 divided doses; >18 years: initially 200 mg bid; may increase weekly as needed by 200 mg/day; usual maintenance 800 mg-1.2 gm/day

Cap: 200, 300 mg ext-rel

Tegretol(G) <6 years: initially 10-20 mg/kg/day in 2 divided doses; increase weekly as needed in 3-4 divided doses; max 35 mg/kg/day in 3-4 divided doses; ≥6 years-12 years: initially 100 mg bid; increase weekly as needed by 100 mg/day in 3-4 divided doses; max 1 gm/day in 3-4 divided doses; >12 years: initially 100 mg bid <u>or</u> 1/2 tsp susp qid; may increase dose by 100 mg q 12 hours <u>or</u> by 1/2 tsp susp q 6 hours; usual maintenance 400-800 mg/day; max 200 mg/day

Tab: 200*mg; *Chew tab:* 100*mg; *Oral susp:* 100 mg/5 ml (450 ml) (citrus-vanilla)

Tegretol XR (G) <6 years: use other forms; 6-12 years: initially 100 mg bid; may increase weekly by 100 mg/day in 2 divided doses; max 1 gm/day; >12 years: initially 200 mg bid; may increase weekly by 200 mg/day in 2 divided doses

Tab: 100, 200, 400 mg ext-rel

▷ *clonazepam* (D)(IV)(G) <10 years, <30 kg: initially 0.1-0.3 mg/kg/day; may increase up to 0.05 mg/kg/day bid-tid; usual maintenance 0.1-0.2 mg/kg/day tid; ≥10 years: initially 0.25 mg bid; increase to 1 mg/day after 3 days

Klonopin *Tab:* 0.5*, 1, 2 mg

Klonopin Wafers dissolve in mouth with <u>or</u> without water

Wafer: 0.125, 0.25, 0.5, 1, 2 mg orally-disint

▷ *divalproex sodium* (D) <10 years: not recommended; ≥10 years: initially 250 mg bid; gradually increase to max 1000 mg/day if needed

Depakene *Cap:* 250 mg; *Syr:* 250 mg/5 ml

Depakote *Tab:* 125, 250 mg

Depakote ER *Tab:* 250, 500 mg ext-rel

Depakote Sprinkle *Cap:* 125 mg

▷ *phenytoin* (D) 400 mg/day in divided doses

Dilantin *Cap:* 30, 100 mg; *Oral susp:* 125 mg/5 ml (8 oz); *Infatab:* 50 mg

Comment: Monitor *phenytoin* serum levels. Therapeutic serum level: 10-20 gm/ml. An ASE is gingival hyperplasia.

▷ *valproic acid* (D) initially 15 mg/kg/day; may increase weekly by 5-10 mg/kg/day; max 60 mg/kg/day <u>or</u> 250 mg/day

Depakene *Cap:* 250 mg; *Syr:* 250 mg/5 ml

TRICYCLIC ANTIDEPRESSANTS (TCAs)

Comment: Co-administration of SSRIs and TCAs requires extreme caution.

➤ *amitriptyline* (C)(G) <12 years: not recommended; ≥12 years: 10-20 mg q HS
   Tab: 10, 25, 50, 75, 100, 150 mg
➤ *amoxapine* (C) <12 years: not recommended; ≥12 years: initially 50 mg bid-tid;
   after 1 week may increase to 100 mg bid-tid; usual effective dose 200-300 mg/day; if
   total dose exceeds 300 mg/day, give in divided doses (max 400 mg/day); may give as
   a single bedtime dose (max 300 mg q HS)
   Tab: 25, 50, 100, 150 mg
➤ *clomipramine* (C)(G) <10 years: not recommended; 10-<16 years: initially 25 mg
   daily in divided doses; gradually increase; max 3 mg/kg or 100 mg, whichever is
   less; >16 years: initially 25 mg daily in divided doses; gradually increase to 100 mg
   during first 2 weeks; max 250 mg/day; total maintenance dose may be given at HS
   Anafranil *Cap:* 25, 50, 75 mg
➤ *desipramine* (C)(G) <12 years: not recommended; ≥12 years: 100-200 mg/day in
   single or divided doses; max 300 mg/day
   Norpramin *Tab:* 10, 25, 50, 75, 100, 150 mg
➤ *doxepin* (C)(G) <12 years: not recommended; ≥12 years: 75 mg/day; max 150
   mg/day
        Cap: 10, 25, 50, 75, 100, 150 mg; *Oral conc:* 10 mg/ml (4 oz w. dropper)
➤ *imipramine* (C)(G) <12 years: not recommended; ≥12 years:
        Tofranil initially 75 mg daily (max 200 mg); adolescents initially 30-40 mg daily
        (max 100 mg/day); if maintenance dose exceeds 75 mg daily, may switch to
        Tofranil PM for divided or bedtime dose
          Tab: 10, 25, 50 mg
        Tofranil PM initially 75 mg daily 1 hour before HS; max 200 mg
          Cap: 75, 100, 125, 150 mg
➤ *nortriptyline* (D)(G) <12 years: not recommended; ≥12 years: initially 25 mg tid-
   qid; max 150 mg/day
        Pamelor *Cap:* 10, 25, 50, 75 mg; *Oral soln:* 10 mg/5 ml (16 oz)
➤ *protriptyline* (C) <12 years: not recommended; ≥12 years: initially 5 mg tid; usual
   dose 15-40 mg/day in 3-4 divided doses; max 60 mg/day
        Vivactil *Tab:* 5, 10 mg
➤ *trimipramine* (C) <12 years: not recommended; ≥12 years: initially 75 mg/day in
   divided doses; max 200 mg/day
        Surmontil *Cap:* 25, 50, 100 mg

PULMONARY TUBERCULOSIS (TB; *MYCOBACTERIUM TUBERCULOSIS*)

SCREENING

➤ *purified protein derivative (PPD)* (C) 0.1 ml intradermally; examine inoculation
   site for induration at 48 to 72 hours.
        Aplisol, Tubersol *Soln:* 5 US units/0.1 ml (1, 5 ml)

PROPHYLACTIC IMMUNIZATION

The only tuberculosis vaccine uses attenuation of the related organism *Mycobacterium bovis* by culture in bile-containing media to create the *Bacillus Calmette-Guerin* (BCG) vaccination strain. It was first used experimentally in 1921 by Albert Calmette and

Camille Guerin and is currently in widespread use outside of the United States. It is not available in the US. The BCG vaccine protects newborns against tuberculosis-related meningitis and other systemic tuberculosis infections, but it has limited protection against active pulmonary disease. Once vaccinated, the patient will be PPD positive.

ANTITUBERCULAR AGENTS

Comment: Avoid *streptomycin* in pregnancy. *Pyridoxine* (*vitamin B₆*) 25 mg once daily x 6 months should be administered concomitantly with *INH* for prevention of side effects. *Rifapentine* produces red-orange discoloration of body tissues and body fluids and may stain contact lenses.

▷ *bedaquiline* (B)(G)
  Sirturo *Tab:* 100 mg
  Comment: *bedaquiline* is a diarylquinoline antimycobacterial ATP synthase for the treatment of pulmonary multidrug resistant TB (MDR-TB).
▷ *ethambutol (EMB)* (B)(G)
  Myambutol *Tab:* 100, 400*mg
▷ *isoniazid (INH)* (C) *Tab:* 300*mg
▷ *pyrazinamide (PZA)* (C) *Tab:* 500*mg
▷ *rifampin (RIF)* (C)(G)
  Rifadin, Rimactane *Cap:* 150, 300 mg
▷ *rifapentine* (C)
  Priftin *Tab:* 150 mg (24, 32 ct pck)
  Comment: The 32-count packs of **Priftin** are intended for patients with active tuberculosis infection (TB). The 24-count packs are intended for patients with latent tuberculosis infection (LTBI) who are at high risk for progression to tuberculosis disease. **Priftin** for active TB is indicated for patients ≥12 years-of-age. **Priftin** for LTBI is indicated for patients ≥2 years-of-age.
▷ *rilpivirine* (C) *Tab:* 25 mg
  Rifabutin *Cap:* 150 mg
▷ *streptomycin (SM)* (C)(G) *Amp:* 1 gm/2.5 ml or 400 mg/ml (2.5 ml)

COMBINATION AGENTS

▷ *rifampin/isoniazid* (C)
  Rifamate *Cap: rif* 300 mg/*iso* 150 mg
▷ *rifampin/isoniazid/pyrazinamide* (C)
  Rifater *Tab: rif* 120 mg/*iso* 50 mg/*pyr* 300 mg

PROPHYLAXIS AFTER EXPOSURE TO TUBERCULOSIS, WITH NEGATIVE PPD

▷ *isoniazid* (C) <12 years: 10-20 mg/kg/day x 9 months; ≥12 years: 300 mg once daily in a single dose x at least 6 months

PROPHYLAXIS AFTER EXPOSURE, WITH NEW PPD CONVERSION

▷ *isoniazid* (C) <12 years: 10-20 mg/kg/day x 9 months; ≥12 years: 300 mg once daily in a single dose x 12 months
  Tab: 100, 300*mg; *Syr:* 50 mg/5 ml; *Inj:* 100 mg/ml
▷ *rifampin* (C) <12 years: *rifampin* 10-20 mg/kg + *isoniazid* 10-20 mg/kg once daily x 4 months; ≥12 years: 600 mg once daily + *isoniazid* 300 mg once daily x 4 months

▷ *rifapentine* (C) <12 years: ≤12 years: Treat x 12 weeks; 10-14 kg: *rifapentine* 300 mg once weekly + *isoniazid* 25 mg/kg (max 900 mg) once weekly; 14.1-25 kg: *rifapentine* 450 mg once weekly + *isoniazid* 25 mg/kg (max 900 mg) once weekly; 25.1-32 kg: *rifapentine* 600 mg once weekly + *isoniazid* 25 mg/kg (max 900 mg) once weekly; 32.1-50 kg: *rifapentine* 750 mg once weekly + *isoniazid* 25 mg/kg (max 900 mg) once weekly; >50 kg: *rifapentine* 900 mg once weekly + *isoniazid* 25 mg/kg (max 900 mg) once weekly; ≥12 years: 600 mg once weekly + *isoniazid* 300 mg once weekly x 12 weeks

TREATMENT REGIMENS, <12 YEARS-OF-AGE

Regimen 1

▷ *rifampin* 10-20 mg/kg + *isoniazid* 10-20 mg/kg + *pyrazinamide* 15-20 mg/kg + *ethambutol* 15-25 mg/kg or *streptomycin* 20-40 mg/kg once daily x 8 weeks; then *isoniazid* 10-20 mg/kg + *rifampin* 10-20 mg/kg once daily x 16 weeks or *isoniazid* 20-40 mg/kg + *rifampin* 10-20 mg/kg 2-3 times/week x 16 weeks

Regimen 2

▷ *rifampin* 10-20 mg/kg + *isoniazid* 10-20 mg/kg + *pyrazinamide* 15-30 mg/kg + *ethambutol* 15-25 mg/kg or *streptomycin* 20-40 mg/kg once daily x 2 weeks; then *rifampin* 10-20 mg/kg + *isoniazid* 20-40 mg/kg + *pyrazinamide* 50-70 mg/kg + *ethambutol* 50 mg/kg or *streptomycin* 25-30 mg/kg 2 times/week x 6 weeks; then *isoniazid* 10-20 mg/kg + *rifampin* 10-20 mg/kg once daily x 16 weeks or *rifampin* 10-20 mg/kg + *isoniazid* 20-40 mg/kg 2 times/week x 16 weeks

Regimen 3

▷ *rifampin* 10-20 mg/kg + *isoniazid* 20-40 mg/kg + *pyrazinamide* 50-70 mg/kg + *ethambutol* 25-30 mg/kg or *streptomycin* 25-30 mg/kg 3 times/week x 6 months

Regimen 4 (When Pyrazinamide Is Contraindicated)

▷ *rifampin* 10-20 mg/kg + *isoniazid* 10-20 mg/kg + *ethambutol* 15-25 mg/kg + *streptomycin* 20-40 mg/kg once daily x 4-8 weeks; then *isoniazid* 10-20 mg/kg + *rifampin* 10-20 mg/kg once daily x 24 weeks or *rifampin* 10-20 mg/kg + *isoniazid* 20-40 mg/kg 2 x/week x 24 weeks

TREATMENT REGIMENS (≥12 YEARS-OF-AGE)

Regimen 1

▷ *rifampin* 600 mg + *isoniazid* 300 mg + *pyrazinamide* 2 gm + *ethambutol* 15-25 mg/kg or *streptomycin* 1 gm once daily x 8 weeks; then *isoniazid* 300 mg + *rifampin* 600 mg once daily x 16 weeks or *isoniazid* 900 mg + *rifampin* 600 mg 2-3 times/week x 16 weeks

Regimen 2

▷ *rifampin* 600 mg + *isoniazid* 300 mg + *pyrazinamide* 2 gm + *ethambutol* 15-25 mg/kg or *streptomycin* 1 gm once daily x 2 weeks; then *rifampin* 600 mg + *isoniazid*

900 mg + *pyrazinamide* 4 gm + *ethambutol* 50 mg/kg or *streptomycin* 1.5 gm 2 times/week x 6 weeks; then *isoniazid* 300 mg + *rifampin* 600 mg once daily x 16 weeks or 2 times/week x 16 weeks *rifampin* 600 mg once daily x 16 weeks or 2 times/week x 16 weeks

Regimen 3

▷ *rifampin* 600 mg + *isoniazid* 900 mg + *pyrazinamide* 3 gm + *ethambutol* 25-30 mg/kg or *streptomycin* 1.5 gm 3 times/week x 6 months

Regimen 4 (Smear and Culture Negative for Pulmonary TB ≥12 Years-of-Age)

▷ Options 1, 2, or 3 x 8 weeks; then *isoniazid* 300 mg + *rifampin* 600 mg once daily x 16 weeks; then *rifampin* 600 mg + *isoniazid* 300 mg + *pyrazinamide* 2 gm + *ethambutol* 15-25 mg/kg or *streptomycin* 1 gm once daily x 8 weeks or 2-3 times/week x 8 weeks

Regimen 5 (smear and culture negative for pulmonary TB ≥12 years-of-age)

▷ *rifapentine* 600 mg twice weekly x 2 months (at least 72 hours between doses) + once daily *isoniazid* 300 mg, *ethambutol* 15-25 mg/kg + *pyrazinamide* 2 g; then *rifapentine* 600 mg once weekly x 4 months + once daily *isoniazid* 300 mg + another appropriate antituberculosis agent for susceptible organisms

Regimen 6 (When Pyrazinamide Is Contraindicated)

▷ *rifampin* 600 mg + *isoniazid* 300 mg + *ethambutol* 15-25 mg/kg + *streptomycin* 1 gm once daily x 4-8 weeks; then *isoniazid* 300 mg + *rifampin* 600 mg once daily x 24 weeks or 2 x/week x 24 weeks

TREATMENT REGIMENS, <12 YEARS-OF-AGE

Regimen 1

▷ *rifampin* 10-20 mg/kg + *isoniazid* 10-20 mg/kg + *pyrazinamide* 15-20 mg/kg + *ethambutol* 15-25 mg/kg or *streptomycin* 20-40 mg/kg once daily x 8 weeks; then *isoniazid* 10-20 mg/kg + *rifampin* 10-20 mg/kg once daily x 16 weeks or *isoniazid* 20-40 mg/kg + *rifampin* 10-20 mg/kg 2-3 times/week x 16 weeks

Regimen 2

▷ *rifampin* 10-20 mg/kg + *isoniazid* 10-20 mg/kg + *pyrazinamide* 15-30 mg/kg + *ethambutol* 15-25 mg/kg or *streptomycin* 20-40 mg/kg once daily x 2 weeks; then *rifampin* 10-20 mg/kg + *isoniazid* 20-40 mg/kg + *pyrazinamide* 50-70 mg/kg + *ethambutol* 50 mg/kg or *streptomycin* 25-30 mg/kg 2 times/week x 6 weeks; then *isoniazid* 10-20 mg/kg + *rifampin* 10-20 mg/kg once daily x 16 weeks or *rifampin* 10-20 mg/kg + *isoniazid* 20-40 mg/kg 2 times/week x 16 weeks

Regimen 3

▷ *rifampin* 10-20 mg/kg + *isoniazid* 20-40 mg/kg + *pyrazinamide* 50-70 mg/kg + *ethambutol* 25-30 mg/kg or *streptomycin* 25-30 mg/kg 3 times/week x 6 months

Regimen 4 (When Pyrazinamide Is Contraindicated)

▷ *rifampin* 10-20 mg/kg + *isoniazid* 10-20 mg/kg + *ethambutol* 15-25 mg/kg + *streptomycin* 20-40 mg/kg once daily x 4-8 weeks; then *isoniazid* 10-20 mg/kg + *rifampin* 10-20 mg/kg once daily x 24 weeks <u>or</u> *rifampin* 10-20 mg/kg + *isoniazid* 20-40 mg/kg 2 x/week x 24 weeks

TYPE 1 DIABETES MELLITUS

Comment: Target glycosylated hemoglobin (HbA1c) is <7%. Addition of daily ACE-I <u>and/or</u> ARB therapy is strongly recommended for renal protection. Insulin may be indicated in the management of Type 2 diabetes with <u>or</u> without concomitant oral antidiabetic agents.

TREATMENT FOR ACUTE HYPOGLYCEMIA

▷ *glucagon (recombinant)* (B) administer SC, IM, <u>or</u> IV; if patient does not respond in 15 minutes, may administer a single dose <u>or</u> 2 divided doses; <20 kg: 0.5 mg <u>or</u> 20-30 mg/kg; ≥20 kg: 1 mg

INHALED INSULIN

Rapid-Acting Inhalation Powder Insulin

▷ *insulin human (inhaled)* (C) <18 years: not established; ≥18 years: one inhaler may be used for up to 15 days, then discard; dose at meal times as follows: *Insulin naïve:* initially 4 units at each meal; adjust according to blood glucose monitoring
Conversion from SC to inhaled mealtime insulin:
    SC 1-4 units: inhal 4 units
    SC 5-8 units: inhal 8 units
    SC 9-12 units: inhal 12 units
    SC 13-16 units: inhal 16 units
    SC 17-20 units: inhal 20 units
    SC 21-24 units: inhal 24 units
Afrezza Inhalation Powder administer at the beginning of the meal; *Mealtime insulin naïve:* initially 4 units at each meal; *Using SC prandial insulin:* convert dose to **Afrezza** using a conversion table (see mfr pkg insert); *Using SC premixed:* divide 1/2 of total daily injected premixed insulin equally among 3 meals of the day; administer 1/2 total injected premixed dose as once daily injected basal insulin dose
    Inhal: 4, 8, 12 unit single-inhalation color-coded cartridges (30, 60, 90/pkg w. 2 disposable inhalers)
Comment: **Afrezza** is not a substitute for long-acting insulin. **Afrezza** must be used in combination with long-acting insulin in patients with T1DM. **Afrezza** is not recommended for the treatment of diabetic ketoacidosis. **Afrezza** is contraindicated with chronic lung disease because of the risk of acute bronchospasm. The use of **Afrezza** is not recommended in patients who smoke <u>or</u> who have recently stopped smoking. Each card contains 5 blister strips with 3 cartridges each (total 15 cartridges). The doses are color-coded. **Afrezza** is contraindicated with chronic respiratory disease (e.g., asthma, COPD) and patients prone to episodes of hypoglycemia.

INJECTABLE INSULINS

Rapid-Acting Insulins

▷ *insulin aspart (recombinant)* **(B)** <2 years: not recommended; 2-4 years: use SC only; >4 years: may use SC or insulin pump (CSII); onset ≤15 minutes; peak 1-3 hours; duration 3-5 hours; administer 5-10 minutes prior to a meal; SC or infusion pump or IV infusion

> **NovoLog** *Vial:* 100 U/ml (10 ml); *PenFill cartridge:* 100 U/ml (3 ml, 5/pck) (zinc, m-cresol)

▷ *insulin glulisine (rDNA origin)* **(C)** <4 years: not recommended; ≥4 years: SC only; may administer via insulin pump; do not dilute or mix with other insulin in pump; onset <15 minutes; peak 1 hour; duration 2-4 hours; administer up to 15 minutes before, or within 20 minutes after starting a meal; use with an intermediate or long-acting insulin

> **Apidra** *Vial:* 100 U/ml (10 ml); *Cartridge:* 100 U/ml (3 ml, 5/pck; m-cresol)

▷ *insulin lispro (recombinant)* **(B)** <3 years: not recommended; ≥3 years: administer up to 15 minutes before, or immediately after, a meal; SC or IV infusion pump only onset ≤15 minutes; peak 1 hour; duration 3.5-4.5 hours

> **Humalog**
> *Vial:* 100 U/ml (10 ml); *Prefilled disposable KwikPen:* 100 U/ml (3 ml, 5/pck) (zinc, m-cresol); *HumaPen Memoir* and *HumaPen Luxura* HD inj device for *Humalog cartridges* (100 U/ml, 3 ml 5/pck) (zinc, m-cresol)

▷ *insulin regular* **(B)**

> **Humulin R U-100 *(human, recombinant)*** **(OTC)** onset 30 minutes; peak 2-4 hours; duration up to 6-8 hours; SC or IV or IM
> *Vial:* 100 U/ml (10 ml)

> **Humulin R U-500 *(human, recombinant)*** onset 30 minutes; peak 1.75-4 hours; duration up to 24 hours; SC only; for in-hospital use only
> *Vial:* 500 U/ml (20 ml) (m-cresol); *KwikPen:* 3 ml (2, 5/carton)
> **Comment:** Humulin R U-500 formulation is 5 times more concentrated than standard U-100 concentration, indicated for patient's ≥18 years-of-age and children who require ≥200 units of insulin/day, allowing patients to inject 80% less liquid to receive the desired dose.

> **Iletin II Regular *(pork)*** **(OTC)** onset 30 minutes; peak 2-4 hours; duration 6-8 hours; SC or IV or IM
> *Vial:* 100 U/ml (10 ml)

> **Novolin R *(human)*** **(OTC)** onset 30 minutes; peak 2.5-5 hours; duration 8 hours; SC or IV or IM
> *Vial:* 100 U/ml (10 ml); *PenFill cartridge:* 100 U/ml (1.5 ml, 5/pck); *Prefilled syringe:* 100 U/ml (1.5 ml, 5/pck)

▷ *pramlintide* (*amylin analog/amylinomimetic*) **(C)** <12 years: not recommended; ≥12 years: administer immediately before major meals (≥250 kcal or ≥30 gm carbo-hydrates); initially 15 mcg; titrate in 15 mcg increments for 3 days if no significant nausea occurs; if nausea occurs at 45 or 60 mcg, reduce to 30 mcg; if not tolerated, consider discontinuing therapy; *Maintenance:* 60 mcg (30 mcg *only* if 60 mcg not tolerated)

> **Symlin** *Vial:* 0.6 mg/ml (5 ml) (m-cresol, mannitol)
> **Comment:** **Symlin** is indicated as adjunct to mealtime insulin with or without a sulfonylurea and blood glucose control is suboptimal despite optimal insulin therapy. Do not mix with insulin. When initiating **Symlin**, reduce preprandial

short/rapid-acting insulin dose by 50% and monitor pre- and postprandial and bedtime blood glucose. Do not use in patients with poor compliance, HgbA1c is >9%, recurrent hypoglycemia requiring assistance in the previous 6 months, or if taking a prokinetic drug. With Type 2 DM, initial therapy is 60 mcg/dose and max is 120 mcg/dose.

RAPID-ACTING AND INTERMEDIATE-ACTING INSULIN

Insulin Aspart Protamine Suspension/Insulin Aspart Combinations

▷ *insulin aspart protamine suspension 70%/insulin aspart 30% (recombinant)* **(B)(G)** <12 years: not recommended; do not mix with other insulin; SC only; onset 15 min; peak 2.4 hours; duration up to 24 hours
> **NovoLog Mix 70/30 (OTC)** *Vial:* 100 U/ml (10 ml)
> **NovoLog Mix 70/30 FlexPen (OTC)** *Prefilled disposable pen:* 100 U/ml (3 ml, 5/pck); *PenFill cartridge:* 100 U/ml (3 ml, 5/pck)

LONG-ACTING INSULINS

▷ *insulin detemir (human)* **(B)** <2 years: not recommended; ≥2 years: administer SC once daily with evening meal or at HS as a basal insulin; may administer twice daily (AM/PM); administer in the deltoid, abdomen, or thigh; onset 1-2 hours; peak 6-8 hours; duration 24 hours; switching from another basal insulin, dose should be the same on a unit-to-unit basis; may need more *insulin detemir* when switching from **NPH;** *Type 1:* starting dose 1/3 of total daily insulin requirements; rapid-acting or short-acting, pre-meal insulin should be used to satisfy the remainder of daily insulin requirements; *Type 2 (inadequately controlled on oral antidiabetic agents):* initially 10 units or 0.1-0.2 units/kg, once daily in the evening or divided twice daily (AM/PM); do not add-mix or dilute *insulin detemir* with other insulins.
> **Levemir** *Vial:* 100 U/ml (10 ml); *FlexPen:* 100 U/ml (3 ml, 5/pck) (zinc, m-cresol)
> **Comment:** Do not mix or dilute *insulin detemir* with other insulins.
▷ *insulin glargine (recombinant)* **(C)** <6 years: not established; ≥6 years: do not mix or dilute with other insulins
> **Basaglar** administer SC once daily, at the same time each day, as a basal insulin in the deltoid, abdomen, or thigh; onset 1-1.5 hours, no pronounced peak, duration 20-24 hours; *T1DM (adults, adolescents, and children >6 years-of-age):* initially 1/3 of total daily insulin dose; administer the remainder of the total dose as short- or rapid-acting preprandial insulin; *T2DM (≥18 years only):* initially 2 units/kilogram or up to 10 units once daily; *Switching from once daily insulin glargine 300 units/ml (i.e., Toujeo) to 100 units/ml:* initially 80% of the insulin glargine 300 units/ml; *Switching from twice daily NPH:* initially 80% of the total daily NPH dose; do not add-mix or dilute *insulin glargine* with other insulins.
>> *Prefilled KwikPen (disposable),* 100 U/ml (3 ml) (5/carton)
> **Lantus** <6 years: not recommended; ≥6 years: administer SC once daily at the same time each day as a basal insulin; onset 1-1.5 hours, no pronounced peak, duration 20-24 hours; initial average starting dose 10 units for insulin-naïve patients; *Switching from once daily NPH or Ultralente insulin:* initial dose of *insulin glargine* should be on a unit-for-unit basis; *Switching from twice daily NPH insulin:* start at 20% lower than the total daily *NPH* dose

Vial: 100 U/ml (10 ml); *Cartridge:* 100 U/ml (3 ml, for use in the *OptiPen One Insulin Delivery Device*) (5/carton) (m-cresol); *SoloStar pen (disposable):* 100 U/ml (3 ml) (5/carton)

Toujeo <18 years: not established; ≥18 years: administer SC once daily at the same time each day as a basal insulin; in the upper arm, abdomen, or thigh; onset of action 6 hours; duration 20-24 hours; *T2DM, insulin naïve:* initially 0.2 units/kg; titrate every 3-4 days; *T1DM, insulin naïve:* initially 1/3-1/2 total daily insulin dose; remainder as short-acting insulin divided between each meal; *Switch from once daily long-* or *intermediate-acting insulin:* on a unit-for-unit basis; *Switching from* **Lantus:** a higher daily dose is expected; *Switching from twice daily NPH:* reduce initial dose by 20% of total daily NPH dose

Soln for SC injection: 300 units/ml prefilled disposable SoloStar Pen (1.5 ml, 3-5/carton)

▷ *insulin isophane suspension (NPH)* (B) <18 years: not recommended; ≥18 years:
Humulin N *(human, recombinant)* (OTC) onset 1-2 hours; peak 6-12 hours; duration 18-24 hours; SC only

Vial: 100 U/ml (10 ml); *Prefilled disposable pen:* 100 U/ml (3 ml, 5/pck)

Novolin N *(recombinant)* (OTC) onset 1.5 hours; peak 4-12 hours; duration 24 hours; SC only

Vial: 100 U/ml (10 ml); *PenFill cartridge:* 1.5 ml (5/pck); *KwikPens:* 1.5 ml (5/pck)

Iletin II NPH *(pork)* (OTC) onset 1-2 hours; peak 6-12 hours; duration 18-26 hours; SC only

Vial: 100 U/ml (10 ml)

▷ *insulin zinc suspension (lente)* (B) <18 years: not recommended; ≥18 years:
Humulin L *(human)* (OTC) onset 1-3 hours; peak 6-12 hours; duration 18-24 hours; SC only

Vial: 100 U/ml (10 ml)

Iletin II Lente *(pork)* (OTC) onset 1-3 hours; peak 6-12 hours; duration 18-26 hours; SC only

Vial: 100 U/ml (10 ml)

Novolin L *(human)* (OTC) onset 2.5 hours; peak 7-15 hours; duration 22 hours; SC only

Vial: 100 U/ml (10 ml)

Ultra Long-Acting Insulin

▷ *insulin degludec (insulin analog)* (C) <1 year: not established; ≥1 year: administer by SC injection once daily at any time of day, with or without food, into the upper arm, abdomen, or thigh; titrate every 3-4 days; *Insulin naïve with type 1 diabetes:* initially 1/3-1/2 of total daily insulin dose, usually 0.2-0.4 units/kg; administer the remainder of the total dose as short-acting insulin divided between each daily meal; *Insulin naive with type 2 diabetes:* initially 10 units once daily; adjust dose of concomitant oral antidiabetic agent; *Already on insulin (type 1 or type 2):* initiate at same unit dose as total daily long- or intermediate-acting insulin unit dose

Tresiba FlexTouch *Pen:* 100 U/ml (3 ml, 5 pens/carton), 200 U/ml (3 ml, 5 pens/carton) (zinc, m-cresol)

Comment: Tresiba U-200 FlexTouch is the only long-acting insulin in a 160-unitpen allowing up to 160 units in a single injection. The U-200 dose counter always shows the desired dose (i.e., no conversion from U/100 to U-200 is required)

▷ *insulin extended zinc suspension (**Ultralente**) (human)* (B) <18 years: not recommended; ≥18 years: SC only; onset 4-6 hours; peak 8-20 hours; duration 24-48 hours
  Humulin U (OTC) *Vial:* 100 U/ml (10 ml)

Insulin Lispro Protamine/Insulin Lispro Combinations

▷ *insulin lispro protamine 75%/insulin lispro 25%* (B) <18 years: not recommended; ≥18 years:
  Humalog Mix 75/25 *(human)* onset 15 minutes; peak 30 minutes to 1 hour; duration 24 hours; SC only
    Vial: 100 U/ml (10 ml); *Prefilled disposable KwikPen:* 100 U/ml (3 ml, 5/ carton) (zinc, m-cresol); *HumaPen Memoir* and *HumaPen Luxura HD* inj device for *Humalog cartridges* (100 U/ml, 3 ml, 5/carton) (zinc, m-cresol)
▷ *insulin lispro protamine 50%/insulin lispro 50%* (B) <18 years: not recommended; ≥18 years:
  Humalog Mix 50/50 *(recombinant)* (B) onset 15 minutes; peak 2.3 hours; range 1-5 hours; SC only
    Vial: 100 U/ml (10 ml); *Prefilled disposable KwikPen:* 100 U/ml (3 ml, 5/ carton) (zinc, m-cresol); *HumaPen Memoir* and *HumaPen Luxura HD* inj device for *Humalog cartridges* (100 U/ml, 3 ml, 5/carton) (zinc, m-cresol)

Insulin Isophane Suspension (NPH)/Insulin Regular Combinations

▷ *NPH 70%/regular 30%* (B) <18 years: not recommended; ≥18 years:
  Humulin 70/30 *(human, recombinant)* (OTC) onset 30 minutes; peak 2-12 hours; duration up to 24 hours; SC only
    Vial: 100 U/ml (10 ml)
  Novolin 70/30 *(recombinant)* (OTC) onset 30 minutes; peak 2-12 hours; duration up to 24 hours; SC only
    Vial: 100 U/ml (10 ml)
▷ *NPH 50%/regular 50%* (B) <18 years: not recommended; ≥18 years:
  Humulin 50/50 *(human)* (OTC) onset 30 minutes; peak 3-5 hours; duration up to 24 hours; SC only
    Vial: 100 U/ml (10 ml)

Insulin Lispro Protamine/Insulin Lispro Combinations

▷ *insulin lispro protamine 75%/insulin lispro 25%* (B) <18 years: not recommended; ≥18 years:
  Humalog Mix 75/25 *(recombinant)* onset 15 minutes; peak 30-90 minutes; duration 24 hours; SC only
    Vial: 100 U/ml (10 ml); *Prefilled disposable KwikPen:* 100 U/ml (3 ml, 5/ carton) (zinc, m-cresol); *HumaPen Memoir* and *HumaPen Luxura HD* inj device for *Humalog cartridges* (100 U/ml, 3 ml 5/carton) (zinc, m-cresol)
▷ *insulin lispro protamine 50%/insulin lispro 50%* (B) <18 years: not recommended; ≥18 years:
  Humalog Mix 50/50 *(recombinant)* onset 15 minutes; peak 1 hour; duration up to 16 hours; SC only
    Vial: 100 U/ml (10 ml); *Prefilled disposable KwikPen:* 100 U/ml (3 ml, 5/ carton) (zinc, m-cresol); *HumaPen Memoir* and *HumaPen LUXURA HD* inj device for *Humalog cartridges* (100 U/ml, 3 ml 5/carton) (zinc, m-cresol);

U/ml (3 ml, 5/pck) (zinc, m-cresol); *HumaPen Memoir* and *HumaPen LUXURA* HD inj device for *Humalog cartridges* (100 U/ml, 3 ml 5/pck) (zinc, m-cresol); (100 U/ml, 3 ml 5/carton (zinc, m-cresol)

Basal insulin/GLP-1 RA Combinations

▷ **insulin degludec (insulin analog)/liraglutide (C)** <18 years: not recommended; ≥18 years: for treatment of type 2 diabetes only in patients inadequately controlled on <50 units of basal insulin daily or <1.8 mg of *liraglutide* daily; administer by SC injection once daily, with or without food, into the upper arm, abdomen, or thigh; titrate every 3-4 days

Xultophy *Prefilled pen:* 100/3.6 U/ml (3 ml, 5 pens/carton)

▷ **insulin glargine (insulin analog)/lixisenatide (C)** <18 years: not recommended; ≥18 years: for treatment of type 2 diabetes only in patients inadequately controlled on <60 units of basal insulin daily or *lixisenatide;* administer by SC injection once daily, with or without food, into the upper arm, abdomen, or thigh; titrate every 3-4 days

Soliqua *Prefilled pen:* 100/33 U/ml (3 ml, 5 pens/carton) covering 15-60 mg *insulin glargine* 100 units/ml and 15-20 mcg of *lixisenatide (m-cresol)*

TYPE 2 DIABETES MELLITUS

Comment: Normal fasting glucose is <100 mg/dL. Impaired glucose tolerance is a risk factor for type 2 diabetes and a marker for cardiovascular disease risk; it occurs early in the natural history of these two diseases. Impaired fasting glucose is ≥100 mg/dL and <125 mg/dL. Impaired glucose tolerance is OGTT, 2 hour post-load 75 gm glucose >140 mg/dL and <200 mg/dL. Target pre-prandial glucose is 80 mg/dL to 120 mg/dL. Target bedtime glucose is 100 mg/dL to 140 mg/dL. Target glycosylated hemoglobin (HbA1c) is <7.0%. Addition of daily ACE-I and/or ARB therapy is strongly recommended for renal protection. Consider diabetes screening at age 25 years for persons in high-risk groups (non-Caucasian, positive family history for DM, obesity). Hypertension and hyperlipidemia are common comorbid conditions. Macrovascular complications include cerebral vascular disease, coronary artery disease, and peripheral vascular disease. Microvascular complications include retinopathy, nephropathy, neuropathy, and cardiomyopathy. Oral hypoglycemics are contraindicated in pregnancy.
Insulins *see Type 1 Diabetes Mellitus page* 417

TREATMENT FOR ACUTE HYPOGLYCEMIA

▷ **glucagon (recombinant) (B)** <20 kg: 0.5 mg or 20-30 mg/kg; ≥20 kg: 1 mg; administer SC or IM or IV; if patient does not respond in 15 minutes, may administer a single or 2 divided doses

SULFONYLUREAS

Comment: Sulfonylureas are secretagogues (i.e., stimulate pancreatic insulin secretion); therefore, the patient taking a sulfonylurea should be alerted to the risk for hypoglycemia. Action is dependent on functioning beta cells in the pancreatic islets.

1st Generation Sulfonylureas

▷ *chlorpropamide* (C)(G) <12 years: not recommended; ≥12 years: initially 250 mg/day with breakfast; max 750 mg
  Diabinese *Tab:* 100*, 250*mg
▷ *tolazamide* (C)(G) <12 years: not recommended; ≥12 years: initially 100-250 mg/day with breakfast; increase by 100-250 mg/day at weekly intervals; maintenance 100 mg 1 gm/day; max 1 gm/day
  Tolinase *Tab:* 100, 250, 500 mg
▷ *tolbutamide* (C) <12 years: not recommended; ≥12 years: initially 1-2 gm in divided doses; max 2 gm/day
  Tab: 500 mg

2nd Generation Sulfonylureas

▷ *glimepiride* (C) <12 years: not recommended; ≥12 years: initially 1-2 mg once daily with breakfast; after reaching dose of 2 mg, increase by 2 mg at 1-2 week intervals as needed; usual maintenance 1-4 mg once daily; max 8 mg/day
  Amaryl *Tab:* 1*, 2*, 4*mg
▷ *glipizide* (C)(G) <12 years: not recommended; ≥12 years:
  Glucotrol initially 5 mg before breakfast; increase by 2.5-5 mg every few days if needed; max 15 mg/day; max 40 mg/day in divided doses
    Tab: 5*, 10* mg
  Glucotrol XL initially 5 mg with breakfast; usual range 5-10 mg/day; max 20 mg/day
    Tab: 2.5, 5, 10 mg ext-rel
▷ *glyburide* (C)(G) <12 years: not recommended; ≥12 years: initially 2.5-5 mg/day with breakfast; increase by 2.5 mg at weekly intervals; maintenance 1.25-20 mg/day in a single or 2 divided doses; max 20 mg/day
  DiaBeta, Micronase *Tab:* 1.25*, 2.5*, 5*mg
▷ *glyburide, micronized* (B) <12 years: not recommended; ≥12 years:
  Glynase PresTab initially 1.5-3 mg/day with breakfast; increase by 1.5 mg at weekly intervals if needed; usual maintenance 0.75-12 mg/day in single or divided doses; max 12 mg/day
    Tab: 1.5*, 3*, 6*mg

ALPHA-GLUCOSIDASE INHIBITORS

Comment: Alpha-glucosidase inhibitors block the enzyme that breaks down carbohydrates in the small intestine, delaying digestion and absorption of complex carbohydrates, and lowering peak postprandial glycemic concentrations. Use as monotherapy or in combination with a sulfonylurea. Contraindicated in inflammatory bowel disease, colon ulceration, and intestinal obstruction. Side effects include flatulence, diarrhea, and abdominal pain.
▷ *acarbose* (B) <12 years: not recommended; ≥12 years: initially 25 mg tid ac, increase at 4-8 week intervals; or initially 25 mg once daily, increase gradually to 25 mg tid; usual range 50-100 mg tid; max 100 mg tid
  Precose *Tab:* 25, 50, 100 mg
▷ *miglitol* (B) <12 years: not recommended; ≥12 years: initially 25 mg tid at the start of each main meal, titrated to 50 mg tid at the start of each main meal; max 100 mg tid
  Glyset *Tab:* 25, 50, 100 mg

BIGUANIDE

Comment: The biguanides decrease gluconeogenesis by the liver in the presence of insulin. Action is dependent on the presence of circulating insulin. Lower hepatic glucose production leads to lower overnight, fasting, and preprandial plasma glucose levels. Common side effects include GI distress, nausea, vomiting, bloating, and flatulence, which usually eventually resolve. May be used as monotherapy (≥12 years only) or with a sulfonylurea or insulin.

➤ *metformin* (B)(G) take with meals

Comment: *metformin* is contraindicated with renal impairment, metabolic acidosis, and ketoacidosis. Suspend *metformin*, prior to, and for 48 hours after, surgery or receiving IV iodinated contrast agents.

Fortamet <17 years: not recommended; ≥17 years: initially 1000 mg once daily; may increase by 500 mg/day at 1 week intervals; max 2.5 gm/day
Tab: 500, 1000 mg ext-rel

Glucophage <10 years: not recommended; 10-16 years: use only as monotherapy; >16 years: initially 500 mg bid; may increase by 500 mg/day at 1 week intervals; max 1 gm bid or 2.5 gm in 3 divided doses; or initially 850 mg once daily in AM; may increase by 850 mg/day in divided doses at 2 week intervals; max 2000 mg/day; take with meals
Tab: 500, 850, 1000*mg

Glucophage XR <10 years: not recommended; 10-16 years: use immediate release form; >16 years: initially 500 mg by mouth every evening; may increase by 500 mg/day at 1 week intervals; max 2 gm/day
Tab: 500, 750 mg ext-rel

Glumetza ER (G) <18 years: not recommended; ≥18 years: initially 1000 mg once daily; may increase by 500 mg/day at weekly intervals; max 2 gm/day
Tab: 500, 1000 mg ext-rel

Riomet XR <10 years: not recommended; ≥10 years: monotherapy only; initially 500 mg once daily; may increase by 500 mg/day at 1 week intervals; max 2 gm/day in divided doses; take with meals
Oral soln: 500 mg/ml (4 oz) (cherry)

MEGLITINIDES

Comment: Meglitinides are secretagogues (i.e., stimulate pancreatic insulin secretion) in response to a meal. Action is dependent on functioning beta cells in the pancreatic islets. Use as monotherapy or in combination with *metformin*.

➤ *nateglinide* (C) <12 years: not recommended; ≥12 years: 60-120 mg tid ac 1-30 minutes prior to start of the meal
Starlix *Tab:* 60, 120 mg

➤ *repaglinide* (C)(G) <12 years: not recommended; ≥12 years: initially 0.5 mg with 2-4 meals/day; take 30 minutes ac; titrate by doubling dose at intervals of at least 1 week; range 0.5-4 mg with 2-4 meals/day; max 16 mg/day
Prandin *Tab:* 0.5, 1, 2 mg

THIAZOLIDINEDIONES (TZDs)

Comment: The TZDs decrease hepatic gluconeogenesis and reduce insulin resistance (i.e., increase glucose uptake and utilization by the muscles). Liver function tests are indicated before initiating these drugs. Do not start if ALT more than 3 times greater than normal. Recheck ALT monthly for the first six months of therapy; then, every two months for the remainder of the first year and periodically thereafter. Liver function tests should be obtained at the first symptoms suggestive of hepatic dysfunction (nausea, vomiting, fatigue, dark urine, anorexia, abdominal pain).

▷ *pioglitazone* (C)(G) <18 years: not recommended; ≥18 years: initially 15-30 mg once daily; max 45 mg/day as a monotherapy; usual max 30 mg/day in combination with *metformin*, insulin, or a sulfonylurea

  Actos *Tab:* 15, 30, 45 mg

▷ *rosiglitazone* (C)(G) <18 years: not recommended; ≥18 years: initially 4 mg/day in a single or 2 divided doses; may increase after 8-12 weeks; max 8 mg/day as a monotherapy or combination therapy with *metformin* or a sulfonylurea; not for use with *insulin*

  Avandia *Tab:* 2, 4, 8 mg

DIPEPTIDYL PEPTIDASE-4 (DPP-4) INHIBITOR/THIAZOLIDINEDIONE COMBINATION

Comment: The FDA has reported that *alogliptin*-containing drugs may increase the risk of heart failure, especially in patients who already have cardiovascular or renal disease. The drug **Oseni** (*alogliptin/pioglitazone*) is in this risk group.

▷ *alogliptin/pioglitazone* (C) <18 years: not recommended; ≥18 years: take 1 dose once daily with first meal of the day; max: *rosiglitazone* 8 mg and max *glimepiride* per day; same precautions as *alogliptin* and *pioglitazone*

  Oseni
  Tab: **Oseni 12.5/15:** *alo* 12.5 mg/*pio* 15 mg
  Oseni 12.5/30: *alo* 12.5 mg/*pio* 30 mg
  Oseni 12.5/45: *alo* 12.5 mg/*pio* 45 mg
  Oseni 25/15: *alo* 25/*pio* 15 mg
  Oseni 25/30: *alo* 25/*pio* 30 mg
  Oseni 25/45: *alo* 25 mg/*pio* 45 mg

2ND GENERATION SULFONYLUREA/BIGUANIDE COMBINATIONS

Comment: **Metaglip** and **Glucovance** are combination secretagogues (sulfonylureas) and insulin sensitizers (biguanides). *Sulfonylurea:* Action is dependent on functioning beta cells in the pancreatic islets; patient should be alerted to the risk for hypoglycemia. Common side effects of the biguanide include GI distress, nausea, vomiting, bloating, and flatulence, which usually eventually resolve. Take with food. *Metformin* is contraindicated with renal impairment, metabolic acidosis, and ketoacidosis. Suspend *metformin*, prior to, and for 48 hours after, surgery or receiving IV iodinated contrast agents.

▷ *glipizide/metformin* (C) <12 years: not recommended; ≥12 years: take with meals; *Primary therapy:* 2.5/250 once daily or if FBS is 280-320 mg/dL, may start at 2.5/250 bid; may increase by 1 tab/day every 2 weeks; max 10/2,000 per day in 2 divided doses; *Second-Line Therapy:* 2.5/500 or 5/500 bid; may increase by up to 5/500 every 2 weeks; max: 20/2000 per day; same precautions as *glipizide* and *metformin*

  Metaglip
  Tab: **Metaglip 2.5/250:** *glip* 2.5 mg/*met* 250 mg
  Metaglip 2.5/500: *glip* 2.5 mg/*met* 500 mg
  Metaglip 5/500: *glip* 5 mg/*met* 500 mg

▶ *glyburide/metformin* (B) <12 years: not recommended; ≥12 years: take with meals;
Primary therapy (initial therapy if HgbA1c <9.0%): initially 1.25/250 once daily; max
glyburide 20 mg and *metformin* 2,000 mg per day; *Primary therapy (initial therapy
if HbA1c >9.0% or FBS >200):* initially 1.25/250 bid; max *glyburide* 20 mg and
metformin 2000 mg per day; *Second-line therapy (initial therapy if HbA1c >7.0%):*
initially 2.5/500 or 5/500 bid; max *glyburide* 20 mg and *metformin* 2,000 mg per
day; *Previously treated with a sulfonylurea and metformin:* dose to approximate total
daily doses of *glyburide* and *metformin* already being taken; max: *glyburide* 20 mg
and *metformin* 2000 mg per day; same precautions as *glyburide* and *metformin*

    Glucovance

      Tab: Glucovance **1.25/250:** *glyb* 1.25 mg/*met* 250 mg

           Glucovance **2.5/500:** *glyb* 2.5 mg/*met* 500 mg

           Glucovance **5/500:** *glyb* 5 mg/*met* 500 mg

Comment: *metformin* is contraindicated with renal impairment, metabolic acidosis,
and ketoacidosis. Suspend *metformin*, prior to, and for 48 hours after, surgery or
receiving IV iodinated contrast agents.

THIAZOLIDINEDIONE/BIGUANIDE COMBINATION

▶ *pioglitazone/metformin* (C) <12 years: not recommended; ≥12 years: take in
divided doses with meals; *Previously on metformin alone:* initially 15 mg/500 mg
or 15 mg/850 mg once or twice daily; *Previously on pioglitazone alone:* initially
15 mg/500 mg bid; *Previously on pioglitazone and metformin:* switch on a mg/mg
basis; may increase after 8-12 weeks; max: *pioglitazone* 45 mg and *metformin* 2000
mg per day; same precautions as *pioglitazone* and *metformin*

    Actoplus Met, Actoplus Met R (G)

      Tab: Actoplus Met **15/500:** *pio* 15 mg/*met* 500 mg

           Actoplus Met **15/850:** *pio* 15 mg/*met* 850 mg

           Actoplus Met XR **15/1000:** *pio* 15 mg/*met* 1000 mg

           Actoplus Met XR **30/1000:** *pio* 30 mg/*met* 1000 mg

Comment: *metformin* is contraindicated with renal impairment, metabolic acidosis,
ketoacidosis. Suspend *metformin*, prior to, and for 48 hours after, surgery or
receiving IV iodinated contrast agents.

▶ *rosiglitazone/metformin* (C) <12 years: not recommended; ≥12 years: take in
divided doses with meals; *Previously on metformin alone:* add *rosiglitazone* 4
mg/day; may increase after 8-12 weeks; *Previously on rosiglitazone alone:* add
metformin 1000 mg/day; may increase after 1-2 weeks; *Previously on rosiglitazone
and metformin:* switch on a mg/mg basis; may increase *rosiglitazone* by 4 mg and/
or *metformin* by 500 mg per day; max: *rosiglitazone* 8 mg and *metformin* 2,000 mg
per day; same precautions as *rosiglitazone* and *metformin*

    Avandamet

      Tab: Avandamet **2/500:** *rosi* 2 mg/*met* 500 mg

           Avandamet **2/1,000:** *rosi* 2 mg/*met* 1,000 mg

           Avandamet **4/500:** *rosi* 4 mg/*met* 500 mg

           Avandamet **4/1,000:** *rosi* 4 mg/*met* 1,000 mg

Comment: *rosiglitazone* has been withdrawn from retail pharmacies. In order to
enroll and receive *rosiglitazone*, health care providers and patients must enroll in
the *Avandia-Rosiglitazone Medicines Access Program.* The program limits the use
of *rosiglitazone* to patients already being treated successfully, and those whose
blood sugar cannot be controlled with other antidiabetic medicines. *Metformin*

is contraindicated with renal impairment, metabolic acidosis, and ketoacidosis. Suspend **metformin**, prior to, and for 48 hours after, surgery or receiving IV iodinated contrast agents.

THIAZOLIDINEDIONE/SULFONYLUREA COMBINATIONS

▷ *pioglitazone/glimepiride* (C) <18 years: not recommended; ≥18 years: take 1 dose daily with first meal of the day; *Previously on sulfonylurea alone:* initially 30 mg/2 mg; *Previously on **pioglitazone** and **glimepiride**:* switch on a mg/mg basis; max: **pioglitazone** 30 mg and **glimepiride** 4 mg per day; Same precautions as **pioglitazone** and **glimepiride**

    Duetact
        Tab: **Duetact 30/2:** *pio* 30 mg/*glim* 2 mg
                Duetact 304: *pio* 30 mg/*glim* 4 mg

▷ *rosiglitazone/glimepiride* (C) <18 years: not recommended; ≥18 years: take 1 dose daily with first meal of the day; max: **rosiglitazone** 8 mg and **glimepiride** 4 mg per day; same precautions as **rosiglitazone** and **glimepiride**

    Avandaryl
        Tab: **Avandaryl 4/1:** *rosi* 4 mg/*glim* 1 mg
                Avandaryl 4/2: *rosi* 4 mg/*glim* 2 mg
                Avandaryl 4/4: *rosi* 4 mg/*glim* 4 mg
                Avandaryl 8/2: *rosi* 8 mg/*glim* 2 mg
                Avandaryl 8/4: *rosi* 8 mg/*glim* 4 mg

GLUCAGON-LIKE PEPTIDE-1 (GLP-1) RECEPTOR AGONISTS

Comment: GLP-1 receptor agonists act as an agonist at the GLP-1 receptors. They have a longer half-life than the native protein allowing them to be dosed once daily. They increase intracellular cAMP resulting in **insulin** release in the presence of increased serum concentration, decrease **glucagon** secretion, and delay gastric emptying, thus, reducing fasting, premeal, and postprandial glucose throughout the day. GLP-1 receptor agonists are not a substitute for **insulin**, not for treatment of DKA, and not for postprandial administration.

▷ *albiglutide* (C) <18 years: not recommended; ≥18 years: administer by SC injection into the upper arm, abdomen, or thigh once daily; initially 30 mg once weekly on the same day; may increase to max 50 mg once weekly

    Tanzeum *Prefilled pen/syringe:* 30, 50 mg/pen pwdr for injection after reconstitution (4/carton) (preservative-free)

▷ *dulaglutide* (C) <18 years: not recommended; ≥18 years: administer by SC injection into the upper arm, abdomen, or thigh once daily; initially 0.6 mg/day for 1 week; then 1.2 mg/day; may increase to max 1.8 mg/day; if more than 3 days since last dose, restart at 0.6 mg/day and titrate as before

    Trulicity *Prefilled pen/syringe:* 0.75, 1.5 mg/0.5 ml single dose (4/carton)

▷ *exenatide* (C) <18 years: not recommended; ≥18 years: administer by SC injection into the upper arm, abdomen, or thigh

    Bydureon administer 2 mg weekly (every 7 days); inject immediately after mixing; if changing from **Byetta**, discontinue and start *Vial:* 2 mg pwdr for reconstitution (1 vial pwdr and 1 syringe prefilled w. diluents, vial connector, and needles, 4/carton)

    Byetta inject within 60 minutes before AM and PM meals; initially 5 mcg/dose; may increase to 10 mcg/dose after one month

Prefilled pen: 250 mcg/ml (5, 10 mcg/dose; 60 doses, needles not included) (m-cresol, mannitol)

▶ *liraglutide* (C) <18 years: not recommended; ≥18 years: administer by SC injection into the upper arm, abdomen, or thigh once daily; initially 0.6 mg/day for 1 week; then 1.2 mg/day; may increase to 1.8 mg/day

Victoza *Prefilled pen:* 6 mg/ml (3 ml; needles not included)

▶ *lixisenatide* (C) <18 years: not established; ≥18 years: administer SC in the upper arm, abdomen, or thigh once daily; initially 10 mcg SC x 14 days; maintenance: 20 mcg beginning on day 15; administer within one hour of the first meal of the day and the same meal of the day

Adlyxin Soln for SC inj; *Starter Pen:* 50 mcg/ml (14 doses of 10 mcg; 3 ml); *Maintenance Pen:* 100 mcg/ml (14 doses of 20 mcg); *Starter Pack:* 1 prefilled starter pen + 1 prefilled maintenance pen; *Maintenance Pack:* 2 prefilled maintenance pens

Comment: **Adlyxin** is indicated as an adjunct to diet and exercise for T2DM. Not indicated for treatment of T1DM. Do not use with **Victoza**, **Saxenda**, other GLP-1 receptor agonists, or insulin. Contraindicated with gastroparesis and GFR <15 mL/min. Poorly controlled diabetes in pregnancy increases the maternal risk for diabetic ketoacidosis, pre-eclampsia, spontaneous abortions, preterm delivery, stillbirth and delivery complications. Poorly controlled diabetes increases the fetal risk for major birth defects, stillbirth, and macrosomia related morbidity. **Adlyxin** should be used during pregnancy only if the potential benefit justifies the potential risk to the fetus. Estimated background risk of major birth defects and miscarriage in clinically recognized pregnancies is 2-4% and 15-20% respectively.

SODIUM-GLUCOSE CO-TRANSPORTER 2 (SGLT2) INHIBITORS

Comment: SGLT2 inhibitors block the SGLT2 protein involved in 90% of glucose reabsorption in the proximal renal tubule, resulting in increased renal glucose excretion (typically >2000 mg/dL), and lower blood glucose levels (low risk of hypoglycemia), modest weight loss, and mild reduction in blood pressure (probably due to sodium loss). These agents probably also increase insulin sensitivity, decrease gluconeogenesis, and improve *insulin* release from pancreatic beta cells. SGLT2 inhibitors are contraindicated in T1DM, and dose is decreased or contraindicated with decreased GFR, increased SCr, renal failure, ESRD, renal dialysis, metabolic acidosis, or diabetic ketoacidosis. The most common side effects are UTI, female genital mycotic infection, and increased urination. These effects may be managed with adequate hydration and genital hygiene. The SGLT2 inhibitors are not recommended in nursing females. There is potential for a hypersensitivity reaction to include angioedema and anaphylaxis. Caution with SGLT2 use due to reports of increased risk of treatment-emergent bone fractures.

▶ *canagliflozin* (C) <18 years: not recommended; ≥18 years: take one tab before the first meal of the day; initially 100 mg; may titrate up to max 300 mg once daily; *GFR <45 mL/min:* do not initiate

Invokana *Tab:* 100, 300 mg

Comment: **Invokana** is contraindicated with GFR <45 *mL/min;* If GFR 45-≤60 *mL/min,* max 100 mg once daily or consider other antihyperglycemic agents.

▶ *dapagliflozin* (C) <18 years: not recommended; ≥18 years: take one tab before the first meal of the day; initially 5 mg; may increase to max 10 mg once daily

Farxiga *Tab:* 5, 10 mg

Comment: **Farxiga** is contraindicated with GFR <60 mL/min.

▶ *empagliflozin* (C) <18 years: not recommended; ≥18 years: take one tab before the first meal of the day; initially 10 mg; may increase to max 25 mg once daily

Jardiance *Tab:* 10, 25 mg

Comment: **Jardiance** is contraindicated with GFR <45 mL/min.

SODIUM-GLUCOSE CO-TRANSPORTER 2 (SGLT2) INHIBITOR/BIGUANIDE COMBINATIONS

Comment: Caution with **SGLT2** use due to reports of increased risk of treatment-emergent bone fractures. *Metformin* is contraindicated with renal impairment, metabolic acidosis, and ketoacidosis. Suspend *metformin*, prior to, and for 48 hours after, surgery or receiving IV iodinated contrast agents.

▶ *canagliflozin/metformin* (C) <18 years: not recommended; ≥18 years: take 1 dose twice daily with meals; max daily dose 300/2000; *GFR 45-≤60 mL/min: canagliflozin* max 100 mg once daily or consider other antihyperglycemic agents; *GFR <45 mL/min:* do not initiate

Invokamet
> *Tab:* **Invokamet 50/500:** *cana* 50 mg/*met* 500 mg
> **Invokamet 50/1,000:** *cana* 50 mg/*met* 1,000 mg
> **Invokamet 150/500:** *cana* 150 mg/*met* 500 mg
> **Invokamet 150/1,000:** *cana* 150 mg/*met* 1,000 mg

▶ *dapagliflozin/metformin* (C) <18 years: not recommended; ≥18 years: swallow whole; do not crush or chew; take once daily first meal of the day; max daily dose 10/2000

Xigduo XR
> *Tab:* **Xigduo XR 5/500:** *dapa* 5 mg/*met* 500 mg ext-rel
> **Xigduo XR 5/1000:** *dapa* 5 mg/*met* 1000 mg ext-rel
> **Xigduo XR 10/500:** *dapa* 10 mg/*met* 500 mg ext-rel
> **Xigduo XR 10/1000:** *dapa* 10 mg/*met* 1000 mg ext-rel

Comment: **Xigduo** is contraindicated with GFR <60 *mL/min*, SCr >1.5 (males) or SCr >1.4 (females)

▶ *empagliflozin/metformin* (C) <18 years: not recommended; ≥18 years: take 1 dose twice daily with meals; max daily dose 25/2000

Synjardy
> *Tab:* **Synjardy 5/500:** *empa* 5 mg/*met* 500 mg
> **Synjardy 5/1000:** *empa* 5 mg/*met* 1000 mg
> **Synjardy 12.5/500:** *empa* 12.5 mg/*met* 500 mg
> **Synjardy 12.5/1000:** *empa* 12.5 mg/*met* 1000 mg

Synjardy XR
> *Tab:* **Synjardy XR 5/1000:** *empa* 5 mg/*met* 1000 mg
> **Synjardy XR 12.5/1000:** *empa* 12.5 mg/*met* 1000 mg
> **Synjardy XR 10/1000:** *empa* 10 mg/*met* 1000 mg
> **Synjardy XR 25/1000:** *empa* 25 mg/*met* 1000 mg

Comment: **Synjardy** is contraindicated with *GFR <45 mL/min, SCr* >1.5 (males), or *SCr* >1.4 (females).

SODIUM-GLUCOSE CO-TRANSPORTER 2 (SGLT2) INHIBITOR/DIPEPTIDYL PEPTIDASE-4 (DPP-4) INHIBITOR COMBINATIONS

Comment: Caution with **SGLT2** use due to reports of increased risk of treatment-emergent bone fractures. DPP-4 inhibitors have been associated with a risk of developing and exacerbating acute pancreatitis.

▶ *dapagliflozin/saxagliptin* (C) <18 years: not established; ≥18 years: initially 5/10 once daily, at any time of day, with or without food; if a dose is missed and it is ≥12 hours until the next dose, the dose should be taken; if a dose is missed and it is <12 hours until the next dose, the missed dose should be skipped and the next dose taken at the usual time.

Qtern *Tab:* dapa 10 mg/*saxa* 5 mg film-coat

Comment: **Qtern** should not be used during pregnancy. If pregnancy is detected, treatment with **Qtern** should be discontinued. It is unknown whether **Qtern** and/or its metabolites are excreted in human milk. Do not use with CrCl <60 mL/min or eGFR <60 mL/min/1.73 m² or ESRD or severe hepatic impairment or history of pancreatitis.

▶ *empagliflozin/linagliptin* (C) <18 years: not recommended; ≥18 years: initially 10/5 once daily with the first meal of the day; max daily dose 25/5; *GFR <45 mL/min:* contraindicated

Glyxambi
Tab: **Glyxambi 10/5:** *empa* 10 mg/*lina* 5 mg
Glyxambi 25/5: *empa* 25 mg/*lina* 5 mg

DIPEPTIDYL PEPTIDASE-4 (DPP-4) INHIBITOR

Comment: DPP-4 is an enzyme that degrades incretin hormones glucagon-like peptide-1 (GLP-1) and glucose-dependent insulinotropic polypeptide (GIP). Thus, DPP-4 inhibitors increase the concentration of active incretin hormones, stimulating the release of **insulin** in a glucose-dependent manner and decreasing the levels of circulating **glucagon**. The FDA has reported that *saxagliptin-* and *alogliptin-* containing drugs may increase the risk of heart failure, especially in patients who already have cardiovascular or renal disease. Drugs in this risk group include **Nesina** (*alogliptin*) and **Onglyza** (*saxagliptin*)

▶ *alogliptin* (B) <18 years: not recommended; ≥18 years: take twice daily with meals; max 25 mg/day
Nesina *Tab:* 6.25, 12.5, 25 mg
▶ *linagliptin* (B) <18 years: not recommended; ≥18 years: 5 mg once daily
Tradjenta *Tab:* 5 mg
▶ *saxagliptin* (B) <18 years: not recommended; ≥18 years: 2.5-5 mg once daily
Onglyza *Tab:* 2.5, 5 mg
▶ *sitagliptin* (B) <18 years: not recommended; ≥18 years: as monotherapy or as combination therapy with metformin or a TZD
Januvia 25-100 mg once daily
Tab: 25, 50, 100 mg

DIPEPTIDYL PEPTIDASE-4 (DPP-4) INHIBITOR/BIGUANIDE COMBINATIONS

Comment: DPP-4 inhibitor/*metformin* combinations are contraindicated with renal impairment (males: SCr ≥1.5 mg/dL; females: SCr ≥1.4 mg/dL) or abnormal CrCl, metabolic acidosis, ketoacidosis, or history of angioedema. Suspend *metformin*, prior to, and for 48 hours after, surgery or receiving IV iodinated contrast agents. Avoid in the malnourished, dehydrated, or with clinical or lab evidence of hepatic disease. For other DPP-4 and/or *metformin* precautions, see mfr pkg insert. The FDA has reported that *saxagliptin*- and *alogliptin*-containing drugs may increase the risk of heart failure, especially in patients who already have cardiovascular or renal disease. These drugs include: **Onglyza** (*saxagliptin*), **Kombiglyze XR** (*saxagliptin/metformin*), **Nesina** (*alogliptin*), **Kazano** (*alogliptin/metformin*), and **Oseni** (*alogliptin/pioglitazone*).

▷ *alogliptin/metformin* (B) <18 years: not recommended; ≥18 years: take twice daily with meals; max *alogliptin* 25 mg/day, max *metformin* 2000 mg/day

    Kazano

        Tab: **Kazano 12.5/500:** *algo* 12.5 mg/*met* 500 mg

           Kazano 2.5/1000: *algo* 12.5 mg/*met* 1000 mg

▷ *linagliptin/metformin* (B) <18 years: not recommended; ≥18 years:

    Jentadueto take twice daily with meals; max *linagliptin* 5 mg/day, max *metformin* 2000 mg/day

        Tab: **Jentadueto 2.5/500:** *lina* 2.5 mg/*met* 500 mg film-coat

           Jentadueto 2.5/850: *lina* 2.5 mg/*met* 850 mg film-coat

           Jentadueto 2.5/1000: *lina* 2.5 mg/*met* 1,000 mg film-coat

    Jentadueto XR *Currently not treated with **metformin**:* initiate **Jentadueto XR 5/1,000** once daily; *Already treated with **metformin**:* initiate **Jentadueto XR** 5 mg *linagliptin* total daily dose and a similar total daily dose of *metformin* once daily; *Already treated with **linagliptin** and **metformin** or **Jentadueto**:* switch to **Jentadueto XR** containing 5 mg of *linagliptin* total daily dose and a similar total daily dose of *metformin* once daily; max *linagliptin 5 mg* and *metformin* 2,000 mg; take as a single dose once daily; take with food; do not crush or chew; *eGFR <30 mL/min:* contraindicated; *eGFR 30-45 mL/min:* not recommended

        Tab: **Jentadueto 2.5/1000:** *lina* 2.5 mg/*met* 1,000 mg film-coat ext-rel

           Jentadueto 5/1000: *lina* 5 mg/*met* 1,000 mg film-coat ext-rel

▷ *saxagliptin/metformin* (B) <18 years: not recommended; ≥18 years: take once daily with meals; max *saxagliptin* 5 mg/day, max *metformin* 2000 mg/day; do not crush or chew

    Kombiglyze XR

        Tab: **Kombiglyze XR 5/500:** *saxa* 5 mg/*met* 500 mg

           Kombiglyze XR 2.5/1000: *saxa* 2.5 mg/*met* 1000 mg

           Kombiglyze XR 5/1000: *saxa* 5 mg/*met* 1000 mg

Comment: The FDA has reported that *saxagliptin*-containing drugs may increase the risk of heart failure, especially in patients who already have cardiovascular or renal disease. The drug **Kombiglyze XR** (*saxagliptin/metformin*) is in this risk group. *Metformin* is contraindicated with renal impairment, metabolic acidosis, and ketoacidosis. Suspend *metformin*, prior to, and for 48 hours after, surgery or receiving IV iodinated contrast agents.

▷ *sitagliptin/metformin* (B) <18 years: not recommended; ≥18 years: take twice daily with meals; max *sitagliptin* 100 mg/day, max *metformin* 2000 mg/day

    Janumet

        Tab: **Janumet 50/500:** *sita* 50 mg/*met* 500 mg

           Janumet 50/1000: *sita* 50 mg/*met* 1000 mg

    Janumet XR

        Tab: **Janumet XR 50/500:** *sita* 50 mg/*met* 500 mg ext-rel

           Janumet XR 50/1000: *sita* 50 mg/*met* 1000 mg ext-rel

Janumet XR 100/1000: *sita* 100 mg/*met* 1000 mg ext-rel

Comment: *metformin* is contraindicated with renal impairment, metabolic acidosis, and ketoacidosis. Suspend *metformin*, prior to, and for 48 hours after, surgery or receiving IV iodinated contrast agents.

MEGLITINIDE/BIGUANIDE COMBINATION

▷ *repaglinide/metformin* (C)(G) <12 years: not recommended; ≥12 years: take in 2-3 divided doses within 30 minutes before food; max 4/1000 per meal and 10/2000 per day

Prandimet
Tab: **Prandimet 1/500:** *repa* 1 mg/*met* 500 mg
Prandimet 2/500: *repa* 2 mg/*met* 500 mg

Comment: *metformin* is contraindicated with renal impairment, metabolic acidosis, and ketoacidosis. Suspend *metformin*, prior to, and for 48 hours after, surgery or receiving IV iodinated contrast agents.

DIPEPTIDYL PEPTIDASE-4 (DPP-4) INHIBITOR/HMG-COA REDUCTASE INHIBITOR COMBINATION

▷ *sitagliptin/simvastatin* (B) <18 years: not recommended; ≥18 years: take once daily in the PM; swallow whole; adjust dose if needed after 4 weeks; *Concomitant verapamil* or *diltiazem*: max 100/10 once daily; *Concomitant amiodarone, amlodipine,* or *ranolazine:* max 100/20 once daily; *HoFH:* max 100/40 once daily; *Chinese patients taking lipid-modifying doses (>1 gm/day niacin) of niacin-containing products:* caution with 100/40 dose; increase risk of myopathy

Juvisync
Tab: **Juvisync 100/10:** *sita* 100 mg/*simva* 10 mg
Juvisync 100/20: *sita* 100 mg/*simva* 20 mg
Juvisync 100/40: *sita* 100 mg/*simva* 40 mg

DOPAMINE RECEPTOR AGONIST

▷ *bromocriptine mesylate* (B) <12 years: not recommended; ≥12 years: take with food in the morning within 2 hours of waking; initially 0.8 mg once daily; may increase by 0.8 mg/week; max 4.8 mg/week; *Severe psychotic disorders:* not recommended
Cycloset *Tab:* 0.8 mg
Comment: **Cycloset** is an adjunct to diet and exercise to improve glycemic control. Contraindicated with syncopal migraines, nursing mothers, and other ergot-related drugs.

Bile Acid Sequestrant

▷ *colesevelam* (B) <12 years: not recommended; ≥12 years: *Monotherapy:* 3 tabs bid or 6 tabs once daily or one 1.875 gm pkt bid or one 3.75 gm pkt once daily
WelChol *Tab:* 625 mg; *Pwdr for oral susp:* 1.875 gm pwdr pkts (60/carton); 3.75 gm pwdr pkts (30/carton) (citrus; phenylalanine)
Comment: *colesevelam* (WelChol) is indicated as an adjunctive therapy to improve glycemic control in older adolescents ≥18 years with type 2 diabetes. It can be added to *metformin*, sulfonylureas, or *insulin* alone or in combination with other antidiabetic agents.

TYPHOID FEVER (*SALMONELLA TYPHI*)

PRE-EXPOSURE PROPHYLAXIS

➤ *typhoid* vaccine, oral, live, attenuated strain

Vivotif Berna <6 years: not recommended; ≥6 years: 1 cap every other day, 1 hour before a meal, with a lukewarm (not > body temperature) or cold drink for a total of 4 doses; do not crush or chew; complete therapy at least 1 week prior to expected exposure; reimmunization recommended every 5 years if repeated exposure

Cap: ent-coat

➤ *typhoid* **Vi polysaccharide** vaccine (C) <2 years: not recommended; ≥2 years:

Typhim Vi 0.5 ml IM in deltoid; reimmunization recommended every 2 years if repeated exposure

Vial: 20, 50 dose; *Prefilled syringe:* 0.5 ml

Comment: Febrile illness may require delaying administration of the vaccine; have *epinephrine* 1:1000 readily available.

TREATMENT

➤ *azithromycin* (B) 8-10 mg/kg/day; max 500 mg/day; *Mild Illness:* treat x 7 days; *Severe Illness:* treat x 14 days; *see page 548 for dose by weight table*

Zithromax *Tab:* 250, 500, 600 mg; *Oral susp:* 100 mg/5 ml (15 ml); 200 mg/5 ml (15, 22.5, 30 ml) (cherry); *Pkt:* 1 gm for reconstitution (cherry-banana)

Zithromax Tri-pak *Tab:* 3 x 500 mg tabs/pck

Zithromax Z-pak *Tab:* 6 x 250 mg tabs/pck

Zmax *Oral susp:* 2 gm ext-rel for reconstitution (cherry-banana) (148 mg Na$^+$)

➤ *cefixime* (B)(G) <6 months: not recommended; 6 months-12 years, <50 kg: 8 mg/kg/day in 1-2 divided doses x 10 days; *see page 552 for dose by weight table;* >12 years, >50 kg: *Mild illness:* 15-20 mg/kg/day x 7-14 days; *Severe illness:* 20 mg/kg/day x 10-14 days

Suprax *Tab:* 400 mg; *Cap:* 400 mg; *Oral susp:* 100, 200, 500 mg/5 ml (50, 75, 100 ml) (strawberry)

➤ *ciprofloxacin* (C) <18 years: not recommended; ≥18 years: 15 mg/kg/day; *Mild illness:* treat x 5-7 days; *Severe illness:* treat x 10-14 days; max 1.5 gm/day

Cipro (G) *Tab:* 250, 500, 750 mg; *Oral susp:* 250, 500 mg/5 ml (100 ml) (strawberry)

Cipro XR *Tab:* 500, 1000 mg ext-rel

ProQuin XR *Tab:* 500 mg ext-rel

Comment: *ciprofloxacin* is contraindicated <18 years-of-age, and during pregnancy and lactation. Risk of tendonitis or tendon rupture.

➤ *ofloxacin* (C) <18 years: not recommended; ≥18 years: 15 mg/kg/day; *Mild Illness:* treat x 5-7 days; *Severe Illness:* treat x 10-14 days

Floxin *Tab:* 200, 300, 400 mg

Comment: *ofloxacin* is contraindicated <18 years-of-age, and during pregnancy and lactation. Risk of tendonitis or tendon rupture.

➤ *cefotaxime* 80 mg/kg/day IM/IV x 10-14 days; max 2 gm/day

Claforan *Vial:* 500 mg; 1, 2 g

➤ *ceftriaxone* (B)(G) 75 mg/kg/day IM/IV x 10-14 days; max 2 gm/day

Rocephin *Vial:* 250, 500 mg; 1, 2 gm

▷ *trimethoprim/sulfamethoxazole* (D)(G)

Bactrim, Septra <12 years: not recommended; ≥12 years: 2 tabs bid x 10 days
Tab: trim 80 mg/*sulfa* 400 mg*
Bactrim DS, Septra DS <12 years: not recommended; ≥12 years: 1 tab bid x 10 days
Tab: trim 160 mg/*sulfa* 800 mg*
Bactrim Pediatric Suspension, Septra Pediatric Suspension <2 months: not recommended; ≥2 months-12 years: 40 mg/kg/day of *sulfamethoxazole* in 2 doses bid; >12 years: use tabs
Oral susp: trim 40 mg/*sulfa* 200 mg per 5 ml (100 ml) (cherry) (alcohol 0.3%)

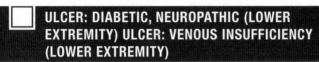

ULCER: DIABETIC, NEUROPATHIC (LOWER EXTREMITY) ULCER: VENOUS INSUFFICIENCY (LOWER EXTREMITY)

NUTRITIONAL SUPPLEMENT

▷ *L-methylfolate calcium (as metafolin)/pyridoxyl 5-phosphate/methylcobalamin* (NE) <12 years: not recommended; ≥12 years: take 1 cap daily

Metanx *Cap:* metafo 3 mg/*pyrid* 35 mg/*methyl* 2 mg (gluten-free, yeast-free, lactose-free)

Comment: Metanx is indicated as adjunct treatment of endothelial dysfunction and/or hyperhomocysteinemia in patients who have lower extremity ulceration.

DEBRIDING/CAPILLARY STIMULANT AGENT

▷ *trypsin/balsam peru/castor oil* (NE) apply at least twice daily; may cover with a wet dressing

Granulex *Aerosol liq:* tryp 0.12 mg/*bal peru* 87 mg/*cast* 788 mg per 0.82 ml

GROWTH FACTOR

▷ *becaplermin* (C) apply once daily with a cotton swab or tongue depressor; then, cover with saline moistened gauze dressing; rinse after 12 hours; then, re-cover with a clean saline dressing

Regranex *Gel:* 0.01% (2, 7.5, 15 gm) (parabens)

Comment: Store in refrigerator; do not freeze. Not for use with wounds that close by primary intention.

ULCER: PRESSURE/DECUBITUS

DEBRIDING/CAPILLARY STIMULANT AGENT

Granulex (*trypsin* 0.1 mg/*balsam peru* 72.5 mg/*castor oil* 650 mg per 0.82 ml) apply at least twice daily; may cover with a wet dressing
Aerosol liq: (2, 4 oz)

GROWTH FACTOR

➤ *becaplermin* (C) apply once daily with a cotton swab <u>or</u> tongue depressor; then cover with saline moistened gauze dressing; rinse after 12 hours; then recover with a clean saline dressing

> **Regranex** *Gel:* 0.01% (2, 7.5, 15 gm) (parabens)

Comment: Store in refrigerator; do not freeze. Not for use in wounds that close by primary intention.

ULCERATIVE COLITIS

Comment: Standard treatment regimen is anti-infective, antispasmodic, and bowel rest; progressing to clear liquids; then to high fiber.

Parenteral Corticosteroids *see page 499*
Oral Corticosteroids *see page 498*

➤ *budesonide micronized* (C)(G) <12 years: not recommended; ≥12 years: 9 mg once daily in the AM for up to 8 weeks; may repeat an 8-week course; *Maintenance of remission:* 6 mg once daily for up to 3 months; taper other systemic steroids when transferring to *budesonide*

> **Entocort EC** *Cap:* 3 mg ent-coat granules
> **Uceris** *Tab:* 9 mg ext-rel

RECTAL CORTICOSTEROIDS

➤ *hydrocortisone* rectal (C) <12 years: not recommended; ≥12 years:

> **Anusol-HC Suppositories** 1 supp rectally 3 times daily <u>or</u> 2 supp rectally twice daily for 2 weeks; max 8 weeks
> > *Rectal supp:* 25 mg (12, 24/pck)
>
> **Cortenema** 1 enema q HS x 21 days <u>or</u> until symptoms controlled
> > *Enema:* 100 mg/60 ml (1, 7/pck)
>
> **Cortifoam** 1 applicator full qd-bid x 2-3 weeks and every 2nd day thereafter until symptoms are controlled
> > *Aerosol:* 80 mg/applicator (14 applications/container)
>
> **Proctocort** 1 supp rectally in AM and PM x 2 weeks; for more severe cases, may increase to 1 supp rectally 3 times daily <u>or</u> 2 supp rectally twice daily; max 4-8 weeks
> > *Rectal supp:* 30 mg (12, 24/pck)

Comment: Use *hydrocortisone* foam as adjunctive therapy in the distal portion of the rectum when *hydrocortisone* enemas cannot be retained.

RECTAL CORTICOSTEROID/ANESTHETIC

Hydrocortisone/Pramoxine

> **Proctofoam HC** apply to anal/rectal area 3-4 times daily; max 4-8 weeks
> > *Rectal foam: hydrocort* 1%/*pram* 1% (10 gm w. applicator)

SALICYLATES

➤ *balsalazide disodium* (B)

> **Colazal** <5 years: not recommended; ≥5 years: 2.25 gm 3 times daily <u>or</u> 750 mg once daily x 8 weeks; swallow whole <u>or</u> sprinkle contents into applesauce

Cap: 750 mg

Comment: *balsalazide* 6.75 gm provides 2.4 gm of *mesalamine* to the colon.

Giazo take <18 years: not established; ≥18 years: 3 tabs bid; max 8 weeks
Tab: 1.1 gm (sodium 126 mg/tab) film-coat

▷ *mesalamine* (B) <12 years: not recommended; ≥12 years:

Apriso take 1.5 gm once daily in the AM for maintenance of remission
Cap: 0.375 gm ext-rel (phenylalanine 0.56 mg/cap)

Asacol HD 1600 mg tid x 6 weeks; maintenance 1.6 gm/day in divided doses; swallow whole; do not crush or chew
Tab: 800 mg del-rel

Canasa 1 gm qid for up to 8 weeks
Rectal supp: 1 gm del-rel (30, 42/pck)

Delzicol 800 mg tid x 6 weeks; maintenance once daily for up to 8 weeks; *Maintenance:* 1.6 gm/day in 2-4 divided doses once daily; swallow whole; do not crush or chew
Cap: 400 mg del-rel

Lialda 2.4-4.8 gm once daily for up to 8 weeks; maintenance 2.4 gm once daily; swallow whole; do not crush or chew
Tab: 1.2 gm del-rel

Pentasa 1 gm qid for up to 8 weeks
Cap: 250, 500 mg cont-rel

Rowasa Suppository 1 supp rectally bid x 3-6 weeks; retain for 1-3 hours or longer
Rectal supp: 500 mg (12, 24/pck)

Sulfite-Free Rowasa Rectal Suspension 4 gm rectally by enema q HS; retain for 8 hours x 3-6 weeks
Enema: 4 gm/60 ml (7, 14, 28/pck; kit, 7, 14, 28/pck w. wipes)

▷ *olsalazine* (C) 1 gm/day in 2 divided doses
Dipentum *Cap:* 250 mg

▷ *sulfasalazine* (B; D in 2nd, 3rd)(G) <2 years: not recommended; 2-16 years: initially 40-60 mg/kg/day in 3 to 6 divided doses; max 30 mg/kg/day in 4 divided doses; max 2 gm/day; >16 years:

Azulfidine initially 1-2 gm/day; increase to 3-4 gm/day in divided doses pc until clinical symptoms controlled; maintenance 2 gm/day; max 4 gm/day
Tab: 500*mg

Azulfidine EN-Tabs initially 500 mg in the PM x 7 days; then 500 mg bid x 7 days; then 500 mg in the AM and 1 gm in the PM x 7 days; then 1 gm bid; max 4 gm/day
Tab: 500 mg ent-coat

TUMOR NECROSIS FACTOR (TNF) BLOCKER

▷ *adalimumab* (B) <18 years: not recommended; ≥18 years: initially 180 mg SC (as 4 injections in 1 day or divided over 2 days) on week 0; then 80 mg at week 2; start 40 mg every other week maintenance at week 4; only continue if evidence of clinical remission by 8 weeks; administer in abdomen or thigh; rotate sites
Humira *Prefilled syringe:* 20 mg/0.4 ml; 40 mg/0.8 ml single dose (2/pck; 2, 6/ starter pck) (preservative-free)

▷ *infliximab* (B) <6 years: not recommended; ≥6 years: administer by IV infusion over 2 hours; 5 mg/kg weeks 0, 2, 6; then once every 8 weeks

Remicade
Vial: 100 mg pwdr for reconstitution for IV infusion (preservative-free)
▷ *vedolizumab* (B) <18 years: not recommended; ≥18 years: administer by IV infusion over 30 minutes; 300 mg at weeks 0, 2, 6; then once every 8 weeks
Entyvio
Vial: 300 mg (20 ml) single dose, pwdr for IV infusion after reconstitution (preservative-free)

ANTIDIARRHEAL AGENTS

▷ *difenoxin/atropine* (C) 2 tabs; then 1 tab after each loose stool or 1 tab q 3-4 hours; max 8 tabs/day x 2 days
Motofen *Tab:* dif 1 mg/*atro* 0.025 mg
▷ *diphenoxylate/atropine* (C)(G) 2 tabs or 10 ml qid
Lomotil *Tab:* diphen 2.5 mg/*atro* 0.025 mg; *Liq:* diphen 2.5 mg/*atro* 0.025 mg/5 ml (2 oz w. dropper)
▷ *loperamide* (B)(G)
Imodium (OTC) 4 mg initially; then 2 mg after each loose stool; max 16 mg/day
Cap: 2 mg
Imodium A-D (OTC) 4 mg initially; then 2 mg after each loose stool; usual max 8 mg/day x 2 days
Cplt: 2 mg; *Liq:* 1 mg/5 ml (2, 4 oz)
▷ *loperamide/simethicone* (B)(G)
Imodium Advanced (OTC) 2 tabs chewed after first loose stool; then 1 after the next loose stool; max 4 tabs/day
Chew tab: loper 2 mg/simeth 125 mg

URETHRITIS: NON-GONOCOCCAL (NGU)

Comment: The following treatment regimens for NGU are published in the **2015 CDC Sexually Transmitted Diseases Treatment Guidelines**. Treatment regimens are for patients ≥18 years-of-age; consult a specialist for treatment of patients <18 years-of-age. Treatment regimens are presented by generic drug name first, followed by information about brands and dose forms. All persons who have confirmed or suspected urethritis should be tested for gonorrhea and chlamydia. Males treated for NGU should be instructed to abstain from sexual intercourse for 7 days after a single-dose regimen or until completion of a 7-day regimen.

RECOMMENDED REGIMEN: UNCOMPLICATED NGU

▷ *azithromycin* 1 gm in a single dose or 100 mg orally bid x 7 days
plus
▷ *doxycycline* 100 mg bid x 7 days

PERSISTENT/RECURRENT NGU

Males Initially Treated With Azithromycin+Doxycycline

▷ *azithromycin* 1 gm PO in a single dose

Males Who Fail a Regimen of Azithromycin

▷ *moxifloxacin* 400 mg PO once daily x 7 days

Heterosexual Males Who Live in Areas Where T. Vaginalis is Highly Prevalent

▷ *metronidazole* 2 gm PO in a single dose
   or
▷ *tinidazole* 2 gm PO in a single dose

ALTERNATIVE REGIMENS

▷ *erythromycin base* 500 mg PO qid x 7 days
   or
▷ *erythromycin ethylsuccinate* 800 mg PO qid x 7 days
   or
▷ *levofloxacin* 500 mg once daily x 7 days
   or
▷ *ofloxacin* 300 mg PO bid x 7 days

DRUG BRANDS AND DOSE FORMS

▷ *azithromycin* (B)
   Zithromax *Tab:* 250, 500, 600 mg; *Oral susp:* 100 mg/5 ml (15 ml); 200 mg/5 ml (15, 22.5, 30 ml) (cherry); *Pkt:* 1 gm for reconstitution (cherry-banana)
   Zithromax Tri-pak *Tab:* 3 x 500 mg tabs/pck
   Zithromax Z-pak *Tab:* 6 x 250 mg tabs/pck
   Zmax *Oral susp:* 2 gm ext-rel for reconstitution (cherry-banana) (148 mg Na$^+$)
▷ *doxycycline* (D)(G)
   Acticlate *Tab:* 75, 150**mg
   Adoxa *Tab:* 50, 75, 100, 150 mg ent-coat
   Doryx *Tab:* 50, 75, 100, 150, 200 mg del-rel
   Monodox *Cap:* 50, 75, 100 mg
   Oracea *Cap:* 40 mg del-rel
   Vibramycin *Tab:* 100 mg; *Cap:* 50, 100 mg; *Syr:* 50 mg/5 ml (raspberry-apple) (sulfites); *Oral susp:* 25 mg/5 ml (raspberry)
   Vibra-Tab *Tab:* 100 mg film-coat
   Comment: *doxycycline* is contraindicated <8 years-of-age, in pregnancy, and lactation (discolors developing tooth enamel). A side effect may be photo-sensitivity (photophobia). Do not take with antacids, calcium supplements, milk or other dairy, or within 2 hours of taking another drug.
▷ *erythromycin base* (B)
   Ery-Tab *Tab:* 250, 333, 500 mg ent-coat
   PCE *Tab:* 333, 500 mg
▷ *erythromycin ethylsuccinate* (B)(G)
   EryPed *Oral susp:* 200 mg/5 ml (100, 200 ml) (fruit); 400 mg/5 ml (60, 100, 200 ml) (banana); *Oral drops:* 200, 400 mg/5 ml (50 ml) (fruit); *Chew tab:* 200 mg wafer (fruit)
   E.E.S. *Oral susp:* 200, 400 mg/5 ml (100 ml) (fruit)
   E.E.S. Granules *Oral susp:* 200 mg/5 ml (100, 200 ml) (cherry)

  E.E.S. 400 Tablets *Tab:* 400 mg
➤ *levofloxacin* (C)
  Levaquin *Tab:* 250, 500, 750 mg; *Oral soln:* 25 mg/ml (480 ml) (benzyl alcohol); *Inj conc:* 25 mg/ml for IV infusion after dilution (20, 30 ml single-use vial) (preservative-free); *Premix soln:* 5 mg/ml for IV infusion (50, 100, 150 ml) (preservative-free)

Comment: *levofloxacin* is contraindicated <18 years-of-age, and during pregnancy and lactation. Risk of tendonitis <u>or</u> tendon rupture.

➤ *metronidazole* (**not for use in 1st; B in 2nd, 3rd**)(G)
  Flagyl *Tab:* 250*, 500*mg
  Flagyl 375 *Cap:* 375 mg
  Flagyl ER *Tab:* 750 mg ext-rel

Comment: Alcohol is contraindicated during treatment with oral *metronidazole* and for 72 hours after therapy due to a possible *disulfiram*-like reaction (nausea, vomiting, flushing, headache).

➤ *moxifloxacin* (C)(G)
  Avelox *Tab:* 400 mg

Comment: *moxifloxacin* is contraindicated <18 years-of-age, and during pregnancy and lactation. Risk of tendonitis <u>or</u> tendon rupture.

➤ *ofloxacin* (C)(G)
  Floxin *Tab:* 200, 300, 400 mg

Comment: *ofloxacin* is contraindicated <18 years-of-age, and during pregnancy and lactation. Risk of tendonitis <u>or</u> tendon rupture.

➤ *tinidazole* (**not for use in 1st; B in 2nd, 3rd**)
  Tindamax *Tab:* 250*, 500*mg

URINARY RETENTION: UNOBSTRUCTIVE

➤ *bethanechol* (C) 10-30 mg tid
  Urecholine *Tab:* 5, 10, 25, 50 mg
  Comment: Contraindicated in presence of urinary obstruction. *Atropine* 0.4 mg administered SC reverses the effects of *bethanechol*.

URINARY TRACT INFECTION (UTI, CYSTITIS: ACUTE)

URINARY TRACT ANALGESIA

➤ *phenazopyridine* (B)(G) <12 years: not recommended; ≥12 years: 95-200 mg q 6 hours prn; max 2 days
  AZO Standard, Prodium, Uristat (OTC) *Tab:* 95 mg
  AZO Standard Maximum Strength (OTC) *Tab:* 97.5 mg
  Pyridium, Urogesic *Tab:* 100, 200 mg

ANTI-INFECTIVES

➤ *amoxicillin/clavulanate* (B)(G)
  Augmentin <40 kg: 40-45 mg/kg/day divided tid x 10 days <u>or</u> 90 mg/kg/day divided bid x 10 days; *see page 545 for dose by weight table;* ≥40 kg: 500 mg tid <u>or</u> bid x 10 days

Tab: 250, 500, 875 mg; *Chew tab:* 125, 250 mg (lemon-lime); 200, 400 mg (cherry-banana) (phenylalanine); *Oral susp:* 125 mg/5 ml (banana), 250 mg/5 ml (75, 100, 150 ml) (orange); 200, 400 mg/5 ml (50, 75, 100 ml) (orange) (phenylalanine)

Augmentin ES-600 <3 months: not recommended; ≥3 months, <40 kg: 90 mg/kg/day divided q 12 hours x 10 days; *see page 546 for dose by weight table;* ≥40 kg: not recommended

Oral susp: 600 mg/5 ml (50, 75, 100, 125, 150, 200 ml) (strawberry cream) (phenylalanine)

Augmentin XR <16 years: use other forms; ≥16 years: 2 tabs q 12 hours x 7-10 days

Tab: 1000*mg ext-rel

➤ *ciprofloxacin* (C) <18 years: 20-40 mg/kg/day divided q 12 hours; ≥18 years: 500 mg bid x 7-10 days; max 1.5 gm/day

Cipro (G) *Tab:* 250, 500, 750 mg; *Oral susp:* 250, 500 mg/5 ml (100 ml) (strawberry)

Cipro XR *Tab:* 500, 1000 mg ext-rel

ProQuin XR *Tab:* 500 mg ext-rel

Comment: *ciprofloxacin* is contraindicated <18 years-of-age, and during pregnancy and lactation. However, in the case of <u>complicated</u> UTI, it is indicated for patients <18 years-of-age and dosed based on mg/kg body weight. Risk of tendonitis <u>or</u> tendon rupture.

➤ *fosfomycin* (B) 1 pkt in 3-4 oz cold water x 1 dose

Monurol *Single-dose pkts:* 1-3 gm (mandarin orange) (sucrose)

➤ *levofloxacin* (C) <18 years: not recommended; ≥18 years: 250 mg once daily x 3 days

Levaquin *Tab:* 250, 500, 750 mg; *Oral soln:* 25 mg/ml (480 ml) (benzyl alcohol); *Inj conc:* 25 mg/ml for IV infusion after dilution (20, 30 ml single-use vial) (preservative-free); *Premix soln:* 5 mg/ml for IV infusion (50, 100, 150 ml) (preservative-free)

Comment: *levofloxacin* is contraindicated <18 years-of-age, and during pregnancy and lactation. Risk of tendonitis <u>or</u> tendon rupture.

➤ *norfloxacin* (C) <18 years: not recommended; ≥18 years: 400 mg once daily x 3 days

Noroxin *Tab:* 400 mg

Comment: *norfloxacin* is contraindicated <18 years-of-age, and during pregnancy and lactation. Risk of tendonitis <u>or</u> tendon rupture.

➤ *ofloxacin* (C)(G) <18 years: not recommended; ≥18 years: 200 mg q 12 hours x 3 days

Floxin *Tab:* 200, 300, 400 mg

Floxin UroPak *Tab:* 200 mg (6/pck)

Comment: *ofloxacin* is contraindicated <18 years-of-age, and during pregnancy and lactation. Risk of tendonitis <u>or</u> tendon rupture.

➤ *trimethoprim* (C)(G)

Primsol <6 months: not recommended; ≥6 months-12 years: 10 mg/kg/day in 2 divided doses x 10 days; >12 years: 100 mg q 12 hours <u>or</u> 200 mg once daily x 10 days

Oral soln: 50 mg/5 ml (bubble gum) (dye-free, alcohol-free)

Proloprim <12 years: not recommended; ≥12 years: 100 mg q 12 hours <u>or</u> 200 mg once daily x 10 days

Tab: 100, 200 mg

Trimpex <12 years: not recommended; ≥12 years: 100 mg q 12 hours or 200 mg once daily x 10 days
Tab: 100 mg

▷ *trimethoprim/sulfamethoxazole* (D)(G)

Bactrim, Septra <12 years: not recommended; ≥12 years: 2 tabs bid x 10 days
Tab: trim 80 mg/*sulfa* 400 mg*

Bactrim DS, Septra DS <12 years: not recommended; ≥12 years: 1 tab bid x 10 days
Tab: trim 160 mg/*sulfa* 800 mg*

Bactrim Pediatric Suspension, Septra Pediatric Suspension <2 months: not recommended; ≥2 months-12 years: 40 mg/kg/day of *sulfamethoxazole* in 2 doses bid; >12 years: use tabs
Oral susp: trim 40 mg/*sulfa* 200 mg per 5 ml (100 ml) (cherry) (alcohol 0.3%)

ANTI-INFECTIVES: STANDARD REGIMEN FOR UTI

▷ *acetyl sulfisoxazole* (C)(G)

Gantrisin <12 years: not recommended; ≥12 years: initially 2-4 gm in a single or divided doses; then 4-8 gm/day in 4-6 divided doses x 7 days
Tab: 500 mg

Gantrisin <2 months: not recommended; ≥2 months: initial dose 75 mg/kg/day; then 150 mg/kg/day in 4-6 divided doses x 7 days; max 6 gm/day
Oral susp: 500 mg/5 ml (4, 16 oz); *Syr:* 500 mg/5 ml (16 oz)

▷ *amoxicillin* (B)(G) <40 kg (88 lb): 20-40 mg/kg/day in 3 divided doses x 10 days or 25-45 mg/kg/day in 2 divided doses x 10 days; *see page 543 for dose by weight table;* ≥40 kg: 500-875 mg bid or 250-500 mg tid x 10 days

Amoxil *Cap:* 250, 500 mg; *Tab:* 875*mg; *Chew tab:* 125, 200, 250, 400 mg (cherry-banana-peppermint) (phenylalanine); *Oral susp:* 125, 250 mg/5 ml (80, 100, 150 ml) (strawberry); 200, 400 mg/5 ml (50, 75, 100 ml) (bubble gum); *Oral drops:* 50 mg/ml (30 ml) (bubble gum)

Moxatag *Tab:* 775 mg ext-rel

Trimox *Tab:* 125, 250 mg; *Cap:* 250, 500 mg; *Oral susp:* 125, 250 mg/5 ml (80, 100, 150 ml) (raspberry-strawberry)

▷ *amoxicillin/clavulanate* (B)(G)

Augmentin <40 kg: 40-45 mg/kg/day divided tid x 10 days or 90 mg/kg/day divided bid x 10 days; *see page 545 for dose by weight table;* ≥40 kg: 500 mg tid or 875 mg bid x 10 days
Tab: 250, 500, 875 mg; *Chew tab:* 125, 250 mg (lemon-lime); 200, 400 mg (cherry-banana) (phenylalanine); *Oral susp:* 125 mg/5 ml (banana), 250 mg/5 ml (75, 100, 150 ml) (orange); 200, 400 mg/5 ml (50, 75, 100 ml) (orange) (phenylalanine)

Augmentin ES-600 <3 months: not recommended; ≥3 months, <40 kg: 90 mg/kg/day divided q 12 hours x 10 days; *see page 546 for dose by weight table;* ≥40 kg: not recommended
Oral susp: 600 mg/5 ml (50, 75, 100, 125, 150, 200 ml) (strawberry cream) (phenylalanine)

Augmentin XR <16 years: use other forms; ≥16 years: 2 tabs q 12 hours x 7-10 days
Tab: 1000*mg ext-rel

▷ *ampicillin* (B) <12 years: 50-100 mg/kg/day in 4 divided doses x 7-14 days; *see page 547 for dose by weight table;* ≥12 years: 500 mg qid x 7-14 days
  Omnipen, Principen *Cap:* 250, 500 mg; *Oral susp:* 125, 250 mg/5 ml (100, 150, 200 ml) (fruit)
▷ *carbenicillin* (B) <12 years: not recommended; ≥12 years: 1-2 tabs qid x 7-14 days
  Geocillin *Tab:* 382 mg
▷ *cefaclor* (B)(G) <1 month: not recommended; 1 month-12 years: 20-40 mg/kg divided bid x 10 days; *see page 549 for dose by weight table;* ≥12 years: 250-500 mg q 8 hours x 10 days; max 2 gm/day
    Tab: 500 mg; *Cap:* 250, 500 mg; *Susp:* 125 mg/5 ml (75, 150 ml) (strawberry); 187 mg/5 ml (50, 100 ml) (strawberry); 250 mg/5 ml (75, 150 ml) (strawberry); 375 mg/5 ml (50, 100 ml) (strawberry)
  Cefaclor Extended Release <16 years: not recommended; ≥16 years: 500 mg bid x 10 days (clinically equivalent to 250 mg immed-rel caps tid); swallow whole; take with meals
    Tab: 375, 500 mg ext-rel
▷ *cefadroxil* (B) <12 years: 30 mg/kg/day in 2 divided doses x 10 days; *see page 550 for dose by weight table;* ≥12 years: 1-2 gm in a single or 2 divided doses x 10 days
  Duricef *Cap:* 500 mg; *Tab:* 1 g; *Oral susp:* 250 mg/5 ml (100 ml); 500 mg/5 ml (75, 100 ml) (orange-pineapple)
▷ *cefixime* (B)(G) <6 months: not recommended; 6 months-12 years, <50 kg: 8 mg/kg/day in 1-2 divided doses x 10 days; *see page 552 for dose by weight table;* >12 years, >50 kg: 400 mg once daily x 10 days
  Suprax *Tab:* 400 mg; *Cap:* 400 mg; *Oral susp:* 100, 200, 500 mg/5 ml (50, 75, 100 ml) (strawberry)
▷ *cefpodoxime proxetil* (B) <2 months: not recommended; 2 months-12 years: 10 mg/kg/day (max 400 mg/dose) or 5 mg/kg/day bid (max 200 mg/dose) x 7 days: *see page 553 for dose by weight table;* ≥12 years: 100 mg bid x 7 days
▷ *cefuroxime axetil* (B)(G) <3 months: not recommended; 3 months-12 years: 20-30 mg/kg/day in 2 divided doses x 7-10 days; *see page 556 for dose by weight table;* ≥12 years: 125-250 mg bid x 7-10 days
  Ceftin *Tab:* 250, 500 mg; *Oral susp:* 125, 250 mg/5 ml (50, 100 ml) (tutti-frutti)
▷ *cephalexin* (B)(G) <12 years: 25-50 mg/kg/day in 4 divided doses x 7-10 days; *see page 557 for dose by weight table;* ≥12 years: 500 mg bid x 7-10 days
  Keflex *Cap:* 250, 333, 500, 750 mg; *Oral susp:* 125, 250 mg/5 ml (100, 200 ml) (strawberry)
▷ *ciprofloxacin* (C) <18 years: not recommended; ≥18 years: 500 mg bid or 1000 mg XR once daily x 3-14 days
  Cipro (G) *Tab:* 250, 500, 750 mg; *Oral susp:* 250, 500 mg/5 ml (100 ml) (strawberry)
  Cipro XR *Tab:* 500, 1000 mg ext-rel
  ProQuin XR *Tab:* 500 mg ext-rel
  Comment: *ciprofloxacin* is contraindicated <18 years-of-age, and during pregnancy and lactation. Risk of tendonitis or tendon rupture.
▷ *doxycycline* (D)(G) <8 years: not recommended; ≥8 years, <100 lb: 2 mg/lb on first day in 2 divided doses, followed by 1 mg/lb/day in a single or 2 divided doses x 7-10 days; ≥8 years, ≥100 lb: 100 mg bid x 7-10 days
  Acticlate *Tab:* 75, 150***mg
  Adoxa *Tab:* 50, 75, 100, 150 mg ent-coat
  Doryx *Tab:* 50, 75, 100, 150, 200 mg del-rel

Monodox *Cap:* 50, 75, 100 mg
Oracea *Cap:* 40 mg del-rel
Vibramycin *Tab:* 100 mg; *Cap:* 50, 100 mg; *Syr:* 50 mg/5 ml (raspberry-apple) (sulfites); *Oral susp:* 25 mg/5 ml (raspberry)
Vibra-Tab *Tab:* 100 mg film-coat

Comment: *doxycycline* is contraindicated <8 years-of-age, in pregnancy, and lactation (discolors developing tooth enamel). A side effect may be photosensitivity (photophobia). Do not take with antacids, calcium supplements, milk or other dairy, or within 2 hours of taking another drug.

➤ *enoxacin* (C) <18 years: not recommended; ≥18 years: 200 mg q 12 hours x 7 days
Penetrex *Tab:* 200, 400 mg

Comment: *enoxacin* is contraindicated <18 years-of-age, and during pregnancy and lactation. Risk of tendonitis or tendon rupture.

➤ *levofloxacin* (C) <18 years: not recommended; ≥18 years: 250 mg once daily x 7-10 days
Levaquin *Tab:* 250, 500, 750 mg; *Oral soln:* 25 mg/ml (480 ml) (benzyl alcohol); *Inj conc:* 25 mg/ml for IV infusion after dilution (20, 30 ml single-use vial) (preservative-free); *Premix soln:* 5 mg/ml for IV infusion (50, 100, 150 ml) (preservative-free)

Comment: *levofloxacin* is contraindicated <18 years-of-age, and during pregnancy and lactation. Risk of tendonitis or tendon rupture.

➤ *lomefloxacin* (C) <18 years: not recommended; ≥18 years: 400 mg once daily x 10 days
Maxaquin *Tab:* 400 mg

Comment: *lomefloxacin* is contraindicated <18 years-of-age, and during pregnancy and lactation. Risk of tendonitis or tendon rupture.

➤ *minocycline* (D)(G) <8 years: not recommended; ≥8 years, <100 lb: 2 mg/lb on first day in 2 divided doses, followed by 1 mg/lb q 12 hours x 9 more days; ≥8 years, >100 lb: 100 mg q 12 hours x 10 days
Dynacin *Cap:* 50, 100 mg
Minocin *Cap:* 50, 75, 100 mg; *Oral susp:* 50 mg/5 ml (60 ml) (custard) (sulfites, alcohol 5%)

Comment: *minocycline* is contraindicated <8 years-of-age, in pregnancy, and lactation (discolors developing tooth enamel). A side effect may be photosensitivity (photophobia). Do not give with antacids, calcium supplements, milk or other dairy, or within two hours of taking another drug.

➤ *nalidixic acid* (B) <3 months: not recommended; ≥3 months-<12 years: 25 mg/lb/day in 4 divided doses x 7-14 days; ≥12 years: 1 gm qid x 7-14 days
NegGram *Tab:* 250, 500 mg; 1 g; *Cap:* 250, 500 mg; *Oral susp:* 250 mg/5 ml

➤ *nitrofurantoin* (B)(G)
Furadantin <1 month: not recommended; ≥1 month-12 years: 5-7 mg/kg/day in 4 divided doses x 7-10 days; *see page 571 for dose by weight table;* >12 years: 50-100 mg qid x 7-10 days
Oral susp: 25 mg/5 ml (60 ml)
Macrobid <12 years: not recommended; ≥12 years: 100 mg q 12 hours x 7-10 days
Cap: 100 mg
Macrodantin <12 years: not recommended; ≥12 years: 50-100 mg qid x 5-7 days; long-term use 50-100 mg q HS

    Cap: 25, 50, 100 mg
➤ *norfloxacin* (C) <18 years: not recommended; ≥18 years: 400 mg x 7-10 days
    Noroxin *Tab:* 400 mg

Comment: *norfloxacin* is contraindicated <18 years-of-age, and during pregnancy and lactation. Risk of tendonitis or tendon rupture.

➤ *ofloxacin* (C)(G) <18 years: not recommended; ≥18 years: 200 mg q 12 hours x 7-10 days
    Floxin *Tab:* 200, 300, 400 mg

Comment: *ofloxacin* is contraindicated <18 years-of-age, and during pregnancy and lactation. Risk of tendonitis or tendon rupture.

➤ *trimethoprim* (C)(G)
    Primsol <6 months: not recommended; ≥6 months-12 years: 10 mg/kg/day in 2 divided doses x 10 days; >12 years: 100 mg q 12 hours or 200 mg once daily x 10 days
      Oral soln: 50 mg/5 ml (bubble gum) (dye-free, alcohol-free)
    Proloprim <12 years: not recommended; ≥12 years: 100 mg q 12 hours or 200 mg once daily x 10 days
      Tab: 100, 200 mg
    Trimpex <12 years: not recommended; ≥12 years: 100 mg q 12 hours or 200 mg once daily x 10 days
      Tab: 100 mg

➤ *trimethoprim/sulfamethoxazole* (D)(G)
    Bactrim, Septra <12 years: not recommended; ≥12 years: 2 tabs bid x 10 days
      Tab: trim 80 mg/*sulfa* 400 mg*
    Bactrim DS, Septra DS <12 years: not recommended; ≥12 years: 1 tab bid x 10 days
      Tab: trim 160 mg/*sulfa* 800 mg*
    Bactrim Pediatric Suspension, Septra Pediatric Suspension <2 months: not recommended; ≥2 months-12 years: 40 mg/kg/day of *sulfamethoxazole* in 2 doses bid; >12 years: use tabs
      Oral susp: trim 40 mg/*sulfa* 200 mg per 5 ml (100 ml) (cherry) (alcohol 0.3%)

PARENTERAL THERAPY

➤ *ertapenem* (B) <18 years: not recommended; ≥18 years: 1 gm once daily; *CrCl <30 mL/min:* 500 mg once daily; treat x 10-14 days; may switch to an oral antibiotic after 3 days if warranted; *IV infusion:* administer over 30 minutes; *IM injection:* reconstitute
    Invanz *Vial:* 1 gm pwdr for reconstitution

LONG-TERM PROPHYLACTIC/SUPPRESSION THERAPY

➤ *methenamine hippurate* (C) <6 years: not recommended; ≥6-12 years: 1/2 tab bid; >12 years: 1 tab bid
    Hiprex, Urex *Tab:* 1 g

URINARY TRACT ANALGESIC/ANTISPASMODICS

➤ *hyoscyamine* (C)(G)
    Anaspaz <2 years: not recommended; 2-12 years: 0.0625-0,125 mg q 4 hours prn; max 0.75 mg/day; >12 years: 1-2 tabs q 4 hours prn; max 12 tabs/day

Tab: 0.125*mg

Levbid <12 years: not recommended; ≥12 years: 1-2 tabs q 12 hours prn; max 4 tabs/day

Tab: 0.375*mg ext-rel

Levsin <6 years: not recommended; 6-12 years: 1 tab q 4 hours prn; ≥12 years: 1-2 tabs q 4 hours prn; max 12 tabs/day

Tab: 0.125*mg

Levsin Drops 3.4 kg: 4 drops q 4 hours prn; max 24 drops/day; 5 kg: 5 drops q 4 hours prn; max 30 drops/day; 7 kg: 6 drops q 4 hours prn; max 36 drops/day; 10 kg: 8 drops q 4 hours prn; max 40 drops/day

Oral drops: 0.125 mg/ml (15 ml) (orange) (alcohol 5%)

Levsin Elixir <10 kg: use drops; 10-19 kg: 1.25 ml q 4 hours prn; 20-39 kg: 2.5 ml q 4 hours prn; 40-49 kg: 3.75 ml q 4 hours prn; 50-60 kg: 5 ml q 4 hours prn; >60 kg: 5-10 ml q 4 hours prn

Elix: 0.125 mg/5 ml (16 oz) (orange) (alcohol 20%)

Levsinex SL <2 years: not recommended; 2-12 years: 1 tab q 4 hours; max 6 tabs/day; >12 years: 1-2 tabs q 4 hours SL <u>or</u> PO; max 12 tabs/day

SL tab: 0.125 mg

Levsinex Timecaps <2 years: not recommended; 2-12 years: 1 cap q 12 hours; max 2 caps/day; >12 years: 1-2 caps q 12 hours; may adjust to 1 cap q 8 hours

Cap: 0.375 mg time-rel

NuLev <2 years: not recommended; 2-12 years: dissolve 1 tab on tongue, with <u>or</u> without water, q 4 hours prn; max 6 tabs/day; >12 years: dissolve 1-2 tabs on tongue, with <u>or</u> without water, q 4 hours prn; max 12 tabs/day

ODT: 0.125 mg (mint) (phenylalanine)

▶ *methenamine/phenyl salicylate/methylene blue/benzoic acid/atropine sulfate/hyoscyamine* (C)(G) <6 years: not recommended; ≥6 years: 2 tabs qid prn

Urised *Tab:* meth 40.8 mg/*phenyl salic* 18.1 mg/*meth blue* 5.4 mg/*benz acid* 4.5 mg/*atro sulf* 0.03 mg/*hyoscy* 0.03 mg

Comment: **Urised** imparts a blue-green color to urine which may stain fabrics.

▶ *methenamine/phenyl salicylate/methylene blue/na phosphate monobasic/hyoscyamine* (C) <6 years: not recommended; ≥6 years: 1 cap qid prn

Uribel *Cap:* meth 118 mg/*phenyl salic* 36 mg/*meth blue* 10 mg/*sod phos mono* 40.8 mg/*hyoscy* 0.12 mg

▶ *methenamine/phenyl salicylate/methylene blue/sod biphosphate/hyoscyamine* (C) <6 years: not recommended; ≥6 years: 1 tab qid prn

Urelle *Cap:* meth 81 mg/*phenyl salic* 32.4 mg/*meth blue* 10.8 mg/*sod biphos* 40.8 mg/*hyoscy* 0.12 mg

▶ *phenazopyridine* (B)(G) <12 years: not recommended; ≥12 years: 95-200 mg q 6 hours prn; max 2 days

AZO Standard, Prodium, Uristat (OTC) *Tab:* 95 mg

AZO Standard Maximum Strength (OTC) *Tab:* 97.5 mg

Pyridium, Urogesic *Tab:* 100, 200 mg

Comment: *phenazopyridine* imparts an orange-red color to urine which may stain fabrics.

PROPHYLACTIC/SUPPRESSION THERAPY

▶ *methenamine hippurate* (C) 6 years: 0.25 gm/30 lb qid; 6-12 years: 25-50 mg/kg/day in 2 divided doses <u>or</u> 0.5-1 gm bid; >12 years: 1 gm bid

Hiprex *Tab:* 1 g; *Oral susp:* 500 mg/5 ml (480 ml)

UROLITHIASIS (RENAL CALCULI, KIDNEY STONES)

Acetaminophen for IV Infusion *see Pain page* 296
Oral Prescription NSAIDs *see page* 490
Other Oral Analgesics *see Pain page* 298
Opioids and Other Analgesics *see page* 298

ANTISPASMODIC

➤ *flavoxate* (B)(G)
   Urispas 100-200 mg tid-qid

PARENTERAL NARCOTICS

Aid to Stone Passage: Alpha-1A Blockers

➤ *alfuzosin* (B)(G) 10 mg once daily taken immediately after the same meal each day
   UroXatral *Tab:* 10 mg ext-rel
➤ *tamsulosin* (B)(G) initially 0.4 mg once daily; may increase to 0.8 mg once daily
   after 2-4 weeks if needed
   Flomax *Cap:* 0.4 mg
   Comment: May take Flomax 0.4 mg with Avodart 0.5 mg once daily as
   combination therapy.
➤ *buprenorphine* (C)
   Buprenex administer <2 years: not recommended; 2-12 years: 2-6 mcg/kg IM/
   IV q 4-6 hours prn; >12-18 years: 0.1-0.2 mg IM or IV q 3-4 hours prn; may
   repeat once (up to 0.3 mg) if required, 30 to 60 minutes after initial dose; >18
   years: 0.3 mg IM or IV q 6 hours prn
      Amp: 0.3 mg/ml (1 ml)
   Comment: Buprenex is approximately equivalent to 10 mg morphine sulfate in
   analgesic and respiratory depressant effects.
➤ *meperidine* (B; D in 2nd, 3rd)(II)(G) <12 years: 0.5-0.8 mg/lb q 3-4 hours prn; ≥12
   years: 50-100 mg IM q 3-4 hours prn
   Demerol *Tubex:* 25, 50, 75, 100 mg/ml (2 ml); *Vial:* 25 mg/ml (1 ml); 50 mg/ml
   (1, 30 ml); 75 mg/ml; (1 ml); 100 mg/ml (1, 20 ml); *Amp:* 25, 50, 75, 100 mg/
   ml (1 ml)
➤ *morphine sulfate* (C)(II)(G) 10-15 mg q 3-4 hours prn
   Vial: 1 mg/ml (1, 60 ml); 5 mg/ml (1 ml); 8 mg/ml (1 ml); 10 mg/ml (1, 2, 10
   ml); 15 mg (1, 20 ml); *Amp:* 8 mg/ml (1 ml); 10 mg/ml (1 ml); 15 mg/ml (1 ml)

PREVENTION OF CALCIUM STONES

➤ *chlorothiazide* (B)(G) 50 mg bid
   Diuril *Tab:* 250*, 500*mg; *Oral susp:* 250 mg/5 ml (237 ml)
➤ *hydrochlorothiazide* (B)(G) 50 mg bid
   Esidrix *Tab:* 25, 50 mg
   Microzide *Cap:* 12.5 mg

PREVENTION OF CYSTINE STONES

➤ *penicillamine* (D) <12 years: not recommended; ≥12 years: 1-4 gm/day
   Cuprimine *Cap:* 125, 250 mg

Depen *Titratable tab:* 250 mg
▷ *potassium citrate* (C)(G)30 mEq qid
    Urocit-K *Tab:* 5, 10, 15 mEq ext-rel
Comment: *potassium citrate* is contraindicated in hyperkalemia.

PREVENTION OF URIC ACID STONES

▷ *allopurinol* (C)(G) <12 years: not recommended; ≥12 years: 200-300 mg in 1-3 doses; max 800 mg/day
    Zyloprim *Tab:* 100*, 300*mg
▷ *potassium citrate* (C)(G) 30 mEq qid
    Urocit-K *Tab:* 5, 10, 15 mEq ext-rel
Comment: *potassium citrate* is contraindicated in hyperkalemia. Encourage patients to limit salt intake and maintain liberal hydration (urine volume should be at least 2 liters/day). Target urine pH is 6.0-7.0 and urine citrate at least 320 mg/day and close to the normal mean of 640 mg/day. Take with food.

URTICARIA: MILD, CHRONIC IDIOPATHIC (CIU), ACUTE

Oral Prescription Drugs for the Management of Allergy, Cough, and Cold Symptoms *see page 523*
Topical Corticosteroids *see page 494*
Oral Corticosteroids *see page 498*
Parenteral Corticosteroids *see page 499*

SECOND GENERATION ANTIHISTAMINES

Comment: Second generation antihistamines are sedating, but much less so than the first generation antihistamines. All antihistamines are excreted into breast milk.
▷ *cetirizine* (C)(OTC)(G) <6 years: not recommended; ≥6-<65 years: initially 5-10 mg once daily; ≥65 years: 5 mg once daily
    Children's Zyrtec Chewable *Chew tab:* 5, 10 mg (grape)
    Children's Zyrtec Allergy Syrup *Syr:* 1 mg/ml (4 oz) (grape, bubble gum) (sugar-free, dye-free)
    Zyrtec *Tab:* 10 mg
    Zyrtec Hives Relief *Tab:* 10 mg
    Zyrtec Liquid Gels *Liq gel:* 10 mg
▷ *desloratadine* (C)
    Clarinex <6 years: not recommended; ≥6 years: 1/2-1 tab once daily
        Tab: 5 mg
    Clarinex RediTabs <6 years: not recommended; 6-12 years: 2.5 mg once daily; ≥12 years: 5 mg once daily
        ODT: 2.5, 5 mg (tutti-frutti) (phenylalanine)
    Clarinex Syrup <6 months: not recommended; 6-11 months: 1 mg (2 ml) once daily; 1-5 years: 1.25 mg (2.5 ml) once daily; 6-11 years: 2.5 mg (5 ml) once daily; ≥12 years: 5 mg (10 ml) once daily
        Tab: 0.5 mg per ml (4 oz) (tutti-frutti) (phenylalanine)
    Desloratadine ODT

▷ *fexofenadine* (C)(OTC)(G) 6 months-2 years: 15 mg bid; *CrCl ≤90 mL/min:* 15 mg once daily; 2-11 years: 30 mg bid; *CrCl ≤90 mL/min:* 30 mg once daily ≥12 years and older: ≥ 12 years: 60 mg once daily-bid <u>or</u> 180 mg once daily; *CrCl <90 mL/ min:* 60 mg once daily **Allegra** *Tab:* 30, 60, 180 mg film-coat
    Allegra Allergy *Tab:* 60, 180 mg film-coat
    Allegra ODT *ODT:* 30 mg (phenylalanine)
    Allegra Oral Suspension *Oral susp:* 30 mg/5 ml (6 mg/ml) (4 oz)
▷ *loratadine* (C)(OTC)(G) <2 years: not recommended; 2-5 years: 5 mg once daily; ≥6 years: 5 mg bid or 10 mg once daily; *Hepatic <u>or</u> Renal Insufficiency:* (see mfr pkg insert)
    Children's Claritin Chewables *Chew tab:* 5 mg (grape) (phenylalanine)
    Children's Claritin Syrup 1 mg/ml (4 oz) (fruit) (sugar-free, alcohol-free, dye-free; sodium 6 mg/5 ml)
    Claritin *Tab:* 10 mg
    Claritin Hives Relief *Tab:* 10 mg
    Claritin Liqui-Gels *Liq gel:* 10 mg
    Claritin RediTabs 12 Hours *ODT:* 5 mg (mint)
    Claritin RediTabs 24 Hours *ODT:* 10 mg (mint)
▷ *levocetirizine* (B)(OTC) administer dose in the PM; *Seasonal Allergic Rhinitis:* <2 years: not recommended; may start at ≥2 years; *Chronic Idiopathic Urticaria (CIU), Perennial Allergic Rhinitis:* <6 months: not recommended; may start at ≥ 6 months; *Dosing by Age:* 6 months-5 years: max 1.25 mg once daily; 6-11 years: max 2.5 mg once daily; ≥12 years: 2.5-5 mg once daily; *Renal Dysfunction <12 years:* contraindicated; *Renal Dysfunction ≥12 years:* CrCl 50-80 ml/min: 2.5 mg once daily; CrCl 30-50 mL/min: 2.5 mg every other day; CrCl: 10-30 mL/min: 2.5 mg twice weekly (every 3-4 days); CrCl <10 mL/min, ESRD <u>or</u> hemodialysis: contraindicated;
    Xyzal *Tab:* 5*mg
    Xyzal Oral Solution *Oral soln:* 0.5 mg/ml (150 ml)

VAGINAL IRRITATION: EXTERNAL

▷ **Replens Vaginal Moisturizer** (NE)(OTC) apply as needed; for external use only *Bottle:* 2 oz
▷ **Vagisil Intimate Moisturizer** (NE)(OTC) apply as needed; for external use *only Bottle:* 2 oz
Comment: **Vagisil** has no effect on condom integrity.

VERTIGO

▷ *meclizine* (B)(G) <12 years: not recommended; ≥12 years: 25-100 mg/day in divided doses
    Antivert *Tab:* 12.5, 25, 50*mg
    Bonine (OTC) *Cap:* 15, 25, 30 mg; *Tab:* 12.5, 25, 50 mg; *Chew tab/Film-coat tab:* 25 mg
    Dramamine II (OTC) *Tab:* 25*mg
    Zentrip *Strip:* 25 mg orally-disint

◻ VITILIGO

REPIGMENTATION ENHANCEMENT

▷ *methoxsalen* (C) <12 years: not recommended; ≥12 years: apply to well-defined area of vitiligo; then expose area to source of UVA (ultraviolet A) or sunlight; initial exposure no more than 1/2 predicted minimal erythemal dose; repeat weekly

Oxsoralen *Lotn:* 1% (30 ml)

Comment: *methoxsalen* may only be applied by a health care provider. Do not dispense to patient.

▷ *trioxsalen* (C) <12 years: not recommended; ≥12 years: 10 mg daily, taken 2-4 hours before ultraviolet light exposure; max 14 days and 28 tabs

Trisoralen *Tab:* 5 mg

Depigmenting Agents *see Hyperpigmentation page* 200

◻ WART: COMMON (VERRUCA VULGARIS)

▷ *salicylic acid* (NE)(G)

Duo Film (OTC) apply daily-bid; max 12 weeks; *Liq:* 17% (1/2 oz w. applicator)

Duo Film Patch for Kids (OTC) apply 1 patch q 48 hours; max 12 weeks
   Patch: 40% (18/pck)

Occlusal HP (OTC) apply daily-bid; max 12 weeks
   Liq: 17% (10 ml w. applicator)

Wart-Off (OTC) apply one drop at a time to sufficiently cover wart, let dry; repeat 1-2 times daily; max 12 weeks
   Liq: 17% (0.45 oz)

◻ WART: PLANTAR (VERRUCA PLANTARIS)

▷ *salicylic acid* (NE)(G)

Duo Plant Gel (OTC) apply daily bid; max 12 weeks
   Gel: 17% (1/2 oz)

Mediplast cut to size of wart and apply; remove q 1-2 days, peel keratin, and reapply; repeat as often as needed

Occlusal-HP (OTC) apply qd-bid; max 12 weeks
   Liq: 17% (10 ml w. applicator)

Wart-Off (OTC) apply one drop at a time to sufficiently cover wart, let dry; repeat 1-2 times daily; max 12 weeks
   Liq: 17% (0.45 oz)

▷ *trichloroacetic acid* (NE) apply after wart is pared and repeat weekly

◻ WART: VENEREAL, HUMAN PAPILLOMAVIRUS (HPV), CONDYLOMA ACUMINATA

Comment: This section contains treatment regimens for genital warts published in the **2015 CDC Sexually Transmitted Diseases Treatment Guidelines** as well as other treatment options. Due to the increased risk of cervical cancer with HPV, Pap smears should be done q 3 months during active disease and then q 3-6 months for the next 2 years.

PATIENT-APPLIED AGENTS

Regimen 1

▷ *imiquimod* (C) <12 years: not recommended; ≥12 years:
 Aldara (G) rub into lesions before bedtime and remove with soap and water 6-10 hours later; treat 3 times per week; max 16 weeks
   Crm: 5% (12 single-use pkts/carton)
 Zyclara rub into lesions before bedtime and remove with soap and water 8 hours later; treat 3 times per week; max 1 packet per treatment; max 8 weeks
   Crm: 3.75% (28 single-use pkts/carton) (parabens)

Regimen 2

▷ *podofilox 0.5% cream* (C) apply bid (q 12 hours) x 3 days; then discontinue for 4 days; may repeat if needed; max 4 treatment cycles
 Condylox *Soln:* 0.5% (3.5 ml); *Gel:* 0.5% (3.5 gm)

Regimen 3

▷ *sinecatechins 15% ointment* (C) apply to each lesion tid for up to 16 weeks
 Veregen *Oint:* 15% (15, 30 gm)

PROVIDER-ADMINISTERED AGENTS

Regimen 1

Cryotherapy with liquid nitrogen <u>or</u> cryoprobe; repeat applications every 1-2 weeks as needed

Regimen 2

▷ *trichloroacetic acid (TCA) 80-90%* (C) apply to warts; repeat weekly if needed
 Comment: TCA is the preferred treatment during pregnancy. Immediate application of sodium bicarbonate paste following treatment decreases pain.

Regimen 3

▷ *podofilox 0.5% cream* (C) apply bid (q 12 hours) x 3 days; then discontinue for 4 days; may repeat if needed; max 4 treatment cycles
 Condylox *Soln:* 0.5% (3.5 ml); *Gel:* 0.5% (3.5 gm)

Regimen 4

▷ *interferon alfa-n3* (C) 0.05 ml injected into base of wart twice weekly for up to 8 weeks; max 0.5 ml/session (20 warts/session)
 Alferon N Vial: 5 million units/ml (1 ml)

Regimen 5

➤ *interferon alfa-2b* (C) 0.1 ml injected into base of wart three times weekly for up to 3 weeks; max 0.5 ml/session (5 warts/session)
　　Intron A Vial: 1 million units/0.1 ml (0.5, 1 ml)

Regimen 6

Surgical removal either by tangential scissor excision, tangential shave excision, curettage, or electrosurgery

WHIPWORM (TRICHURIASIS)

ANTHELMINTICS

➤ *albendazole* (C) take with a meal; may crush and mix with food; may repeat in 3 weeks if needed; <2 years: 200 mg once daily x 3 days; 2-12 years: 400 mg once daily x 3 days; >12 years: 400 mg as bid x 3 days;
　　Albenza *Tab:* 200 mg
➤ *mebendazole* (C)(G) take with a meal; may crush and mix with food; may repeat in 3 weeks if needed; <2 years: not recommended; ≥2 years: 100 mg bid x 3 days
　　Emverm *Chew tab:* 100 mg
　　Vermox (G) *Chew tab:* 100 mg
➤ *pyrantel pamoate* (C) take with a meal; may open capsule and sprinkle or mix with food; treat x 3 days; 11 mg/kg/dose; max 1 gm/dose; 25-37 lb: 1/2 tsp/dose; 38-62 lb: 1 tsp/dose; 63-87 lb: 1 tsp/dose; 88-112 lb: 2 tsp/dose; 113-137 lb: 2 tsp/dose; 138-162 lb: 3 tsp/dose; 163-187 lb: 3 tsp/dose; >187 lb: 4 tsp/dose
　　Antiminth (OTC) *Cap:* 180 mg; *Liq:* 50 mg/ml (30 ml); 144 mg/ml (30 ml); *Oral susp:* 50 mg/ml (60 ml)
　　Pin-X (OTC) *Cap:* 180 mg; *Liq:* 50 mg/ml (30 ml); 144 mg/ml (30 ml); *Oral susp:* 50 mg/ml (30 ml)
➤ *thiabendazole* (C) take with a meal; may crush and mix with food; treat x 7 days; max 1.5 gm/dose; max 3 g/day; <30 lb: consult mfr pkg insert; ≥30 lb: 25 mg/kg/dose bid; 30-50 lb: 250 mg bid meals; >50 lb: 10 mg/lb/dose bid
　　Mintezol *Chew tab:* 500*mg (orange); *Oral susp:* 500 mg/5 ml (120 ml) (orange)
Comment: *thiabendazole* is not for prophylaxis. May impair mental alertness. May not be available in the US.

WOUND: INFECTED, NON-SURGICAL, MINOR

TETANUS PROPHYLAXIS

Previously Immunized (within previous 5 years)

➤ *tetanus toxoid* vaccine (C) 0.5 ml IM x 1 dose
　　Vial: 5 Lf units/0.5 ml (0.5, 5 ml); *Prefilled syringe:* 5 Lf units/0.5 ml (0.5 ml)

Not Previously Immunized

see Tetanus *page 398*

TOPICAL ANTI-INFECTIVES

▷ *mupirocin* (B)(G) <12 years: not recommended; ≥12 years: apply to lesions bid
  Bactroban *Oint:* 2% (22 gm); *Crm:* 2% (15, 30 gm)
  Centany *Oint:* 2% (15, 30 gm)

ORAL ANTI-INFECTIVES

▷ *azithromycin* (B) <12 years: 10 mg/kg x 1 dose on day 1, then 5 mg/kg/day on days
  2-5; *see page 548 for dose by weight table;* max 500 mg/day; ≥12 years: 500 mg x 1
  dose on day 1, then 250 mg daily on days 2-5 or 500 mg daily x 3 days or Zmax 2
  gm in a single dose
  Zithromax *Tab:* 250, 500, 600 mg; *Oral susp:* 100 mg/5 ml (15 ml); 200 mg/5 ml
  (15, 22.5, 30 ml) (cherry); *Pkt:* 1 gm for reconstitution (cherry-banana)
  Zithromax Tri-pak *Tab:* 3 x 500 mg tabs/pck
  Zithromax Z-pak *Tab:* 6 x 250 mg tabs/pck
  Zmax *Oral susp:* 2 gm ext-rel for reconstitution (cherry-banana) (148 mg Na+)
▷ *amoxicillin/clavulanate* (B)(G)
  Augmentin <40 kg: 40-45 mg/kg/day divided tid x 10 days or 90 mg/kg/day
  divided bid x 10 days; *see page 545 for dose by weight table;* ≥40 kg: 500 mg tid
  or 875 mg bid x 10 days
    Tab: 250, 500, 875 mg; *Chew tab:* 125, 250 mg (lemon-lime); 200, 400 mg
    (cherry-banana) (phenylalanine); *Oral susp:* 125 mg/5 ml (banana), 250
    mg/5 ml (75, 100, 150 ml) (orange); 200, 400 mg/5 ml (50, 75, 100 ml)
    (orange) (phenylalanine)
  Augmentin ES-600 <3 months: not recommended; ≥3 months, <40 kg: 90 mg/
  kg/day divided q 12 hours x 10 days; *see page 546 for dose by weight table;* ≥40
  kg: not recommended
    Oral susp: 600 mg/5 ml (50, 75, 100, 125, 150, 200 ml) (strawberry cream)
    (phenylalanine)
  Augmentin XR <16 years: use other forms; ≥16 years: 2 tabs q 12 hours x 7-10
  days
    Tab: 1000*mg ext-rel
▷ *cefaclor* (B)(G) <1 month: not recommended; 1 month-12 years: 20-40 mg/kg
  divided bid x 10 days; *see page 549 for dose by weight table;* max 1 gm/day; ≥12
  years: 250-500 mg q 8 hours x 10 days; max 2 gm/day
    Tab: 500 mg; *Cap:* 250, 500 mg; *Susp:* 125 mg/5 ml (75, 150 ml) (strawberry);
    187 mg/5 ml (50, 100 ml) (strawberry); 250 mg/5 ml (75, 150 ml) (straw-
    berry); 375 mg/5 ml (50, 100 ml) (strawberry)
  Cefaclor Extended Release <16 years: not recommended; ≥16 years: 500 mg bid
  x 10 days (clinically equivalent to 250 mg immed-rel caps tid); swallow whole;
  take with meals
    Tab: 375, 500 mg ext-rel
▷ *cefadroxil* <12 years: 30 mg/kg/day in 2 divided doses x 10 days; *see page 550 for
  dose by weight table;* ≥12 years: 1-2 gm in a single or 2 divided doses x 10 days
    Duricef *Cap:* 500 mg; *Tab:* 1 g; *Oral susp:* 250 mg/5 ml (100 ml); 500 mg/5 ml
    (75, 100 ml) (orange-pineapple)
▷ *cefdinir* (B) <6 months: not recommended; 6 months-12 years: 14 mg/kg/day in 1-2
  divided doses x 10 days; *see page 551 for dose by weight table;* ≥12 years: 300 mg bid
  x 10 days or 600 mg daily x 10 days
    Omnicef *Cap:* 300 mg; *Oral susp:* 125 mg/5 ml (60, 100 ml) (strawberry)

➤ *cefpodoxime proxetil* (B) <2 months: not recommended; 2 months-12 years: 10 mg/kg/day (max 400 mg/dose) <u>or</u> 5 mg/kg/day bid (max 200 mg/dose) x 7-14 days; *see page 553 for dose by weight table;* >12 years: 400 mg bid x 7-14 days

➤ *cefprozil* (B) <2 years: not recommended; 2-12 years: 7.5 mg/kg-15 mg/kg q 12 hours x 10 days; *see page 554 for dose by weight table;* >12 years: 250-500 mg q 12 hours <u>or</u> 500 mg daily x 10 days

    Cefzil *Tab:* 250, 500 mg; *Oral susp:* 125, 250 mg/5 ml (50, 75, 100 ml) (bubble gum, phenylalanine)

➤ *cephalexin* (B)(G) <12 years: 50 mg/kg/day in 4 divided doses x 10 days; *see page 557 for dose by weight table;* ≥12 years: 2 gm 1 hour before procedure

    Keflex *Cap:* 250, 333, 500, 750 mg; *Oral susp:* 125, 250 mg/5 ml (100, 200 ml) (strawberry)

➤ *clarithromycin* (C)(G) <6 months: not recommended; ≥6 months-12 years: 7.5 mg/kg bid x 7-10 days; *see page 558 for dose by weight table;* >12 years: 500 mg bid <u>or</u> 500 mg ext-rel daily x 7-10 days

    Biaxin *Tab:* 250, 500 mg

    Biaxin Oral Suspension *Oral susp:* 125, 250 mg/5 ml (50, 100 ml) (fruit punch)

    Biaxin XL *Tab:* 500 mg ext-rel

➤ *dirithromycin* (C)(G) <12 years: not recommended; ≥12 years: 500 mg daily x 7 days

    Dynabac *Tab:* 250 mg

➤ *erythromycin base* (B)(G) <45 kg: 30-50 mg in 2-4 divided doses x 7 days; ≥45 kg: 500 mg q 6 hours x 7 days

    Ery-Tab *Tab:* 250, 333, 500 mg ent-coat

    PCE *Tab:* 333, 500 mg

➤ *erythromycin ethylsuccinate* (B)(G) 30-50 mg/kg/day in 4 divided doses x 7 days; may double dose with severe infection; max 100 mg/kg/day <u>or</u> 400 mg qid; *see page 563 for dose by weight table*

    EryPed *Oral susp:* 200 mg/5 ml (100, 200 ml) (fruit); 400 mg/5 ml (60, 100, 200 ml) (banana); *Oral drops:* 200, 400 mg/5 ml (50 ml) (fruit); *Chew tab:* 200 mg wafer (fruit)

    E.E.S. *Oral susp:* 200, 400 mg/5 ml (100 ml) (fruit)

    E.E.S. Granules *Oral susp:* 200 mg/5 ml (100, 200 ml) (cherry)

    E.E.S. 400 Tablets *Tab:* 400 mg

➤ *gemifloxacin* (C)(G) <18 years: not recommended; ≥18 years: 320 mg once daily x 5-7 days

    Factive *Tab:* 320*mg

Comment: *gemifloxacin* is contraindicated <18 years-of-age, and during pregnancy and lactation. Risk of tendonitis <u>or</u> tendon rupture.

➤ *levofloxacin* (C) <18 years: not recommended; ≥18 years: *Uncomplicated:* 500 mg daily x 7 days; *Complicated:* 750 mg daily x 7 days

    Levaquin *Tab:* 250, 500, 750 mg

Comment: *levofloxacin* is contraindicated <18 years-of-age, and during pregnancy and lactation. Risk of tendonitis <u>or</u> tendon rupture.

➤ *loracarbef* (B) <12 years: 15 mg/kg/day in 2 divided doses x 7 days; *see page 570 for dose by weight table;* ≥12 years: 200 mg bid x 7 days

    Lorabid *Pulvule:* 200, 400 mg; *Oral susp:* 100 mg/5 ml (50, 100 ml); 200 mg/5 ml (50, 75, 100 ml) (strawberry bubble gum)

➤ *ofloxacin* (C)(G) <18 years: not recommended; ≥18 years: 400 mg bid x 10 days

    Floxin *Tab:* 200, 300, 400 mg

Comment: *ofloxacin* is contraindicated <18 years-of-age, and during pregnancy and lactation. Risk of tendonitis or tendon rupture.

XEROSIS

MOISTURIZING AGENTS

Aquaphor Healing Ointment (OTC) *Oint:* 1.75, 3.5, 14 oz (alcohol)
Eucerin Daily Sun Defense (OTC) *Lotn:* 6 oz (fragrance-free)
  Comment: **Eucerin Daily Sun Defense** is a moisturizer with SPF-15 sunscreen.
Eucerin Facial Lotion (OTC) *Lotn:* 4 oz
Eucerin Light Lotion (OTC) *Lotn:* 8 oz
Eucerin Lotion (OTC) *Lotn:* 8, 16 oz
Eucerin Original Creme (OTC) *Crm:* 2, 4, 16 oz (alcohol)
Eucerin Plus Creme (OTC) *Crm:* 4 oz
Eucerin Plus Lotion (OTC) *Lotn:* 6, 12 oz
Eucerin Protective Lotion (OTC) *Lotn:* 4 oz (alcohol)
  Comment: **Eucerin Protective** is a moisturizer with SPF-25 sunscreen.
Lac-Hydrin Cream (OTC) *Crm:* 280, 385 g
Lac-Hydrin Lotion (OTC) *Lotn:* 225, 400 g
Lubriderm Dry Skin Scented (OTC) *Lotn:* 6, 10, 16, 32 oz
Lubriderm Dry Skin Unscented (OTC) *Lotn:* 3.3, 6, 10, 16 oz (fragrance-free)
Lubriderm Sensitive Skin Lotion (OTC) *Lotn:* 3.3, 6, 10, 16 oz (lanolin-free)
Lubriderm Dry Skin (OTC) *Lotn:* 2.5, 6, 10, 16 oz (scented); 1, 2.5, 6, 10, 16 oz (fragrance-free)
Lubriderm Bath & Shower Oil (OTC) 1-2 capfuls in bath or rub onto wet skin as needed, then rinse
  Oil: 8 oz
Moisturel apply as needed
  Crm: 4, 16 oz; *Lotn:* 8, 12 oz; *Clnsr:* 8.75 oz

Topical Oil

▶ *fluocinolone acetamide* 0.01% topical oil (C) <6 years: not recommended; ≥6 years: apply sparingly bid for up to 4 weeks
  Derma-Smoothe/FS Topical Oil apply sparingly tid
    Topical oil: 0.01% (4 oz; peanut oil)

ZOLLINGER–ELLISON SYNDROME

PROTON PUMP INHIBITORS

Comment: If hepatic impairment, or if patient is Asian, consider reducing the PPI dose.
▶ *dexlansoprazole* (B)(G) <18 years: not recommended; ≥18 years: 30-60 mg daily for up to 4 weeks
  Dexilant *Cap:* 30, 60 mg ent-coat del-rel granules; may open and sprinkle on applesauce; do not crush or chew granules

Dexilant SoluTab *Tab:* 30 mg del-rel orally-disint

▷ *esomeprazole* (B)(OTC)(G) <1 year: not recommended; 1-11 years, <20 kg: 10 mg; >20 kg: 10-20 mg once daily; 12-17 years: 20-40 mg once daily; >17 years: 20-40 mg daily; max 8 weeks; take 1 hour before food; swallow whole or mix granules with food or juice and take immediately; do not crush or chew granules; max 8 weeks

Nexium *Cap:* 20, 40 mg ent-coat del-rel pellets

Nexium for Oral Suspension *Oral susp:* 10, 20, 40 mg ent-coat del-rel granules/ pkt; mix in 2 tbsp water and drink immediately; 30 pkt/carton

▷ *esomeprazole/aspirin* (D) <18 years: not recommended; ≥18 years: take one dose daily; max 8 weeks; take 1 hour before food

Yosprala

Tab: **Yosprala 40/81** *esom* 40 mg/*asp* 81 mg del-rel

Yosprala 40/325 *esom* 40 mg/*asp* 325 mg del-rel

▷ *lansoprazole* (B)(OTC)(G) <1 year: not recommended; 1-11 years, <30 kg: 15 mg once daily; >11 years: 15-30 mg daily for up to 8 weeks; may repeat course; take before eating

Prevacid *Cap:* 15, 30 mg ent-coat del-rel granules; swallow whole or mix granules with food or juice and take immediately; do not crush or chew granules; follow with water

Prevacid for Oral Suspension *Oral susp:* 15, 30 mg ent-coat del-rel granules/pkt; mix in 2 tbsp water and drink immediately; 30 pkt/carton (strawberry)

Prevacid SoluTab *ODT:* 15, 30 mg (strawberry; phenylalanine)

Prevacid 24HR *Oral granules:* 15 mg ent-coat del-rel granules; swallow whole or mix granules with food or juice and take immediately; do not crush or chew granules; follow with water

▷ *omeprazole* (C)(OTC)(G) <1 year: not recommended; 5-<10 kg: 5 mg daily; 10-<20 kg: 10 mg daily; ≥20 kg: 20-40 mg daily; take before eating; swallow whole or mix granules with applesauce and take immediately; do not crush or chew; follow with water

Prilosec *Cap:* 10, 20, 40 mg ent-coat del-rel granules

Prilosec *Tab:* 20 mg del-rel (regular, wild berry)

▷ *pantoprazole* (B) <12 years: not recommended; ≥12 years: initially 40 mg bid

Protonix (G) *Tab:* 40 mg ent-coat del-rel

Protonix for Oral Suspension *Oral susp:* 40 mg ent-coat del-rel granules/ pkt; mix in 1 tsp apple juice for 5 seconds or sprinkle on 1 tsp applesauce, and swallow immediately; do not mix in water or any other liquid or food; take approximately 30 minutes prior to a meal; 30 pkt/carton any other liquid or food; take approximately 30 minutes prior to a meal; 30 pkt/carton

▷ *rabeprazole* (B)(OTC)(G) <12 years: not recommended; ≥12-18 years: 20 mg once daily; max 8 week; >18 years: initially 20 mg daily; then titrate; may take 10 mg daily in divided doses or 60 mg bid

AcipHex *Tab:* 20 mg ent-coat del-rel

AcipHex Sprinkle *Cap:* 5, 10 mg del-rel

SECTION II

APPENDICES

APPENDIX A: U.S. FDA PREGNANCY CATEGORIES

Comment: For drugs FDA-approved *after June 30, 2015*, the 5-letter categories are no longer used and there is no replacement (categorical nomenclature) at this time. Rather, information regarding special populations, including pregnant and breastfeeding females, is addressed in a structured narrative format. Prescribers should refer to the drug's FDA labeling (https://www.fda.gov/Drugs/default.htm) or the manufacturer's package insert for this information. Prescription drugs submitted for FDA approval after June 30, 2015 use the new format immediately, while labeling for prescription drugs approved on or after June 30, 2015 are phased in gradually. Although drugs approved prior to June 29, 2015 are not subject to the FDA's **Pregnancy and Lactation Labeling** Final Rule (PLLR), the *pregnancy letter category must be removed by June 29, 2018*. Labeling for over-the-counter (OTC) medicines will not change, as OTC drugs are not affected by the new FDA pregnancy labeling. For a more detailed explanation of the final rule **and** new narrative format, **visit** https://www.drugs.com/pregnancy-categories.html.

Category	Description
A	Controlled studies in women have failed to demonstrate risk to the fetus in the first trimester of pregnancy and there is no evidence of risk in later trimesters.
B	Animal reproduction studies have not demonstrated risk to the fetus, but there are no controlled studies in pregnant women, or animal studies have demonstrated an adverse effect, but controlled studies in pregnant women have not documented risk to the fetus in the first trimester of pregnancy and there is no evidence of risk in later trimesters.
C	Risk to the fetus cannot be ruled out. Animal reproduction studies have demonstrated adverse effects on the fetus (i.e., teratogenic or embryocidal effects or other) but there are no controlled studies in pregnant women or controlled studies in women and animals are not available.
D	There is positive evidence of human fetal risk, but benefits from use by pregnant women may be acceptable despite the potential risk (e.g., if the drug is needed in a life-threatening situation or for a serious disease for which safer drugs cannot be used or are ineffective.
X	Studies in animals or humans have demonstrated fetal abnormalities or there is evidence of fetal risk based on human experience, or both, and the risk of using the drug in pregnant women clearly outweighs any possible benefit. The drug is contraindicated in women who are pregnant or who may become pregnant.

(continued)

APPENDIX B: U.S. SCHEDULE OF CONTROLLED SUBSTANCES

Schedule	Description
I	High potential for abuse and of no currently accepted medical use. Not obtainable by prescription, but may be legally procured for research, study, or instructional use (examples: *heroin, LSD, marijuana, mescaline, peyote*).
II	High abuse potential and high liability for severe psychological or physical dependence potential. Prescription required and cannot be refilled. Prescription must be written in ink or typed and signed. A verbal prescription may be allowed in an emergency by the dispensing pharmacist, but must be followed by a written prescription within 72 hours. Includes opium derivatives, other opioids, and short-acting barbiturates.
III	Potential for abuse is less than that for drugs in schedules I and II. Moderate to low physical dependence and high psychological dependence potential. Prescription required. May be refilled up to 5 times in 6 months. Prescription may be verbal (telephone) or written. Includes certain stimulants and depressants not included in the above schedules, and preparations containing limited quantities of certain opioids.
IV	Lower potential for abuse than Schedule III drugs. Prescription required. May be refilled up to 5 times in 6 months. Prescription may be verbal (telephone) or written.
V	Abuse potential less than that for Schedule IV drugs. Preparations contain limited quantities of certain narcotic drugs. Generally intended for antitussive and antidiarrheal purposes and may be distributed without a prescription provided that: • Such distribution is made only by a pharmacist. • Not more than 240 ml or not more than 48 solid dosage units of any substance containing opium, nor more than 120 ml or not more than 24 solid dosage units of any other controlled substance may be distributed at retail to the same purchaser in any given 48-hour period without a valid prescription order. • The purchaser is at least 18 years-of-age. • The pharmacist knows the purchaser or requests suitable identification. • The pharmacist keeps an official written record of: name and address of purchaser, name and quantity of controlled substance purchased, date of sale, initials of dispensing pharmacist. This record is to be made available for inspection and copying by the U.S. officers authorized by the Attorney General. • Other federal, state, or local laws do not require a prescription order. Under jurisdiction of the Federal Controlled Substances Act. Refillable up to 5 times within 6 months.

APPENDIX C: JNC-8* AND ASH** HYPERTENSION EVALUATION AND TREATMENT RECOMMENDATIONS

APPENDIX C.1: BLOOD PRESSURE CLASSIFICATION (≥18 YEARS)¶

Classification	SBP mmHg		DBP mmHg
Normal	<120	and	<80
Prehypertension	120-139	or	80-89
Hypertension, Stage 1	140-159	or	90-99
Hypertension, Stage 2	≥160	or	≥100

¶Adapted from PL Detail-Document. (2014, February). Treatment of hypertension: JNC 8 and more. *Pharmacist's Letter/Prescriber's Letter*. Retrieved from https://www.scribd.com/doc/290772273/JNC-8-guideline-summary

APPENDIX C.2: BLOOD PRESSURE RECOMMENDATIONS (>18 YEARS)

Classification	SBP mmHg	DBP mmHg
Optimal	<120	<80
Normal	<130	<85
High normal	130-139	85-89

APPENDIX C.2.A: BLOOD PRESSURE CLASSIFICATION (<18 YEARS)¶

Age Group	Significant		Severe	
	SBP	DBP	SBP	DBP
Newborn <7 days	>96		>106	
Newborn 8-30 days	>104		>110	
Infant 30 days-2 years	>112	>74	>118	>82
Children 3-5 years	>116	>76	>124	>84
Children 6-9 years	>122	>78	>130	>86
Children 10-12 years	>126	>82	>134	>90
Adolescents 13-15 years	>136	>86	>144	>92
Adolescents 16-18 years	>142	>92	>150	>98

¶Adapted from American Pharmacists Association. (2015). *Pediatric and neonatal dosage handbook: A universal resource for clinicians treating pediatric and neonatal patients* (22nd ed.). Hudson, Ohio: Lexicomp.

APPENDIX C.3: IDENTIFIABLE CAUSES OF HYPERTENSION (JNC-8)

• Obstructive sleep apnea • Chronic kidney disease • Primary aldosteronism • Renovascular disease • Excess sodium ingestion • Herbal supplements • Coarctation of the aorta • Pheochromocytoma • Thyroid disease • Parathyroid disease • Cushing's syndrome	• *Prescription Drugs:* oral contraceptives, sympathomimetics, *venlafaxine,* **bupropion, clozapine, buspirone, bromocriptine, carbamazepine, metoclopramide** • *Illicit, Over-the-Counter Drugs, and Herbal Products:* excess alcohol consumption, alcohol withdrawal, anabolic steroids, cocaine, cocaine withdrawal, phenylpropanolamine analogs, ephedra alkaloids, ergot-containing herbal products, St. John's wart, nicotine withdrawal

APPENDIX C.4: CVD RISK FACTORS (JNC-8)

• Hypertension • Obesity (BMI ≥30 kg/m²) • Dyslipidemia • Diabetes mellitus • Cigarette smoking • Physical inactivity	• Microalbuminuria, GFR <60 mL/min • Age (men >55 yrs, women >65 yrs) • Family history of premature CVD (men <55 yrs, women <65 yrs)

APPENDIX C.5: DIAGNOSTIC WORKUP OF HYPERTENSION (JNC-8)

- Assess risk factors and comorbidities
- Reveal identifiable causes of hypertension
- Assess for presence of target organ damage
- History and physical examination
- Urinalysis, blood glucose, hematocrit, lipid panel, potassium, creatinine, calcium, (*optional:* urine albumin/Cr ratio), EKG

APPENDIX C.6: BLOOD PRESSURE MEASUREMENT RECOMMENDATIONS (JNC-8)

- Blood pressure should be measured after the patient has emptied his or her bladder and has been seated for 5 minutes with back supported and legs resting on the ground (not crossed)
- Arm used for measurement should rest on a table, at heart level
- Use a sphygmomanometer/stethoscope <u>or</u> automated electronic device (preferred) with the correct size arm cuff
- Take two readings one to two minutes apart, and average the readings (preferred)
- Measure blood pressure in both arms at initial valuation; use the higher reading for measurements thereafter
- Confirm the diagnosis of HTN at a subsequent visit one to four weeks after the first
- If blood pressure is very high (e.g., systolic 180 mmHg <u>or</u> higher), <u>or</u> timely follow-up unrealistic, treatment can be started after just one set of measurements

APPENDIX C.7: PATIENT-SPECIFIC FACTORS TO CONSIDER WHEN SELECTING DRUG THERAPY(IES) (JNC-8* AND ASH**)

JNC-8:
- Non-Black, including those with diabetes: thiazide, CCB, ACEI, or ARB
- African American, including those with diabetes: thiazide or CCB
- CKD; regimen should include an ACEI or ARB (including African Americans)
- Can initiate with two agents, especially if systolic >20 mmHg above goal or diastolic >10 mmHg above goal
- If goal not reached: stress adherence to medication and lifestyle, increase dose or add a second or third agent from one of the recommended classes
- Choose a drug outside of the classes recommended above only if these options have been exhausted. Consider specialist referral.

ASH:
- **Non-Black <60 years-of-age:** *First-line:* ACEI or ARB; *Second-line (add-on):* CCB or thiazide; *Third-line:* CCB plus ACEI or ARB plus thiazide
- **Non-Black 60 years-of-age and older:** *First-line:* CCB or thiazide preferred, ACEI, or ARB; *Second-line (add-on):* CCB, thiazide, ACEI, or ARB (do not use ACEI plus ARB); *Third-line:* CCB plus ACEI or ARB plus thiazide
- **African American:** *First-line:* CCB or thiazide; *Second-line (add-on):* ACEI or ARB. *Third-line:* CCB plus ACEI or ARB plus thiazide

Comorbidities (ASH):
- **Diabetes:** *First-line:* ACEI or ARB (can start with CCB or thiazide in African Americans); *Second-line:* add CCB or thiazide (can add ACEI or ARB in African Americans); *Third-line:* CCB plus ACEI or ARB plus thiazide
- **CKD:** *First-line:* ARB or ACEI (ACEI for African Americans); *Second-line (add-on):* CCB or thiazide; *Third-line:* CCB plus ACEI or ARB plus thiazide
- **CAD:** *First-line:* BB plus ARB or ACEI; *Second-line (add-on):* CCB or thiazide; *Third-line:* BB plus ARB or ACEI plus CCB plus thiazide
- **Stroke history:** *First-line:* ACEI or ARB; *Second-line:* add CCB or thiazide; *Third-line:* CCB plus ACEI or ARB plus thiazide
- **Heart failure:** ACEI or ARB plus BB plus diuretic plus aldosteronism antagonist. **Amlodipine** can be added for additional BP control (Start with ACEI, BB, diuretic. Can add BB even before ACE-I optimized. Use diuretic to manage fluid.)
- In patients 60 years of age or older who do not have diabetes or chronic kidney disease, the goal blood pressure level is now <150/90 mmHg
- In patients 18 to 59 years-of-age without major comorbidities, and in patients 60 years-of-age or older who have diabetes, chronic kidney disease, or both conditions, the new goal blood pressure level is <140/90 mmHg

APPENDIX C.8: BLOOD PRESSURE MANAGEMENT CHANGES FROM JNC VII TO JNC-8[¶]

- First-line and later-line treatments should now be limited to 4 classes of medications: thiazide-type diuretics, calcium channel blockers (CCBs), ACEIs, and ARBs
- Second- and third-line alternatives included higher doses <u>or</u> combinations of ACEIs, ARBs, thiazide type diuretics, and CCBs
- Several medications are now designated as later-line alternatives, including the following:
- Beta-blockers
- Alpha-blockers
- Alpha1/beta-blockers (e.g., *carvedilol*)
- Vasodilating beta-blockers (e.g., *nebivolol*)
- Central alpha2-adrenergic agonists (e.g., *clonidine*)
- Direct vasodilators (e.g., *hydralazine*)
- Loop diuretics (e.g., *furosemide*)
- Aldosterone antagonists (e.g., *spironolactone*)
- Peripherally acting adrenergic antagonists (e.g., *reserpine*)
- When initiating therapy, patients of African descent without chronic kidney disease should use CCBs and thiazides instead of ACEIs
- Use of ACEIs and ARBs is recommended in all patients with chronic kidney disease regardless of ethnic background, either as first-line therapy <u>or</u> in addition to first-line therapy
- ACEIs and ARBs should not be used in the same patient simultaneously
- CCBs and thiazide-type diuretics should be used instead of ACEIs and ARBs in patients over the age of 75 with impaired kidney function due to the risk of hyperkalemia, increased creatinine, and further renal impairment

[¶]Adapted from PL Detail-Document. (2014, February). Treatment of hypertension: JNC 8 and more. *Pharmacist's Letter/Prescriber's Letter*. Retrieved from https://www.scribd.com/doc/290772273/JNC-8-guideline-summary

APPENDIX D: ATP-IV TARGET LIPID RECOMMENDATIONS[¶]

APPENDIX D.1: TARGET TC, TG, HDL-C, NON-HDL-C

Total cholesterol	<200 mg/dL
Triglyceride	<150 mg/dL
High-density lipoprotein (HDL)	>40 mg/dL (male) >50 mg/dL (female)
Non-high-density lipoprotein (Non-HDL-C)	<130 mg/dL; 30 mg/dL above the LDL-treatment target

[¶]Adapted from the National Cholesterol Education Program Expert Panel on Detection, Evaluation, and Treatment of High Blood Cholesterol in Adults (Adult Treatment Panel IV, 2012)

APPENDIX D.2: TARGET LDL-C†

Risk Assessment††	LDL Target	Initiate TLC†††	Initiate Drug Therapy
0-1	<160 mg/dL	≥160 mg/dL	≥190 mg/dL (optional at 160-189 mg/dL)
2 or more plus 10-year risk <10%	<130 mg/dL	≥130 mg/dL	≥160 mg/dL
2 or more plus 10-year risk <20%	<130 mg/dL <100 mg/dL (optional)	≥130 mg/dL	≥130 mg/dL
CHD or CHD risk equivalents 10-year risk >20%	<100 mg/dL <70 mg/dL (optional)	≥100 mg/dL	≥100 mg/dL

†Treatment decisions based on LDL cholesterol.
††Risk factors include age (men ≥45 years and women ≥55 years).
†††Therapeutic lifestyle changes (e.g., exercise, weight loss, low fat diet).

APPENDIX D.3: NON-HDL-C¶

Desirable	<130 mg/dL	Non-HDL-C is calculated as total cholesterol minus HDL-C. The addition of non-HDL-C to the Lipid Panel reflects the recognition of this calculated value as a predictive factor in cardiovascular disease based on the National Cholesterol Education III studies. The reference ranges for non-HDL-C are based on National Cholesterol Education III guidelines: Non-HDL-C is thought to be a better predictor of CVD than LDL-C; treatment goal for non-HDL-C is usually 30 mg/dL above the LDL-C treatment target. For example, if the LDL-C treatment goal is <70 mg/dL, then Non-HDL-C treatment target would be <100 mg/dL.
Borderline high	139-159 mg/dL	
High	160-189 mg/dL	
Very high	≥190 mg/dL	

¶Adapted from the National Cholesterol Education Program Expert Panel on Detection, Evaluation, and Treatment of High Blood Cholesterol in Adults (Adult Treatment Panel IV, 2012).

APPENDIX E: EFFECTS OF SELECTED DRUGS ON INSULIN ACTIVITY

Hyper- and Hypoglycemic Drug Effects	
Drugs That May Cause Hyperglycemia	Drugs That May Cause Hypoglycemia
Calcium channel blockers	Alcohol
Thiazide diuretics	Beta-blockers
Corticosteroids	MAO inhibitors
Nicotinic acid	Salicylates
Oral contraceptives	NSAIDs
phenytoin	*warfarin*
Sympathomimetics diazoxide	*phenylbutazone*

APPENDIX F: GLYCOSYLATED HEMOGLOBIN (HgbA1c) AND AVERAGE BLOOD GLUCOSE EQUIVALENT

HbA1c and Average Blood Glucose Equivalent			
HbA1c (%)	GLU	HbA1c (%)	GLU
4	60 mg/dL	14	360 mg/dL
5	90 mg/dL	15	390 mg/dL
6	120 mg/dL	16	420 mg/dL
7	150 mg/dL	17	450 mg/dL
8	180 mg/dL	18	480 mg/dL
9	210 mg/dL	19	510 mg/dL
10	240 mg/dL	20	540 mg/dL
11	270 mg/dL	21	570 mg/dL
12	300 mg/dL	22	600 mg/dL
13	330 mg/dL	23	630 mg/dL

APPENDIX G: ROUTINE IMMUNIZATION RECOMMENDATIONS

- Prior to 1 year-of-age, administer IM vaccinations in the vastus lateralis muscle
- After 1 year-of-age, administer vaccinations in the posterolateral upper arm
- Influenza vaccine should be administered annually for all ages ≥6 months of age
- Inactivated vaccines (e.g., pneumococcal, meningococcal, and inactivated influenza vaccines) are generally acceptable and live vaccines are generally avoided, in persons with immune deficiencies or immunocompromising conditions
- Additional information about routine vaccinations, unknown vaccination status, travel vaccinations, vaccinations in pregnancy, and other vaccines, is available at:
- **www.cdc.gov/vaccines/hcp/acip-recs/index.html**
- **wwwnc.cdc.gov/travel/destinations/list**
- **DTaP** (diphtheria-tetanus-toxoid, acellular pertussis); minimum age 6 wks
- **DTaP** should not be administered at or after the 7th birthday
- The 4th dose of **DTaP** vaccine can be administered as early as age 12 months, provided that the interval between doses 3 and 4 is at least 6 months
- **DTaP** and **IPV** should be administered at or before school entry
- **HAV** (*hepatitis A vaccine*) is recommended for all children at 1 year (12-23 months) of age
- **HAV** 2-dose series should be administered at least 6 months apart
- **HBV** (*hepatitis B vaccine*) is a 3-dose series initiated at birth; administer 2nd dose at 1-2 months; administer the 3rd dose at age 6 months (not before ≥24 weeks)
- **HBV** should be offered to all children who have not received the full series
- Infants born to HBsAg-positive mothers should be tested for HBsAG and antibody to HBsAg after completion of the **HBV** series (at age 9-18 months)
- **Hib** (*Haemophilus influenza* type b conjugate vaccine) minimum age 6 months
- **Hib** is not recommended if age >5 years
- **HPV** (*human papillomavirus vaccine*) vaccine should be administered anytime between 11 and 12 years-of-age
- **HPV** is a 3-series vaccine administered at months 0, 1, 6; females may receive HPV/4 or HPV/2; males should receive HPV/2
- **HPV** if not previously received at 11 or 12 years-of-age, may be initiated at anytime between 13 and 26 years-of-age
- **IIV** (*inactivated influenza vaccine*) can be administered >6 months (use age-appropriate formulation), pregnant women, and persons with hives-only allergy to eggs
- **IHD** (*influenza high dose*) (**Fluzone High Dose**) may be recommended to persons ≥65 years of age
- **IPV** (inactivated poliovirus vaccine) minimum age 4 weeks
- An all-**IPV** schedule is recommended to eliminate the risk of vaccine-associated

(*continued*)

(*continued*)

paralytic polio (VAPP) associated with **OPV** (*oral poliovirus vaccine*)

- **LAIV** (*live attenuated influenza vaccine*) may be administered intranasally (**FluMist**)
- **Men** (*meningococcal vaccine*) should be administered to all children at the 11-12 year old visit as well as to unvaccinated adolescents 15 years-of-age (usually at high school entry)
- **Men** should be administered to all college freshmen living in dormitories
- Use MPSV4 for children aged 2-10 years and MCV4 for older children, although MPSV4 is an acceptable alternative for prophylaxis in men
- **MMR** (*mumps-measles-rubella*) should be administered at age 12 months in high-risk areas; if indicated, tuberculin testing can be done at the same visit
- **MMR** should be administered at age 11-12 years unless 2 doses were given after the first birthday; the interval between doses should be at least 4 weeks
- **MMR** adults born <1957 are generally considered immune to measles and mumps; all adults born ≥1957 should have documentation of at least 1 dose of MMR vaccine unless there is a medical contraindication <u>or</u> laboratory evidence of immunity to each of the 3 disease components; documentation of provider-diagnosed diseases <u>not</u> acceptable evidence of immunity to any of the 3 disease components
- **PCV-13** (*pneumococcal vaccine*) does <u>not</u> replace 23-valent pneumococcal polysaccharide in children age ≥24 months
- **PCV-13** when PCV-13 and PCV-23 are indicated, administer PCV-13 first; do <u>not</u> administer PCV-13 and PCV-23 in the same visit
- **PCV-13** adults ≥65 years-of-age, who have <u>not</u> received PCV-13 <u>or</u> PCV-23, should receive PCV-13 followed by PCV-23 6-12 months later
- **PCV-23** (pneumococcal vaccine 23 trivalent) minimum age 6 weeks
- **PCV-23** adults ≥65 years of age, who have received **PCV-23**, but <u>not</u> received PCV-13, should receive. **PCV-13** at least I year later; adults ≥65 years of age, who have <u>not</u> received **PCV-23**, should receive
- **PCV-13** followed by **PCV-23** 6-12 months later
- **RIV** (*recombinant influenza vaccine*; **FluBlok**) may be administered to any adult >18 years-of-age, including pregnant women
- **RIV** does <u>not</u> contain any egg protein; can be administered to anyone with egg allergy at any severity
- Older infants and children previously vaccinated with **PCV** should receive 3 doses (if age 7-11 months), 2 doses (if age 12-23 months), <u>or</u> 1 dose (if age >24 months)
- **Rot** (*rotavirus vaccine*) is a live attenuated oral vaccine for infants aged >6 weeks <u>or</u> <32 weeks *only*; administer the 1st dose at 6-12 weeks-of-age; administer 2nd and 3rd doses at 4-10-week intervals for a total of 3 doses
- **Rot** If an incomplete dose is administered, *<u>do not</u>* administer a replacement dose, but continue with the remaining doses in the recommended series
- **Td** (*tetanus-diphtheria vaccine*) should be repeated every 10 years throughout life (<u>or</u> if at-risk injury ≥5 years after previous dose)

(*continued*)

(*continued*)

- **Td** should <u>not</u> be administered until minimum age ≥7 years
- **TdaP** (*tetanus-diphtheria-acellular pertussis*) administer 1 dose to pregnant women during each pregnancy, preferably during 27-36 weeks gestation, regardless of interval since prior Td <u>or</u> TdaP
- **TdaP** persons ≥11 years-of-age who have <u>not</u> received **TdaP** vaccine <u>or</u> for whom vaccine status is unknown, should receive 1 dose of **TdaP** followed by a **Td** booster every 10 years
- **Var** should be administered to children at age 11-12 years who have <u>not</u> had chickenpox <u>or</u> who report having had chickenpox but do <u>not</u> have laboratory documentation of immunity
- **Var** If <u>not</u> received between age 11 and 12 years, administer 2 doses at least 4 weeks apart anytime after 12 years-of-age <u>or</u> a 2nd dose if previously only received 1 dose
- **VarZ** (*herpes zoster vaccine*) should be administered in a single dose once at ≥60 years-of-age, whether <u>or</u> not the person reports a prior episode of active herpes zoster infection
- **VarZ** is contraindicated in pregnancy and immune deficiency
- **DTaP** and **IPV** can be initiated as early as 4 weeks in areas of high endemicity <u>or</u> outbreak.

¶Adapted from DHHS CDC 2015.

APPENDIX G.1: CONTRAINDICATIONS TO VACCINES¶

All vaccines	Previous anaphylactic reaction to the vaccine Moderate <u>or</u> severe illness with <u>or</u> without fever
TdaP/DTaP, Td	Encephalopathy within 7 days of administration of previous dose
Hib	Previous anaphylactic reaction to the vaccine Moderate <u>or</u> severe illness with <u>or</u> without fever
HBV	Anaphylactic reaction to baker's yeast
HAV	Previous anaphylactic reaction to the vaccine Moderate <u>or</u> severe illness with <u>or</u> without fever
Influenza	Allergy to eggs (*except* **FluBlok,** which does <u>not</u> contain any egg protein)
IPV	Anaphylactic reaction to neomycin <u>or</u> streptomycin
Pneumococcal	Hypersensitivity to diphtheria toxoid
MMR	Pregnancy, immunodeficiency, anaphylactic reaction to eggs <u>or</u> neomycin
Meningococcal	Encephalopathy within 7 days of administration of previous dose
Rotavirus	<6 months <u>or</u> >32 months

(*continued*)

(*continued*)

HPV	Pregnancy; pregnancy testing is not required; however, if administered, defer the remaining dose(s) until completion or termination of pregnancy
Varicella	Pregnancy
Herpes zoster	Pregnancy

[¶]Adapted from DHHS CDC 2015.

APPENDIX G.2: ROUTE OF ADMINISTRATION AND DOSE OF VACCINES[¶]

Vaccine	Route	Dose
Single Vaccines		
Diphtheria-Tetanus-Pertussis (DTaP, Dtap, DT)	IM	0.5 ml
Haemophilus influenza type b (Hib)	IM	0.5 ml
Hepatitis A vaccine (HAV)	IM	0.5 ml: age <18 yrs 1.0 ml: age ≥19 yrs
Hepatitis B vaccine (HBV)	IM	0.5 ml: age <18 yrs 1.0 ml: age ≥19 yrs
Human Papillomavirus (HPV)	IM	0.5 ml
Influenza **(Fluzone Intradermal)**	ID	0.5 ml
Influenza, inactivated (IIV), recombinant (RIV)	IM	0.25 ml: age 6-35 months 0.5 ml: age ≥3 yrs
Influenza, live attenuated (LAIV)	NS	0.2 ml; 0.1 ml in each nostril
Meningococcal conjugate	IM	0.5 ml
Vaccine	Route	Dose
Meningococcal polysaccharide (MPSV)	SC	0.5 ml
Meningococcal serogroup B (Men B)	IM	0.5 ml
Mumps-Measles-Rubella (MMR)	SC	0.5 ml
Pneumococcal conjugate (PCV)	IM	0.5 ml
Pneumococcal polysaccharide (PPSV)	IM/SC	0.5 ml
Polio, Inactivated (IPV)	IM/SC	0.5 ml

(*continued*)

(*continued*)

Rotavirus (**Rotarix**)	PO	1 ml
Rotavirus (**Rotateq**)	PO	2 ml
Tetanus (Td)	IM	0.5 ml
Varicella	SC	0.5 ml
Herpes Zoster	SC	0.65 ml: age ≥60 yrs
Combination Vaccines		
MMR-Var (**ProQuad**)	SC	0.5 ml: age ≤12 yrs
HBV-HAV (**Twinrix**)	IM	1 ml: >18 yrs
DTaP-HBV-IPV (**Pediarix**)	IM	0.5 ml
DTaP-IPV-Hib (**Pentacel**)	IM	0.5 ml
DTaP-IPV (**Kinrix, Quadracel**)	IM	0.5 ml
Hib-HBV (**Comvax**)	IM	0.5 ml
Hib-MenCY (**MenHibrix**)	IM	0.5 ml

¶Adapted from DHHS CDC 2015.

APPENDIX G.3: ADVERSE REACTIONS TO VACCINES¶

Vaccine	Signs and Symptoms	Treatment
Inactivated antigens: DTP, Dtap, DTaP, Td, IPV, influenza inactivated (IIV) recombinant (RIV) Live attenuated viruses: MMR, Meningococcal, rotavirus, varicella, herpes zoster	Local tenderness Erythema Swelling Low-grade fever Drowsiness Fretfulness Decreased appetite Prolonged crying Unusual cry	*acetaminophen* or *ibuprofen* for age and/or weight; *aspirin* and *aspirin*-containing products are contraindicated

¶Adapted from DHHS CDC 2015.

APPENDIX G.4: MINIMUM INTERVALS BETWEEN VACCINE DOSES¶

Type	#1 to #2	#2 to #3	#3 to #4	#4 to #5
HBV	4 weeks	5 months		
HAV	6 months			

(*continued*)

(*continued*)

Type	#1 to #2	#2 to #3	#3 to #4	#4 to #5
DTaP	4 weeks	4 weeks	6 months	6 months
IPV	4 weeks	4 weeks	4 weeks	
MMR	4 weeks			
Var	4 weeks			
Rotavirus	4 weeks	4 weeks; do not administer >32 weeks of age		
PCV-13	4 weeks (if #1 at age <12 months and current age <24 months); 8 weeks (as last dose if #1 at age>12 months or current age 24-59 months); No more doses needed if healthy and #1 at age ≥24 months	4 weeks if age <12 months; 8 weeks (as last dose if age ≥12 months); No more doses needed if healthy and previous dose at age ≥24 months	8 weeks (as last dose; only necessary for age 12 months to 5 years who received 3 doses before age 12 months)	
Hib	4 weeks (if #1 at age <12 months); 8 weeks (as last dose if #1 at age 12-14 months); No more doses needed if healthy and #1 at age ≥15 months	4 weeks if age 12 months; 8 weeks (as last dose if age ≥12 months); No more doses needed if previous dose at age ≥15 months	8 weeks (as last dose; only necessary for age 12 months to 2 years who received 3 doses before age 12 months)	
HPV	4 weeks	20 weeks (24 weeks after #1		

[¶]Adapted from DHHS CDC 2015.

APPENDIX G.5: RECOMMENDED CHILDHOOD IMMUNIZATION SCHEDULE[¶]

Type	Birth	1 month	2 months	4 months	6 months	6-18 months	12-15 months	15-18 months	4-6 years	11-12 years
HBV	●	●			●					
DTaP			●	●	●		●		●	
IPV			●	●		●	●		●	
Hib			●	●	●		●			
Rotavirus			●	●						
MMR							●		●	
TdaP										●
Varicella			●	●	●		●		●	
PVC-13			●	●			●			
HAV							●	●		
Meningitis										●
HPV●										●●●

[¶]Adapted from DHHS CDC 2015.

●Shaded box = immunization due.

●●●HPV 3-dose series, months 0, 1, 6.

APPENDIX G.6: RECOMMENDED CHILDHOOD IMMUNIZATION CATCH-UP SCHEDULE[¶]

Vaccine	Minimum Interval Between Doses			
	#1 to #2	#2 to #3	#3 to #4	#4 to #5
HBV	4 weeks	8 weeks (16 weeks after #1)		
DTaP	4 weeks	4 weeks	6 months	6 months
IPV	4 weeks	4 weeks	4 weeks	
MMR	4 weeks			
Var	4 weeks			
Rotavirus	4 weeks	4 weeks; do not administer >32 weeks of age		
PCV	2 months	2 months	2 months	6-15 months
HPV	4 weeks	20 weeks (24 weeks after #1		

[¶]Adapted from DHHS CDC 2015.

APPENDIX G.7: RECOMMENDED ADULT IMMUNIZATION SCHEDULE[¶]

Type	19-21 yrs	22-26 yrs	27-49 yrs	50-59 yrs	60-65 yrs	≥65 yrs
Influenza	1 dose annually					
HBV	3 dose series: months 0, 1, 6					
Td/TdaP	Substitute Tdap for Td one time; then continue Td once every 10 years					
MMR*	Born >1957: 2 doses					
Varicella*	Without evidence of immunity: 2 doses, 4 weeks apart					
Herpes zoster*					1 time dose	
PVC-13/ PVC-23					1 time dose	
HAV	Single antigen, 2 doses: months 0, 6-12 (Havrix); 0, 6-18 (Vaqta)					
Meningitis	1 or more doses					

(continued)

(*continued*)

Type	19-21 yrs	22-26 yrs	27-49 yrs	50-59 yrs	60-65 yrs	≥65 yrs
HPV (female)*β	3 doses; months 0, 1, 6					
HPV (male)β	3 doses; months 0, 1, 6					

¶Adapted from DHHS CDC 2015.
*Contraindicated in pregnancy.
βOnly if <u>not</u> previously vaccinated between 11-12 years-of-age.

APPENDIX H: CONTRACEPTIVES: CONTRAINDICATIONS AND RECOMMENDATIONS

- All contraceptives are pregnancy category X
- No non-barrier contraceptives protect against STDs
- **Absolute Contraindications:**
  - HTN >35 years-of-age
  - DM >35 years-of-age
  - LDL-C >160 <u>or</u> TG >250
  - Known <u>or</u> suspected pregnancy
  - Known <u>or</u> suspected carcinoma of the breast
  - Known <u>or</u> suspected carcinoma of the endometrium
  - Known <u>or</u> suspected estrogen-dependent neoplasia
  - Undiagnosed abnormal genital bleeding
  - Cerebral vascular <u>or</u> coronary artery disease
  - Cholestatic jaundice of pregnancy <u>or</u> jaundice with prior use
  - Hepatic adenoma <u>or</u> carcinoma <u>or</u> benign liver tumor
  - Active <u>or</u> past history of thrombophlebitis <u>or</u> thromboembolic disorder
- **Relative Contraindications:**
  - Lactation
  - Asthma
  - Ulcerative colitis
  - Migraine <u>or</u> vascular headache
  - Cardiac <u>or</u> renal dysfunction
  - Gestational diabetes, prediabetes, diabetes mellitus
  - Diastolic BP 90 mmHg <u>or</u> greater <u>or</u> hypertension by any other criteria
  - Psychic depression
  - Varicose veins
  - Smoker >35 years-of-age
  - Sickle-cell <u>or</u> sickle-hemoglobin C disease
  - Cholestatic jaundice during pregnancy, active gallbladder disease
  - Hepatitis <u>or</u> mononucleosis during the preceding year

(*continued*)

(*continued*)

- First-order family history of fatal <u>or</u> non-fatal rheumatic CVD <u>or</u> diabetes prior to age 50 years
- Drug(s) with known interaction(s)
- Elective surgery <u>or</u> immobilization within 4 weeks
- Age >50 years
- **Recommendations:**
  - Start the first pill on the first Sunday after menses begins. Thereafter, each new pill pack will be started on a Sunday.
  - Take each daily pill in the same 3-hour window (e.g., 9A-12N, 12N-3P; a 4-hour window prior to bedtime is not recommended).
  - If 1 pill is missed, take it as soon as possible and the next pill at the regular time.
  - If 2 pills are missed, take both pills as soon as possible and then two pills the following day. A barrier method should be used for the remainder of the pill pack.
  - If 3 pills are missed before 10th cycle day, resume taking OCs on a regular schedule and take precautions.
  - If 3 pills are missed after the 10th cycle day, discard the current pill pack and begin a new one 7 days after the last pill was taken.
  - If very low-dose OCs are used <u>or</u> if combination OCs are begun after the 5th day of the menstrual cycle, an additional method of birth control should be used for the first 7 days of OC use.
  - If nausea occurs as a side effect, select an OC with *lower **estrogen*** content.
  - If breakthrough bleeding occurs during the first half of the cycle, select an OC with *higher **progesterone*** content.
  - Symptoms of a serious nature include loss of vision, diplopia, unilateral numbness, weakness, <u>or</u> tingling, severe chest pain, severe pain in left arm <u>or</u> neck, severe leg pain, slurring of speech, and abdominal tenderness <u>or</u> mass.

APPENDIX H.1: 28-DAY ORAL CONTRACEPTIVES

Comment: **Beyaz, Loryna, Syeda, Safyral, Yasmin,** and **Yaz** are contraindicated with renal and adrenal insufficiency. Monitor k$^+$ level during the first cycle if the patient is at risk for hyperkalemia for any reason. If the patient is taking drugs that increase potassium (e.g., ACEIs, ARBS, NSAIDs, K$^+$ sparing diuretics), the patient is at risk for hyperkalemia.

Combined Oral Contraceptive	Estrogen (mcg)	Progesterone (mg)
Alesse-21, Alesse-28 (X)(G) *ethinyl estradiol/levonorgestrel*	20	0.1
Altavera (X) *ethinyl estradiol/levonorgestrel*	30	0.15
Apri (X)(G) *ethinyl estradiol/desogestrel*	30	0.15

(*continued*)

(*continued*)

Combined Oral Contraceptive	Estrogen (mcg)	Progesterone (mg)
Aranelle (X)(G) *ethinyl estradiol/norethindrone*	35	0.5 1 0.5
Aviane (X)(G) *ethinyl estradiol/levonorgestrel*	20	0.1
Balziva (X)(G) *ethinyl estradiol/norethindrone*	35	0.4
Beyaz (X)(G) *ethinyl estradiol/drospirenone* plus levomefolate calcium 0.451 mcg (28 tabs)	20	3
Blisovi 24 Fe (X)(G) *ethinyl estradiol/norethindrone* plus *ferrous fumarate* 75 mg (4 tabs)	20	1
Brevicon-21, Brevicon-28 (X)(G) *ethinyl estradiol/norethindrone*	35	0.5
Camrese (X) *ethinyl estradiol/levonorgestrel*	30 10	0.15
Camrese Lo (X) *ethinyl estradiol/levonorgestrel*	20 10	0.1
Cesia (X)(G) *ethinyl estradiol/desogestrel*	25 25 25	0.1 0.125 0.15
Cryselle (X)(G) *ethinyl estradiol/norgestrel*	30	0.3
Cyclessa (X)(G) *ethinyl estradiol/desogestrel*	25 25 25	0.1 0.125 0.15
Demulen 1/35-21, Demulen 1/35-28 (X)(G) *ethinyl estradiol/ethynodiol diacetate*	35	1
Demulen 1/50-21, Demulen 1/50-28 (X)(G) *ethinyl estradiol/ethynodiol diacetate*	50	1
Desogen (X)(G) *ethinyl estradiol/desogestrel diacetate*	30	0.15

(*continued*)

(*continued*)

Combined Oral Contraceptive	Estrogen (mcg)	Progesterone (mg)
Enpresse (X)(G) *ethinyl estradiol/levonorgestrel*	30 40 30	0.05 0.075 0.125
Estrostep Fe (X) *ethinyl estradiol/norethindrone* plus *ferrous fumarate* 75 mg	20 30 35	1 1 1
Femcon Fe (X)(G) *ethinyl estradiol/norethindrone* plus *ferrous fumarate* 75 mg	35	0.4
Generess Fe Chew tab (X)(G) *ethinyl estradiol/norethindrone* plus *ferrous fumarate* 75 mg	25	0.8
Genora (X)(G) *ethinyl estradiol/norethindrone*	35 35 35	0.5 1 0.5
Gianvi (X)(G) *ethinyl estradiol/drospirenone*	20	3
Gildess 1.5/30 (X)(G) *ethinyl estradiol/norethindrone*	30	1.5
Introvale (X) *ethinyl estradiol/levonorgestrel*	30	0.15
Jenest-28 (X) *ethinyl estradiol/norethindrone*	35 35	0.5 1
Jolessa (X)(G) *ethinyl estradiol/levonorgestrel*	30	0.15
Junel 1/20 (X)(G) *ethinyl estradiol/norethindrone*	20	1
Junel 1.5/30 (X)(G) *ethinyl estradiol/norethindrone*	30	1.5
Junel Fe 1/20 (X)(G) *ethinyl estradiol/norethindrone* plus *ferrous fumarate* 75 mg	20	1
Junel Fe 1.5/30 (X)(G) *ethinyl estradiol/norethindrone* plus *ferrous fumarate* 75 mg	30	1.5

(*continued*)

(*continued*)

Combined Oral Contraceptive	Estrogen (mcg)	Progesterone (mg)
Kaitlib Fe Chew Tab (X)(G) *ethinyl estradiol/norethindrone* plus *ferrous fumarate* 75 mg	25	0.8
Kariva (X)(G) *ethinyl estradiol/desogestrel*	20 10	0.15 0.15
Kelnor 1/35 (X)(G) *ethinyl estradiol/ethynodiol diacetate*	35	1
Leena (X) *ethinyl estradiol/norethindrone*	35 35 35	0.5 1 0.5
Lessina 28 (X)(G) *ethinyl estradiol/levonorgestrel*	20	0.1
Levlen 21, Levlen 28 (X)(G) *ethinyl estradiol/levonorgestrel*	30	0.15
Levlite 28 (X)(G) *ethinyl estradiol/levonorgestrel*	20	0.1
Levora-21, Levora-28 (X)(G) *ethinyl estradiol/levonorgestrel*	30	0.15
Loestrin 21 1/20 (X)(G) *ethinyl estradiol/norethindrone*	20	1
Loestrin 21 1.5/30 (X)(G) *ethinyl estradiol/norethindrone*	30	1.5
Loestrin Fe 1/20 (X)(G) *ethinyl estradiol/norethindrone* plus *ferrous fumarate* 75 mg	20	1
Loestrin Fe 1.5/30 (X)(G) *ethinyl estradiol/norethindrone* plus *ferrous fumarate* 75 mg (4 tabs)	30	1.5
Loestrin 24 Fe (X)(G) *ethinyl estradiol/norethindrone* plus *ferrous fumarate* 75 mg (4 tabs)	20	1
Lo Loestrin Fe (X) *ethinyl estradiol/norethindrone* plus *ferrous fumarate* 75 mg (2 tabs)	10	1

(*continued*)

(*continued*)

Combined Oral Contraceptive	Estrogen (mcg)	Progesterone (mg)
Lomedia 24 Fe (X)(G) *ethinyl estradiol/norethindrone* <u>plus</u> *ferrous fumarate* 75 mg	20	1
Lo/Ovral-21, Lo/Ovral-28 (X)(G) *ethinyl estradiol/norgestrel*	30	0.3
Loryna (X) *ethinyl estradiol/drospirenone*	20	3
Low-Ogestrel-21, **Low-Ogestrel-28 (X)(G)** *ethinyl estradiol/norgestrel*	30	0.3
Lutera (X)(G) *ethinyl estradiol/levonorgestrel*	20	0.1
Lybrel (X) *ethinyl estradiol/levonorgestrel*	20	0.09
Mibelas 24 FE (X)(G) *ethinyl estradiol/norethindrone* <u>plus</u> *ferrous fumarate* 75 mg	20	1
Microgestin 1/20 (X)(G) *ethinyl estradiol/norethindrone*	20	1
Microgestin Fe 1/20 (X)(G) *ethinyl estradiol/norethindrone* plus *ferrous fumarate* 75 mg	20	1
Microgestin 1.5/30 (X)(G) *ethinyl estradiol/norethindrone*	30	1.5
Microgestin Fe 1.5/30 (X)(G) *ethinyl estradiol/norethindrone* plus *ferrous fumarate* 75 mg	30	1.5
Minastrin 24 FE (X)(G) *ethinyl estradiol/norethindrone* plus *ferrous fumarate* 75 mg	20	1
Mircette (X)(G) *ethinyl estradiol/desogestrel diacetate*	20 10	0.15
Modicon 0.5/35-28 (X)(G) *ethinyl estradiol/norethindrone*	35	0.5

(*continued*)

(*continued*)

Combined Oral Contraceptive	Estrogen (mcg)	Progesterone (mg)
MonoNessa (X)(G) *ethinyl estradiol/norgestimate*	35	0.25
Natazia (X)(G) *estradiol valerate/dienogest*	30 20 20 10	— 2 3 —
Necon 0.5/35-21, Necon 0.5/35-28 (X)(G) *ethinyl estradiol/norethindrone*	35	0.5
Necon 1/35-21, Necon 1/35-28 (X)(G) *ethinyl estradiol/norethindrone*	35	0.5
Necon 10/11-21, Necon 10/11-28 (X)(G) *ethinyl estradiol/norethindrone*	35 35	0.5 1
Necon 1/50-21, Necon 1/50-28 (X)(G) *mestranol/norethindrone*	50	1
Nelova 0.5/35-21, Nelova 0.5/35-28 (X)(G) *ethinyl estradiol/norethindrone*	35	0.5
Nelova 1/35-21, Nelova 1/35-28 (X)(G) *ethinyl estradiol/norethindrone*	35	1
Nelova 10/11-21, Nelova 10/11-28 (X)(G) *ethinyl estradiol/norethindrone*	35 35	0.5 1
Nelova 1/50-21, Nelova 1/50-28 (X)(G) *mestranol/norethindrone*	50	1
Neocon 7/7/7 (X)(G) *ethinyl estradiol/norethindrone*	35 35 35	0.5 0.75 1
Nordette-21, Nordette-28 (X)(G) *ethinyl estradiol/levonorgestrel*	30	0.15
Norinyl 1+35-21, Norinyl 1+35-28 (X)(G) *ethinyl estradiol/norethindrone*	35	1
Norinyl 1+50-21, Norinyl 1+50-28 (X)(G) *mestranol/norethindrone*	50	1
Nortrel 0.5/35 (X)(G) *ethinyl estradiol/norethindrone*	35	0.5

(*continued*)

(*continued*)

Combined Oral Contraceptive	Estrogen (mcg)	Progesterone (mg)
Nortrel 1/35-21, Nortrel 1/35-28 (X)(G) *ethinyl estradiol/norethindrone*	35	1
Nortrel 7/7/7-28 (X)(G) *ethinyl estradiol/norethindrone*	35 35 35	0.5 0.75 1
Ocella (X)(G) *ethinyl estradiol/drospirenone*	30	3
Ortho-Cept 28 (X)(G) *ethinyl estradiol/desogestrel*	30	0.15
Ortho-Cyclen 28 (X)(G) *ethinyl estradiol/norgestimate*	35	0.25
Ortho-Novum 1/35-21, Ortho-Novum 1/35-28 (X)(G) *ethinyl estradiol/norethindrone*	35	1
Ortho-Novum 1/50-21, Ortho-Novum 1/50-28 (X)(G) *mestranol/norethindrone*	50	1
Ortho-Novum 7/7/7-28 (X)(G) *ethinyl estradiol/norethindrone*	35 35 35	0.5 0.75 1
Ortho-Novum 10/11-28 (X) *ethinyl estradiol/norethindrone*	35 35	0.5 1
Ortho Tri-Cyclen 21, Ortho Tri-Cyclen 28 (X)(G) *ethinyl estradiol/norgestimate*	35 35 35	0.18 0.215 0.25
Ortho Tri-Cyclen Lo (X)(G) *ethinyl estradiol/norgestimate*	25 25 25	0.18 0.215 0.25
Ovcon 35 Fe (X)(G) *ethinyl estradiol/norethindrone plus ferrous fumarate* 75 mg (4 tabs)	35	0.4
Ovcon 50-28, Ovcon 50-28 (X)(G) *ethinyl estradiol/norethindrone*	50	1
Ovral-21, Ovral-28 (X)(G) *ethinyl estradiol/norgestrel*	50	0.5

(*continued*)

(continued)

Combined Oral Contraceptive	Estrogen (mcg)	Progesterone (mg)
Portia (X)(G) *ethinyl estradiol/levonorgestrel*	30	0.15
Previfem (X) *ethinyl estradiol/norgestimate*	35	0.25
Quasense (X) *ethinyl estradiol/levonorgestrel*	30	0.15
Reclipsen (X)(G) *ethinyl estradiol/desogestrel* plus *ferrous fumarate* 75 mg (4 tabs)	30	0.15
Safyral (X) *ethinyl estradiol/drospirenone* plus *levomefolate calcium* 0.451 mg	30	3
Sprintec 28 (X)(G) *ethinyl estradiol/norgestimate*	35	0.25
Syeda (X) *ethinyl estradiol/drospirenone*	30	3
Tarina Fe 1/20 (X)(G) *ethinyl estradiol/norethindrone* plus *ferrous fumarate* 75 mg (7 tabs)	20	1
Taytulla Fe 1/20 (X)(G) (Softgel caps) *ethinyl estradiol/norethindrone* plus *ferrous fumarate* 75 mg (4 Softgel caps)	20	1
Tilia Fe (X)(G) *ethinyl estradiol/norethindrone* plus *ferrous fumarate* 75 mg (7 tabs)	20 30 35	1 1 1
Tri-Legest 21 (X)(G) *ethinyl estradiol/norethindrone*	20 30 35	1 1 1
Tri-Legest Fe (X)(G) *ethinyl estradiol/norethindrone* plus *ferrous fumarate* 75 mg (7 tabs)	20 30 35	1 1 1
Tri-Levlen 21, Tri-Levlen 28 (X)(G) *ethinyl estradiol/levonorgestrel*	30 40 30	0.05 0.075 0.125

(continued)

(*continued*)

Combined Oral Contraceptive	Estrogen (mcg)	Progesterone (mg)
Tri-Lo-Estarylla (X)(G) *ethinyl estradiol/norgestimate*	25 25 25	0.18 0.215 0.25
Tri-Lo-Sprintec (X)(G) *ethinyl estradiol/norgestimate*	25 25 25	0.18 0.215 0.25
TriNessa (X)(G) *ethinyl estradiol/norgestimate*	35 35 35	0.18 0.215 0.25
Tri-Norinyl 21, Tri-Norinyl 28 (X)(G) *ethinyl estradiol/norethindrone*	35 35 35	0.5 1 0.5
Triphasil-21, Triphasil-28 (X)(G) *ethinyl estradiol/levonorgestrel*	30 40 30	0.050 0.075 0.125
Tri-Previfem (X)(G) *ethinyl estradiol/norgestimate*	35 35 35	0.18 0.215 0.25
Tri-Sprintec (X)(G) *ethinyl estradiol/norgestimate*	35 35 35	0.18 0.215 0.25
Trivora (X)(G) *ethinyl estradiol/levonorgestrel*	30 40 30	0.05 0.075 0.125
Velivet (X)(G) *ethinyl estradiol/desogestrel*	25 25 25	0.1 0.125 0.15
Yasmin (X)(G) *ethinyl estradiol/drospirenone*	30	3
Yaz (X)(G) *ethinyl estradiol/drospirenone*	20	3
Zovia 1/35E-28 (X)(G) *ethinyl estradiol/ethynodiol diacetate*	35	1
Zovia 1/50E-28 (X)(G) *ethinyl estradiol/ethynodiol diacetate*	50	1

APPENDIX H.2: EXTENDED-CYCLE ORAL CONTRACEPTIVES

91 Day
▷ *ethinyl estradiol/levonorgestrel* (X) 1 tab daily x 91 days; repeat (no tablet-free days)

Ashlyna (G) *Tab: levonorgest* 15 mcg/*eth est* 30 mcg (84) + *eth est* 10 mcg (7) (91 tabs/pck)

Jolessa (G) *Tab: levonorgest* 15 mcg/*eth est* 30 mcg (84) + inert tabs (7) (91 tabs/pck)

LoSeasonique *Tab: levnorgest* 0.1 mcg/*eth est* 20 mcg (84) + *eth est* 10 mcg (7) (91 tabs/pck)

Quartette (G) *Tab: levonorgest* 15 mcg/*eth est* 30 mcg (84) + *eth est* 10 mcg (7) (91 tabs/pck)

Quasense (G) *Tab: levonorgest* 15 mcg/*eth est* 30 mcg (84) + inert tabs (7) (91 tabs/pck)

Seasonale (G) *Tab: levonorgest* 15 mcg/*eth est* 30 mcg (84) + inert tabs (7) (91 tabs/pck)

Seasonique (G) *Tab: levnorgest* 15 mcg/*eth est* 30 mcg (84) + *eth est* 10 mcg (7) (91 tabs/pck)

365 Day
▷ *ethinyl estradiol/levonorgestrel* (X) 1 tab daily x 28 days; repeat (no tablet-free days)

Lybrel *Tab: levnorgest* 0.09 mcg/*eth est* 20 mcg (28 tabs/pck)

APPENDIX H.3: PROGESTERONE-ONLY ORAL CONTRACEPTIVES ("MINI-PILL")

Brand	Progesterone	mcg
Comment: Take progestin-only pills at the same time each day (within a 3-hour time window). If a pill is missed, another method of contraception should be used for the remainder of the pill pack.		
Camila (X)(G)	*norethindrone*	35
Errin (X)(G)	*norethindrone*	35
Jolivette (X)(G)	*norethindrone*	35
Micronor (X)(G)	*norethindrone*	35
Nora-BE (X)(G)	*norethindrone*	35
Nor-QD (X)(G)	*norethindrone*	35
Ovrette (X)	*norgestrel*	7.5

APPENDIX H.4: INJECTABLE CONTRACEPTIVES

APPENDIX H.4.1: Injectable Progesterone

90 Days
Comment: Administer first dose within 5 days of onset of normal menses, within 5 days postpartum if not breastfeeding, or at 6 weeks postpartum if breastfeeding exclusively. Do not use for >2 years unless other methods are inadequate.

➤ *medroxyprogesterone* (X)(G)
  Depo-Provera 150 mg deep IM q 3 months
    Vial: 150 mg/ml (1 ml); *Prefilled syringe:* 150 mg/ml
  Depo-SubQ 104 mg SC q 3 months
    Prefilled syringe: 104 mg/ml (0.65 ml) (parabens)

APPENDIX H.5: TRANSDERMAL CONTRACEPTIVE

Ethinyl Estradiol/Norelgestromin
Comment: Apply the transdermal patch to the abdomen, buttock, upper-outer arm, or upper torso. *Do* not apply the transdermal patch to the breast. Rotate the site (however, may use the same anatomical area).

➤ *ethinyl estradiol/norelgestromin* (X)(G) apply one patch once weekly x 3 weeks; then 1 patch-free week; then repeat sequence
  Ortho Evra
    Transdermal patch: *eth est* 20 mcg/*norel* 150 mcg per day (1, 3/pck)

APPENDIX H.6: CONTRACEPTIVE VAGINAL RINGS

Ethinyl Estradiol/Etonogestrel
Comment: The vaginal ring should be inserted prior to, or on 5th day, of the menstrual cycle. Use of a backup method is recommended during the first week. When switching from oral contraceptives, the vaginal ring should be inserted anytime within 7 days after the last active tablet and no later than the day a new pill pack would have been started (no backup method is needed). If the ring is accidently expelled for less than 3 hours, it should be rinsed with cool to lukewarm water and reinserted promptly. If ring removal lasts for more than 3 hours, an additional contraceptive method should be used. If the ring is lost, a new ring should be inserted and the regimen continued without alteration.

➤ *etonogestrel/ethinyl estradiol* (X) insert 1 ring vaginally and leave in place for 3 weeks; then remove for 1 ring-free week; then repeat
  NuvaRing *Vag ring:* *eth est* 15 mcg/*eton* 120 mcg per day (1, 3/pck)

APPENDIX H.7: SUBDERMAL CONTRACEPTIVES

Comment: Implants must be inserted within 7 days of the onset of menses. A complete physical examination is required annually. Remove if pregnancy, thromboembolic disorder including thrombophlebitis, jaundice, visual

(*continued*)

(continued)

---

disturbances. Not for use by patients with hypertension, diabetes, hyperlipidemia, impaired liver function, epilepsy, asthma, migraine, depression, cardiac or renal insufficiency, thromboembolic disorder including thrombophlebitis, prolonged immobilization, or who are smokers.

▷ *etonogestrel* (X) implant rod subdermally in the upper inner non-dominant arm; remove and replace at the end of 3 years

Implanon, Nexplanon
   Implantable rod: 68 mg implant for subdermal insertion (w. insertion device; latex-free)

▷ *levonorgestrel* (X) implant rods subdermally in the upper inner non-dominant arm; remove and replace at the end of 5 years

Norplant
   Implantable rods: 6-36 mg implants (total 216 mg) for subdermal insertion (1 kit w. sterile supplies)

APPENDIX H.8: INTRAUTERINE CONTRACEPTIVES

Comment: Indicated in females who have had at least one child and who are in a stable, mutually monogamous relationship. Re-examine after menses within 3 months (recommend 4-6 weeks) to check placement.

▷ *levonorgestrel* (X)
   Kyleena *IUD:* 19.5 mg (replace at least every 5 years)
   Liletta *IUD:* 52 mg (replace at least every 3 years)
   Mirena *IUD:* 52 mg (replace at least every 5 years)
   Skyla *IUD:* 13.5 mg (replace at least every 3 years)

APPENDIX H.9: EMERGENCY CONTRACEPTION

Comment: Emergency contraception must be started within 72 hours after unprotected intercourse following a negative urine hCG pregnancy test. If vomiting occurs within 1 hour of taking a dose, repeat the dose.

▷ *ethinyl estradiol/levonorgestrel* (X) premenarchal: not applicable; 2 tabs as soon as possible after unprotected intercourse or contraceptive failure, then 2 more 12 hours after first dose

Preven
   Tab: eth est 50 mcg/*lev* 250 mcg (4/pck) + *Pregnancy test:* 1 hCG home pregnancy test
Yuzpe Regimen
   Tab: eth est 50 mcg/*lev* 250 mcg (4/pck)

▷ *levonorgestrel* (X)(OTC)(G) *Premenarchal:* not applicable; <17 years-of-age (prescription required; ≥17 years of age (OTC)
   My Way take 1 tab as soon as possible, within 72 hours, after unprotected sex or suspected contraceptive failure

---

(continued)

(*continued*)

> Tab: 1.5 mg
> **Plan B One Step** take 1 tab as soon as possible, within 72 hours, after unprotected sex or suspected contraceptive failure
> Tab: 1.5 mg
> **EContra EZ** take 1 tab within 72 hours after unprotected sex or suspected contraceptive failure
> Tab: 1.5 mg

▷ *uliprista* **(X)(G)** *Premenarchal:* not applicable
  Ella 1 tab as soon as possible within 120 hours (5 days) after unprotected sex or contraceptive failure; may repeat dose if vomiting occurs within 3 hours
    Tab: 30 mg

APPENDIX I: ANESTHETIC AGENTS FOR LOCAL INFILTRATION AND DERMAL/ MUCOSAL MEMBRANE APPLICATION

Agents and Indications	
Brand/*generic*	**Indication(s)**
AnaMantle HC *lidocaine 3%/hydrocortisone 0.5%*	Local anesthetic/steroid; for hemorrhoids, pruritus ani, anal fissure
Decadron Phosphate with Xylocaine *dexamethasone 4 mg/lidocaine 10 mg/ml (5 ml)*	Local anesthetic/steroid; infiltration by injection
Dyclone *dyclonine 0.5%, 0.1%*	Local anesthetic; infiltration by injection
Duranest (B) *etidocaine 1% (30 ml)* **Duranest (B) w. Epinephrine** *Inj: etido 1.5%/epi 1:200,000 (30 ml) Dental Cartridge: etido 1.5%/epi 1:200,000 (1.8 ml)*	Nerve block and local anesthetic; mouth, pharynx, larynx, trachea, esophagus, anogenital area, urethra Local anesthetic: dental procedures
Ela-Max 4% Cream (B) *lidocaine 4%* **Ela-Max 5% Cream (B)** *lidocaine 5%*	Local dermal anesthetic and for anorectal irritation and pain

(*continued*)

(*continued*)

Agents and Indications	
Brand/*generic*	**Indication(s)**
Emla Cream (B) (5, 30 g) **Emla Anesthetic Disc (B)** (2 discs/box) *lidocaine 2.5%/prilocaine 2.5%*	Local dermal anesthetic; preparation for phlebotomy, PIV starts, injections
Flector Patch (C/D) (30/box) *diclofenac epolamine 180 mg*	Local dermal NSAID analgesic
Exparel (B) *Vial:* 13.3 mg/ml (20 ml) *bupivacaine liposome 1.3% susp for inj*	Surgical site injection for post-op pain management
LidaMantle (B) cream (1, 2 oz) **LidaMantle (B)** lotion (177 ml) **Lidoderm** cream **(B)** (85 g) *lidocaine 3%* **Lidoderm (B)(G)** adhesive patch (10 cm x 14 cm; 30/box) *lidocaine 5%*	Local dermal anesthetic lotion, cream, and adhesive patch
Ophthaine (B) (15 ml) *proparacaine 0.5% ophthalmic solution*	Ophthalmic anesthetic for examination/removal of foreign body (eye)
Pliaglis Cream (B) (30 g) *lidocaine 7%/tetracaine 7%*	Local dermal anesthetic for superficial dermatological procedures
Qutenza (B) (1, 2 patches, each *with 50 g tube of cleansing gel*) *capsaicin 8% patch*	Local dermal NSAID analgesic for postherpetic neuralgia
Synera Topical Patch (B) (2, 10/pck) *lidocaine 70 mg/tetracaine 70 mg*	Local dermal anesthetic for venous access or skin lesion removal
Tetracaine Ophthalmic Solution (B) (15 ml) *proparacaine 0.5% ophthalmic solution*	Ophthalmic anesthetic for examination/removal of foreign body (eye)
Xylocaine Jelly (B) (5, 10, 20, 30 ml) *lidocaine 2% aqueous*	For procedures of the urethra, painful urethritis, and endotracheal intubation
Xylocaine Ointment (B) (3.5, 35 g) *lidocaine 5% water miscible*	For procedures of the urethra, painful urethritis, and endotracheal intubation

(*continued*)

(*continued*)

Agents and Indications	
Brand/*generic*	Indication(s)
Xylocaine Topical Solution (B) (100 ml) *lidocaine 2% solution* **Xylocaine Viscous (B)** (50 ml) *lidocaine 2% viscous solution*	Anesthetic for the nasal and oropharyngeal mucosa and the proximal portions of the GI tract
Zingo *lidocaine monohydrate 0.5 mg*	Hand-held, needle-free device, helium-powered delivery system that numbs site in 1-3 minutes, delivers 0.5 mg sterile lidocaine HCL for intradermal injection for the management of venous access pain
Zostrix (B) (0.7, 1.5, 3 oz) *capsaicin 0.025% cream* **Zostrix HP (B)** (1, 2 oz) *capsaicin 0.075% emollient cream*	Local dermal NSAID analgesic

APPENDIX J: ORAL PRESCRIPTION NSAIDs

Comment: NSAIDs should be taken with food to decrease gastric upset. Dosing of NSAIDs should be scheduled rather than PRN for maximal benefit. NSAIDs are contraindicated with sulfonamide or *aspirin* allergy, 3rd trimester pregnancy (causes premature closure of the ductus arteriosus), and coronary artery bypass graft (CABG) surgery. Concomitant use of *misoprostol* (**Cytotec**) with NSAIDs reduces gastric upset and potential for ulceration; however, *misoprostol* is pregnancy category X. Administration of *misoprostol* in pregnancy can cause spontaneous abortion, premature birth, birth defects, and uterine rupture (beyond the 8th week of pregnancy). NSAIDs and *warfarin* (**Coumadin**) are synergistic. With all patients, use the lowest effective dose for the shortest time necessary. NSAIDs should be taken with food to reduce the risk of gastrointestinal adverse side effects (GIASE).

GI ADVERSE SIDE EFFECTS:
(+) MILD; (++) FREQUENT; (+++) MORE FREQUENT/SEVERE

➤ *celecoxib* (C/D)(G)(+) <2 years: not recommended; 2-12 years, >10-<25 kg: 50 mg bid;≥25 kg: 100 mg once daily; >12 years: 100 mg bid or 200 mg once daily or 200 mg bid or 400 mg once daily; <50 kg, start at lowest dose
Celebrex *Cap:* 50, 100, 200, 400 mg

(*continued*)

(continued)

➤ *diclofenac sodium* (D)(+++)<12 years: not recommended; ≥12 years:
  Dyloject administer 37.5 mg IV bolus over 15 seconds q 6 hours; max 150 mg/day
    Vial: 37.5 mg/ml (25/box)
  Pennsaid 1% in 10 drop increments, dispense and rub into front, side, and back of knee: usually 40 drops (40 mg) qid
    Topical soln: 1.5% (150 ml)
  Pennsaid 2% apply 2 pump actuations (40 mg) and rub into front, side, and back of knee bid
    Topical soln: 2% (20 mg/pump actuation; 112 gm)
  Solaraze Gel apply to affected areas bid
    Gel: 3% (30 mg (100 gm)
  Voltaren 50 mg bid <u>or</u> qid <u>or</u> 75 mg bid <u>or</u> 25 mg qid with an additional 25 mg at HS if necessary
    Tab: 25, 50, 75 mg ent-coat
  Voltaren XR 100 mg once daily; rarely, 100 mg bid may be used
    Tab: 100 mg ext-rel
  Zorvolex 35 mg tid
    Gelcap: 18, 35 mg ext-rel

➤ *diclofenac potassium* (C/D)(G)(+++) <12 years: not recommended; ≥12 years: 50 mg tid <u>or</u> qid <u>or</u> 25 mg tid <u>or</u> qid and may add 25 mg at HS
  Cataflam *Tab:* 50 mg
  Zipsor *Gel cap:* 25 mg

➤ *diclofenac sodium* <u>plus</u> *misoprostol* (X)(++) <12 years: not recommended; ≥12 years:
  Arthrotec *Tab:* 50, 75 mg

➤ *diflunisal* (C/D)(G)(+++) <12 years: not recommended; >12 years: initially 1 gm as a single dose followed by 500 mg q 8-12 hours <u>or</u> 500 mg as a single dose followed by 250 mg q 8-12 hours
  Dolobid *Tab:* 500*mg

➤ *etodolac* (C/D)(G)(+) <12 years: not recommended; ≥12 years:
  Lodine initially 600 mg to 1 gm/day in 2-3 divided doses; usual max 1 gm/day in divided doses; may increase to 1.2 gm/day when needed
    Tab: 400, 500 mg; *Cap:* 200, 300 mg
  Lodine XL 400 mg to 1 gm once daily; max 1.2 gm/day
    Tab: 400, 500, 600 mg ext-rel

➤ *fenoprofen* (B/D)(++) <12 years: not recommended; ≥12 years: 300-600 mg tid-qid; max 3.2 gm/day
  Nalfon *Tab:* 200 mg

➤ *flurbiprofen* (B/D)(G)(++) <12 years: not recommended; ≥12 years: 200-300 mg/day in 2-4 divided doses; max single dose 100 mg; reduce dosage for renal impairment
  Ansaid *Tab:* 50, 100 mg

(continued)

> ***ibuprofen/famotidine*** (B/D)(++) <12 years: not recommended; ≥12 years: 1 tab tid; swallow whole; use lowest effective dose for the shortest duration
>   **Duexis** *Tab: ibu* 800 mg/*fam* 26.6 mg

> ***indomethacin*** (B/D)(G)(+++) <14 years: not recommended; ≥14 years: 75-100 mg daily in 3-4 divided doses; max 200 mg/day
>   **Indocin** *Cap:* 25, 50 mg; *Rectal supp:* 50 mg; *Oral susp:* 25 mg/5 ml; *Vial:* 1 mg pwdr for reconstitution and IV infusion
>   **Indocin SR** *Cap:* 75 mg ext-rel
>   **Tivorbex** *Cap:* 20, 40 mg

> ***ketoprofen*** (C/D)(G)(++) <18 years: not recommended; ≥18 years: 75 mg tid <u>or</u> 50 mg qid; max 300 mg/day
>   **Orudis** *Cap:* 50, 75 mg
>   **Oruvail** *Cap:* 100, 150, 200 mg ext-rel

> ***ketorolac tromethamine*** (C/D)(G)(+++)
>   **Sprix** <17 years: not recommended; ≥17 years: 1 spray each nostril (total dose 31.5 mg) every 6-8 hours prn; max 4 doses/24 hours (total daily dose 126 mg); *renal impairment* <u>or</u> *<50 kg:* 1 spray in one nostril (total dose 15.75 mg) every 6-8 hours; max 4 doses/24 hours (63 mg); discard used bottle after 24 hours
>   *Nasal spray:* 15.75 mg/100 mcl nasal spray (8 sprays, 1.7 gm)
>   **Toradol** <17 years: not recommended; ≥17 years: 60 mg as a single IM dose; max 30 mg as a single IV dose; may administer 30 mg IV and 30 mg IM as a single dose; oral dosing is indicated <u>only</u> as continuation therapy to IM <u>or</u> IV dosing; oral formulation should <u>never</u> be administered as an initial dose; initiate oral dosing at 20 mg followed by 10 mg q 4-6 hours prn; max oral dosing 40 mg/day; the combined duration of IV/IM/PO dosing is not to exceed 5 days
>   *Tab:* 10 mg; *Inj* 15, 30, 60 mg/ml

> ***magnesium chol salicylate*** (C/D)(G)(+) <12 kg: not recommended; 12-37 kg: 50 mg/kg/day in 2 divided doses; >37 kg: 2.25 gm/day in 2 divided doses; ≥18 years: 3 gm daily at bedtime <u>or</u> in 2 divided doses
>   **Trilisate** *Tab:* 500*, 750*mg; 1*gm; *Oral susp:* 5 mg/5 ml (cherry cordial)

> ***meclofenamate sodium*** (B/D)(G)(++) <14 years: not recommended; ≥14 years: 50-100 mg q 4-6 hours <u>or</u> 300-400 mg/day in 3-4 equal doses; max 400 mg/day
>   **Meclofen** *Cap:* 50, 100 mg

> ***mefenamic acid*** (C)(G)(++) <14 years: not recommended; ≥14 years: 500 mg once; then, 250 mg q 6 hours
>   **Ponstel** *Cap:* 250 mg

> ***meloxicam*** (C/D)(G)(+) <2 years: not recommended; 2-<12 years: 0.125 mg/kg; max 7.5 mg once daily; ≥12 years: 7.5 mg once daily; max 15 mg/day; *Hemodialysis:* max 7.5 mg/day
>   **Mobic** *Tab:* 7.5, 15 mg; *Oral susp:* 7.5 mg/5 ml (100 ml) (raspberry)
>   **Relafen** *Tab:* 500, 750 mg

(continued)

▷ *nabumetone* (C/D)(G)(+) <12 years: not recommended; ≥12 years: 1-2 gm/day in a single dose <u>or</u> 2 divided doses; max 2 gm/day; <50 kg: max 1 gm/day

▷ *naproxen* (B)(G)(++) <2 years: not recommended; ≥2-12 years: 5 mg/kg bid; max 15 mg/kg/day has been used; use suspension; 275-550 mg bid <u>or</u> 275 mg every 6-8 hours; max 1.375 gm first day; then, max 1.1 gm/day; *Acute gout:* 825 mg once, then 275 mg every 8 hours
    Naprosyn *Tab:* 250, 375, 500 mg
    Naprosyn Suspension *Oral susp:* 125 mg/5 ml

▷ *naproxen/esomeprazole (as magnesium trihydrate)* (C/D)(++)(G) <18 years: not recommended; ≥18 years: one 375/20 <u>or</u> one 500/20 tab bid; take at least 30 minutes before meals; take lowest effective dose
    Vimovo 375/20 *Tab:* nap 375 mg/*eso* 20 mg
    Vimovo 500/20 *Tab:* nap 500 mg/*eso* 20 mg

▷ *oxaprozin* (C/D)(++) <6 years: not recommended; 6-16 years, 21-31 kg: 600 mg once daily; 32-54 kg: 900 mg once daily; ≥55 kg: 1.2 gm once daily; >16 years: 1.2 gm once daily; max 1.8 gm <u>or</u> 26 mg/kg, whichever is less, in divided doses; low body weight, milder disease, <u>or</u> on dialysis: initially 600 mg once daily; max 1.2 gm/day
    Daypro *Tab:* 600*

▷ *piroxicam* (C/D)(G)(+++) <12 years: not recommended; ≥12 years: 20 mg once daily
    Feldene *Cap:* 10, 20 mg

Comment: Because of the long half-life, steady state blood levels of *piroxicam* are not reached for 7-12 days. Therefore, there is a progressive response over several weeks.

▷ *salsalate* (C/D)(G)(+) <12 years: not recommended; ≥12 years: 1.5 gm bid <u>or</u> 1 gm tid
    Disalcid *Tab:* 500*, 750*mg; *Cap:* 500 mg

▷ *sulindac* (B/D)(G)(+++) 150-200 mg bid; max 400 mg/day; usually x 7-14 days
    Clinoril *Tab:* 150*, 200*mg
    Tolectin DS *Cap:* 400 mg
    Tolectin 600 *Tab:* 600 mg film-coat

▷ *tolmetin* (C/D)(G)(+++) <2 years: not recommended; 2-<12 years: 20 mg/kg divided tid to qid; usual range 15-30 mg/kg/day divided tid-qid: max 30 mg/kg/day; ≥12 years: initially 400 mg tid; usual range 600 mg to 1.8 gm/day in divided doses tid-qid; max 1,800 mg/day
    Tolectin *Tab:* 200*mg

▷ *nabumetone* (C/D)(G)(+) <12 years: not recommended; ≥12 years: 1-2 gm/day in a single dose <u>or</u> 2 divided doses; max 2 gm/day; <50 kg: max 1 gm/day

▷ *naproxen* (B)(G)(++) <2 years: not recommended; ≥2 years: 5 mg/kg bid; max 15 mg/kg/day has been used; use suspension; 275-550 mg bid <u>or</u> 275 mg q 6-8

(*continued*)

> hours; max 1.375 gm first day, then, max 1.1 gm/day; *Acute gout attack:* 825 mg once, then 275 mg every 8 hours
>> **Naprosyn** *Tab:* 250, 375, 500 mg
>> **Naprosyn Suspension** *Oral susp:* 125 mg/5 ml

▷ *naproxen/esomeprazole (as magnesium trihydrate)* **(C/D)(++)(G)** <18 years: not recommended; ≥18 years: 1 x 375/20 or 1 x 500/20 tab bid; take at least 30 minutes before meals; use lowest effective dose
>> **Vimovo 375/20** *Tab: nap* 375 mg/*eso* 20 mg
>> **Vimovo 500/20** *Tab: nap* 500 mg/*eso* 20 mg

▷ *oxaprozin* **(C/D)(++)** <6 years: not recommended; 6-16 years, 21-31 kg: 600 mg once daily; 32-54 kg: 900 mg once daily; ≥55 kg: 1.2 gm once daily; >16 years: 1.2 gm once daily; max 1.8 gm or 26 mg/kg/day, whichever is less, in divided doses; *Low body weight, milder disease, or on dialysis:* initially 600 mg once daily; max 1.2 gm daily
>> **Daypro** *Tab:* 600*

▷ *piroxicam* **(C/D)(G)(+++)** <12 years: not recommended; ≥12 years: 20 mg once daily
>> **Feldene** *Cap:* 10, 20 mg

Comment: Because of the long half-life, steady state blood levels of *piroxicam* are not reached for 7-12 days. Therefore, there is a progressive response over several weeks.

▷ *salsalate* **(C/D)(G)(+)** <12 years: not recommended; ≥12 years: 1.5 gm bid or 1 gm tid
>> **Disalcid** *Tab:* 500*, 750*mg; *Cap:* 500 mg
>> **Tolectin 600** *Tab:* 600 mg film-coat

APPENDIX K: TOPICAL CORTICOSTEROIDS BY POTENCY

Comment: All topical, oral, and parenteral corticosteroids are pregnancy category C. Use with caution in infants and children. Steroids should be applied sparingly and for the shortest time necessary. Do not use in the diaper area. Do not use an occlusive dressing. Systemic absorption of topical corticosteroids can induce reversible hypothalamic-pituitary-adrenal (HPA) axis suppression with the potential for clinical glucocorticoid insufficiency.

Potency guide:
- Face: Low potency
- Ears/scalp margin: Intermediate potency
- Eyelids: Hydrocortisone in ophthalmic ointment base 1%
- Chest/back: Intermediate potency
- Skin folds: Low potency

Generic	Brand/Formulation/Frequency	Strength/Volume
Low Potency		
alclometasone dipropionate (C)	**Aclovate** Crm bid-tid **Aclovate** Oint bid-tid	0.05% (15, 45, 60 gm) 0.05% (15, 45, 60 gm)
fluocinolone acetonide (C)	**Synalar** Crm bid-qid	0.025% (15, 60 gm)
hydrocortisone base or acetate (C)(G)	**Anusol-HC** Crm bid-qid **Hytone** Crm bid-qid **Hytone** Oint bid-qid **Hytone** Lotn bid-qid **Hytone** Crm bid-qid **Hytone** Oint bid-qid **Hytone** Lotn bid-qid **U-cort** Crm bid-qid	2.5% (30 gm) 1% (1, 2 oz) 1% (1 oz) 1% (2 oz) 2.5% (1, 2 oz) 2.5% (1 oz) 2.5% (1 oz) 1% (7, 28, 35 gm)
triamcinolone acetonide (C)(G)	**Kenalog** Crm bid-qid **Kenalog** Lotn bid-qid **Kenalog** Oint bid-qid	0.025% (15, 80 gm) 0.025% (60 ml) 0.025% (15, 60, 80 gm)
Intermediate Potency		
betamethasone valerate (C)(G)	**Luxiq** Foam bid	0.12% (100 gm)
clocortolone pivalate (C)	**Cloderm** Crm tid	0.1% (30, 45, 75, 90 gm)
desonide (C)(G)	**Desonate** Gel/Formulation bid-tid **DesOwen** Crm bid-tid **DesOwen** Lotn bid-tid **DesOwen** Oint bid-tid **Tridesilon** Crm bid-qid **Tridesilon** Oint bid-qid **Verdeso** Foam	0.05% (15, 60 gm) 0.05% (15, 60 gm) 0.05% (2, 4 fl oz) 0.05% (15, 60 gm) 0.05% (15, 60 gm) 0.05% (15, 60 gm)
desoximetasone (C)(G)	**Topicort-LP** Emol Crm bid	0.05% (15, 60 gm, 4 oz)
fluocinolone acetonide (C)(G)	**Capex** Shampoo **Derma-Smoothe/FS** Oil tid **Derma-Smoothe/FS** Shampoo **Synalar** Crm bid-qid **Synalar** Oint bid-qid	0.01% (4 oz) 0.01% (4 oz) 0.01% (4 oz) 0.025% (15, 30, 60 gm) 0.025% (15, 60 gm)

(*continued*)

(continued)

Generic	Brand/Formulation/Frequency	Strength/Volume
flurandrenolide (C)	**Cordran-SP** Crm bid to tid	0.025% (30, 60 gm)
	Cordran Oint bid-tid	0.025% (30, 60 gm)
	Cordran-SP Crm bid-tid	0.05% (15, 30, 60 gm)
	Cordran Lotn bid-tid	0.05% (15, 60 ml)
	Cordran Oint bid-tid	0.05% (15, 30, 60 gm)
fluticasone propionate (C)(G)	**Cutivate** Oint bid	0.005% (15, 30, 60 gm)
	Cutivate Crm qd-bid	0.05% (15, 30, 60 gm)
	Cutivate Lotn qd-bid	0.05%
hydrocortisone probutate (C)	**Pandel** Crm qd-bid	0.1% (15, 45 gm)
hydrocortisone butyrate (C)(G)	**Locoid** Crm bid-tid	0.1% (15, 45 g)
	Locoid Oint bid-tid	0.1% (15, 45 gm)
	Locoid Soln bid-tid	0.1% (30, 60 ml)
hydrocortisone valerate (C)(G)	**Westcort** Crm bid-tid	0.2% (15, 45, 60, 120 gm)
	Westcort Oint bid-tid	0.2% (15, 45, 60 gm)
mometasone furoate (C)	**Elocon** Crm qd	0.1% (15, 45 gm)
	Elocon Lotn qd	0.1% (30, 60 ml)
	Elocon Oint qd	0.1% (15, 45 gm)
prednicarbate (C)	**Dermatop** Emol Crm bid	0.1% (15, 60 gm)
	Dermatop Oint bid	
triamcinolone acetonide (C)(G)	**Kenalog** Crm bid-tid	0.1% (15, 60, 80 gm)
	Kenalog Lotn bid-tid	0.1% (60 ml)
	Kenalog Emul Spray bid-tid	0.2% (63, 100 gm)
High Potency		
amcinonide (C)(G)	Crm bid-tid	0.1% (15, 30, 60 gm)
	Lotn bid	0.1% (20, 60 ml)
	Oint bid	0.1% (15, 30, 60 gm)
betamethasone dipropionate (C)	**Sernivo Spray** Emul Spray bid	0.05% (60, 120 ml)
betamethasone dipropionate, augmented (C)	**Diprolene AF** Emol Crm qd-bid	0.05% (15, 50 gm)
	Diprolene Lotn qd-bid	0.05% (30, 60 ml)

(continued)

(*continued*)

Generic	Brand/Formulation/Frequency	Strength/Volume
desoximetasone (C)(G)	**Topicort** Spray bid **Topicort** Gel bid **Topicort** Emol Crm bid **Topicort** Oint bid	0.25% (30, 50, 100 ml) 0.05% (15, 60 gm) 0.25% (15, 60 gm) 0.25% (15, 60 gm)
diflorasone diacetate (C)	**Psorcon e** Emol Crm bid **Psorcon e** Emol Oint qd-tid	0.05% (15, 30, 60 gm) 0.05% (15, 30, 60 gm)
fluocinonide (C)	**Lidex** Crm bid-qid **Lidex** Gel bid-qid **Lidex** Oint bid-qid **Lidex** Soln bid-qid **Lidex-E** Emol Crm bid-qid	0.05% (15, 30, 60, 120 gm) 0.05% (15, 30, 60 gm) 0.05% (15, 30, 60, 120 gm) 0.05% (20, 60 ml) 0.05% (15, 30, 60 gm)
flurandrenolide (C)	**Cordran** Oint bid-tid **Cordran** Crm bid-tid	0.05% (15, 30, 60 gm) 0.025% (30, 60, 120 gm) 0.05% (15, 30, 60, 120 gm)
halcinonide (C)	**Halog** Crm bid-tid **Halog** Oint bid-tid **Halog** Soln bid-tid **Halog-E** Emol Crm qd-tid	0.1% (15, 30, 60, 240 gm) 0.1% (15, 30, 60, 120 gm) 0.1% (20, 60 ml) 0.1% (15, 30, 60 gm)
triamcinolone acetonide (C)(G)	**Kenalog** Crm bid-tid	0.5% (20 gm)
Super High Potency		
betamethasone dipropionate, augmented (C)	**Diprolene** Oint qd-bid **Diprolene** Gel qd-bid	0.05% (15, 50 gm) 0.05% (15, 50 gm)
clobetasol propionate (C)(G)	**Clobex** Shampoo daily **Clobex** Spray bid **Cormax** Oint bid **Cormax** Scalp App **Olux** Foam **Olux E** Foam **Temovate** Crm bid **Temovate** Gel bid **Temovate** Oint bid **Temovate Scalp** App bid **Temovate-E** Emol Crm bid	0.05% (4 oz) 0.05% (2, 4.5 oz) 0.05% (15, 45 gm) 0.05% (15, 45 gm) 0.05% (50, 100 gm) 0.05% (50, 100 gm) 0.05% (15, 30, 45, 60 gm) 0.05% (15, 30, 60 gm) 0.05% (15, 30, 45, 60 gm) 0.05% (25, 50 ml) 0.05% (15, 30, 60 gm)

(*continued*)

(*continued*)

Generic	Brand/Formulation/Frequency	Strength/Volume
fluocinonide (C)	**Vanos** Oint qd-tid	0.1% (30, 60, 120 gm)
flurandrenolide (C)	**Cordran** Tape q 12 hours	4 mcg/sq cm (roll of 3″ x 80″)
halobetasol propionate (C)	**Ultravate** Crm qd-bid **Ultravate** Oint qd to bid	0.05% (15, 45 gm) 0.05% (15, 45 gm)

APPENDIX L: ORAL CORTICOSTEROIDS

Comment: Systemic corticosteroids increase glucose intolerance, reduce the action of insulin and oral hypoglycemic agents, reduce adrenal cortex activity, decrease immunity, mask signs of infection, impair wound healing, suppress growth in children, and promote osteoporosis, fluid retention, and weight gain. Use systemic steroids with caution, using the lowest possible dose to affect clinical response, and withdraw (wean) gradually in tapering doses to avoid adrenal insufficiency. The American Academy of Rheumatology (AAR) recommends the following daily doses of calcium and vitamin D for anyone on a chronic systemic corticosteroid regimen: Calcium 1,200-1,500 mg/day and vitamin D 800-1,000 IU/day.

▷ *betamethasone* (C)(G) initially 0.6-7.2 mg daily
   Celestone *Tab:* 0.6 mg; *Syr:* 0.6 mg/5 ml (120 ml)

▷ *cortisone* (D)(G) <12 years: not recommended; ≥12 years: initially 25-300 mg daily <u>or</u> every other day
   Cortone Acetate *Tab:* 25 mg

▷ *dexamethasone* (C)(G)<12 years: not recommended; ≥12 years: initially 0.75-9 mg/day
   Decadron *Tab:* 0.5*, 0.75*, 4*mg; *Syr:* 0.5 mg/5 ml (100 ml)
   Decadron 5-12 Pak *Tabs:* 0.75*mg (12/pck)

▷ *hydrocortisone* (C)(G) <12 years: 2-8 mg/day; ≥12 years: 20-240 mg/daily
   Cortef *Tab:* 5, 10, 20 mg; *Oral susp:* 10 mg/5 ml
   Hydrocortone *Tab:* 10 mg

▷ *methylprednisolone* (C)(G) 4-48 mg/day
   Medrol *Tab:* 2*, 4*, 8*, 16*, 24*, 32*mg
   Medrol Dosepak *Dosepak:* 4*mg tabs (21/pck, 42 pck)

▷ *prednisolone* (C)(G) <12 years: 0.14-2 mg/kg/day in 3-4 doses x 3-5 days; ≥12 years: initially 5-60 mg/day in 1-2 doses x 3-5 days
   Flo-Pred *Susp:* 5, 15 mg/5 ml
   Orapred *Soln:* 15 mg/5 ml (grape) (dye-free, alcohol 2%)

(*continued*)

(*continued*)

> **Orapred ODT** *Tab:* 10, 15, 30 mg orally disint (grape)
> **Pediapred** *Soln:* 5 mg/5 ml (raspberry) (sugar-, alcohol-, dye-free)
> **Prelone** *Syr:* 15 mg/5 ml

Comment: **Flo-Pred** does not require refrigeration or shaking prior to use.

➤ *prednisone* (C)(G) <12 years: 0.14-2 mg/kg/day in 3-4 doses x 3-5 days; >12
  years: initially 5-60 mg/day in 1-2 doses x 3-5 days
      Deltasone *Tab:* 2.5*, 5*, 10*, 20*, 50*mg

➤ *prednisone (delayed release)* (C) <12 years: 0.14-2 mg/kg/day in 3-4 divided
  doses x 3-5 days; ≥12 years: initially 5-60 mg/day in 1-2 doses x 3-5 days
      RAYOS *Tab:* 1, 2, 5 mg del-rel

➤ *triamcinolone* (C)(G) <12 years: 0.14-2 mg/kg/day in 3-4 divided doses x 3-5
  days; ≥12 years: initially 4-48 mg/day in 1-2 divided doses x 3-5 days
      Aristocort *Tab:* 4*mg
      Aristocort Forte *Susp:* 40 mg/ml (benzoyl alcohol)
      Aristocort Aristopak *Tab:* 4*mg (16/pck)

APPENDIX M: PARENTERAL CORTICOSTEROID THERAPY

Comment: Systemic glucocorticosteroids increase glucose intolerance, reduce
the action of insulin and oral hypoglycemic agents, reduce adrenal cortex activity,
decrease immunity, mask signs of infection, impair wound healing, suppress
growth in children, and promote osteoporosis, fluid retention, and weight gain.
Use systemic steroids with caution, using the lowest possible dose to affect clinical
response, and withdraw (wean) gradually in tapering doses to avoid adrenal
insufficiency. The American Academy of Rheumatology (AAR) recommends the
following daily doses for anyone on a chronic systemic corticosteroid regimen:
Calcium 1,200-1,500 mg/day and vitamin D 800-1,000 IU/day.

➤ *betamethasone* (C)(G)
      Celestone 0.5-9 mg IM/IV x 1 dose
          Vial: 3 mg/ml (10 ml)
      Celestone Sol span 0.5-9 mg IM/IV x 1 dose; usual IM dose 6 mg
          Vial: 6 mg/ml (10 ml)

➤ *cortisone* (D)(G) <12 years: not recommended; ≥12 years: 20-300 mg IM
      Cortone Acetate *Vial:* 50 mg/ml (10 ml)

➤ *dexamethasone* (C)(G) initially 0.5-9 mg IM/IV daily
      Dalalone D.P. *Vial:* 16 mg/ml (1, 5 ml)
      Decadron *Vial:* 4, 24 mg/ml for IM use (5 ml) (sulfites)
      Decadron-LA *Vial:* 8 mg/ml (1, 5 ml)

(*continued*)

(continued)

> *hydrocortisone* **(C)(G)** <12 years: 2-8 mg/kg loading dose (max 250 mg); then 8 mg/kg/day; >12 years: initially 100-500 mg IM/IV daily
>> **Hydrocortone** *Vial:* 50 mg/ml (5 ml)
>> **Solu-Cortef** *Vial:* 100 mg (2 ml); 250 mg (2 ml); 500 mg (4 ml); 1 g (8 ml)

> *hydrocortisone phosphate* **(C)(G)** for IM, IV, and SC injection
>> **Hydrocortone** *Vial:* 50 mg/ml (2 ml)

> *methylprednisolone* **(C)(G)** 40-120 mg IM/week for 1-4 weeks
>> **Depo-Medrol** *Vial:* 20 mg/ml (5 ml); 40 mg/ml (5, 10 ml); 80 mg/ml (5 ml)

> *methylprednisolone sodium succinate* **(C)(G)** <12 years: 1-2 mg/kg loading dose; then 1.6 mg/kg/day in divided doses at least 6 hours apart; ≥12 years: 10-40 mg IV initially; then, IM <u>or</u> IV
>> **Solu-Medrol** *Vial:* 40 mg (1 ml), 125 mg (2 ml), 500 mg (4 ml); 1 gm (8 ml); 2 gm (8 ml)

> *triamcinolone* **(C)(G)** 40 mg IM/week
>> **Aristocort** *Vial:* 25 mg/ml (5 ml)
>> **Aristocort Forte** *Vial:* 40 mg/ml (1, 5 ml) *(do not administer IV)*
>> **Aristospan** *Vial:* 5 mg/ml (5 ml); 20 mg/ml (1, 5 ml)
>> **TAC-3** *Vial:* 3 mg/ml (5 ml) for intralesional and intradermal use

INJECTABLE CORTICOSTEROID/ANESTHETIC

> *dexamethasone/lidocaine* **(C)** 0.1-0.75 ml into painful area
>> **Decadron Phosphate with Xylocaine** *Vial: dexa* 4 mg/*lido* 10 mg per ml (5 ml)

APPENDIX N: INHALATIONAL CORTICOSTEROID THERAPY

Comment: Inhaled corticosteroids are indicated for the long-term control of asthma. Inhaled corticosteroids are not indicated for exercise induced asthma <u>or</u> for relief of acute symptoms (i.e., "rescue"). Low doses are indicated for mild persistent asthma, medium doses are indicated for moderate persistent asthma, and high doses are reserved for severe cases. Titrate to lowest effective dose. To reduce the potential for adverse effects with inhalers, the patient should use a spacer <u>or</u> holding chamber and rinse the mouth and spit after every inhalation treatment. Linear growth should be monitored in children. When inhaled doses exceed 1,000 mcg/day, consider supplements of calcium (1-1.5 g/day), vitamin D (400 IU/day).

> *beclomethasone* **(C)**
>> **Beclovent** <6 years: not recommended; 6-12 years: 1-2 inhalations tid-qid <u>or</u> 4 inhalations bid; max 10 inhalations/day; >12 years: 2 inhalations tid-qid <u>or</u> 4 inhalations bid; max 20 inhalations/day
>>> *Inhaler:* 42 mcg/actuation (6.7 g, 80 inh); 16.8 g (200 inh)

(continued)

(*continued*)

Qvar <12 years: not recommended; ≥12 years: *Previously using only bronchodilators:* initiate 40-80 mcg bid; max 320 mcg/day; *Previously using an inhaled corticosteroid:* initiate 40-160 mcg bid; max 320 mcg/day; *Previously taking a systemic corticosteroid:* attempt to wean off the systemic drug after approximately 1 week after initiating **Qvar**
   Inhaler: 40, 80 mcg/actuation metered-dose aerosol w. dose counter (8.7 g, 120 inh) (CFC-free)
Vanceril <6 years: not recommended; 6-12 years: 1-2 inhalations tid-qid; >12 years: 2 inhalations tid to qid <u>or</u> 4 inhalations bid
   Inhaler: 42 mcg/actuation (16.8 g, 200 inh)
Vanceril Double Strength <6 years: not recommended; 6-12 years: 1-2 inhalations bid; >12 years: 2 inhalations bid
   Inhaler: 84 mcg/actuation (12.2 g, 120 inh)

➤ *budesonide* (B)(G)
Pulmicort Respules use turbuhaler; <12 months: not recommended; ≥12 months-8 years: *Previously using only bronchodilators:* initiate 0.5 mg/day once daily <u>or</u> in 2 divided doses; may start at 0.25 mg/day; *Previously using inhaled corticosteroids:* initiate 0.5 mg/day daily <u>or</u> in 2 divided doses; max 1 mg/day; *Previously using oral corticosteroids:* initiate 1 mg/day daily <u>or</u> in 2 divided doses
   Inhal susp: 0.25 mg/2 ml (30/box)
Pulmicort Turbuhaler <6 years: not recommended; ≥6-12 years: 1-2 inhalations bid; >12 years: 1-2 inhalations bid; *Previously on oral corticosteroids:* 2-4 inhalations bid
   Turbuhaler: 200 mcg/actuation (200 inh)

➤ *flunisolide* (C)(G)
AeroBid, AeroBid M <6 years: not recommended; 6-15 years: 2 inhalations bid; ≥16 years: initially 2 inhalations bid; max 8 inhalations/day
   Inhaler: 250 mcg/actuation (7 g, 100 inh)

➤ *fluticasone* (C)(G)
Flovent HFA use Rotadisk: initially 50-88 mcg inh bid; <4 years: not recommended; 4-11 years: initially 50-88 mcg bid; >11 years: initially 100 mcg bid; *If previously using an inhaled corticosteroid:* initially 100-200 mcg bid; *Previously taking an oral corticosteroid:* initially 1000 mcg bid
   Inhaler: 44 mcg/actuation (7.9 g, 60 inh; 13 g, 120 inh); 110 mcg/actuation (13 gm, 120 inh); 220 mcg/actuation (13 g, 120 inh)
Rotadisk ≥11 years: initially 88 mcg bid; *If previously using an inhaled corticosteroid:* initially 88-220 mcg bid; *If previously taking an oral corticosteroid;* initially 880 mcg/day
   Rotadisk: 50 mcg/actuation (60 blisters/disk); 100 mcg/actuation (60 blisters/disk); 250 mcg/actuation (60 blisters/disk)

➤ *mometasone furoate* (C) <12 years: not recommended; ≥12 years: *Previously using a bronchodilator <u>or</u> inhaled corticosteroid:* 220 mcg q PM <u>or</u> bid; max 440 mcg q PM <u>or</u> 220 mcg bid; *Previously using an oral corticosteroid:* 440 mcg bid; max 880 mcg/day
Asmanex Twisthaler
   Inhaler: 220 mcg/actuation (6.7 g, 80 inh); 16.8 g (200 inh)

APPENDIX O: ORAL ANTIARRHYTHMIA DRUGS

Antiarrhythmics by Classification With Dose Forms		
Brand/*generic* **Pregnancy Category**	Class/Indication(s)	Dose Form(s)
Betapace *sotalol* (B)	*Class:* Class II and III Antiarrhythmic *Indications:* Documented life-threatening ventricular arrhythmias	*Tab:* 80*, 120*, 160*, 240*mg
Betapace AF *sotalol* (B)	*Class:* Class II and III Antiarrhythmic *Indications:* Maintenance of normal sinus rhythm in patients with highly symptomatic atrial fibrillation <u>or</u> atrial flutter who are currently in sinus rhythm	*Tab:* 80*, 120*, 160*mg
Calan *verapamil* (C)(G)	*Class:* Calcium Channel Blocker *Indications:* Control (with *digitalis*) of ventricular rate in patients with chronic atrial fibrillation <u>or</u> atrial flutter; prophylaxis of repetitive paroxysmal supraventricular tachycardia	*Tab:* 40, 80*, 120*mg
Cordarone *amiodarone* (D)(G)	*Class:* Class III Antiarrhythmic *Indications:* Documented life-threatening recurrent refractory ventricular fibrillation <u>or</u> hemodynamically unstable ventricular tachycardia	*Tab:* 200*mg
Quinidex *quinidine sulfate* (C)(G)	*Class:* Class I Antiarrhythmic *Indications:* Atrial and ventricular arrhythmias	*Tab:* 300 mg ext-rel
Inderal *propranolol* (C)(G) **Inderal XL** *propranolol ext-rel* (C)(G) **InnoPran XL** *propranolol ext-rel* (C)	*Class:* Beta-Blocker *Indications:* Atrial and ventricular arrhythmias; tachyarrhythmias due to *digitalis* intoxication; reduce mortality and risk of reinfarction in stabilized patients after myocardial infarction	*Tab:* 10*, 20*, 40*, 60*, 80*mg *Cap:* 60, 80, 120, 160 mg sust-rel *Cap:* 80, 120 mg ext-rel
Mexitil *mexiletine* (C)	*Class:* Class IB Antiarrhythmic *Indications:* Documented life-threatening ventricular arrhythmias	*Cap:* 150, 200, 250 mg

(continued)

(continued)

Antiarrhythmics by Classification With Dose Forms		
Brand/*generic* Pregnancy Category	Class/Indication(s)	Dose Form(s)
Multaq *dronedarone* (C)	*Class:* IB Antiarrhythmic *Indications:* Paroxysmal <u>or</u> persistent atrial fibrillation <u>or</u> atrial flutter	*Tab:* 400 mg
Norpace *disopyramide* (C)	*Class:* Class I Antiarrhythmic *Indications:* Documented life-threatening ventricular arrhythmias	*Cap:* 100, 150 mg
Procanbid *procainamide* (C)(G)	*Class:* Class IA Antiarrhythmic *Indications:* Life-threatening ventricular arrhythmias	*Tab:* 500, 1000 mg ext-rel
Quinaglute *quinidine gluconate* (C)(G)	*Class:* Class I Antiarrhythmic *Indications:* Atrial and ventricular arrhythmias	*Tab:* 324 mg ext-rel
Rythmol *propafenone* (C)(G)	*Class:* Class IC Antiarrhythmic *Indications:* Documented life-threatening ventricular arrhythmias; prolonged recurrence of paroxysmal atrial fibrillation <u>and/or</u> atrial flutter <u>or</u> paroxysmal supraventricular tachycardia associated with disabling symptoms in patients without structural heart disease	*Tab:* 150*, 225*, 300*mg *Cap:* 225, 325, 425 mg ext-rel
Sectral *acebutolol* (B)(G)	*Class:* Beta-Blocker *Indications:* Ventricular arrhythmias	*Cap:* 200, 400 mg
Sotylize *sotalol* (B)	*Class:* Class II and III Antiarrhythmic *Indications:* Documented life-threatening ventricular arrhythmias, and highly symptomatic AFlutter/AFib	*Oral soln:* 5 mg/ml
Tambocor *flecainide acetate* (C) (G)	*Class:* Class IC Antiarrhythmic *Indications:* Documented life-threatening ventricular arrhythmias; paroxysmal atrial fibrillation <u>and/or</u> atrial flutter <u>or</u> paroxysmal supraventricular tachycardia in patients without structural heart disease	*Tab:* 50, 100*, 150* mg

(continued)

(continued)

Antiarrhythmics by Classification With Dose Forms		
Brand/*generic* Pregnancy Category	Class/Indication(s)	Dose Form(s)
Tenormin *atenolol* (C)(G)	*Class:* Beta-Blocker *Indications:* Reduce mortality and in stabilized patients after myocardial infarction	*Tab:* 25, 50, 100 mg *Inj:* 5 mg/ml (10 ml) for IV administration
timolol maleate (C)(G)	*Class:* Beta-Blocker *Indications:* Reduce mortality and in stabilized patients after myocardial infarction	*Tab:* 5, 10*, 20*mg
dofetilide (C)(G)	*Class:* Class III Antiarrhythmic *Indications:* Maintenance of normal sinus rhythm in patients with atrial fibrillation or atrial flutter of >1 week duration who were converted to normal sinus rhythm (only for highly symptomatic patients); conversion to normal sinus rhythm	*Cap:* 125, 250, 500 mcg
Tonocard *tocainide* (C)(G)	*Class:* Class I Antiarrhythmic *Indications:* Documented life-threatening ventricular arrhythmias	*Tab:* 400*, 600*mg
Toprol XL *metoprolol* (C)(G)	*Class:* Beta-Blocker *Indications:* Ischemic, hypertensive, or cardiomyopathic heart failure	*Tab:* 25*, 50*, 100*, 200*mg

APPENDIX P: ORAL ANTINEOPLASIA DRUGS

Antineoplastics With Classification With Dose Forms		
Brand/*generic* Pregnancy Category	Class/Indications	Dose Forms
Alkeran *melphalan* (D)	Alkylating Agent	*Tab:* 2*mg
Arimidex *anastrozole* (D)	Aromatase Inhibitor	*Tab:* 1 mg
Aromasin *exemestane* (D)	Aromatase Inactivator	*Tab:* 25 mg

(continued)

(*continued*)

Antineoplastics With Classification With Dose Forms		
Brand/*generic* Pregnancy Category	**Class/Indications**	**Dose Forms**
Arranon *nelarabine* (D)	Nucleoside Analog	*Vial:* 250 mg for IV infusion
Casodex *bicalutamide* (X)	Antiandrogen	*Tab:* 50 mg
Cytoxan *cyclophosphamide* (D)	Alkylating Agent	*Tab:* 25, 50 mg
Eligard *leuprolide acetate* (X)	GnRH Analog	*Inj:* 7.5 mg ext-rel per monthly SC injection
Eulexin *flutamide* (D)	Antiandrogen	*Cap:* 125 mg
Faslodex *fulvestrant* (D)(G)	Estrogen Receptor Antagonist	*Prefilled syringe for IM inj:* 50 mg/ml (2.5, 5 ml/syringe)
Femara *letrozole* (D)	Aromatase Inhibitor	*Tab:* 2.5
Gleevec *imatinib mesylate* (D)	Signal Transduction Inhibitor	*Cap:* 100 mg
Hydrea *hydroxyurea* (D)(G)	Substituted Urea	*Cap:* 500 mg
Iressa *gefitinib* (D)	Epidermal Growth Factor receptor tyrosine kinase inhibitor	*Tab:* 250 mg
Leukeran *chlorambucil* (D)(G)	Alkylating Agent	*Tab:* 2 mg
Lupron *leuprolide* (X)	GnRH Analog	*Susp for IM inj:* 1 mg (daily); 7.5 mg depot (monthly); 22.5 mg depot (every 3 months); 30 mg depot (every 4 months)
Megace, Megace Oral Suspension, Megace ES, *megestrol acetate* (D)(G)	Progestin	*Tab:* 20*, 40*mg; *Susp:* 40 mg/ml; ES concentrate: 125 mg/ml, 625 mg/5 ml

(*continued*)

(*continued*)

Antineoplastics With Classification With Dose Forms		
Brand/*generic* **Pregnancy Category**	Class/Indications	Dose Forms
Nexavar *sorafenib* (**D**)	Multikinase Inhibitor	*Tab:* 200 mg
Nolvadex *tamoxifen citrate* (**D**) (**G**)	Anti-estrogen	*Tab:* 10, 20 mg
Tarceva *erlotinib* (**D**)	Kinase Inhibitor	*Tab:* 25, 100, 150 mg
Velcade *bortezomib* (**D**)	Proteasome Inhibitor	*Vial:* 3.5 mg (pwdr for IV injection after reconstitution)
Viadur *leuprolide acetate* (**X**)	GnRH Analog	*SC implant:* 65 mg depot (replace every 12 months)
Xeloda *capecitabine* (**D**)	Fluoropyrimidine (prodrug of 5-fluorouracil)	*Tab:* 150, 500 mg
Zoladex *goserelin acetate* (**D**)	GnRH Analog	*SC implant:* 3.6 mg depot (28 days), 10.8 mg depot (3-month)
Zometa *zoledronic acid* (**D**)	Bisphosphonate	*Vial:* 4 mg pwdr for reconstitution for IV infusion, single dose

APPENDIX Q: ORAL AND DEPOT ANTIPSYCHOTIC DRUGS

ANTIPSYCHOTIC DRUGS WITH DOSE FORMS

Comment: Patients receiving an antipsychotic agent should be monitored closely for the following adverse side effects: neuroleptic malignant syndrome, extrapyramidal reactions, tardive dyskinesia, blood dyscrasias, anticholinergic effects, drowsiness, hypotension, photo-sensitivity, retinopathy, and lowered seizure threshold. Use lower doses for elderly or debilitated patients. Prescriptions should be written for the smallest practical amount. Foods and beverages containing alcohol are contraindicated for patients receiving any psychotropic drug. *Neuroleptic Malignant Syndrome* (NMS) and *Tardive Dyskinesia* (TD) are adverse side effects (ASEs) most often associated with the older antipsychotic drugs. Risk is decreased with

(*continued*)

(*continued*)

the newer "atypical" antipsychotic drugs. However, these syndromes can develop, although much less commonly, after relatively brief treatment periods at low doses. Given these considerations, antipsychotic drugs should be prescribed in a manner that is most likely to minimize the occurrence. NMS, a potentially fatal symptom complex, is characterized by hyperpyrexia, muscle rigidity, altered mental status and evidence of autonomic instability (irregular pulse or blood pressure, tachycardia, diaphoresis, and cardiac dysrhythmia). Additional signs may include elevated creatine phosphokinase (CPK), myoglobinuria (rhabdomyolysis), and acute renal failure (ARF). TD is a syndrome consisting of potentially irreversible, involuntary, dyskinetic movements that can develop in patients with antipsychotic drugs. Characteristics include repetitive involuntary movements, usually of the jaw, lips and tongue, such as grimacing, sticking out the tongue and smacking the lips. Some affected people also experience involuntary movement of the extremities or difficulty breathing. The syndrome may remit, partially or completely, if antipsychotic treatment is withdrawn. If signs and symptoms of NMS and/or TD appear in a patient, management should include immediate discontinuation of antipsychotic drugs and other drugs not essential to concurrent therapy, intensive symptomatic treatment, medical monitoring, and treatment of any concomitant serious medical problems. The risk of developing NMS and/or TD, and the likelihood that either syndrome will become irreversible, is believed to increase as the duration of treatment and the total cumulative dose of antipsychotic drugs administered to the patient increase. The first and only FDA-approved treatment for TD is *valbenazine* (**Ingrezza**) (*see page* 395).

➤ *aripiprazole* (C)(G)
  Abilify *Tab:* 2, 5, 10, 15, 20, 30 mg; *Oral soln:* 1 mg/ml (150 ml) (orange cream) (parabens)
  Abilify Discmelt *Tab:* 15 mg orally disintegrating (vanilla) (phenylalanine)
  Abilify Maintena *Vial:* 300, 400 mg ext-rel pwdr for IM injection after reconstitution; 300, 400 mg single-dose prefilled dual chamber syringes w. supplies

➤ *asenapine* (C)
  Saphris *SL tab:* 2.5, 5, 10 mg

➤ *brexpiprazole* (C)
  Rexulti *Tab:* 0.25, 0.5, 1, 2, 3, 4 mg

➤ *bupropion* (C)
  Forfivo XL *Tab:* 450 mg ext-rel

➤ *cariprazine* (NE)
  Vraylar *Cap:* 1.5, 3, 4.5, 6 mg

➤ *chlorpromazine* (C)(G)
  Thorazine *Tab:* 10, 25, 50, 100, 200 mg; *Cap:* 30, 75, 150 mg sust-rel; *Syr:* 10 mg/5 ml (4 oz, orange-custard); *Vial/Amp:* 25 mg/ml (1, 2 ml) (sulfites)

➤ *clozapine* (B)(G)
  Clozapine ODT (G) *ODT:* 150, 200 mg
  Clozaril (G) *Tab:* 25*, 100* mg; *ODT:* 150, 200 mg
  FazaClo ODT (G) *ODT:* 12.5, 25, 100, 150, 200 mg (phenylalanine)
  Versacloz *Oral susp:* 50 mg/ml (100 ml)

(*continued*)

(*continued*)

▷ *fluphenazine* (C)(G)
  Prolixin *Tab:* 1, 2.5, 5*, 10 mg (tartrazine); *Conc:* 5 mg/ml (4 oz w. calib dropper) (alcohol 14%); *Elix:* 5 mg/ml (2 oz w. calib dropper) (alcohol 14%); *Vial:* 25 mg/ml (10 ml)

▷ *fluphenazine decanoate* (C)(G)
  Prolixin Decanoate *Vial:* 25 mg/ml (5 ml) (benzyl alcohol)

▷ *fluphenazine* (C)(G)
  Prolixin Ethanate *Vial:* 25 mg (5 ml) (benzyl alcohol)

▷ *fluphenazine decanoate* (C)(G)
  Prolixin Decanoate *Vial:* 25 mg/ml (5 ml) (benzyl alcohol)

▷ *haloperidol* (B)(G)
  Haldol *Tab:* 0.5*, 1*, 2*, 5*, 10*, 20 mg

▷ *iloperidone* (C)(G)
  Fanapt *Tab:* 1, 2, 4, 6, 8, 10, 12 mg

▷ *loxapine* (C)
  Adasuve *Oral inhal pwdr:* 10 mg single-use disposable inhaler (5/box)

▷ *lurasidone* (B)
  Latuda *Tab:* 20, 40, 80 mg

▷ *olanzapine fumarate* (C)(G)
  Zyprexa *Tab:* 2.5, 5, 7.5, 10, 15, 20 mg
  Zyprexa Zydis *ODT:* 5, 10, 15, 20 mg (phenylalanine)

▷ *paliperidone palmitate* (C)(G)
  Invega *Tab:* 3, 6, 9 mg ext-rel
  Invega Sustenna *Prefilled syringe:* 39, 78, 117, 156, 234 mg ext-rel suspension w. needle
  Invega Trinza *Prefilled syringe:* 273, 410, 546, 819 mg ext-rel suspension

▷ *prochlorperazine* (C)(G)
  Compazine *Tab:* 5, 10 mg; *Cap:* 10, 15 mg sus-rel; *Syr:* 5 mg/5 ml (4 oz) (fruit); *Supp:* 2.5, 5, 25 mg

▷ *quetiapine* (C)(G)
  Seroquel *Tab:* 25, 100, 200, 300 mg
  Seroquel XR *Tab:* 50, 150, 200, 300, 400 mg ext-rel

▷ *risperidone* (C)(G)
  Risperdal *Tab:* 0.25, 0.5, 1, 2, 3, 4 mg; *Soln:* 1 mg/ml (30 ml w. pipette); *Consta (Inj):* 25, 37.5, 50 mg
  Risperdal M-Tabs *M-tab:* 0.5, 1, 2, 3, 4 mg orally-disint (phenylalanine)

▷ *thioridazine* (C)(G) *Tab:* 10, 25, 50, 100 mg

▷ *trifluoperazine* (C)(G)
  Stelazine *Tab:* 1, 2, 5, 10 mg; *Conc:* 10 mg/ml; (2 oz w. calib dropper (banana-vanilla) (sulfites); *Vial:* 2 mg/ml (10 ml)

▷ *ziprasidone* (C)(G)
  Geodon *Cap:* 20, 40, 60, 80 mg

APPENDIX R: ORAL ANTICONVULSANT DRUGS

ANTICONVULSANT DRUGS WITH DOSE FORMS

▷ *brivaracetam* (C)
  Briviact *Tab:* 10, 25, 50, 75, 100 mg; *Oral soln:* 10 mg/ml (300 ml); *Vial:* 50 mg/5 ml single dose for IV inj

▷ *carbamazepine* (D)(G)
  Carbatrol *Cap:* 200, 300 mg ext-rel
  Equetro *Cap:* 100, 200, 300 mg ext-rel
  Tegretol *Tab:* 100*, 200*mg; *Chew tab:* 100*mg
  Tegretol Suspension *Oral susp:* 100 mg/5 ml (450 ml)(citrus vanilla) (sorbitol)
  Tegretol-XR *Tab:* 100, 200, 400 mg ext-rel

▷ *clobazam* (C)(IV)
  Onfi *Tab:* 10*, 20*mg
  Onfi Oral Suspension *Oral susp:* 2.5 mg/ml (120 ml w. 2 dosing syringes)(berry)

▷ *clonazepam* (D)(IV)(G)
  Clonazepam ODT *ODT:* 0.125, 0.25, 0.5, 1, 2, oral-dis
  Klonopin *Tab:* 0.5*, 1, 2 mg

▷ *diazepam* (D)(IV)(G)
  Diastat *Rectal gel delivery system:* 2.5 mg
  Diastat AcuDial *Rectal gel delivery system:* 10, 20 mg
  Valium *Tab:* 2*, 5*, 10*mg
  Valium Injectable *Vial:* 5 mg/ml (10 ml); *Amp:* 5 mg/ml (2 ml); *Prefilled syringe:* 5 mg/ml (5 ml)
  Valium Intensol *Conc oral soln:* 5 mg/ml (30 ml w. dropper) (alcohol 19%)
  Valium Oral Solution *Oral soln:* 5 mg/5 ml (500 ml) (winter green-spice)

▷ *divalproex sodium* (D)(G)
  Depakene *Cap:* 250 mg; *Syr:* 250 mg/5 ml (16 oz)
  Depakote *Tab:* 125, 250, 500 mg
  Depakote ER *Tab:* 250, 500 mg ext-rel
  Depakote Sprinkle *Cap:* 125 mg

▷ *eslicarbazepine* (C)
  Aptiom *Tab:* 200*, 400, 600*, 800* mg

▷ *ethosuccimide* (C)(G)
  Zarontin *Cap:* 250 mg; *Oral soln:* 250 mg/5 ml (raspberry)

▷ *ezogabine* (C)
  Potiga *Tab:* 50, 200, 300, 400 mg

▷ *felbamate* (C)(G)
  Felbatol *Tab:* 400*, 600*mg
  Felbatol Oral Suspension *Oral susp:* 600 mg/5 ml (4, 8, 32 oz)
  Peganone *Tab:* 250, 500 mg

(continued)

(*continued*)

▷ *gabapentin* (C)
    Horizant *Tab:* 300, 600 ext-rel
    Neurontin (G) *Cap:* 100, 300, 400 mg; *Tab:* 600*, 800*mg
    Neurontin Oral Solution *Oral soln:* 250 mg/5 ml (480 ml) (strawberry-anise)

▷ *lacosamide* (C)(V)(G)
    Vimpat *Tab:* 50, 100, 150, 200 mg; *Oral soln:* 10 mg/ml (200, 465 ml); *Vial:* 10 mg/ml soln for IV infusion, single use (20 ml)

▷ *lamotrigine* (C)(G)
    Lamictal *Tab:* 25*, 100*, 150*, 200*mg
    Lamictal Chewable Dispersible Tab *Chew tab:* 2, 5, 25, 50 mg (black current)
    Lamictal ODT *ODT:* 25, 50, 100, 200 mg oral-dis
    Lamictal XR *Tab:* 25, 50, 100, 200, 250, 300 mg ext-rel

▷ *levetiracetam* (C)
    Elepsia *Tab:* 1000, 1500 mg ext-rel
    Keppra *Tab:* 250*, 500*, 750*, 1000*mg
    Keppra Oral Solution *Oral soln:* 100 mg/ml (16 oz) (grape) (dye-free)
    Keppra XR *Tab:* 500, 750 mg ext-rel
    Levetiracetam IV (G) *Premixed:* 500, 1,000, 1,500 mg for IV infusion (100 ml)

▷ *mephobarbital* (D)(II)
    Mebaral *Tab:* 32, 50, 100 mg

▷ *methsuximide* (C)
    Celontin Kapseals *Cap:* 150, 300 mg

▷ *oxcarbazepine* (C)(G)
    Trileptal *Tab:* 150, 300, 600 mg; *Oral susp:* 300 mg/5 ml (lemon) (alcohol)
    Oxtellar XR *Tab:* 150, 300, 600 mg ext-rel

▷ *perampanel* (C)(III)
    Fycompa *Tab:* 2, 4, 6, 8, 10, 12 mg
    Fycompa Oral Suspension *Oral susp:* 0.5 mg/ml (340 ml w. dosing syringe)

▷ *phenytoin* (D)(G), *primidone* (D)(G) **Dilantin** *Cap:* 30, 100 mg ext-rel
    Dilantin Infatabs *Chew tab:* 50 mg
    Dilantin Oral Suspension *Oral susp:* 125 mg/5 ml (237 ml) (alcohol 6%)
    Phenytek *Cap:* 200, 300 mg ext-rel

▷ *pregabalin* (C)(V)
    Lyrica *Cap:* 25, 50, 75, 100, 200, 225, 300 mg
    Lyrica Oral Solution *Oral soln:* 20 mg/ml

▷ *primidone* (C)
    Mysoline *Tab:* 50*, 250*mg
    Mysoline Oral Solution *Oral susp:* 250 mg/5 ml (8 oz)

▷ *rufinamide* (C)(G)
    Banzel *Tab:* 200*, 400*mg
    Banzel Oral Solution *Susp:* 40 mg/ml (orange) (lactose-free, gluten-free, dye-free)

(*continued*)

(*continued*)

> *tiagabine* (C)(G)
>   **Gabitril** *Tab*: 2, 4, 12, 16 mg

> *topiramate* (D)(G)
>   **Topamax** *Tab*: 25, 50, 100, 200 mg
>   **Topamax Sprinkle Caps** *Cap*: 15, 25, 50 mg
>   **Trokendi XR** *Cap*: 100, 200 mg ext-rel
>   **Qudexy** *Tab*: 25, 50, 100, 150, 200 mg ext-rel
>   **Qudexy XR** *Cap*: 25, 50, 100, 150, 200 mg ext-rel

> *vigabatrin* (C)
>   **Sabril** *Tab*: 500 mg
>   **Sabril for Oral Solution** 500 mg/pkt pwdr for reconstitution

> *zonisamide* (C)
>   **Zonegran** *Cap*: 25, 50, 100 mg

APPENDIX S: ORAL ANTI-HIV DRUGS WITH DOSE FORMS

Aptivus (C) *tipranavir*

Gel cap: 250 mg (alcohol); *Oral soln*: 100 mg/ml (95 ml w. dosing syringe) (Vit E 116 IU/ml) (buttermint-butter, toffee)

Comment: *valganciclovir* is indicated for the treatment of AIDS-related cytomegalovirus (CMV) retinitis.

Atripla (D) *efavirenz/emtricitabine/tenofovir disoproxil*

Tab: *efa* 600 mg/*emtri* 200 mg/*teno diso* 300 mg

Combivir (C)(G) *lamivudine/zidovudine*

Tab: *lami* 150/*zido* 300 mg

Complera (B) *emtricitabine/tenofovir disoproxil fumarate/rilpivirine*

Tab: *emtri* 200 mg/*teno diso* 300 mg/*rilpiv* 25 mg

Crixivan (C) *indinavir sulfate*

Cap: 100, 200, 333, 400 mg

Cytovene (C)(G) *ganciclovir*

Cap: 250, 500 mg; *Vial*: 50 mg/ml single dose (500 mg, 10 ml)

Descovy (D) *emtricitabine/tenofovir alafenamide/rilpivirine*

Tab: *emtri* 200 mg/*teno ala* 25 mg

(*continued*)

(*continued*)

Edurant (B) *rilpivirine*

   Tab: 25 mg

Emtriva (B) *emtricitabine*

   Cap: 200 mg; *Oral soln:* 10 mg/ml (170 ml) (cotton candy)

Epivir (C)(G) *lamivudine*

   Tab: 150*, 300 mg; *Oral soln:* 10 mg/ml (240 ml) (strawberry-banana) (sucrose 3 gm/15 ml)

Epzicom (B) *abacavir sulfate/lamivudine*

   Tab: aba 600 mg/*lami* 300 mg

Evotaz (B) *atazanavir/cobicistat*

   Tab: ataz 300/*cobi* 150 mg

Fortovase (B) *saquinavir*

   Soft gel cap: 200 mg

Fuzeon (B) *enfuvirtide*

   Vial: 90 mg/ml pwdr for SC inj after reconstitution (1 ml, 60 vials/kit) (preservative-free)

Genvoya (B) *elvitegravir/cobicistat/emtricitabine/tenofovir alafenamide (TAF)*

   Tab: elv 150 mg/*cob* 150 mg/*emtri* 200 mg/*teno alafen* 10 mg

Intelence (C) *etravirine*

   Tab: 25*, 100, 200 mg

Invirase (B) *saquinavir mesylate*

   Hard gel cap: 200 mg

Isentress (C) *raltegravir (potassium)*

   Tab: 400 mg film-coat; *Chew tab:* 25, 100*mg (orange-banana) (phenylalanine); *Oral susp:* 100 mg/pkt pwdr for oral susp (banana)

Kaletra (C)(G) *lopinavir* <u>*plus*</u> *ritonavir*

   Cap: lopin 100 mg/*riton* 25 mg, *lopin* 200 mg/*riton* 50 mg; *Oral soln:* lopin 80 mg/ riton 20 mg per ml (160 ml w. dose cup) (cotton candy) (alcohol 42%) *Hard gel cap:* 200 mg

---

(*continued*)

(*continued*)

Lexiva (C)(G) *fosamprenavir*

   Tab: 700 mg; *Oral soln:* 50 mg/ml (grape, bubble gum) (peppermint)

Norvir (B) *ritonavir*

   Soft gel cap: 100 mg (alcohol); *Oral soln:* 80 mg/ml (8 oz) (peppermint-caramel) (alcohol)

Odefsey (D) *emtricitabine/rilpivirine/tenofovir alafenamide*

   Tab: emtri 200 mg/rilpiv 25 mg/tenof alafen 25 mg

Prezcobix (B) *darunavir/cobicistat*

   Tab: daru 800 mg/cobi 150 mg

Prezista (C) *darunavir*

   Tab: 75, 150, 600, 800 mg; *Oral susp:* 100 mg/ml (200 ml) (strawberry cream)

Rescriptor (C) *delavirdine mesylate*

   Tab: 100, 200 mg

Retrovir (C)(G) *zidovudine*

   Tab: 300 mg; *Cap:* 100 mg; *Syr:* 50 mg/5 ml (240 ml) (strawberry); *Vial:* 10 mg/ml (20 ml for IV infusion) (preservative-free)

Reyataz (B) *atazanavir*

   Cap: 100, 150, 200, 300 mg

Selzentry (B) *maraviroc*

   Tab: 150, 300 mg

Stribild (B) *elvitegravir/cobicistat/emtricitabine/tenofovir disoproxil fumarate*

   Tab: elv 150 mg/cob 150 mg/emtri 200 mg/teno diso fumar 300 mg

Sustiva (C) *efavirenz*

   Tab: 75, 150, 600, 800 mg; *Cap:* 50, 200 mg

Tivicay (B) *dolutegavir*

   Tab: 10, 25, 50 mg

Triumeq (C) *abacavir sulfate/dolutegravir/lamivudine*

   Tab: aba 600 mg/dilu 50 mg/lami 300 mg

Trizivir (C)(G) *abacavir sulfate/lamivudine/zidovudine*

   Tab: aba 300 mg/lami 150 mg/zido 300 mg

(*continued*)

(*continued*)

Truvada (B) *emtricitabine/tenofovir disoproxil fumarate*

Tab: emt 100 mg/*teno* 150 mg, 133 mg/*teno* 200 mg, *emt* 167 mg/*teno* 250 mg, *emt* 200 mg/*teno* 300 mg

Valcyte (C)(G) *valganciclovir*

Tab: 450 mg

Videx EC (C)(G) *didanosine*

Cap: 125, 200, 250, 400 mg ent-coat del-rel; *Chew tab:* 25, 50, 100, 150, 200 mg (mandarin orange) (buffered with calcium carbonate and magnesium hydroxide, phenylalanine); *Pwdr for oral soln:* 2 gm (120 ml), 4 gm (240 ml)

Videx Pediatric Pwdr for Oral Solution (C) *didanosine*

Pwdr for oral soln: 2 gm (120 ml), 4 gm (240 ml)

Viracept (B) *nelfinavir mesylate*

Tab: 250, 625 mg; *Pwdr for oral soln:* 50 mg/gm (144 gm) (phenylalanine)

Viramune (C)(G) *nevirapine*

Tab: 200*mg; *Oral susp:* 50 mg/5 ml (240 ml)

Viramune XR (C) *nevirapine*

Tab: 100, 400 mg ext-rel

Viread (C) *tenofovir disoproxil fumarate*

Tab: 150, 200, 250, 300 mg; *Oral pwdr:* 40 mg/1 gm pwdr (60 gm w. dosing scoop)

Vistide (C) *cidofovir*

Inj: 75 mg/ml (5 ml vials for IV infusion) (preservative-free)
Comment: *cidofovir* is indicated for the treatment of AIDS-related cytomegalovirus (CMV) retinitis.

Vitekta (C) *elvitegravir*

Inj: 75 mg/ml (5 ml vials for IV infusion) (preservative-free)
Comment: *cidofovir* is indicated for the treatment of AIDS-related cytomegalovirus (CMV) retinitis.

Zerit (C)(G) *stavudine*

Cap: 15, 20, 30, 40 mg; *Oral soln:* 1 mg/ml pwdr for reconstitution (200 ml) (fruit) (dye-free)

Ziagen (C)(G) *abacavir sulfate*

Tab: 300*mg; *Oral soln:* 20 mg/ml (240 ml) (strawberry-banana) (parabens, propylene glycol)

APPENDIX T: COUMADIN (WARFARIN)

APPENDIX T.1: COUMADIN TITRATION AND DOSE FORMS

▷ *warfarin* (X)(G) <18 years: not recommended; ≥18 years: dosage initially 2-5 mg/day; usual maintenance 2-10 mg/day; adjust dosage to maintain INR in therapeutic range:
Venous thrombosis: 2.0-3.0
Atrial fibrillation: 2.0-3.0
Post MI: 2.5-3.5
Mechanical and bioprosthetic heart valves: 2.0-3.0 for 12 weeks after valve insertion, then 2.5-3.5 long-term
Coumadin *Tab*: 1*, 2*, 2.5*, 3*, 4*, 5*, 6*, 7.5*, 10*mg
Coumadin for Injection *Vial*: 2 mg/ml (2.5 ml)
Comment: **Coumadin for Injection** is for peripheral IV administration only.

APPENDIX T.2: COUMADIN OVER-ANTICOAGULATION REVERSAL

▷ *phytonadione (vitamin K)* (G) 2.5-10 mg PO or IM; max 25 mg
    AquaMEPHYTON
      Vial: 1 mg/0.5 ml (0.5 ml), 10 mg/ml (1, 2.5, 5 ml)
    Mephyton
      Tab: 5 mg

APPENDIX T.3: AGENTS THAT INHIBIT COUMADIN'S ANTICOAGULATION EFFECTS

Increase Metabolism	Decrease Absorption	Other Mechanism(s)
azathioprine	*azathioprine*	coenzyme Q10
carbamazepine	*cholestyramine*	estrogen
dicloxacillin	*colestipol*	*griseofulvin*
ethanol	*sucralfate*	oral contraceptives
griseofulvin		*ritonavir*
nafcillin		*spironolactone*
pentobarbital		*trazodone*
phenobarbital		vitamin C (high dose)
phenytoin		vitamin K
primidone		
rifabutin		
rifampin		

APPENDIX U: LOW MOLECULAR WEIGHT HEPARINS

Comment: Administer by subcutaneous injection *only*, in the abdomen, and rotate sites. Avoid concomitant drugs that affect hemostasis (e.g., oral anticoagulants and platelet aggregation inhibitors, including *aspirin*, NSAIDs, *dipyridamole, sulfinpyrazone, ticlopidine*). Not recommended <18 years-of-age.

▷ *dalteparin* (B)
  Fragmin *Prefilled syringe:* 2500 IU/0.2 ml, 5000 IU/0.2 ml (10/box) (preservative-free); *Multidose vial:* 1,000 IU/ml (95,000 IU, 9.5 ml) (benzyl alcohol)

▷ *danaparoid* (B)
  Orgaran *Amp:* 750 anti-Xa units/0.6 ml (0.6 ml, 10/box); *Prefilled syringe:* 750 anti-Xa units/0.6 ml (0.6 ml, 10/box) (sulfites)

▷ *enoxaparin* (B)(G)
  Lovenox *Prefilled syringe:* 30 mg/0.3 ml, 40 mg/0.4 ml, 60 mg/0.6 ml, 80 mg/0.8 ml (100 mg/ml) (preservative-free); *Vial:* 100 mg/ml (3 ml)

▷ *tinzaparin* (B)
  Innohep *Vial:* 20,000 *anti-Factor Xa* IU/ml (2 ml) (sulfites, benzyl alcohol)

APPENDIX V: FACTOR XA INHIBITOR THERAPY

▷ *apixaban* (C) <12 years: not recommended; >12 years: 5 mg bid; reduce to 2.5 mg bid if any two of the following: ≥80 years, ≤60 kg, serum Cr ≥1.5
  Eliquis *Tab:* 2.5, 5 mg
  Comment: **Eliquis** is indicated to reduce the risk of stroke and systemic embolism in patients with non-valvular atrial fibrillation (NVAF).

▷ *edoxaban* (C) <12 years: not recommended; ≥12 years: transition to and from **Savaysa**; assess CrCl prior to initiation: *NVAF CrCl >50 mL/min:* 60 mg once daily; *CrCl 15-50 mL/min:* 30 mg once daily; *DVT/PE CrCl >50 mL/min:* 60 mg once daily following initial parental anticoagulant; *CrCl 15-50 mL/min, <60 kg, or concomitant Pgp inhibitors:* 30 mg once daily
  Savaysa *Tab:* 15, 30, 60 mg
  Comment: **Savaysa** is indicated to reduce the risk of stroke and systemic embolism in patients with non-valvular atrial fibrillation (NVAF), treatment of DVT and pulmonary embolism (PE) following 5-10 days of initial therapy with parenteral anticoagulant. Not for use in persons with NVAF with *CrCl >95 mL/min*.

▷ *fondaparinux* (B) <12 years: not established; ≥12 years: administer SC; administer first dose no earlier than 6-8 hours after hemostasis is achieved, start warfarin usually within 72 hours of last dose of *fondaparinux*

(continued)

(continued)

> *Post-op:* 2.5 mg once daily x 5-9 days; *Hip/Knee Replacement:* once daily x 11 days *Hip Fracture:* once daily x 32 days; *Abdominal Surgery:* once daily x 10 days *Prophylaxis:* do not use <50 kg; *Treatment:* once daily for at least 5 days until INR = 2-3 (usually 5-9 days); max 26 days; <50 kg: 5 mg; 50-100 kg: 7.5 mg; >100 kg: 10 mg
>
> **Arixtra** *Soln for SC inj:* 2.5 mg/0.5 ml, 5 mg/0.4 ml, 7.5 mg/0.6 ml, 10 mg/0.8 ml *prefilled syringe* (10/box) (preservative-free)

▷ *prasugrel* (B) <12 years: not recommended; ≥12 years: *Loading dose:* 60 mg once in a single dose; *Maintenance:* 10 mg once daily; <60 kg: consider 5 mg once daily; take with *aspirin* 75-325 mg once daily

> **Effient** *Tab:* 5, 10 mg
>
> **Comment:** *Effient* is indicated to reduce the risk of thrombotic cardiovascular events in persons with acute coronary syndrome (ACS) who are to be managed with percutaneous coronary intervention (PCI) including unstable angina, non-ST elevation myocardial infarction (NSTEMI) and STEMI. Do not start if active pathological bleeding (e.g., peptic ulcer, intracranial hemorrhage), prior TIA or stroke, or if patient likely to undergo urgent CABG. Discontinue 7 days before surgery and if TIA or stroke occurs.

▷ *rivaroxaban* (C) take with food; <12 years: not recommended; ≥12 years: *Treatment of DVT or PE:* 15 mg twice daily for the first 21 days; then 20 mg once daily
Reduction in risk of DVT or PE recurrence: 20 mg once daily with the evening meal; *CrCl <30 mL/min:* avoid
Prophylaxis of DVT: take 6-10 hours after surgery when hemostasis established, then 20 mg once daily with the evening meal; *CrCl 30-50 mL/min:* 10 mg; *CrCl <30 mL/min:* avoid; discontinue if acute renal failure develops; monitor closely for blood loss
Hip: treat for 35 days; *Knee:* treat for 12 days
Non-valvular AF: take once daily with the evening meal; *CrCl >50 mL/min:* 20 mg; *CrCl 15-50 mL/min:* 15 mg; *CrCl >15 mL/min:* avoid

> **Xarelto** *Cap:* 10, 15, 20 mg
>
> **Comment:** **Xarelto** is indicated to reduce the risk of stroke and systemic embolism in non-valvular atrial fibrillation (AF), to treat deep vein thrombosis (DVT) and pulmonary embolism (PE), to reduce the risk of recurrence of DVT and/or PE following 6 months treatment for DVT and/or PE, and prophylaxis of DVT which may lead to PE in patients undergoing knee or hip replacement surgery. **Xarelto** eliminates the need for bridging with heparin or LMWH; no need for routine monitoring of INR or other coagulation parameters; no need for dose adjustments for age, weight, or gender; no known dietary restrictions. Switching from *warfarin* or other anticoagulant, see mfr pkg insert.

APPENDIX W: DIRECT THROMBIN INHIBITOR THERAPY

▷ *aspirin* (D) <12 years: not recommended; ≥12 years: one single dose once daily
Durlaza *Cap:* 162.5 mg 24-hr ext-rel (30, 90/bottle)
Comment: Presently there is only one reversal agent for this drug class.
idarucizumab (**Praxbind**) is a specific reversal agent for *dabigatran* (**Pradaxa**).
It is a humanized monoclonal antibody fragment (Fab) that binds to *dabigatran*
and its acylglucuronide metabolites with higher affinity than the binding affinity
of *dabigatran* to thrombin, neutralizing its anticoagulant effects.

IDARUCIZUMAB REVERSAL AGENT: HUMANIZED MONOCLONAL ANTIBODY FRAGMENT (FAB)

▷ *idarucizumab* (NE) <12 years: not established; ≥12 years: administer 5 g (2 vials)
IV drip or push; administer within 1 hour of removal from vial
Praxbind *Vial:* 2.5 gm/50 ml, single use (preservative-free)
Comment: Presently, there is inadequate human and animal data to assess
risk of *idarucizumab* (**Praxbind**) use in pregnancy. Risk/benefit should be
considered prior to use.

▷ *dabigatran etexilate mesylate* (C) <12 years: not recommended; ≥12 years: swallow whole; *CrCl >30 mL/min:* 150 mg bid; *CrCl 15-30 mL/min:* 75 mg bid; *CrCl
<15 mL/min:* not recommended
Pradaxa *Cap:* 75, 150 mg
Comment: **Pradaxa** is indicated to reduce the risk of stroke and systemic
embolism in non-valvular AF, DVT prophylaxis, PE prophylaxis in patients
who have undergone hip replacement surgery, treatment of DVT and PE in
patients who have been treated with a parenteral anticoagulant for 5-10 days,
and to reduce the risk of recurrent DVT and PE in patients who have been
previously treated. **Pradaxa** is contraindicated in patients with a mechanical
prosthetic heart valve.

▷ *desirudin (recombinant hirudin)* (C) <12 years: not recommended; ≥12 years:
15 mg SC every 12 hours, preferably in the abdomen or thigh, starting up to 5-15
minutes before surgery (after induction of regional block anesthesia, if used);
may continue for 9-12 days post-op; *CrCl <60 mL/min:* reduce dose (see mfr pkg
insert)
Iprivask *Pwdr for SC inj after reconstitution:* 15 mg/single-use vial (10/box)
(preservative-free, diluent contains mannitol)
Comment: **Iprivask** is indicated for DVT prophylaxis in patients undergoing
hip replacement surgery. It is not interchangeable with other hirudins.

APPENDIX X: PLATELET AGGREGATION INHIBITOR THERAPY

▷ *cilostazol* (B) <12 years: not recommended; ≥12 years: 100 mg bid
Pletal *Tab:* 50, 100 mg
Comment: **Pletal** is an (antiplatelet/vasodilator [PDE III inhibitor]).

▷ *clopidogrel* (B) <12 years: not recommended; ≥12 years: 75 mg once daily
Plavix *Tab:* 75, 300 mg
Comment: **Plavix** is indicated for the reduction of atherosclerotic events in recent MI or stroke, established PAD, non-ST-segment elevation acute coronary syndrome (unstable angina/non-STEMI), or STEMI.

▷ *dipyridamole* (B)(G) <12 years: not recommended; ≥12 years: 75-100 mg qid
Persantine *Tab:* 25, 50, 75 mg
Comment: *dipyridamole* is indicated as an adjunct to oral anticoagulants after cardiac valve replacement surgery to prevent thromboembolism.

▷ *dipyridamole/aspirin* (B)(G) <12 years: not recommended; ≥12 years: swallow whole; one cap bid
Aggrenox *Cap: dipyr* 200 mg/*asa* 25 mg

▷ *pentoxifylline* (C) (hemorrhologic [xanthine]) <12 years: not recommended; ≥12 years:
Trental *Tab:* 400 mg sust-rel

▷ *prasugrel* (C) <12 years: not recommended; ≥12 years:
Effient *Tab:* 5, 10 mg
Comment: **Effient** is indicated to reduce the risk of cardiovascular events in patients with acute coronary syndrome (ACS) who are to be managed with percutaneous coronary intervention (unstable angina or non-STEMI), and STEMI when managed with either primary or delayed PCI.

▷ *ticagrelor* (C) <12 years: not recommended; ≥12 years: initiate 180 mg loading dose once in a single dose with aspirin 325 mg loading dose in a single dose; maintenance 90 mg twice daily with aspirin 75-100 mg once daily; ACS patients may start *ticagrelor* after a loading dose of *clopidogrel*
Brilinta *Tab:* 90 mg
Comment: **Effient** is indicated to reduce the risk of cardiovascular events in patients with acute coronary syndrome (ACS) (unstable angina, non-ST elevation (NSTEMI), myocardial infarction, or STEMI).

▷ *ticlopidine* (B) <12 years: not recommended; ≥12 years: 250 mg bid
Ticlid *Tab:* 250 mg
Comment: **Ticlid** is indicated to reduce the risk of thrombotic stroke in selected patients intolerant of aspirin.

APPENDIX Y: PROTEASE-ACTIVATED RECEPTOR-1 (PAR-1) INHIBITOR THERAPY

▷ *vorapaxar* (B) <12 years: not established; ≥12 years: administer 2.08 mg once daily; use with *aspirin* or *clopidogrel*
Zontivity *Tab:* 2.08 mg (equivalent to 2.5 mg *vorapaxar sulfate*)
Comment: **Zontivity** is indicated to reduce thrombotic cardiovascular events in patients with a history of myocardial infarction or with peripheral arterial disease (PAD). Contraindicated with active pathological bleeding (e.g., peptic ulcer, intracranial hemorrhage), prior TIA or stroke. Not recommended with severe hepatic impairment.

APPENDIX Z: PRESCRIPTION PRENATAL VITAMINS

Comment: It is recommended that prenatal vitamins be started at least 3 months prior to conception to improve preconception nutritional status, and continued throughout pregnancy and the postnatal period, in lactating and non-lactating women, and throughout the childbearing years.

▷ **CitraNatal 90 DHA** take 1 tab* and 1 DHA cap daily
Tab: thiamine 3 mg, riboflavin 3.4 mg, niacinamide 20 mg, pyridoxine HCL 20 mg, folic acid 1 mg, Vit C 120 mg, Vit D₃ 400 IU, Vit E 30 IU, calcium (as citrate) 160 mg, copper (as oxide) 2 mg, iodine (as potassium iodide) 150 mcg, iron (as carbonyl) 90 mg, zinc (as oxide) 25 mg, docusate sodium 50 mg
Cap: docosahexaenoic acid (DHA) 300 mg

▷ **CitraNatal Assure** take 1 tab and 1 DHA cap daily
Tab: thiamine 3 mg, riboflavin 3.4 mg, niacinamide 20 mg, pyridoxine HCL 25 mg, folic acid 1 mg, Vit C 120 mg, Vit D3 400 IU, Vit E 30 IU, calcium (as citrate) 125 mg, copper (as oxide) 2 mg, iodine (as potassium oxide) 150 mcg, iron (as carbonyl and ferrous gluconate) 35 mg, zinc (as oxide) 25 mg, docusate sodium 50 mg
Cap: docosahexaenoic acid (DHA) 300 mg

▷ **CitraNatal B-Calm** take 1 tab every 8 hours; begin with tab #1.
Tab: pyridoxine HCL 25 mg, folic acid 1 mg, Vit C 120 mg, Vit D3 400 IU, calcium (as citrate) 120 mg, iron (as carbonyl) 20 mg
Tab: pyridoxine 25 mg
Comment: **Citranatal B-Calm** may be used as an adjunct treatment to help minimize pregnancy-related nausea and vomiting.

▷ **CitraNatal DHA** take 1 tab and 1 DHA cap daily
Tab: thiamine 3 mg, riboflavin 3.4 mg, niacinamide 20 mg, pyridoxine HCL 20 mg, folic acid 1 mg, Vit C 120 mg, Vit D3 400 IU, Vit E 30 IU, calcium (as citrate) 125 mg, copper (as oxide) 2 mg, iodine (as potassium oxide) 150 mcg, iron (as carbonyl and gluconate) 27 mg, zinc (as oxide) 25 mg, docusate sodium 50 mg
Cap: docosahexaenoic acid (DHA) 250 mg

(*continued*)

(continued)

▷ **CitraNatal Harmony** take 1 gelcap daily
Gelcap: pyridoxine HCL 25 mg, folic acid 1 mg, Vit D3 400 IU, Vit E 30 IU, calcium (as citrate) 104 mg, iron (as carbonyl and ferrous fumarate) 27 mg, docusate sodium 50 mg, docosahexaenoic acid (DHA) 260 mg

▷ **CitraNatal Rx** take 1 tab* and 1 DHA cap daily
Tab: thiamine 3 mg, riboflavin 3.4 mg, niacinamide 20 mg, pyridoxine HCL 20 mg, folic acid 1 mg, Vit C 120 mg, Vit D3 400 IU, Vit E 30 IU, calcium (as citrate) 125 mg, copper (as oxide) 2 mg, iodine (as potassium iodide) 150 mcg, iron (as carbonyl and gluconate) 27 mg, zinc (as oxide) 25 mg, docusate sodium 50 mg

▷ **Duet DHA Balanced** take 1 tab and 1 gelcap daily
Tab: Vit A (as beta carotene) 2800 IU, thiamine 1.5 mg, riboflavin 2 mg, niacinamide 20 mg, pyridoxine HCL 50 mg, Vit B$_{12}$ 12 mcg, folic acid 1 mg, Vit C 120 mg, Vit D3 640 IU, Vit E 15 IU, calcium (as carbonate) 215 mg, iron (as polysaccharide iron complex and sodium iron EDTA, ferrazone) 25 mg, copper (as oxide) 1.8 mg, magnesium (as oxide) 25 mg, zinc (as oxide) 25 mg, iodine (as potassium iodide) 210 mcg, selenium 65 mcg, choline (as bitartrate) 55 mg
Gelcap: omega 3 fatty acids 267 mg (includes docosahexaenoic acid [DHA], eicosapentaenoic acid [EPA], alpha-linolenic acid [ALA], docosapentaenoic acid [DPA]) (gelatin, gluten-free)

▷ **Duet DHA Complete** take 1 tab and 1 gelcap daily
Tab: Vit A (as beta carotene) 3000 IU, thiamine 1.8 mg, riboflavin 4 mg, niacinamide 20 mg, pyridoxine HCL 50 mg, Vit B12 12 mcg, folic acid 1 mg, Vit C 120 mg, Vit D3 800 IU, Vit E 3 mg, calcium (as carbonate) 230 mg, iron (as polysaccharide iron complex and sodium iron EDTA, ferrazone) 27 mg, copper (as oxide) 2 mg, magnesium (as oxide) 25 mg, zinc (as oxide) 25 mg, iodine 220 mcg
Gelcap: omega 3 fatty acids ≥430 mg (as docosahexaenoic acid (DHA) ≥295 mg, as other omega-3 fatty acids ≥135 mg (eicosapentaenoic acid (EPA), docosapentaenoic acid (DHA) (gluten-free)

▷ **Natachew** take 1 chew tab daily
Chew tab: Vit A 1000 IU (as beta carotene), thiamine 2 mg, riboflavin 3 mg, niacinamide 20 mg, pyridoxine HCL 10 mg, B12 12 mcg, folic acid 1 mg, Vit C 120 mg, Vit D3 400 IU, Vit E 11 IU, iron (as ferrous fumarate) 29 mg (wild berry)

▷ **Natafort** take 1 tab daily
Tab: Vit A 1000 IU (as acetate and beta carotene), thiamine 2 mg, riboflavin 3 mg, niacinamide 20 mg, pyridoxine HCL 10 mg, B12 12 mcg, folic acid 1 mg, Vit C 120 mg, Vit D3 400 IU, Vit E 11 IU, iron (as carbonyl and sulfate) 60 mg

▷ **Neevo DHA** take 1 cap daily
Cap: l-methylfolate (as Metafolin) 1.3 mg, thiamin 1.4 mg, riboflavin 1.4 mg, niacinamide 18 mg, pyridoxine HCL 25 mg, B12 1 mg, Vit C 85 mg, Vit D3, 5 mcg, Vit E 15 IU, calcium (as carbonate) 110 mg, iron (ferrous fumarate) 27 mg, iodine (as potassium iodide) 220 mcg, magnesium (as oxide) 60 mg, docosahexaenoic acid (DHA, vegetarian source (algal oil) 581.92 mg (soy, gelatin, sorbitol, glycerin)

(continued)

(*continued*)

> Comment: **Neevo DHA** is indicated as a nutritional supplement during pregnancy, and the prenatal and postnatal periods, in women with dietary needs for the biologically active form of folate, who are at risk for hyperhomocysteinemia, impaired folic acid absorption, and/or impaired folic acid metabolism due to 667C >T mutations in the MTHFR gene.

▷ **Nexa Plus** take 1 cap daily
Cap: pyridoxine HCL 25 mg, folic acid 1.25 mg, Vit C 28 mg, Vit D3 800 IU, Vit E 30 IU, biotin 250 mcg, calcium (as carbonate [158 mg] + docusate calcium[2 mg] 160 mg, iron (as ferrous fumarate) 29 mg, docosahexaenoic acid (DHA, plant-based source [algal oil]) 350 mg (soy)

▷ **Nexa Select** take 1 soft gel cap daily
Soft gel cap: pyridoxine HCL 25 mg, folic acid 1.25 mg, Vit C 28 mg, Vit D3 800 IU, Vit E 30 IU, calcium (as phosphate) 160 mg, iron (as ferrous fumarate) 29 mg, docosahexaenoic acid (DHA) plant-based source (algal oil) 325 mg, docusate sodium 55 mg (soy)

▷ **Prenate AM** take 1 tab daily
Tab: pyridoxine HCL 75 mg, folate (as folic acid 400 mcg + Quatrefolic 1.1 mg [equivalent to 600 mcg folic acid]) 1 mg, Vit B12 12 mcg, calcium (as carbonate) 200 mg, ginger extract 500 mg, lingon-berry 25 mg

▷ **Prenate Chewable** take 1 chew tab daily
Chew tab: pyridoxine HCL 10 mg, Vit B12 125 mcg, calcium (as carbonate) 500 mg, Vit D3 300 IU, biotin 280 mcg, boron amino acid chelate 250 mcg, folate (as Quatrefolic) 1 mg, magnesium (as oxide) 50 mg, blueberry extract 25 mg (Dutch chocolate)

▷ **Prenate DHA** take 1 gel cap daily
Gelcap: pyridoxine HCL 26 mg, folate (as folic acid) 400 mcg + Quatrefolic 1.1 mg [equivalent to 600 mcg folic acid]) 1 mg, Vit B12 13 mcg, Vit C 90 mg, Vit D3 220 IU, Vit E 10 IU, calcium (as carbonate) 145 mg, iron (as ferrous fumarate) 28 mg, magnesium (as oxide) 50 mg, docosahexaenoic acid (DHA) 300 mg (fish oil, soy, gelatin)

▷ **Prenate Elite** take 1 gel cap daily
Gelcap: Vit A (as beta-carotene) 2600 IU, thiamine 3 mg, riboflavin 3.5 mg, pyridoxine HCl 21 mg, niacinamide 21 mg, pantothenic acid 6 mg, folate (as folic acid 400 mcg + Quatrefolic 1.1 mg [equivalent to 600 mcg folic acid]) 1 mg, Vit B12 13 mcg, Vit C 75 mg, Vit D3 450 IU, Vit E 10 IU, biotin 330 mcg, calcium (as carbonate) 100 mg, iron (as ferrous fumarate) 27 mg, magnesium (as oxide) 25 mg, copper (as oxide) 1.5 mg, iodine 150 mcg, iron (as ferrous fumarate) 26 mg, zinc (as oxide) 15 mg

▷ **Prenate Enhance** take 1 gel cap daily
Gelcap: pyridoxine HCL 25 mg, folate (as folic acid 400 mcg + Quatrefolic 1.1 mg[equivalent to 600 mcg folic acid]) 1 mg, Vit B12 12 mcg, Vit C 85 mg, Vit D3

(*continued*)

(continued)

1000 IU, Vit E 10 IU, biotin 500 mcg, calcium (as carbonate + Formical) 155 mg, iodine (as potassium) 150 mcg, iron (as ferrous fumarate) 28 mg, magnesium (as oxide) 50 mg, docosahexaenoic acid (DHA) 400 mg (soy, gelatin)

▷ **Prenate Essential** take 1 gel cap daily
Gelcap: pyridoxine HCL 26 mg, folate (as folic acid 400 mcg + Quatrefolic 1.1 mg [equivalent to 600 mcg folic acid]) 1 mg, Vit B12 13 mcg, Vit C 90 mg, Vit D3 220 IU, Vit E 10 IU, biotin 280 mcg, calcium (as carbonate) 145 mg, iodine (as potassium iodide) 150 mcg, iron (as ferrous fumarate) 29 mg, magnesium (as oxide) 50 mg, docosahexaenoic acid (DHA) 300 mg, eicosapentaenoic acid (EPA) 40 mg (fish oil, soy, gelatin)

▷ **Prenate Mini** take 1 gel cap daily
Gelcap: pyridoxine HCL 26 mg, folate (as folic acid) 400 mcg + Quatrefolic 1.1 mg [equivalent to 600 mcg folic acid]) 1 mg, Vit B12 13 mcg, Vit C 60 mg, Vit D3 220 IU, Vit E 10 IU, calcium (as carbonate) 100 mg, iron (as carbonyl iron) 29 mg, iodine (as potassium iodide) 150 mcg, biotin 280 mcg, magnesium (as oxide) 25 mg, docosahexaenoic acid (DHA) 300 mg, blueberry extract 25 mg (fish oil, soy, gelatin)

▷ **Prenate Restore** take 1 gel cap daily
Gelcap: pyridoxine HCL 25 mg, folate (as folic acid 400 mcg + Quatrefolic 1.1 mg [equivalent to 600 mcg folic acid]) 1 mg, Vit B12 12 mcg, Vit C 85 mg, Vit D3 1000 IU, Vit E 10 IU, biotin 500 mcg, calcium (as carbonate + Formical) 155 mg, iron (as ferrous fumarate) 27 mg, magnesium (as oxide) 45 mg, docosahexaenoic acid (DHA) 400 mg, *Bacillus coagulans* 150 million CFU (as lactospore) 10 mg (soy, gelatin)

▷ **Prenexa** take 1 gel cap daily
Gelcap: pyridoxine HCL 25 mg, folic acid 1.25 mg, Vit C 28 mg, Vit D3 400 IU, Vit E 30 IU, calcium (as phosphate) 160 mg, iron (as ferrous fumarate) 27 mg, docosahexaenoic acid (DHA) plant-based source (algal oil) 300 mg, docusate sodium 55 mg (soy)

APPENDIX AA: ORAL PRESCRIPTION DRUGS FOR THE MANAGEMENT OF ALLERGY, COUGH, AND COLD SYMPTOMS

Prescription drugs for the management of allergy symptoms, cough, and symptoms of the common cold are listed in alphabetical order by brand name.

Legend:	*acriv*	*acrivastine*
	benzo	*benzonatate*
	brom	*brompheniramine*

(continued)

(*continued*)

	carb	**carbinoxamine**
	carbeta	**carbetapentane**
	chlor	**chlorpheniramine**
	cod	**codeine**
	cypro	**cyproheptadine**
	deslorat	**desloratadine**
	dexchlo	**chlorpheniramine**
	dextro	**dextromethorphan**
	diphen	**diphenhydramine**
	guaiac	**potassium guaiacosulfonate**
	guaif	**guaifenesin**
	homat	**homatropine**
	hydro	**hydrocodone**
	hydrox	**hydroxyzine**
	meth	**methscopolamine**
	phenyle	**phenylephrine**
	prometh	**promethazine**
	pseud	**pseudoephedrine**
	pyril	**pyrilamine tannate**

➤ **Allerex (C)** <12 years: not recommended; ≥12 years: 1 AM tab in the morning and 1 PM tab in the evening prn
AM tab: meth 2.5 mg/pseud 120 mg ext-rel; PM tab: meth 2.5 mg/chlor 8 mg/phenyle 10 mg* ext-rel (Dose Pack 20: 10 AM tabs+10 PM tabs; Dose Pack 60:30 AM tabs+30 PM tabs)

➤ **Allerex DF (C)** <12 years: not recommended; ≥12 years: 1 AM tab in the morning and 1 PM tab in the evening prn
AM tab: meth 2.5 mg/chlor 4 mg/PM tab: meth 2.5 mg/chlor 8 mg* (Dose Pack 20:10 AM tabs+10 PM tabs; Dose Pack 60: 30 AM tabs+30 PM tabs)

➤ **Allerex PE (C)** <12 years: not recommended; ≥12 years: 1 AM tab in the morning and 1 PM tab in the evening prn

(*continued*)

(continued)

AM tab: meth 2.5 mg/*phenyle* 40 mg; *PM tab: meth* 8 mg/*phenyle* 10 mg* (*Dose Pack 20:* 10 AM tabs+10 PM tabs; *Dose Pack 60:* 30 AM tabs+30 PM tabs)

➤ **Allerex Suspension (C)** <6 years: not recommended; 6-12 years: 2.5-5 ml q 12 hours prn; ≥12 years: 15 ml q 12 hours prn
Susp: chlor 3 mg/*phenyle* 7.5 mg ext-rel (raspberry)

➤ **Atarax (B)(G)** <2 years: not recommended; 2-6 years: 6.25 mg q 4-6 hours prn; 6-12 years: 12.5-25 mg q 4-6 hours prn; ≥12 years: 25 mg tid or qid prn
Tab: hydrox 10, 25, 50, 100 mg; *Syr:* 10 mg/5 ml (alcohol 0.5%)

➤ **Bromfed DM (C)(G)** <2 years: not recommended; 2-6 years: 1/2 tsp q 4 hours prn; 6-12 years: 1 tsp q 4 hours prn; ≥12 years: 2 tsp q 4 hours prn: max 6 doses/day
Susp: brom 2 mg/*pseudo* 30 mg/*dextro* 10 mg per 5 ml (butterscotch) (alcohol 0.95%)

➤ **Bromfed DM Sugar-Free (C)(G)** <2 years: not recommended; 2-6 years: 1/2 tsp q 4 hours prn; 6-12 years: 1 tsp q 4 hours prn; >12 years: 2 tsp q 4 hours prn: max 6 doses/day

➤ **Clarinex (C)** <6 years: not recommended; ≥6 years: 1/2-1 tab once daily
Tab: deslorat 5 mg

➤ **Clarinex RediTabs (C)** <6 years: not recommended; 6-12 years: 2.5 mg once daily; ≥12 years: 5 mg once daily
ODT: deslorat 2.5, 5 mg (tutti-frutti) (phenylalanine)

➤ **Clarinex Syrup (C)** <6 months: not recommended; 6-11 months: 1 mg (2 ml) once daily; 1-5 years: 1.25 mg (2.5 ml) once daily; 6-11 years: 2.5 mg (5 ml) once daily; ≥12 years: 5 mg (10 ml) once daily
Tab: deslorat 0.5 mg per ml (4 oz) (tutti-frutti) (phenylalanine)

➤ **Duratuss AC 12 (C)** <2 years: not recommended; 2-6 years: 1/2 tsp q 12 hrs prn; >6-12 years: 1 tsp q 12 hours prn; >12 years: 1-2 tsp q 12 hours prn
Susp: diphen 12.5 mg/*dextro* 15 mg/*phenyle* 15 mg per 5 ml (strawberry banana) (sugar-free, alcohol-free, phenylalanine)

➤ **Duratuss DM (C)** <2 years: not recommended; 2-6 years: 1/4 tsp q 4 hrs prn; >6-12 years: 1/2 tsp q 4 hours prn; >12 years: 1 tsp q 4 hours prn; max 6 doses/day
Susp: dextro 25 mg/*guaif* 225 mg per 5 ml (grape) (sugar-free, alcohol-free)

➤ **Duratuss DM 1/2 (C)** <2 years: not recommended; 2-6 years: 1/2 tsp q 12 hrs prn; >6-12 years: 1/2-1 tsp q 12 hours prn; >12 years: 1-2 tsp q 12 hours prn; max 2 doses/day
Susp: dextro 15 mg/*guaif* 225 mg per 5 ml (grape) (sugar-free, alcohol-free)

➤ **Flowtuss Oral Solution (C)(II)(G)** <6 years: not recommended; 6-12 years: 1/2 tsp q 4-6 hours prn; max 15 ml/day; >12 years: 1-2 tsp q 4-6 hours prn; max 6 tsp/24 hours
Oral soln: hydro 2.5 mg/*guaif* 200 mg per 5 ml (black raspberry)
Comment: *hydrocodone* is known to be excreted in breast milk.

➤ **Hycodan (C)(III)** <6 years: not recommended; 6-12 years: 1/2 tab q 4-6 hours prn; max 3 tabs/day; >12 years: 1 tab q 4-6 hours prn; max 6 tabs/day
Tab: hydro 5 mg/*homat* 1.5 mg
Comment: *hydrocodone* is known to be excreted in breast milk.

➤ **Hycodan Syrup (C)(II)(G)** <6 years: not recommended; 6-12 years: 1/2 tsp q 4-6 hours prn; max 15 ml/day; >12 years: 1 tsp q 4-6 hours prn
Syr: hydro 5 mg/*homat* 1.5 mg per 5 ml
Comment: *hydrocodone* is known to be excreted in breast milk.

(continued)

(*continued*)

▷ **Hycofenix Oral Solution (C)(II)** <6 years: not recommended; 6-12 years: 1/2 tsp q 4-6 hours prn; max 15 ml/day; >12 years: 1 tsp q 4-6 hours prn
Oral soln: hydro 2.5 mg/*pseudo* 30 mg/*guaif* 200 mg per 5 ml (black raspberry)
Comment: *hydrocodone* is known to be excreted in breast milk.

▷ **Obredon Oral Solution (C)(II)** <18 years: not recommended: 10 ml q 4-6 hours prn cough; max 60 ml/day
Oral soln: hydro 2.5 mg/*guaif* 200 mg per 5 ml
Comment: **Obredon** is indicated only for short-term treatment of cough due to the common cold. **Obredon** is <u>not</u> indicated for persistent <u>or</u> chronic cough such as occurs with smoking, asthma, chronic bronchitis, <u>or</u> emphysema, <u>or</u> where cough is accompanied by excessive phlegm. Use with caution in patients with diabetes, thyroid disease, Addison's disease, BPH <u>or</u> urethral stricture, and asthma. **Obredon** is contraindicated with paralytic ileus, anticholinergics, TCAs, and within 14 days of an MAOI. *Hydrocodone* is known to be excreted in human milk. There is <u>no</u> FDA-approved generic form of ***hydrocodone/guaifenesin.***

▷ **Palgic (C)** <2 year: not recommended; 2-3 years: 2 mg tid <u>or</u> qid prn <u>or</u> 0.2-0.4 mg/kg/day divided tid <u>or</u> qid; 3-6 years: 2-4 mg daily prn <u>or</u> 0.2-0.4 mg/kg/day divided tid <u>or</u> qid; >6 years: 4 mg daily prn; max 24 mg/day in divided doses 6-8 hours apart
Tab: carb 4*mg; *Syr: carb* 4 mg per 5 ml (bubble gum)

▷ **Periactin (B)(G)** <2 years: not recommended; 2-6 years: 2 mg bid-tid; max 12 mg/day; 7-14 years: 4 mg bid-tid; max 16 mg/day; >14 years: initially 4 mg tid prn, then adjust as needed; usual range 12-16 mg/day; max 32 mg/day
Tab: cypro 4*mg; *Syr: cypro* 2 mg per 5 ml

▷ **Prolex-DH (C)(III)** <3 years: not recommended; 3-6 years: 1/4-1/2 tsp qid prn; 6-12 years: 1/2-1 tsp qid prn; >12 years: 1-1½ tsp qid prn
Liq: hydro 4.5 mg/*pot guaiac* 300 mg per 5 ml (tropical fruit punch) (alcohol-free, sugar-free)
Comment: *hydrocodone* is known to be excreted in breast milk.

▷ **Phenergan (C)(G)** <2 years: not recommended; 2-6 years: 2 years: 0.5 mg/lb <u>or</u> 6.25-25 mg po <u>or</u> rectally q 6 hours prn; 6-12 years: 12.5 mg tid prn; >12 years: 25 mg po <u>or</u> rectally tid ac and HS prn
Tab: 12.5*, 25*, 50 mg; *Syr: prom* 6.25 mg per 5 ml; *Syr fortis: prom* 25 mg per 5 ml; *Rectal supp: prom* 12.5, 25, 50 mg

▷ **Promethazine DM (C)(V)(G)** <6 years: not recommended; 6-12 years: 1/2-1 tsp q 4-6 hours prn; >12 years: 1 tsp q 4-6 hours prn; *Syr: prometh* 6.25 mg/*dex* 15 mg per 5 ml (alcohol 7%)
Comment: Contraindicated with asthma.

▷ **Promethazine VC (C)(V)(G)** 2-6 years: 1.25 ml q 4-6 hours prn; max 7.5 ml/day; 6-12 years: 2.5 ml q 4-6 hours prn; max 15 ml/day; >12 years: 1 tsp q 4-6 hours prn; max 30 ml/day
Syr: prometh 6.25 mg/*phenyle* 5 mg per 5 ml (alcohol 7%)
Comment: Contraindicated with asthma.

▷ **Promethazine VC w. Codeine (C)(V)(G)** <12 years: not recommended; 12-<18: use extreme caution; not recommended for children and adolescents with asthma or other chronic breathing problems; ≥18 years: 1 tsp q 4-6 hours prn; max 30 ml/day
Syr: prometh 6.25 mg/*phenyle* 5 mg/cod 10 mg per 5 ml (alcohol 7%)

(*continued*)

(*continued*)

Comment: *Codeine* is known to be excreted in breast milk. <12 years: not recommended; 12-<18: use extreme caution; not recommended for children and adolescents with asthma or other chronic breathing problem. The FDA and the European Medicines Agency (EMA) are investigating the safety of using *codeine* containing medications to treat pain, cough and colds, in children 12-<18 years because of the potential for serious side effects, including slowed or difficult breathing.

▷ **Promethazine w. Codeine (C)(V)(G)** <12 years: not recommended; 12-<18: use extreme caution; not recommended for children and adolescents with asthma or other chronic breathing problems; ≥18 years: 1 tsp q 4-6 hours prn
Liq: prometh 6.25 mg/*cod* 10 mg per 5 ml (alcohol 7%)
Comment: *Codeine* is known to be excreted in breast milk. <12 years: not recommended; 12-<18: use extreme caution; not recommended for children and adolescents with asthma or other chronic breathing problem. The FDA and the European Medicines Agency (EMA) are investigating the safety of using *codeine* containing medications to treat pain, cough and colds, in children 12-<18 years because of the potential for serious side effects, including slowed or difficult breathing.

▷ **Rynatan (C)** <12 years: not recommended; ≥12 years: 1-2 tabs q 12 hours prn
Tab: chlor 9 mg/*phenyle* 25 mg

▷ **Rynatan Pediatric Suspension (C)** <2 years: not recommended; 2-6 years: 1/2-1 tsp q 12 hours prn; >6-12 years: 1-2 tsp q 12 hours prn
Susp: chlor 4.5 mg/*phenyle* 5 mg

▷ **Ryneze (C)** <6 years: not recommended; 6-12 years: 1/2 tab q 12 hours prn; >12 years: 1 tab q 12 hours prn
Tab: chlor 8 mg/*meth* 2.5 mg

▷ **Robitussin AC (C)(III)(G)** <12 years: not recommended; 12-<18: use extreme caution; not recommended for children and adolescents with asthma or other chronic breathing problems; ≥18 years: 2 tsp q 4 hours prn; max 60 ml/day
Liq: cod 10 mg/*guaif* 100 mg per 5 ml
Comment: *Codeine* is known to be excreted in breast milk. <12 years: not recommended; 12-<18: use extreme caution; not recommended for children and adolescents with asthma or other chronic breathing problem. The FDA and the European Medicines Agency (EMA) are investigating the safety of using *codeine* containing medications to treat pain, cough and colds, in children 12-<18 years because of the potential for serious side effects, including slowed or difficult breathing.

▷ **Rondec Syrup (C)(G)** <2 years: not recommended; 2-5 years: 1/4 tsp q 4-6 hours prn; max 7.5 ml/day; 6-11 years: 1/2 tsp q 4-6 hours prn; max 15 ml/day; >11 years: 1 tsp qid prn; max 30 ml/day
Syr: phenyle 12.5 mg/*chlor* 4 mg per 5 ml (bubblegum) (sugar-free, alcohol-free)

▷ **Semprex-D (B)** <12 years: not recommended; ≥12 years: 1 cap q 4-6 hours prn; max 4 doses/day
Cap: acriv 8 mg/*pseud* 60 mg

▷ **Tanafed DMX (C)(G)** <2 years: not recommended; 2-6 years: 1/2-1 tsp q 12 hours prn; 6-12 years: 1-2 tsp q 12 hours prn; >12 years: 2-4 tsp q 12 hours prn
Susp: dexchlor 2.5 mg/*pseud* 75 mg/*dextro* 25 mg per 5 ml (cotton candy) (alcohol-free)

(*continued*)

(*continued*)

▷ **Tessalon Caps (C)** <10 years: not recommended; ≥10 years: 100-200 mg tid prn; max 600 mg/day
Cap: benzo 200 mg
Comment: Swallow whole with a large glass of water. Do not suck or chew.

▷ **Tessalon Perles (C)** <10 years: not recommended; >10 years: 100-200 mg tid prn; max 600 mg/day
Perles: benzo 100 mg
Comment: Swallow whole with a large glass of water. Do not suck or chew.

▷ **Tussi-12 D Tablets (C)** <6 years: use susp; 6-11 years: 1/2-1 tab q 12 hours prn; >11 years: 1-2 tabs q 12 hours prn
Tab: carbeta 60 mg/*pyril* 40 mg/*phenyle* 10*mg

▷ **Tussi-12 DS (C)** <2 years: individualize; 2-6 years: 1/2-1 tsp q 12 hours prn; 6-12 years: 1-2 tsp q 12 hours prn; >12 years: 1-2 tsp q 12 hours prn
Liq: carbeta 30 mg/*pyril* 30 mg/*phenyle* 5 mg per 5 ml (strawberry-currant) (tartrazine)

▷ **TussiCaps 5 mg/4 mg (C)(III)** <6 years: not recommended; 6-11 years: 1 cap q 12 hours prn; max 2 caps/day; >11 years: 2 caps q 12 hours prn; max 4 caps/day
Cap: hydro 5 mg/*chlor* 4 mg ext-rel (alcohol)
Comment: *hydrocodone* is known to be excreted in breast milk.

▷ **TussiCaps 10 mg/8 mg (C)(III)** <12 years: not recommended; ≥12 years: 1 cap q 12 hours prn; max 2 caps/day
Cap: hydro 10 mg/*chlor* 8 mg ext-rel (alcohol)
Comment: *hydrocodone* is known to be excreted in breast milk.

▷ **Tussionex (C)(III)** <6 years: not recommended; 6-12 years: 1/2 tsp q 12 hours prn; >12 years: 1 tsp q 12 hours prn
Susp: hydro 10 mg/*chlor* 8 mg per 5 ml ext-rel
Comment: *hydrocodone* is known to be excreted in breast milk.

▷ **Tussi-Organidin DM NR Liquid (C)(III)** <6 months: not recommended; 6-23 months: 0.6 ml q 4 hours prn; max 3.7 ml/day; 2-5 years: 1.25 ml q 4 hours prn; max 7.5 ml/day; 6-11 years: 2.5 ml q 4 hours prn; max 15 ml/day; ≥12 years: 5 ml q 4 hours prn; max 40 ml/day
Liq: dextro 10 mg/*guaif* 300 mg per 5 ml (grape; sugar-free, alcohol-free)
Comment: *hydrocodone* is known to be excreted in breast milk.

▷ **Tussi-Organidin NR (C)(V)** <12 years: not recommended; 12-<18: use extreme caution; not recommended for children and adolescents with asthma or other chronic breathing problems; ≥18 years: 1 tsp q 4 hours prn; max 40 ml/day
Liq: guaif 300 mg per 5 ml (grape; sugar-free, alcohol-free)

▷ **Tuzistra XR (C)(III)** <18 years: not recommended; ≥18 years: 1-2 tsp q 12 hours prn; max 20 ml/day
Liq: cod 14.7 mg/*chlor* 2.8 mg per 5 ml (cherry)
Comment: *Codeine* is known to be excreted in breast milk. <12 years: not recommended; 12-<18: use extreme caution; not recommended for children and adolescents with asthma or other chronic breathing problem. The FDA and the European Medicines Agency (EMA) are investigating the safety of using *codeine* containing medications to treat pain, cough and colds, in children 12-<18 years because of the potential for serious side effects, including slowed or difficult breathing.

▷ **Vistaril (C)(G)** <6 years: 50 mg/day divided tid-qid prn; 6-12 years: 50-100 mg daily prn divided tid or qid; >6 years: 100 mg divided tid or qid prn
Cap: hydrox 25, 50, 100 mg; *Susp: hydrox* 25 mg/5 ml (lemon)

APPENDIX BB: SYSTEMIC ANTI-INFECTIVE DRUGS

- Adverse effects of aminoglycosides include nephrotoxicity and ototoxicity.
- Use cephalosporins with caution in persons with penicillin allergy due to potential cross allergy.
- Sulfonamides are contraindicated with sulfa allergy and G6PD deficiency. A high fluid intake is indicated during sulfonamide therapy.
- Tetracyclines should be taken on an empty stomach to facilitate absorption. Tetracyclines should not be taken with milk (binds to calcium).
- Tetracyclines are contraindicated during pregnancy and breastfeeding, and in children <8 years-of-age, due to the risk of developing tooth enamel discoloration.
- Systemic quinolones and fluoroquinolones are contraindicated in pregnancy and children <18 years-of-age due to the risk of joint dysplasia.

Anti-infectives by Class With Dose Forms		
Generic Name	Brand Name	Dose Form/Volume
Amebicide		
chloroquine phosphate (C)	Aralen	*Tab:* 500 mg; *Inj:* 50 mg/ml (5 ml)
iodoquinol (C)	Yodoxin	*Tab:* 210, 650 mg
metronidazole (not for use in 1st; B in 2nd, 3rd)(G)	Flagyl	*Tab:* 250*, 500* mg
	Flagyl 375	*Cap:* 375 mg
	Flagyl ER	*Tab:* 750 mg ext-rel
tinidazole (C)	Tindamax	*Tab:* 250*, 500* mg
Anthelmintic		
albendazole (C)(G)	Albenza	*Tab:* 200 mg
ivermectin (C)(G)	Stromectol	*Tab:* 3 mg
mebendazole (C)(G)	Emverm, Vermox	*Chew tab:* 100 mg
praziquantel (B)	Biltricide	*Tab:* 600 mg film-coat (scored for half or quarter dose)
pyrantel pamoate (C)(G)	Antiminth, Pin-X	*Cap:* 180 mg; *Liq:* 50 mg/ml (30 ml); 144 mg/ml (30 ml); *Oral susp:* 50 mg/ml (30 ml) (caramel) (sodium benzoate, tartrazine-free)

(*continued*)

(*continued*)

Anti-infectives by Class With Dose Forms		
Generic Name	Brand Name	Dose Form/Volume
Thiabendazole (C)(G)	**Mintezol** (currently not available in the United States)	*Chew tab:* 500*mg (orange); *Oral susp:* 500 mg/5 ml (120 ml) (orange)
Antifungal		
atovaquone (C)	**Mepron**	*Susp:* 750 mg/5 ml (210 ml)
clotrimazole (B)(G)	**Mycelex Troche**	10 mg (70, 40/bottle)
fluconazole (C)(G)	**Diflucan**	*Tab:* 50, 100, 150, 200 mg; *Oral susp:* 10, 40 mg/ml (35 ml) (orange)
griseofulvin, microsize (C)	**Grifulvin V**	*Tab:* 250, 500 mg; *Oral susp:* 125 mg/5 ml (120 ml) (alcohol 0.02%)
	Gris-PEG	*Tab:* 125, 250 mg
itraconazole (C)	**Sporanox**	*Cap:* 100 mg; *Soln:* 10 mg/ml (150 ml); *Pulse Pack:* 100 mg caps (7/pck)
ketoconazole (C)(G)	**Nizoral**	*Tab:* 200 mg
nystatin (C)(G)	**Mycostatin**	*Pastille:* 200,000 units/pastille (30 pastilles/pck); *Oral susp:* 100,000 units/ml (60 ml w. dropper)
terbinafine (B)(G)	**Lamisil**	*Tab:* 250 mg
voriconazole (D)(G)	**Vfend**	*Tab:* 50, 200 mg
Antimalarial		
atovaquone/proguanil (C)	**Malarone**	*Tab: atov* 250 mg/*proq* 100 mg
	Malarone Pediatric	*Tab: atov* 62.5 mg/*proq* 25 mg
chloroquine (C)(G)	**Aralen**	*Tab:* 500 mg; *Amp:* 50 mg/ml (5 ml)
doxycycline (D)(G)	**Acticlate**	*Tab:* 75, 150**mg
	Adoxa	*Tab:* 50, 75, 100, 150 mg ent-coat
	Doryx	*Cap:* 100 mg; *Tab:* 50, 75, 100, 150, 200 mg
	Monodox	*Cap:* 50, 75, 100 mg

(*continued*)

(*continued*)

Anti-infectives by Class With Dose Forms		
Generic Name	**Brand Name**	**Dose Form/Volume**
	Oracea	*Cap:* 40 mg del-rel
	Vibramycin	*Cap:* 50, 100 mg; *Syr:* 50 mg/5 ml (raspberry-apple) (sulfites); *Oral susp:* 25 mg/5 ml (raspberry)
	Vibra-Tab	*Tab:* 100 mg film-coat
hydroxychloroquine (C)(G)	Plaquenil	*Tab:* 200 mg
mefloquine (C)	Lariam	*Tab:* 250 mg
Antiprotozoal/Antibacterial		
metronidazole (**not for use in 1st; B in 2nd, 3rd**)(G)	Flagyl, Protostat	*Tab:* 250*, 500* mg
	Flagyl 375	*Cap:* 375 mg
	Flagyl ER	*Tab:* 750 mg ext-rel
nitazoxanide (C) (G)	Alinia	*Tab:* 500 mg; *Oral susp:* 100 mg/5 ml (60 ml) (strawberry)
tinidazole (C)	Tindamax	*Tab:* 250*, 500*mg
Antiviral (for HIV-specific antiviral drugs see page 511)		
acyclovir (C)(G)	Zovirax	*Cap:* 200 mg; *Tab:* 400, 800 mg; *Oral susp:* 200 mg/5 ml (banana)
amantadine (C)(G)	Symmetrel	*Tab:* 100 mg; *Syr:* 50 mg/5 ml (16 oz) (raspberry)
famciclovir (B)	Famvir	*Tab:* 125, 250, 500 mg
lamivudine (C)	Epivir-HBV	*Tab:* 100 mg; *Oral soln:* 5 mg/ml (240 ml) (strawberry-banana)
oseltamivir (C)	Tamiflu	*Cap:* 75 mg
rimantadine (C)	Flumadine	*Tab:* 100 mg
valacyclovir (B)	Valtrex	*Tab:* 500 mg; 1 g
zanamivir	Relenza	*Tab: lami* 150/*zido* 300 mg
Antitubercular		
ethambutol (EMB) (B)(G)	Myambutol	*Tab:* 100, 400*mg

(*continued*)

(*continued*)

Anti-infectives by Class With Dose Forms		
Generic Name	Brand Name	Dose Form/Volume
isoniazid (INH)(C)(G)	*generic only*	*Tab:* 100, 300*mg; *Syr:* 50 mg/5 ml; *Inj:* 100 mg/ml
pyrazinamide (PZA) (C)	*generic only*	*Tab:* 500*mg
rifampin (C)(G)	**Priftin**	*Tab:* 150 mg
	Rifadin	*Cap:* 150, 300 mg
rifampin/isoniazid (C)	**Rifamate**	*Cap:* rif 300 mg/iso 150 mg
rifampin/isoniazid/ pyrazinamide (C)	**Rifater**	*Tab:* rif 120 mg/iso 50 mg/pyr 300 mg
Aminoglycoside		
amikacin (C)	**Amikin**	*Vial:* 500 mg, 1 g (2 ml)
gentamicin (C)(G)	**Garamycin**	*Vial:* 20, 80 mg/2 ml
streptomycin (D)(G)	**Streptomycin**	*Amp:* 1 g/2.5 ml <u>or</u> 400 mg/ml (2.5 ml)
Cephalosporin		
First-Generation Cephalosporin		
cefadroxil (B)	**Duricef**	*Cap:* 500 mg; *Tab:* 1 g; *Oral susp:* 250 mg/5 ml (100 ml); 500 mg/5 ml (75, 100 ml) (orange-pineapple)
cefazolin (B)	**Ancef, Zolicef**	*Vial:* 500 mg; 1, 10 g
cephalexin (B)	**Keflex**	*Cap:* 250, 333, 500, 750 mg; *Oral susp:* 125, 250 mg/5 ml (100, 200 ml)
Second-Generation Cephalosporin		
cefaclor (B)(G)	*generic only*	*Tab:* 500 mg; *Cap:* 250, 500 mg; *Susp:* 125 mg/5 ml (75, 150 ml) (strawberry); 187 mg/5 ml (50, 100 ml) (strawberry); 250 mg/5 ml (75, 150 ml) (strawberry); 375 mg/5 ml (50, 100 ml) (strawberry)
	Cefaclor Extended Release	*Tab:* 375, 500 mg ext-rel

(*continued*)

(*continued*)

Anti-infectives by Class With Dose Forms		
Generic Name	**Brand Name**	**Dose Form/Volume**
cefamandole (B)	Mandol	*Vial:* 1, 2 g
cefotetan (B)(G)	Cefotan	*Vial:* 1, 2 g
cefoxitin (B)	Mefoxin	*Vial:* 1, 2 g
cefprozil (B)(G)	Cefzil	*Tab:* 250, 500 mg; *Oral susp:* 125, 250 mg/5 ml (50, 75, 100 ml) (bubble gum) (phenylalanine)
ceftaroline (B)	Teflaro	*Vial:* 400, 600 mg
cefuroxime axetil (B) (G)	Ceftin	*Tab:* 250, 500 mg; *Oral susp:* 125, 250 mg/5 ml (50, 100 ml) (tutti-frutti)
cefuroxime sodium (B)(G)	Zinacef	*Vial:* 750 mg; 1.5 g
loracarbef (B)	Lorabid	*Pulvule:* 200, 400 mg; *Oral susp:* 100 mg/5 ml (50, 100 ml); 200 mg/5 ml (50, 75, 100 ml) (strawberry bubble gum)
Third-Generation Cephalosporin		
cefoperazone (B)	Cefobid	*Vial:* 1, 2 g pwdr for reconstitution
cefotaxime (B)	Claforan	*Vial:* 500 mg; 1, 2 g pwdr for reconstitution
cefpodoxime (B)	Vantin	*Tab:* 100, 200 mg; *Oral susp:* 50, 100 mg/5 ml (50, 75, 100 ml) (lemon creme)
ceftazidime (B)	Ceftaz	*Vial:* 1, 2 g pwdr for reconstitution
	Fortaz	*Vial:* 500 mg; 1, 2 g pwdr for reconstitution
	Tazicef	*Vial:* 1, 2 g pwdr for reconstitution
	Tazidime	*Vial:* 1, 2 g pwdr for reconstitution
ceftazidime/ avibactam (B)	Avycaz	*Vial:* 2.5 g pwdr for reconstitution
ceftibuten (B)	Cedax	*Cap:* 400 mg; *Oral susp:* 90 mg/5 ml (30, 60, 90, 120 ml); 180 mg/5 ml (30, 60, 120 ml) (cherry)

(*continued*)

(*continued*)

Anti-infectives by Class With Dose Forms		
Generic Name	Brand Name	Dose Form/Volume
Third/Fourth-Generation Cephalosporin		
cefdinir (B)	Omnicef	*Cap:* 300 mg; *Oral susp:* 125 mg/5 ml (60, 100 ml) (strawberry)
cefditoren pivoxil (C)	Spectracef	*Tab:* 200 mg
cefepime (B)(G)	Maxipime	*Vial:* 1 g pwdr for reconstitution
cefixime (B)	Suprax	*Tab/Cap:* 400 mg; *Oral Susp:* 100 mg/5 ml (50, 75, 100 ml)(strawberry)
ceftaroline (B)	Teflaro	*Vial:* 400, 600 mg
ceftriaxone (B)(G)	Rocephin	*Vial:* 250, 500 mg; 1, 2 g
ceftolozane/ tazobactam (B)	Zerbaxa	*Vial:* 1.5 g pwdr for reconstitution
Fluoroquinolone and Quinolone		
First-Generation Quinolone		
enoxacin (C)	Penetrex	*Tab:* 200, 400 mg
Second-Generation Fluoroquinolone		
ciprofloxacin (C)(G)	Cipro	*Tab:* 250, 500, 750 mg; *Oral susp:* 250, 500 mg/5 ml (100 ml) (strawberry) *IV conc:* 10 mg/ml after dilution (20, 40 ml); *IV premix:* 2 mg/ml (100, 200 ml)
	Cipro XR	*Tab:* 500, 1000 mg ext-rel
	ProQuin XR	*Tab:* 500 mg ext-rel
lomefloxacin (C)	Maxaquin	*Tab:* 400 mg
norfloxacin (C)(G)	Noroxin	*Tab:* 400 mg
ofloxacin (C)(G)	Floxin	*Tab:* 200, 300, 400 mg
Third-Generation Fluoroquinolone		
levofloxacin (C)(G)	Levaquin	*Tab:* 250, 500, 750 mg

(*continued*)

(continued)

Anti-infectives by Class With Dose Forms		
Generic Name	Brand Name	Dose Form/Volume
Fourth-Generation Fluoroquinolone		
gemifloxacin (C)(G)	Factive	*Tab:* 320*mg
moxifloxacin (C)(G)	Avelox	*Tab:* 400 mg
Ketolide		
telithromycin (C)	Ketek	*Tab:* 300, 400 mg
Macrolides		
azithromycin (B)	Zithromax	*Tab:* 250, 500, 600 mg; *Pkt:* 1 g for reconstitution (cherry-banana)
	oral susp generic only	*Oral susp:* 100 mg/5 ml, (15 ml); 200 mg/5 ml (15, 22.5, 30 ml) (cherry)
	Zithromax Tri-Pak	*Tab:* 3 x 500 mg tabs/pck
	Zithromax Z-Pak	*Tab:* 6 x 250 mg tabs/pck
	Zmax	Pkt: 2 g for reconstitution (cherry-banana)
clarithromycin (C)(G)	Biaxin	*Tab:* 250, 500 mg; *Oral susp:* 125, 250 mg/5 ml (50, 100 ml)(fruit punch)
	Biaxin XL	*Tab:* 500 mg ext-rel
dirithromycin (C)(G)	generic only	*Tab:* 250 mg
erythromycin base (B)(G)	Ery-Tab	*Tab:* 250, 333, 500 mg ent-coat
	PCE	*Tab:* 333, 500 mg
erythromycin estolate (B)(G)	Ilosone	*Pulvule:* 250 mg; *Tab:* 500 mg; *Liq:* 125, 250 mg/5 ml (100 ml)
erythromycin ethylsuccinate (B)(G)	E.E.S.	*Tab:* 400 mg; *Oral susp:* 200 mg/5 ml (100, 200 ml) (cherry); 200, 400 mg/5 ml (100 ml)(fruit)
	EryPed	*Oral susp:* 200 mg/5 ml (100, 200 ml) (fruit); 400 mg/5 ml (60, 100, 200 ml) (banana); *Oral drops:* 200, 400 mg/5 ml (50 ml) (fruit); *Chew tab:* 200 mg wafer (fruit)

(continued)

(*continued*)

Anti-infectives by Class With Dose Forms		
Generic Name	Brand Name	Dose Form/Volume
erythromycin stearate (B)(G)	Erythrocin	*Film tab:* 250, 500 mg
Penicillin		
amoxicillin (B)(G)	Amoxil	*Cap:* 250, 500 mg; *Tab:* 500, 875* mg; *Chew tab:* 125, 200, 250, 400 mg (cherry-banana-peppermint) (phenylalanine); *Oral susp:* 125, 250 mg/ml (80, 100, 150 ml) (bubble gum); 200, 400 mg/5 ml (50, 75, 100 ml) (bubble gum); *Oral drops:* 50 mg/ml (30 ml) (bubble gum)
	Moxatag	*Tab:* 775 mg ext-rel
	Trimox	*Cap:* 250, 500 mg; *Oral susp:* 125, 250 mg/5 ml (80, 100, 150 ml) (raspberry-strawberry)
amoxicillin/clavulanate (B)(G)	Augmentin	*Tab:* 250, 500, 875 mg; *Chew tab:* 125, 250 mg (lemon lime); 200, 400 mg (cherry-banana; phenylalanine); *Oral susp:* 125 mg/5 ml (banana), 250 mg/5 ml (orange) (75, 100, 150 ml); 200, 400 mg/5 ml (50, 75, 100 ml) (orange)
	Augmentin ES-600	*Oral susp:* 600 mg/5 ml (50, 75, 100, 125, 150, 200 ml) (strawberry cream) (phenylalanine)
	Augmentin XR	*Tab:* 1000*mg ext-rel
ampicillin (B)(G)	Omnipen	*Cap:* 250, 500 mg; *Oral susp:* 125, 250 mg/ml (100, 150, 200 ml)
	Principen	*Cap:* 250, 500 mg; *Syr:* 125, 250 mg/5 ml
ampicillin/ sulbactam (B)(G)	Unasyn	*Vial:* 1.5, 3 g
carbenicillin (B)	Geocillin	*Tab:* 382 mg film-coat

(*continued*)

(*continued*)

Anti-infectives by Class With Dose Forms		
Generic Name	Brand Name	Dose Form/Volume
dicloxacillin (B)(G)	**Dynapen**	*Cap:* 125, 250, 500 mg; *Oral susp:* 62.5 mg/5 ml (80, 100, 200 ml)
ertapenem (B)	**Invanz**	*Vial:* 1 g pwdr for reconstitution
meropenem (B)(G)	**Merrem**	*Vial:* 500 mg; 1 g pwdr for reconstitution (sodium 3.92 mEq/g)
penicillin G benzathine (B)(G)	**Bicillin LA, Bicillin C-R**	*Cartridge-needle unit:* 600,000 million units (1 ml); 1.2 million units (2 ml); 2.4 million units (4 ml)
	Permapen	*Prefilled syringe:* 1.2 million units
penicillin G procaine (B)(G)	*generic only*	*Prefilled syringe:* 1.2 million units
penicillin v potassium (B)(G)	**Pen-Vee K**	*Tab:* 250, 500 mg; *Oral soln:* 125 mg/5 ml (100, 200 ml); 250 mg/5 ml (100, 150, 200 ml)
piperacillin/ tazobactam (B)(G)	**Zosyn**	*Vial:* 2, 3, 4 g pwdr for reconstitution
Sulfonamide		
sulfamethoxazole (B/D)(G)	**Gantrisin Pediatric**	*Oral susp:* 500 mg/5 ml; *Syr:* 500 mg/5 ml
trimethoprim (C)(G)	**Primsol**	*Oral soln:* 50 mg/5 ml (bubble gum) (dye-free, alcohol-free)
	Trimpex	*Tab:* 100 mg
	Proloprim	*Tab:* 100, 200 mg
trimethoprim/ sulfamethoxazole (C) (G)	**Bactrim, Septra**	*Tab: trim* 80 mg/*sulfa* 400 mg*
	Bactrim DS, Septra DS	*Tab: trim* 160 mg/*sulfa* 800 mg*; *Oral susp: trim* 40 mg/*sulfa* 200 mg per 5 ml (100 ml) (cherry) (alcohol 0.3%)
Tetracycline		
demeclocycline (D)	**Declomycin**	*Tab:* 300 mg

(*continued*)

(*continued*)

Anti-infectives by Class With Dose Forms		
Generic Name	Brand Name	Dose Form/Volume
doxycycline (D)(G)	**Adoxa**	*Tab:* 50, 100 mg ent-coat
	Doryx	*Cap:* 100 mg
	Monodox	*Cap:* 50, 100 mg
doxycycline (D)(G)	**Vibramycin**	*Cap:* 50, 100 mg; *Syr:* 50 mg/5 ml; (raspberry) (sulfites); *Oral susp:* 25 mg/5 ml (raspberry-apple); *IV conc:* *doxy* 100 mg/*asc acid* 480 mg after dilution; *doxy* 200 mg/*asc acid* 960 mg after dilution
	Vibra-Tab	*Tab:* 100 mg film-coat
minocycline (D)(G)	**Dynacin**	*Cap:* 50, 100 mg
	Minocin	*Cap:* 50, 100 mg; *Oral susp:* 50 mg/5 ml (60 ml) (custard) (sulfites, alcohol 5%); *Vial:* 100 mg soln for inj:
tetracycline (D)(G)	**Achromycin V**	*Cap:* 250, 500 mg
	Sumycin	*Tab:* 250, 500 mg; *Oral susp:* 125 mg/5 ml (fruit) (sulfites)
Macrolide/Sulfisoxazole		
erythromycin ethylsuccinate/ sulfisoxazole (C)(G)	**Pediazole**	*Oral susp: eryth* 200 mg/*sulf* 600 mg per 5 ml (100, 150, 200 ml) (strawberry-banana)
Miscellaneous		
aztreonam (B)	**Cayston**	*Vial:* 75 mg pwdr for reconstitution (preservative-free)
chloramphenicol (C)(G)	**Chloromycetin**	*Vial:* 1 gm
clindamycin (B)(G)	**Cleocin**	*Cap:* 75 (tartrazine), 150 (tartrazine), 300 mg; *Oral susp:* 75 mg/5 ml (100 ml) (cherry); *Vial:* 150 mg/l (2, 4 ml) (benzyl alcohol)

(*continued*)

(*continued*)

Anti-infectives by Class With Dose Forms		
Generic Name	Brand Name	Dose Form/Volume
dalbavancin (C)	Dalvance	*Vial:* 500 mg pwdr for IV infusion (preservative-free)
daptomycin (B)(G)	Cubicin	*Vial:* 500 mg pwdr for reconstitution
doripenem (B)	Doribax	*Vial:* 500 mg pwdr for reconstitution
fosfomycin (B)	Monurol	*Sachet:* 3 gm single dose (mandarin orange; sucrose)
imipenem/cilastatin (C)(G)	Primaxin	*Vial: imip* 500 mg/*cila* 500 mg; *imip* 750 mg/*cila* 750 mg pwdr for reconstitution
lincomycin (B)(G)	Lincocin	*Vial:* 300 mg/ml (10 ml)
linezolid (C)(G)	Zyvox	*Tab:* 400, 600 mg; *Oral susp:* 100 mg/5 ml (orange) (phenylalanine); *IV:* 2 mg ml (100, 200, 300 ml)
meropenem (B)	Merrem	*Vial:* 500 mg; 1 g (sodium 3.92 mEq/g)
nitrofurantoin (B)(G)	Furadantin	*Oral susp:* 25 mg/5 ml (60 ml)
	Macrobid	*Cap:* 100 mg
	Macrodantin	*Cap:* 25, 50, 100 mg
quinupristin/ dalfopristin (B)	Synercid	*Vial:* 150 mg/350 mg, 180 mg/420 mg
tigecycline (D)(G)	Tygacil	*Vial:* 50 mg pwdr for reconstitution
rifaximin (C)	Xifaxan	*Tab:* 200, 550 mg
telavancin (C)	Vibativ	*Vial:* 250, 750 mg pwdr for reconstitution for IV infusion (preservative-free)
vancomycin (C)(G)	Vancocin	*Cap:* 125, 250 mg; *Vial:* 500 mg, 1 g pwdr for reconstitution for IV infusion

APPENDIX CC: POUNDS/KILOGRAMS CONVERSION TABLE

1 Kg = 2.2 Lbs					
Lb = Kg		Lb = Kg		Lb = Kg	
1	0.45	70	31.75	140	63.5
5	2.27	75	34.02	145	65.77
10	4.54	80	36.29	150	68.04
15	6.8	85	38.56	155	70.31
20	9.07	90	40.82	160	72.58
25	11.34	95	43.09	165	74.84
30	13.61	100	45.36	170	77.11
35	15.88	105	47.63	175	79.38
40	18.14	110	49.9	180	81.65
45	20.41	115	52.16	185	83.92
50	22.68	120	54.43	190	86.18
55	24.95	125	56.7	195	88.45
60	27.22	130	58.91	200	90.72
65	29.48	135	61.24		

¶Adapted from American Pharmacists Association. (2015). *Pediatric and neonatal dosage handbook: A universal resource for clinicians treating pediatric and neonatal patients* (22nd ed.). Hudson, OH: Lexicomp.

APPENDIX DD.1: *ACYCLOVIR* (ZOVIRAX SUSPENSION)

Weight												
Pounds	15	20	25	30	35	40	45	50	55	60	65	70
Kilograms	6.8	9	11.4	13.6	15.9	18.2	20.5	22.7	25	27.3	29.5	31.8
Single Dose (ml)/Frequency/Strength/5-Day Volume (ml)												
20 mg/kg/d ml/dose qid	3.5	4.5	5.5	6.5	8	9	10	11.5	12.5	13.5	14.5	16
mg/5ml	200	200	200	200	200	200	200	200	200	200	200	200
Volume (ml)	70	90	110	130	160	180	200	230	250	270	290	320

Zovirax Oral Suspension <2 years: not recommended; >2 years, <40 kg: 20 mg/kg dosed qid x 5 days; ≥2 years, >40 kg: 800 mg dosed qid x 5 days; *Oral susp:* 200 mg/5 ml (banana).

APPENDIX DD.2: *AMANTADINE* (SYMMETREL SYRUP)

Weight												
Pounds	15	20	25	30	35	40	45	50	55	60	65	70
Kilograms	6.8	9	11.4	13.6	15.9	18.2	20.5	22.7	25	27.3	29.5	31.8
Single Dose (ml)/Frequency/Strength/10-Day Volume (ml)												
4 mg/kg/d ml/dose bid	3	4	5	6	7	8	9	10	11	12	13	14
mg/5ml	50	50	50	50	50	50	50	50	50	50	50	50
Volume (ml)	30	40	50	60	70	80	90	100	110	120	130	140
8 mg/lb/d ml/dose bid	6	8	10	12								
mg/5ml	50	50	50	50								
Volume (ml)	60	80	100	60								

Symmetrel Suspension (C)(G) Symmetrel <1 year: not recommended; 1-8 years: max 150 mg/day; 9-12 years: 2 tsp bid; >12 years: 100 mg bid or 200 mg once daily; Syr: 50 mg/5 ml (raspberry).

APPENDIX DD.3: *AMOXICILLIN* (AMOXIL SUSPENSION, TRIMOX SUSPENSION)

Weight

Pounds	15	20	25	30	35	40	45	50	55	60	65	70
Kilograms	6.8	9	11.4	13.6	15.9	18.2	20.5	22.7	25	27.3	29.5	31.8
Single Dose (ml)/Frequency/Strength/10-Day Volume (ml)												
20 mg/kg/d ml/dose tid	2	2.5	3	3.5	4	5	5.5	6	7	7.5	8	9
mg/5 ml	125	125	125	125	125	125	125	125	125	125	125	125
Volume (ml)	60	75	90	105	120	150	165	180	210	225	240	270
30 mg/kg/d ml/dose tid	3	3.5	2.5	3	3	3.5	4	4.5	5	5.5	6	6.5
mg/5 ml	125	125	250	250	250	250	250	250	250	250	250	250
Volume (ml)	90	105	75	90	90	105	120	135	150	165	180	195
40 mg/kg/d ml/dose bid	5	7	4.5	5	6	7	8	9	10	11	12	13
mg/5 ml	125	125	250	250	250	250	250	250	250	250	250	250
Volume (ml)	100	140	90	100	120	140	160	180	200	220	240	250
45 mg/kg/d ml/dose bid	4	2.5	3	4	4.5	5	6	6.5	7	7.5	8.5	9

(continued)

APPENDIX DD.3: *AMOXICILLIN* (AMOXIL SUSPENSION, TRIMOX SUSPENSION) (continued)

mg/5 ml	200	400	400	400	400	400	400	400	400	400	400	400	400	400	400
Volume (ml)	80	50	60	80	90	100	120	130	140	150	170	180			
90 mg/kg/d ml/dose bid	8	5	6	7	9	10	12	13	14	15	17	18			
mg/5 ml	200	400	400	400	400	400	400	400	400	400	400	400			
Volume (ml)	160	100	120	140	180	200	240	260	280	300	340	360			

<40 kg (88 lb): 20–30 mg/kg/day in 3 divided doses or 40–90 mg/kg/day in 2 divided doses.
Amoxil Suspension (B)(G) 125, 250 mg/5 ml (80, 100, 150 ml) (strawberry); 200, 400 mg/5 ml (50, 75, 100 ml) (bubble gum).
Trimox Suspension (B)(G) 125, 250 mg/5 ml (80, 100, 150 ml) (raspberry-strawberry).

APPENDIX DD.4: AMOXICILLIN/CLAVULANATE (AUGMENTIN SUSPENSION)

Weight												
Pounds	15	20	25	30	35	40	45	50	55	60	65	70
Kilograms	6.8	9	11.4	13.6	15.9	18.2	20.5	22.7	25	27.3	29.5	31.8
Single Dose (ml)/Frequency/Strength/10-Day Volume (ml)												
40 mg/kg/d ml/dose bid	5.5	7	4.5	5.5	6.5	7	8	9	10	11	12	13
mg/5 ml	125	125	250	250	250	250	250	250	250	250	250	250
Volume (ml)	110	140	90	110	130	140	160	180	200	220	240	260
45 mg/kg/d ml/dose bid	3	4	5	6	7	8	9	10	11.5	12.5	13.5	14.5
mg/5 ml	250	250	250	250	250	250	250	250	250	250	250	250
Volume (ml)	60	80	100	120	140	160	180	200	230	250	270	290
45 mg/kg/d ml/dose bid	4	2.5	3	4	4.5	5	6	6.5	7	7.5	8.5	9
mg/5 ml	200	400	400	400	400	400	400	400	400	400	400	400
Volume (ml)	80	50	60	80	90	100	120	130	140	150	170	180
90 mg/kg/d ml/dose bid	4	5	6.5	8	9	10	11.5	13	14	15.5	16.5	18
mg/5 ml	400	400	400	400	400	400	400	400	400	400	400	400
Volume (ml)	80	100	130	160	180	200	240	260	280	300	340	360

Augmentin Suspension (B)(G) 40–45 mg/kg/day divided tid or 90 mg/kg/day divided bid; 125 mg/5 ml (75, 100, 150 ml) (banana); 250 mg/5 ml (75, 100, 150 ml) (orange); 200, 400 mg/5 ml (50, 75, 100 ml) (orange-raspberry) (phenylalanine).

APPENDIX DD.5: *AMOXICILLIN/CLAVULANATE* (AUGMENTIN ES 600 SUSPENSION)

Weight												
Pounds	15	20	25	30	35	40	45	50	55	60	65	70
Kilograms	6.8	9	11.4	13.6	15.9	18.2	20.5	22.7	25	27.3	29.5	31.8
Single Dose (ml)/Frequency/Strength/10-Day Volume (ml)												
40 mg/kg/d ml/dose bid	1	1.5	2	2	2.5	3	3.5	4	4	4.5	5	5
mg/5 ml	600	600	600	600	600	600	600	600	600	600	600	600
Volume (ml)	30	40	40	40	50	60	70	80	80	90	100	100
45 mg/kg/d ml/dose bid	1.25	1.5	2	2.5	3	3.5	4	4.5	5	5	5.5	6
mg/5 ml	600	600	600	600	600	600	600	600	600	600	600	600
Volume (ml)	25	30	40	50	60	70	80	90	100	100	110	120
90 mg/kg/d ml/dose bid	2.5	3.5	4	5	6	7	8	8.5	9.5	10	11	12
mg/5 ml	600	600	600	600	600	600	600	600	600	600	600	600
Volume (ml)	50	70	80	100	120	140	160	170	190	200	220	240

Augmentin ES 600 Suspension (B) <3 months: not recommended; ≥3 months; <40 kg: 90 mg/kg/day in 2 divided doses; ≥40 kg: not recommended; 600 mg/5 ml (50, 75, 100, 125, 150, 200 ml) (strawberry cream) (phenylalanine).

APPENDIX DD.6: *AMPICILLIN* (OMNIPEN SUSPENSION, PRINCIPEN SUSPENSION)

Weight													
Pounds	15	20	25	30	35	40	45	50	55	60	65	70
Kilograms	6.8	9	11.4	13.6	15.9	18.2	20.5	22.7	25	27.3	29.5	31.8
Single Dose (ml)/Frequency/Strength/10-Day Volume (ml)												
50 mg/kg/d ml/dose q6h	3.5	4.5	3	3.5	4	4.5						
mg/5 ml	125	125	250	250	250	250						
Volume (ml)	140	180	120	140	160	180						
100 mg/kg/d ml/dose q6h	3.5	4.5	6	7	8	9						
mg/5 ml	250	250	250	250	250	250						
Volume (ml)	140	180	240	280	320	360						

Omnipen Suspension, Principen Suspension (B)(G) >20 kg: 250-500 mg q 6 h 125, 250 mg/5 ml (100, 150, 200 ml) (fruit).

APPENDIX DD.7: *AZITHROMYCIN* (ZITHROMAX SUSPENSION, ZMAX SUSPENSION)

Weight									
Pounds	11	22	33	44	55	66	77	88	
Kilograms	5	10	15	20	25	30	35	40	
Single Dose (ml)/Frequency/Strength/Volume (ml)									
3-Day Regimen									
10 mg/kg qd	2.5	5	7.5	5	6	7.5	9	10	
mg/5 ml	100	100	100	200	200	200	200	200	
Volume (ml)	7.5	15	22.5	15	18	22.5	27	30	
5-Day Regimen									
10 mg/kg qd									
Day 1	2.5	5	7.5	5	6	7.5	7.5	10	
Days 2–5	1.25	2.5	4	2.5	3	4	4	5	
mg/5 ml	100	100	100	200	200	200	200	200	
Volume (ml)	10	15	23.5	15	18	23.5	23.5	30	

Zithromax ES 600 Suspension (B)(G) 100 mg/5 ml (15 ml), 200 mg/5 ml (15, 22.5, 30 ml) (cherry-vanilla-banana).

APPENDIX DD.8: *CEFACLOR* (CECLOR SUSPENSION)

Weight												
Pounds	15	20	25	30	35	40	45	50	55	60	65	70
Kilograms	6.8	9	11.4	13.6	15.9	18.2	20.5	22.7	25	27.3	29.5	31.8
Single Dose (ml)/Frequency/Strength/10-Day Volume (ml)												
20 mg/kg/d ml/dose tid	2	2.5	3	3.5	4	5	5.5	6	7	7.5	8	8.5
mg/5 ml	125	125	125	125	125	125	125	125	125	125	125	125
Volume (ml)	60	75	90	105	120	150	165	180	210	225	240	255
20 mg/kg/d ml/dose tid	1.5	1.5	2	2.5	3	3	4	4	4.5	5	5.5	6
mg/5 ml	187	187	187	187	187	187	187	187	187	187	187	187
Volume (ml)	45	45	60	75	90	90	105	120	135	150	165	180
40 mg/kg/d ml/dose tid	2	2.5	3	3.5	4	5	5.5	6	6.5	7	8	8.5
mg/5 ml	250	250	250	250	250	250	250	250	250	250	250	250
Volume (ml)	60	75	90	105	120	150	165	180	195	210	240	255
40 mg/kg/d ml/dose tid	1.5	1.5	2	2.5	3	3	3.5	4	4.5	5	5	5.5
mg/5 ml	375	375	375	375	375	375	375	375	375	375	375	375
Volume (ml)	45	45	60	75	90	90	105	120	135	150	150	165

Ceclor Suspension **(B)** <6 months: not recommended; 125, 250 mg/5 ml (75, 150 ml) (strawberry); 187, 375 mg/5 ml (50, 100 ml) (strawberry).

APPENDIX DD.9: *CEFADROXIL* (DURICEF SUSPENSION)

Weight												
Pounds	15	20	25	30	35	40	45	50	55	60	65	70
Kilograms	6.8	9	11.4	13.6	15.9	18.2	20.5	22.7	25	27.3	29.5	31.8
Single Dose (ml)/Frequency/Strength/10-Day Volume (ml)												
30 mg/kg/d ml/dose bid	2	3	3.5	4	5	5.5	6	7	7.5	8	9	9.5
mg/5 ml	250	250	250	250	250	250	250	250	250	250	250	250
Volume (ml)	40	60	75	80	100	110	120	140	150	160	180	190
30 mg/kg/d ml/dose qd	2	3	3.5	4	5	5.5	6	7	7.5	8	9	9.5
mg/5 ml	500	500	500	500	500	500	500	500	500	500	500	500
Volume (ml)	20	30	35	40	50	55	60	70	75	80	90	95

Duricef Suspension (B) 250 mg/5 ml (100 ml) (orange-pineapple); 500 mg/5 ml (75, 100 ml) (orange-pineapple).

APPENDIX DD.10: *CEFDINIR* (OMNICEF SUSPENSION)

Weight

Pounds	15	20	25	30	35	40	45	50	55	60	65	70
Kilograms	6.8	9	11.4	13.6	15.9	18.2	20.5	22.7	25	27.3	29.5	31.8

Single Dose (ml)/Frequency/Strength/10-Day Volume (ml)

	15	20	25	30	35	40	45	50	55	60	65	70
7 mg/kg/d ml/dose bid	2	2.5	3	4	4.5	5	6	6.5	7	7.5	8	9
mg/5 ml	125	125	125	125	125	125	125	125	125	125	125	125
Volume (ml)	40	50	60	80	90	100	120	130	140	150	160	180
14 mg/kg ml/dose bid	4	5	6	8	9	10	12	13	14	15	16	18
mg/5 ml	125	125	125	125	125	125	125	125	125	125	125	125
Volume (ml)	40	50	60	80	90	100	120	130	140	150	160	180

Omnicef Suspension (B) <6 months: not recommended; 125 mg/5 ml (60, 100 ml) (strawberry).

APPENDIX DD.11: *CEFIXIME* (SUPRAX ORAL SUSPENSION)

Weight												
Pounds	15	20	25	30	35	40	45	50	55	60	65	70
Kilograms	6.8	9	11.4	13.6	15.9	18.2	20.5	22.7	25	27.3	29.5	31.8
Single Dose (ml)/Frequency/Strength/10-Day Volume (ml)												
8 mg/kg/d ml/dose bid	1.3	1.8	2.2	2.5	3.1	3.5	4	4.5	5	5.5	6	6.5
mg/5 ml	100	100	100	100	100	100	100	100	100	100	100	100
8 mg/kg/d ml/dose qd	2.7	3.6	4.5	5.5	6.3	7.2	8.2	9	10	11	12	13
mg/5 ml	100	100	100	100	100	100	100	100	100	100	100	100
Volume (ml)	27	36	45	55	65	70	80	90	100	110	120	130

Supra Oral Suspension (B)(G) <6 months: not recommended; 100 mg/5 ml (50, 75, 100 ml) (strawberry).

APPENDIX DD.12: CEFPODOXIME PROXETIL

Weight												
Pounds	15	20	25	30	35	40	45	50	55	60	65	70
Kilograms	6.8	9	11.4	13.6	15.9	18.2	20.5	22.7	25	27.3	29.5	31.8
Single Dose (ml)/Frequency/Strength/10-Day Volume (ml)												
5 mg/kg/d ml/dose bid	3.5	4.5	5.5	7	8	9	10	11	12.5	13.5	15	16
mg/5 ml	50	50	50	50	50	50	50	50	50	50	50	50
Volume (ml)	70	90	110	140	160	180	200	220	250	270	300	320
5 mg/kg/d ml/dose bid	2	2	3	3.5	4	4.5	5	5.5	6	7	7.5	8
mg/5 ml	100	100	100	100	100	100	100	100	100	100	100	100
Volume (ml)	40	40	60	70	80	90	100	110	120	140	150	160

Vantin Suspension (B) <2 months: not recommended; 50, 100 mg/5 ml (50, 75, 100 ml) (lemon-crème).

APPENDIX DD.13: *CEFPROZIL* (CEFZIL SUSPENSION)

Weight												
Pounds	15	20	25	30	35	40	45	50	55	60	65	70
Kilograms	6.8	9	11.4	13.6	15.9	18.2	20.5	22.7	25	27.3	29.5	31.8
Single Dose (ml)/Frequency/Strength/10-Day Volume (ml)												
7.5 mg/kg/d ml/dose bid	2	3	3.5	4	5	5.5	6	7	7.5	4	4.5	5
mg/5 ml	125	125	125	125	125	125	125	125	125	250	250	250
Volume (ml)	40	60	70	80	100	110	120	140	150	80	90	100
15 mg/kg/d ml/dose bid	2	3	3.5	4	5	5	6	7	7.5	8	9	9.5
mg/5 ml	250	250	250	250	250	250	250	250	250	250	250	250
Volume (ml)	40	60	70	80	100	100	120	140	150	160	180	190
20 mg/kg/d ml/dose qd	3	3.5	4.5	5.5	6.5	7	8	9	10	11	12	13
mg/5 ml	250	250	250	250	250	250	250	250	250	250	250	250
Volume (ml)	60	70	90	110	130	140	160	180	200	220	240	260

Cefzil Suspension (B) ≤6 months: not recommended; 2–12 years: 7.5–20 mg/kg bid >12 years: 250–500 mg bid or 500 mg once daily; 125, 250 mg/5 ml (50, 75, 100 ml) (bubble gum) (phenylalanine).

APPENDIX DD.14: *CEFTIBUTEN* (CEDAX SUSPENSION)

Weight

Pounds	15	20	25	30	35	40	45	50	55	60	65	70
Kilograms	6.8	9	11.4	13.6	15.9	18.2	20.5	22.7	25	27.3	29.5	31.8
Single Dose (ml)/Frequency/Strength/10-Day Volume (ml)												
9 mg/kg/d ml/dose qd	3.5	4.5	6	7	8	9	10	11.5	12.5	13.5	15	16
mg/5 ml	90	90	90	90	90	90	90	90	90	90	90	90
Volume (ml)	35	45	60	70	80	90	100	115	125	135	150	160
9 mg/kg/d ml/dose qd	1.75	2.3	3	3.5	4	4.5	5	5.4	6.2	6.6	7.5	8
mg/5 ml	180	180	180	180	180	180	180	180	180	180	180	180
Volume (ml)	20	25	30	35	40	45	50	55	60	65	70	80

Cefzil Suspension (B) 90 mg/5 ml (30, 60, 90, 120 ml) (cherry); 180 mg/5 ml (30, 60, 120 ml) (cherry).

APPENDIX DD.15: *CEFUROXIME AXETIL* (CEFTIN SUSPENSION)

Weight												
Pounds	15	20	25	30	35	40	45	50	55	60	65	70
Kilograms	6.8	9	11.4	13.6	15.9	18.2	20.5	22.7	25	27.3	29.5	31.8
Single Dose (ml)/Frequency/Strength/10-Day Volume (ml)												
20 mg/kg/d ml/dose bid	2.5	3.5	4.5	3	3	3.5	4	4.5	5	5.5	6	6.5
mg/5 ml	125	125	125	250	250	250	250	250	250	250	250	250
Volume (ml)	50	70	90	60	60	70	80	90	100	110	120	130
30 mg/kg/d ml/dose bid	2	3	3.5	4	5	5.5	6	7	7.5	8	9	9.5
mg/5 ml	250	250	250	250	250	250	250	250	250	250	250	250
Volume (ml)	40	60	70	80	100	110	120	140	150	160	180	190

Ceftin Suspension (B) 125, 250 mg/5 ml (50, 100 ml) (tutti-frutti).

APPENDIX DD.16: *CEPHALEXIN* (KEFLEX SUSPENSION)

Weight												
Pounds	15	20	25	30	35	40	45	50	55	60	65	70
Kilograms	6.8	9	11.4	13.6	15.9	18.2	20.5	22.7	25	27.3	29.5	31.8
Single Dose (ml)/Frequency/Strength/10-Day Volume (ml)												
25 mg/kg/d ml/dose tid	1	1.5	2	2	3	3	3.5	4	4	4.5	5	5
mg/5 ml	125	125	125	125	125	125	125	125	125	125	125	125
Volume (ml)	30	45	60	60	90	90	105	120	120	135	150	150
25 mg/kg/d ml/dose qid	1	1	1.5	2	2	2.5	2.5	3	3	3.5	4	4
mg/5 ml	250	250	250	250	250	250	250	250	250	250	250	250
Volume (ml)	40	40	60	80	80	100	100	120	120	140	160	160
50 mg/kg/d ml/dose tid	2	3	4	4.5	5	6	7	7.5	8	9	10	10.5
mg/5 ml	250	250	250	250	250	250	250	250	250	250	250	250
Volume (ml)	60	90	120	135	150	180	210	225	240	270	300	315
50 mg/kg/d ml/dose qid	2	2	3	3.5	4	4.5	5	6	6	7	7.5	8
mg/5 ml	250	250	250	250	250	250	250	250	250	250	250	250
Volume (ml)	80	80	120	140	160	180	200	240	240	280	300	320

Keflex Suspension (B)(G) <2 months: not recommended; 125, 250 mg/5 ml (100, 200 ml) (strawberry).

APPENDIX DD.17: *CLARITHROMYCIN* (BIAXIN SUSPENSION)

Weight												
Pounds	15	20	25	30	35	40	45	50	55	60	65	70
Kilograms	6.8	9	11.4	13.6	15.9	18.2	20.5	22.7	25	27.3	29.5	31.8
Single Dose (ml)/Frequency/Strength/10-Day Volume (ml)												
7.5 mg/kg/d ml/dose bid	2	3	3.5	4	5	5.5	6	7	7.5	8	9	10
mg/5 ml	125	125	125	125	125	125	125	125	125	125	125	125
Volume (ml)	40	60	70	80	100	110	120	140	150	160	180	200
7.5 mg/kg/d ml/dose bid	1	1.5	2	2	2.5	3	3	3.5	4	4	4.5	5
mg/5 ml	250	250	250	250	250	250	250	250	250	250	250	250
Volume (ml)	20	30	40	40	50	60	60	70	80	80	90	100

Biaxin Suspension (B) <6 months: not recommended; 125, 250 mg/5 ml (50, 100 ml) (fruit punch).

APPENDIX DD.18: *CLINDAMYCIN* (CLEOCIN PEDIATRIC GRANULES)

Weight												
Pounds	15	20	25	30	35	40	45	50	55	60	65	70
Kilograms	6.8	9	11.4	13.6	15.9	18.2	20.5	22.7	25	27.3	29.5	31.8
Single Dose (ml)/Frequency/Strength/10-Day Volume (ml)												
8 mg/kg/d ml/dose tid	1	1.5	2	2.5	3	3	3.5	4	4.5	5	5	5.5
mg/5 ml	75	75	75	75	75	75	75	75	75	75	75	75
Volume (ml)	30	45	60	75	90	90	105	120	135	150	150	165
16 mg/kg/d ml/dose tid	2.5	3	4	5	5.5	6.5	7	8	9	9.5	10.5	11
mg/5 ml	75	75	75	75	75	75	75	75	75	75	75	75
Volume (ml)	75	90	120	150	165	105	210	240	270	285	315	330

Cleocin Pediatric Granules (B)(G) 75 mg/5 ml (100 ml) (cherry).

APPENDIX DD.19: *DICLOXACILLIN* (DYNAPEN SUSPENSION)

Weight												
Pounds	15	20	25	30	35	40	45	50	55	60	65	70
Kilograms	6.8	9	11.4	13.6	15.9	18.2	20.5	22.7	25	27.3	29.5	31.8
Single Dose (ml)/Frequency/Strength/10-Day Volume (ml)												
12.5 mg/kg/d ml/dose qid	2	2.5	3	3.5	4	4.5	5	6	6	7	7.5	8
mg/5 ml	62.5	62.5	62.5	62.5	62.5	62.5	62.5	62.5	62.5	62.5	62.5	62.5
Volume (ml)	80	100	120	140	160	180	200	240	240	280	300	320
25 mg/kg/d ml/dose qid	3.5	4.5	6	7	8	9	10	11.5	12.5	13.5	15	16
mg/5 ml	62.5	62.5	62.5	62.5	62.5	62.5	62.5	62.5	62.5	62.5	62.5	62.5
Volume (ml)	140	180	240	280	320	360	400	460	500	540	600	640

Dynapen Suspension (B)(G) 6.25 mg/5 ml (80, 100 ml) (raspberry-strawberry).

APPENDIX DD.20: *DOXYCYCLINE* (VIBRAMYCIN SYRUP/SUSPENSION)

Weight												
Pounds	15	20	25	30	35	40	45	50	55	60	65	70
Kilograms	6.8	9	11.4	13.6	15.9	18.2	20.5	22.7	25	27.3	29.5	31.8
Single Dose (ml)/Frequency/Strength/10-Day Volume (ml)												
1 mg/lb/d ml/dose qd	1.5	2	2.5	3	3.5	4	4.5	5	5.5	6	6.5	7
50 mg/5 ml	50	50	50	50	50	50	50	50	50	50	50	50
Volume (ml)	15	20	25	30	35	40	45	50	55	60	65	70
1 mg/lb/d ml/dose qd	3	4	5	6	7	8	9	10	11	12	13	14
25 mg/5 ml	25	25	25	25	25	25	25	25	25	25	25	25
Volume (ml)	30	40	50	60	70	80	90	100	110	120	130	140

Vibramycin Syrup (B)(G) <8 years: not recommended; double dose first day; 50 mg/5 ml (80, 100, ml) (raspberry-apple) (sulfites).
Vibramycin Suspension (B)(G) <8 years: not recommended; double dose first day; 25 mg/5 ml (80, 100, ml) (raspberry).

APPENDIX DD.21: *ERYTHROMYCIN ESTOLATE* (ILOSONE SUSPENSION)

Weight												
Pounds	15	20	25	30	35	40	45	50	55	60	65	70
Kilograms	6.8	9	11.4	13.6	15.9	18.2	20.5	22.7	25	27.3	29.5	31.8
Dose/Volume (10 days) in ml												
10 mg/kg/d ml/dose bid	3	3.5	4.5	5.5	6	7	8	9	10	5.5	6	6.5
mg/5 ml	125	125	125	125	125	125	125	125	125	250	250	250
Volume (ml)	60	70	90	110	120	140	160	180	200	110	120	130
15 mg/kg/d ml/dose bid	4	5.5	7	8	9.5	5.5	6	7	7.5	8	9	9.5
mg/5 ml	125	125	125	125	125	250	250	250	250	250	250	250
Volume (ml)	80	110	140	160	190	110	120	140	150	160	180	190
20 mg/kg/d ml/dose bid	3	3.5	4.5	5.5	6.5	7	8	9	10	11	12	13
mg/5 ml	250	250	250	250	250	250	250	250	250	250	250	250
Volume (ml)	60	70	90	110	120	140	160	180	200	220	240	260
25 mg/kg/d ml/dose bid	3.5	4.5	5.5	7	8	9	10	11.5	12.5	13.5	15	16
mg/5 ml	250	250	250	250	250	250	250	250	250	250	250	250
Volume (ml)	70	90	110	140	160	180	200	230	250	280	300	320

Ilosone Suspension (B)(G) 125, 250 mg/5 ml (100 ml).

APPENDIX DD.22: *ERYTHROMYCIN ETHYLSUCCINATE* (E.E.S. SUSPENSION, ERY-PED DROPS/SUSPENSION)

Weight												
Pounds	15	20	25	30	35	40	45	50	55	60	65	70
Kilograms	6.8	9	11.4	13.6	15.9	18.2	20.5	22.7	25	27.3	29.5	31.8
Single Dose (ml)/Frequency/Strength/10-Day Volume (ml)												
30 mg/kg/d ml/dose qid	1.5	2	2	2.5	3	3.5	4	4	4.5	5	5.5	6
mg/5 ml	200	200	200	200	200	200	200	200	200	200	200	200
Volume (ml)	60	80	80	100	120	140	160	160	180	200	220	240
30 mg/kg/d ml/dose qid			1	1.5	1.5	2	2	2	2.5	2.5	3	3
mg/5 ml			400	400	400	400	400	400	400	400	400	
Volume (ml)			60	60	80	80	80	100	100	120	120	
50 mg/kg/d ml/dose qid	2	3	3.5	4.5	5	5.5	6.5	7	8	8.5	9	10
mg/5 ml	200	200	200	200	200	200	200	200	200	200	200	200
Volume (ml)	80	120	140	180	200	220	260	280	320	340	360	400

(continued)

APPENDIX DD.22: *ERYTHROMYCIN ETHYLSUCCINATE (E.E.S. SUSPENSION, ERY-PED DROPS/SUSPENSION) (continued)*

50 mg/kg/d ml/dose qid	1	1.5	2	2	2.5	3	3	3.5	4	4.5	4.5	5
mg/5 ml	400	400	400	400	400	400	400	400	400	400	400	400
Volume (ml)	40	60	80	80	100	120	140	140	160	180	180	200

Ery-Ped Drops/Suspension (B)(G) 200 mg/5 ml (100, 200 ml) (fruit); 400 mg/5 ml (60, 100, 200 ml) (banana); Oral drops: 200, 400 mg/5 ml (50 ml) (fruit).

E.E.S. Suspension (B)(G) 200 mg/5 ml, 400 mg/5 ml (100 ml) (fruit).

E.E.S. Granules (B)(G) 200 mg/5 ml (100, 200 ml) (cherry).

APPENDIX DD.23: *ERYTHROMYCIN/SULFAMETHOXAZOLE (ERYZOLE, PEDIAZOLE)*

Weight												
Pounds	15	20	25	30	35	40	45	50	55	60	65	70
Kilograms	6.8	9	11.4	13.6	15.9	18.2	20.5	22.7	25	27.3	29.5	31.8
Single Dose (ml)/Frequency/Strength/10-Day Volume (ml)												
10 mg/kg/d ml/dose bid	3	4	5	6	6.5	7.5	8.5	9.5	10	11	12	13.5
mg/5 ml	200	200	200	200	200	200	200	200	200	200	200	200
Volume (ml)	90	120	150	180	200	225	255	285	300	330	360	400

Eryzole (C)(G) <2 months: not recommended; *eryth* 200 mg/*sulf* 600 mg/5 ml (100, 150, 200, 250 ml).
Pediazole (C)(G) <2 months: not recommended; *eryth* 200 mg/*sulf* 600 mg/5 ml (100, 150, 200 ml) (strawberry-banana).

APPENDIX DD.24: *FLUCONAZOLE* (DIFLUCAN SUSPENSION)

Weight												
Pounds	15	20	25	30	35	40	45	50	55	60	65	70
Kilograms	6.8	9	11.4	13.6	15.9	18.2	20.5	22.7	25	27.3	29.5	31.8
Single Dose (ml)/Frequency/Strength/21-Day Volume (ml)												
3 mg/kg/d ml/dose qd	2	3	3.5	4	5	5.5	6	7	7.5	8	9	9.5
mg/ml	10	10	10	10	10	10	10	10	10	10	10	10
Volume (ml)	44	66	77	88	110	121	132	154	165	176	198	209
6 mg/kg/d ml/dose qd	4	5.5	2	2	2.5	3	3	3.5	4	4	4.5	5
mg/ml	10	10	40	40	40	40	40	40	40	40	40	40
Volume (ml)	88	121	44	44	55	66	66	77	88	88	99	110

Diflucan Suspension (B)(G) double dose first day; 10, 40 mg/5 ml (35 ml) (orange).

APPENDIX DD.25: *FURAZOLIDONE* (FUROXONE LIQUID)

Weight													
Pounds	15	20	25	30	35	40	45	50	55	60	65	70
Kilograms	6.8	9	11.4	13.6	15.9	18.2	20.5	22.7	25	27.3	29.5	31.8
Single Dose (ml)/Frequency/Strength/7-Day Volume (ml)													
5 mg/kg/d ml/dose qid	2.5	3.5	4	5	6	7	8	8.5	9.5	10	11	12
mg/15 ml	50	50	50	50	50	50	50	50	50	50	50	50
Vol	100	140	160	200	240	280	320	340	380	400	440	480

Furoxone Liquid (C)(G) double dose first day; 50 mg/15 ml (35 ml).

APPENDIX DD.26: *GRISEOFULVIN, MICROSIZE* (GRIFULVIN V SUSPENSION)

Weight												
Pounds	15	20	25	30	35	40	45	50	55	60	65	70
Kilograms	6.8	9	11.4	13.6	15.9	18.2	20.5	22.7	25	27.3	29.5	31.8
Single Dose (ml)/Frequency/Strength/30-Day Volume (ml)												
5 mg/lb/d ml/dose day	3	4	5	6	7	8	9	10	11	12	13	14
mg/5 ml	125	125	125	125	125	125	125	125	125	125	125	125
Volume (ml)	90	120	150	180	210	240	270	300	330	360	390	420

Grifulvin V Suspension (C)(G) double dose first day; 125 mg/5 ml (120 ml) (orange) (alcohol 0.02%).

APPENDIX DD.27: *ITRACONAZOLE* (SPORANOX SOLUTION)

Weight

Pounds	15	20	25	30	35	40	45	50	55	60	65	70
Kilograms	6.8	9	11.4	13.6	15.9	18.2	20.5	22.7	25	27.3	29.5	31.8

Single Dose (ml)/Frequency/Strength/7-Day Volume (ml)

	15	20	25	30	35	40	45	50	55	60	65	70
5 mg/kg/d ml/dose qd	3.5	4.5	6	7	8	9	10	11.5	12.5	14	15	16
mg/ml	10	10	10	10	10	10	10	10	10	10	10	10
Volume (ml)	25	32	42	49	56	63	70	71	88	98	105	112

Sporanox V Solution (C)(G) double dose first day; 10 mg/ml (150 ml) (cherry-caramel).

APPENDIX DD.28: *LORACARBEF* (LORABID SUSPENSION)

Weight												
Pounds	15	20	25	30	35	40	45	50	55	60	65	70
Kilograms	6.8	9	11.4	13.6	15.9	18.2	20.5	22.7	25	27.3	29.5	31.8
Single Dose (ml)/Frequency/Strength/10-Day Volume (ml)												
15 mg/kg/d ml/dose bid	2.5	3.5	4	5	3	3.5	4	4	5	5	5.5	6
mg/5 ml	100	100	100	100	200	200	200	200	200	200	200	200
Volume (ml)	50	70	80	100	60	70	80	80	100	100	110	120
30 mg/kg/d ml/dose bid	2.5	3.5	4	5	6	7	8	8.5	9.5	10	11	12
mg/5 ml	200	200	200	200	200	200	200	200	200	200	200	200
Volume (ml)	50	70	80	100	120	140	160	170	190	200	220	240

Lorabid Suspension (B) 100 mg/5 ml (50, 100 ml) (strawberry bubble gum); 200 mg/5 ml (50, 75, 100 ml) (strawberry bubble gum).

APPENDIX DD.29: *NITROFURANTOIN* (FURADANTIN SUSPENSION)

Weight												
Pounds	15	20	25	30	35	40	45	50	55	60	65	70
Kilograms	6.8	9	11.4	13.6	15.9	18.2	20.5	22.7	25	27.3	29.5	31.8
Single Dose (ml)/Frequency/Strength/10-Day Volume (ml)												
5 mg/kg ml/dose qid	1.5	2.5	3	3.5	4	4.5	5	5.5	6	7	7.5	8
mg/5 ml	25	25	25	25	25	25	25	25	25	25	25	25
Volume (ml)	60	100	120	140	160	190	200	220	240	280	300	320

Furadantin Suspension (B)(G) 25 mg/5 ml (60 ml).

APPENDIX DD.30: *PENICILLIN V POTASSIUM* (PEN-VEE K SOLUTION, VEETIDS SOLUTION)

Weight												
Pounds	15	20	25	30	35	40	45	50	55	60	65	70
Kilograms	6.8	9	11.4	13.6	15.9	18.2	20.5	22.7	25	27.3	29.5	31.8
Single Dose (ml)/Frequency/Strength/10-Day Volume (ml)												
25 mg/kg/d ml/dose qid	2	2.5	3	3.5	4	4.5	5	5.5	6	7	7.5	8
mg/5 ml	125	125	125	125	125	125	125	125	125	125	125	125
Volume (ml)	80	90	120	140	160	180	200	220	240	280	300	320
25 mg/kg/d ml/dose qid	1	1	1.5	2	2	2.5	2.5	3	3	3.5	4	4
mg/5 ml	250	250	250	250	250	250	250	250	250	250	250	250
Volume (ml)	40	40	60	80	80	100	100	120	120	140	160	160
50 mg/kg/d ml/dose qid	2	2.5	3	3.5	4	4.5	5	6	6.5	7	7.5	8
mg/5 ml	250	250	250	250	250	250	250	250	250	250	250	250
Volume (ml)	80	100	120	140	160	180	200	240	260	280	300	320

Pen-Vee K Solution (B)(G) 125 mg/5 ml (100, 200 ml); 250 mg/5 ml (100, 150, 200 ml).
Veetids Solution (B)(G) 125, 250 mg/5 ml (100, 200 ml).

APPENDIX DD.31: *RIMANTADINE* (FLUMADINE SYRUP)

Weight												
Pounds	15	20	25	30	35	40	45	50	55	60	65	70
Kilograms	6.8	9	11.4	13.6	15.9	18.2	20.5	22.7	25	27.3	29.5	31.8
Single Dose (ml)/Frequency/Strength/10-Day Volume (ml)												
5 mg/kg/d ml/dose qd	3.5	4.5	6	7	8	9	10	11.5	12.5	13.5	15	16
mg/5 ml	50	50	50	50	50	50	50	50	50	50	50	50
Volume (ml)	35	45	60	70	80	90	100	115	125	135	150	160

Flumadine Syrup (B) 50 mg/5 ml (2, 8, 16 oz) (raspberry).

APPENDIX DD.32: *TETRACYCLINE* (SUMYCIN SUSPENSION)

Weight

Pounds	15	20	25	30	35	40	45	50	55	60	65	70
Kilograms	6.8	9	11.4	13.6	15.9	18.2	20.5	22.7	25	27.3	29.5	31.8

Single Dose (ml)/Frequency/Strength/10-Day Volume (ml)

	15	20	25	30	35	40	45	50	55	60	65	70
25 mg/kg/d ml/dose qid	1.5	2.5	3	3.5	4	4.5	5	6	6.5	7	7.5	8
mg/5 ml	125	125	125	125	125	125	125	125	125	125	125	125
Volume (ml)	60	100	120	140	160	180	200	240	260	280	300	320
50 mg/kg/d ml/dose qid	3.5	4.5	6	7	8	9	10	11.5	12.5	13.5	15	16
mg/5 ml	125	125	125	125	125	125	125	125	125	125	125	125
Volume (ml)	140	180	240	280	320	360	400	460	500	540	600	640

Sumycin Suspension (D)(G) <8 years: not recommended; 125 mg/5 ml (100, 200 ml) (fruit) (sulfites).

APPENDIX DD.33: *TRIMETHOPRIM* (PRIMSOL SUSPENSION)

Weight												
Pounds	15	20	25	30	35	40	45	50	55	60	65	70
Kilograms	6.8	9	11.4	13.6	15.9	18.2	20.5	22.7	25	27.3	29.5	31.8
Single Dose (ml)/Frequency/Strength/10-Day Volume (ml)												
5 mg/kg/d ml/dose bid	3.5	4.5	6	7	8	9	10	11.5	12.5	13.5	15	16
mg/5 ml	50	50	50	50	50	50	50	50	50	50	50	50
Volume (ml)	70	90	120	140	160	180	200	230	250	270	300	320

Primsol Suspension (C)(G) 50 mg/5 ml (50 mg/5 ml) (bubble gum) (dye-free, alcohol-free).

APPENDIX DD.34: *TRIMETHOPRIM/SULFAMETHOXAZOLE* (BACTRIM SUSPENSION, SEPTRA SUSPENSION)

Weight												
Pounds	15	20	25	30	35	40	45	50	55	60	65	70
Kilograms	6.8	9	11.4	13.6	15.9	18.2	20.5	22.7	25	27.3	29.5	31.8
Single Dose (ml)/Frequency/Strength/10-Day Volume (ml)												
10 mg/kg/d ml/dose bid	2	2	3	3.5	4	4.5	5	5.5	6	7	7.5	8
mg/5 ml	200	200	200	200	200	200	200	200	200	200	200	200
Volume (ml)	40	40	60	70	80	90	100	110	120	140	150	160
20 mg/kg/d ml/dose bid	4	4	6	7	8	9	10	11	12	14	15	16
mg/5 ml	200	200	200	200	200	200	200	200	200	200	200	200
Volume (ml)	80	80	120	140	160	180	200	220	240	280	300	320

Bactrim Pediatric Suspension, Septra Pediatric Suspension (C)(G) *trim* 40 mg/*sulfa* 200 mg/5 ml (100 ml) (cherry) (alcohol 0.3%).

APPENDIX DD.35: *VANCOMYCIN* SOLUTION

Weight												
Pounds	15	20	25	30	35	40	45	50	55	60	65	70
Kilograms	6.8	9	11.4	13.6	15.9	18.2	20.5	22.7	25	27.3	29.5	31.8
Single Dose (ml)/Frequency/Strength/10-Day Volume (ml)												
40 mg/kg/d ml/dose tid	2	2.5	3	3.5	4.5	5	5.5	6	7	7.5	8	8.5
mg/5 ml	250	250	250	250	250	250	250	250	250	250	250	250
Volume (ml)	60	75	90	105	135	150	165	180	210	225	240	255
40 mg/kg/d ml/dose qid	1.5	2	2.5	3	3	3.5	4	4.5	5	5.5	6	6.5
mg/5 ml	250	250	250	250	250	250	250	250	250	250	250	250
Volume (ml)	60	80	100	120	120	140	160	180	200	220	240	260
40 mg/kg/d ml/dose tid	1	1	1.5	2	2	2.5	3	3	3.5	3.5	4	4
mg/5 ml	500	500	500	500	500	500	500	500	500	500	500	500
Volume (ml)	30	30	45	60	60	75	90	90	105	105	120	120

(continued)

APPENDIX DD.35: *VANCOMYCIN* SOLUTION *(continued)*

40 mg/kg/d ml/dose qid	1	1	1.5	1.5	1.5	2	2	2.5	2.5	3	3	3.5
mg/5 ml	500	500	500	500	500	500	500	500	500	500	500	500
Volume (ml)	40	40	60	60	60	80	80	100	100	120	120	140

Vancomycin Suspension (C)(G) Suspension or solution currently not available in the United States.; however, a **Vancomycin** oral solution compounding kit is available and a solution may be prepared by pharmacist on request; <12 years: not established; >12 years: usually 40 mg/kg/day in 3-4 divided doses; max 2 gm/day; ≥40 kg: 500 mg to 2 gm in 3-4 divided doses; max 2 gm/day.

ACR Guidelines on Prevention & Treatment of Glucocorticoid-induced Osteoporosis [press release, June 7, 2017]. Atlanta, GA. American College of Rheumatology. https://www.rheumatology.org/About-Us/Newsroom/Press-Releases/ID/812/ACR-Releases-Guideline-on-Prevention-Treatment-of-Glucocorticoid-Induced-Osteoporosis

Advance for Nurse Practitioners http://nurse-practitioners.advanceweb.com

Advanced Practice Education Associates www.apea.com

American Association of Nurse Practitioners www.aanp.org

American Academy of Pediatrics (AAP) http://aapexperience.org/

American College of Cardiology. Then and now: ATP III vs. IV: Comparison of ATP III and ACC/AHA guidelines http://www.acc.org/latest-in-cardiology/articles/2014/07/18/16/03/then-and-now-atp-iii-vs-iv

American Diabetes Association (ADA), Professional Diabetes Resources Online http://professional.diabetes.org/content/clinical-practice-recommendations/?loc=rp- slabnav

American diabetes association standards of medical care. *Diabetes Care 2016, 38*(Suppl. 1). http://care.diabetesjournals.org/content/38/Supplement_1

American Family Physician http://www.aafp.org/online/en/home.html

American Headache Society www.americanheadachesociety.org

American Pain Society http://americanpainsociety.org/

American Pharmacists Association. (2015). *Pediatric and neonatal dosage handbook: A universal resource for clinicians treating pediatric and neonatal patients (22nd ed.).* Lexicomp.

CDC: Morbidity and Mortality Weekly Report (MMWR)
    http://www.cdc.gov/mmwr/mmwr_wk.html

CDC 2015 Sexually Transmitted Diseases Treatment Guidelines
    http://www.cdc.gov/std/tg2015/default.htm

Centers for Disease Control and Prevention
    www.cdc.gov

Centers for Disease Control and Prevention. (2016). *Facts about ADHD.*
    www.cdc.gov/ncbddd/adhd/facts.html

American Trypanosomiasis Centers for Disease Control and Prevention.
*Parasites—American Trypanosomiasis (also known as Chagas disease). Resources
for health professionals.*

Chow, A. W., Benninger, M. S., Brook, I., Brozek, J. L., Goldstein, E. J., Hicks, L.
A., . . . File, T. M., Jr., Infectious Disease Society of America. (2012). IDSA clinical
practice guideline for acute and bacterial rhinosinusitis in children and adults.
Clinical Infectious Diseases, 54(8), e72–e112.

Clinician Reviews
    http://www.clinicianreviews.com/

Consultant 360
    http://www.consultant360.com/home

Daily Med: NIH. US Library of Medicine
    https://dailymed.nlm.nih.gov/dailymed/index.cfm

Domino, F. J., Baldor, R. A., Golding, J., & Stephens, M. B. (2016). *The 5-minute clinical
consult standard 2016.* Philadelphia, PA: Wolters Kluwer.

DRUGS.COM
    www.drugs.com

DRUGS at FDA: FDA Approved Drug Products
    http://www.accessdata.fda.gov/scripts/cder/drugsatfda/index.cfm

Engorn, B., & Flerlage, J. (Eds.). (2015). *The Harriet Lane handbook: A handbook for
pediatric house officers* (20th ed.). Philadelphia, PA: Elsevier.

epocrates
    https://online.epocrates.com/drugs

eMPR: Monthly Prescribing Reference (new FDA approved products, new generics,
new drug withdrawals, safety alerts)
    http://www.empr.com

FDA: Recalls, Market Withdrawals, and Safety alerts
http://www.fda.gov/Safety/Recalls/default.htm

Garber, A. J., Abrahamson, M. J., Barzilay, J. I., Blonde, L., Bloomgarden, Z. T., Bush, M. A., . . . Umpierrez, G. E. (2017). Consensus statement by the American Association of Clinical Endocrinologists and American College of Endocrinology on the comprehensive type 2 diabetes management algorithm – 2017 executive summary. *Endocrine Practice, 23*(2), 207–238. doi:10.4158/ep161682.cs

Gilbert, D. N., Chambers, H. F., Eliopoulos, Saag, M., & Pavia, A. (2016). *The Sanford guide to antimicrobial therapy, 2016* (46th ed.). Sperryville, VA: Antimicrobial Therapy.

Handbook of Antimicrobial Therapy (20th ed.). (2015). New Rochelle, NY: The Medical Letter.

International Diabetes Federation (IDF) Clinical Practice Guidelines
http://www.idf.org/guidelines

JNC 8 Guideline Summary. *Pharmacist's Letter/Prescriber's Letter*
https://www.scribd.com/doc/290772273/JNC-8-guideline-summary

Journal of the American Academy of Nurse Practitioners
https://www.aanp.org/publications/jaanp

Journal of the American Medical Association (JAMA) Internal Medicine
http://archinte.jamanetwork.com/journal.aspx

Lieberthal, A. S., Carroll, A. E., Chonmaitree, T., Ganiats, T. G., Hoberman, A., Jackson, M. A., & Tunkel, D. E. (2013). The diagnosis and management of acute otitis media. *Pediatrics, 131*(3), e964–e999.

Mandell, G. L., Bennett, J. E., & Dolin, R. (Eds.). (2014). *Principles and practices of infectious diseases* (8th ed.). Philadelphia, PA: Elsevier Churchill Livingstone.

Mandell, L. A. Wunderink, R. G., Anzueto, A., Bartlett, J. G., Campbell, G. D., Dean, N. C., . . . Whitney, C. G. (2007). Infectious Diseases Society of America/American Thoracic Society consensus guidelines on the management of community-acquired pneumonia in adults. *Clinical Infectious Diseases, 44*(Suppl. 2), S27–S72.
https://enp-network.s3.amazonaws.com/NPA_Long_Island/pdf/Pneumonia.pdf

McDonald, J., & Mattingly, J. (2016). Chagas disease: Creeping into family practice in the United States. *Clinician Reviews, 26*(11), 38–45.

McMillan, J.A., Lee, C.K.K., Siberry, G.K., & Carroll, K.C. (2013). *The Harriet Lane handbook of pediatric antimicrobial therapy*. Philadelphia, PA: Elsevier Saunders.

MedlinePlus
https://www.nlm.nih.gov/medlineplus/ency/article/000165.htm

MedPage Today
http://www.medpagetoday.com/

Medscape
http://www.medscape.com/

National Academy of Medicine
http://nam.edu/

National Heart, Lung, and Blood Institute (NHLBI)
http://www.nhlbi.nih.gov/

New England Journal of Medicine (NEJM) Journal Watch General Medicine
http://www.jwatch.org/general-medicine

Pharmacist's Letter
www.pharmacistsletter.com

Physicians' Desk Reference (PDR)
http://www.pdr.net/

PLR Requirements for Prescribing Information
https://www.fda.gov/Drugs/GuidanceComplianceRegulatoryInformation/
LawsActsandRules/ucm084159.htm

Pregnancy and Lactation Labeling Final Rule (PLLR)
https://www.drugs.com/pregnancy-categories.html

Prescriber's Letter
http://prescribersletter.therapeuticresearch.com/pl/sample.aspx?cs=&s=PRL&
AspxAutoDetectCookieSupport=1

Psychopharmacology
http://link.springer.com/journal/213

RxLIST
http://www.rxlist.com/script/main/hp.asp

RxLIST: Drugs A-Z
http://www.rxlist.com/drugs/alpha_a.htm

Sanford Guide Web Edition
https://webedition.sanfordguide.com

Solutions for Safer ER/LA Opioid Prescribing in a New Era of Health Care. American
Nurses Credentialing Center, Post Graduate Institute of Medicine
www.cmeuniversity.com

Taketomo, C. K., Hodding, J. H., Kraus, & D. M. (2015). *Pediatric and neonatal dosage handbook: A universal resource for clinicians treating pediatric and neonatal patients* (22nd ed.). Wolters Kluwer.

The American Congress of Obstetrics and Gynecology (ACOG)
http://www.acog.org/

The Handbook of Antimicrobial Therapy (20th ed.). The Medical Letter

The Journal for Nurse Practitioners
www.elsevier.com/locate/tjnp

The Medical Letter on Drugs and Therapeutics
http://secure.medicalletter.org/

The Nurse Practitioner Journal
www.tnpj.com

Treatment Guidelines [Annual Volume]: The Medical Letter

Updated CDC guidance: Superbugs threaten hospital patients. *Medscape Education Clinical Briefs* (March 31, 2016).
http://www.medscape.org/viewarticle/859361?nlid=105320_2713&src=wnl_cmemp_160523_mscpedu_nurs&impID=1106718&faf=1

U.S. Pharmacist Weekly Newsletter
http://www.uspharmacist.com

Wald, E. R., Applegate, K. E., Bordley, C., Darrow, D. H., Glode, M. P., Marcy, S. M., . . . Weinberg, S. T., American Academy of Pediatrics. (2013). Clinical practice guidelines for the diagnosis and management of acute bacterial sinusitis in children 1 to 18 years. *Pediatrics, 132*(1), e262–280.
http://www.ncbi.nlm.nih.gov/pubmed/23796742

WebMD: Drugs and Medications A to Z. Latest Drug News
http://www.webmd.com/drugs/

See **Appendix A** for descriptions of FDA pregnancy categories
See **Appendix B** for descriptions of controlled drug categories
NE = not established <u>or</u> not rated

Drug	Page Numbers	FDA Pregnancy Category	DEA Schedule
abacavir, **Ziagen**	191, 414	C	
A/B Otic, *antipyrine/benzocaine/ glycerin*	290, 294	C	
abatacept, **Orencia**	369	C	
Abilify, *aripiprazole*	44, 48, 102, 507	C	
Abreva, *docosanol*	185	NE	
Abstral, *fentanyl citratesublingual tablet*	307	C	
acamprosate, **Campral**	10	C	
Acanya, *clindamycin/benzoyl peroxide gel*	5, 143	C	
acarbose, **Precose**	23	B	
Accolate, *zafirlukast*	27, 372	B	
Accuneb, *albuterol*	33	C	
Accupril, *quinapril*	169, 206	D	
Accuretic, *quinapril/ hydrochlorothiazide*	211	D	
Accutane, *isotretinoin, retinoic acid*	7	X	
acebutolol, **Sectral**	201, 503	B	
Aceon, *perindopril*	205	D	
Acetadote, *acetylcysteine*	3	B	
acetaminophen, **Feverall, Ofirmev, Panadol, Tempra, Tylenol**	137	B	

Drug	Page Numbers	FDA Pregnancy Category	DEA Schedule
amantadine, **Symmetrel**	531, 542	C	
Amaryl, *glimeperide*	423	C	
Ambien, Ambien CR, *zolpidem tartrate*	141, 234	B	IV
ambrisentan, **Letairis**	360	X	
ambrosia artemisiifolia 12 amb a, **Ragwitek**	371	C	
Amerge, *naratriptan*	161	C	
Americaine, Americaine Otic, *benzocaine*	290, 294	C	
Amevive, *alefacept*	354	B	
amikacin, **Amikin**	532	C	
Amikin, *amikacin*	532	C	
amiloride, **Midamor**	170, 203	B	
amiodarone, **Cordarone**	502	D	
amitriptyline	22, 99, 114, 133, 140, 164, 166, 238, 242, 275, 312, 338, 341, 346, 413	C	
amlodipine, **Norvasc**	14, 207	C	
Amnesteem, *isotretinoin, retinoic acid*	7	X	
amoxapine	22, 100, 114, 133, 164, 166, 238, 242, 276, 312, 338, 341, 346, 413	C	
amoxicillin, **Amoxil, Moxatag, Trimox**	38, 54, 65, 85, 121, 227, 249, 291, 324, 330, 331, 332, 383, 387, 408, 441, 536, 543, 544	B	
Amoxil, *amoxicillin*	38, 54, 65, 85, 121, 227, 249, 291, 324, 330, 331, 332, 383, 387, 408, 441, 536, 543, 544	B	

Drug	Page Numbers	FDA Pregnancy Category	DEA Schedule
Anturane, *sulfinpyrazone*	155	C	
Anusol HC, *hydrocortisone*	174, 435, 495	C	
Anzemet, *dolasetron*	270	B	
Apidra, *insulin glulisine (rDNA origin)*	418	B	
apixaban, **Eliquis**	516	C	
Aplenzin, *bupropion hydrobromide*	100, 406	C	
apraclonidine, **Iopidine**	149	C	
apremilast, **Otezla**	358	C	
aprepitant, **Emend**	270	B	
Apri, *ethinyl estradiol/desogestrel*	476	X	
Apriso, *mesalamine*	436	B	
Aptivus, *tipranavir*	195, 511	C	
AquaMEPHYTON, *phytonadione, vitamin k*	515	C	
Aralen, *chloroquine*	254, 530	C	
Aranelle, *ethinyl estradiol/ norethindrone*	477	X	
Aranesp, *darbepoetin alpha*	13	C	
Arava, *leflunomide*	366	X	
ardeparin, **Normiflo**	496	C	
Arimidex, *anastrozole*	504	D	
aripiprazole, **Abilify**	44, 48, 102, 507	C	
Aristocort, *triamcinolone*	499, 500	C	
Aristocort Forte, *triamcinolone diacetate*	499, 500	C	
Arixtra, *fondaparinux sodium*	517	B	
armodafinil, **Nuvigil**	266, 390	C	IV

Drug	Page Numbers	FDA Pregnancy Category	DEA Schedule
cephalexin, **Keflex**	39, 56, 66, 228, 251, 255, 292, 315, 325, 362, 380, 388, 409, 442, 453, 532, 557	B	
certolizumab, **Cimzia**	94, 367	B	
Cerumenex, *triethanolamine*	68	A	
Cesamet, *nabilone*	268	C	
Cetamide, *sulfacetamide*	83	C	
cetirizine, **Zyrtec, Zyrtec Chewable Tablets**	80, 102, 106, 109, 370, 375, 447	B	
cevimeline, **Evoxac**	385	C	
Chantix, *varenicline*	406	C	
Chemet, *succimer*	239, 247	C	
Children'sNasalCrom, *cromolyn sodium*	374	B	
chlorambucil, **Leukeran**	505	D	
Children's Xyzal Allergy 24HR, *levocetirizine*	103, 107, 109, 371, 379, 448	B	
chlordiazepoxide, **Librium**	9, 21, 314	D	IV
chlorhexidine gluconate, **Peridex, PerioGard**	148	B	
chloroquine, **Aralen**	254, 530	C	
chlorothiazide, **Diuril**	130, 170, 203, 446	B	
chloroxine, **Capitrol**	110	C	
chlorpromazine, **Thorazine**	49, 186, 269, 507	C	
chlorpropamide, **Diabinese**	423	C	
chlorthalidone, **Thalitone**	130, 203	B	
chlorzoxazone, **Parafon Forte**	262	C	
cholestyramine, **Questran, Questran Light**	119, 128	C	
chorionic gonadotropin, **Pregnyl**	11	C	

Drug	Page Numbers	FDA Pregnancy Category	DEA Schedule
Corzide, *nadolol/ bendroflumethiazide*	213	C	
Cosopt, *dorzolamide/timolol*	151	C	
Cotazym, Cotazym S, *pancrelipase*	309	C	
Coumadin, *warfarin*	490, 515	D	
Covera-HS, *verapamil*	15, 163, 208	C	
Cozaar, *losartan*	206	D	
Creon, *pancrelipase*	309	C	
Crestor, *rosuvastatin*	126, 219	X	
crisaborole, Eucrisa	104		
Crixivan, *indinavir*	194, 511	C	
crofelemer, **Fulyzaq**, Mytesi	117, 119	C	
Crolom, *cromolyn sodium*	79, 246	B	
cromolyn sodium, **Children's NasalCrom, Crolom, Intal, Nasal Crom**	374	B	
crotamiton, **Eurax**	380	C	
Cryselle, *ethinyl estradiol/ norgestrel*	477	X	
Cubicin, *daptomycin*	539	B	
Cuprimine, *penicillamine*	367, 446	D	
Cutivate, *fluticasone propionate*	496	C	
cyanocobalamin, vitamin b-12, **Nascobal Gel**	14	C	
Cyclessa, *ethinyl estradiol/ desogestrel*	477	X	
cyclobenzaprine, **Amrix, Fexmid, Flexeril**	140, 262	B	
cyclophosphamide, **Cytoxan**	505	D	
Cycloset, *bromocriptine*	432	B	

Drug	Page Numbers	FDA Pregnancy Category	DEA Schedule
Genvoya, *elvitegravir/cobicistat/ emtricitabine/tenofovir alafenamide (AF)*	196, 512	B	
Geodon, *ziprasidone*	45, 50, 508	C	
Gianvi, *ethinyl estradiol/ drospirenone*	478	X	
Gilenya, *fingolimod*	260	C	
glatiramer acetate, **Copaxone**	260	B	
Gleevec, *imatinib mesylate*	505	D	
glimeperide, **Amaryl**	423	C	
glipizide, **Glucotrol, Glucotrol XL**	423	C	
glucagon, **Glucagon**	143	B	
Glucagon, *glucagon*	143	B	
Glucophage, Glucophage XR, *metformin*	424	B	
Glucotrol, Glucotrol XL, *glipizide*	423	C	
Glucovance, *glyburide/metformin*	426	B	
Glumetza, *metformin*	424	B	
glyburide, **DiaBeta, Glynase, Micronase**	423	B	
Glycet, *miglitol*	423	B	
GlycoLax, *polyethylene glycol*	88	C	
glycopyrrolate, **Robinul**	319	B	
glycopyrrolate, **Seebri Neohaler**	33	C	
Glynase, *glyburide*	423	B	
Gly-Oxide, *carbamide peroxide*	25	NE	
Glyquin, *hydroquinone/padimate o/oxybenzone/octyl methoxycin- namate*	201	C	

Drug	Page Numbers	FDA Pregnancy Category	DEA Schedule
Humulin U, *insulin extended zinc suspension (ultralente)*	421	B	
Hyal, *sodium hyaluronate*	284, 370	B	
Hyalgan, *sodium hyaluronate*	284, 370	B	
Hycet, *hydrocodone bitartrate/ acetaminophen*	300	C	II
Hycodan, Hycodan Syrup, *hydrocodone/homatropine*	525	C	II
hydralazine	17, 210	C	
Hydrea, *hydroxyurea*	505	D	
hydrochlorothiazide, **Esidrix, Microzide**	130, 170, 203, 446	B	
hydrocodone **bitartrate, Hysingla ER,** *Vantrela ER,* **Zohydro ER**	300	C	II
hydrocortisone, **Anusol-HC, Cortaid, Cortef, Cortifoam, Hydrocortone, Hytone, Proctocort, Texacort**	174, 435, 495	C	
hydrocortisone acetate, **U-Cort**	495	C	
hydrocortisone butyrate, **Locoid**	496	C	
hydrocortisone phosphate, **Hydrocotone Phosphate**	500	C	
hydrocortisone probutate, **Pandel**	496	C	
hydrocortisone retention enema, **Cortenema**	435	C	
hydrocortisone sodium succinate, **Solu-Cortef**	500	C	
hydrocortisone valerate, **Westcort**	496	C	
Hydrocortone, *hydrocortisone*	498, 500	C	
Hydrocotone Phosphate, *hydrocortisone phosphate*	500	C	
hydroflumethiazide, **Saluron**	130	B	

Drug	Page Numbers	FDA Pregnancy Category	DEA Schedule
Iletin II NPH, *insulin isophane suspension*	420	B	
Iletin II Regular, *insulin regular*	418	B	
iloperidone, Fanapt	508	C	
Ilotycin, *erythromycin gluceptate*	53, 82, 277, 378, 392	B	
imatinib mesylate, Gleevec	505	D	
Imdur, *isosorbide mononitrate*	16	B	
imipramine, Tofranil, Tofranil PM	22, 100, 114, 133, 164, 166, 238, 242, 276, 313, 338–339, 341–342, 346, 413	C	
imiquimod, Aldara, Zyclara	8, 450	B	
Imitrex, Imitrex Injectable, Imitrex Nasal Spray, *sumatriptan*	161	C	
Imodium, *loperamide*	118, 119, 240, 437	B	
Imodium AD, *loperamide/ simethicone*	118, 119, 240, 437	B	
Impavido, *miltefosine*	248	D	
Implanon, *etonogestrel*	487	X	
Imuran, *azathioprine*	92, 366	D	
Increlex, *mecasermin*	159	B	
indapamide, Lozol	132, 171, 204	B	
Inderal LA, *propranolol*	16, 163, 202, 217, 258, 345	C	
Inderide, Inderide LA, *propranolol/hydrochlorothiazide*	213	C	
indinavir, Crixivan	194, 511	C	
Indocin, *indomethacin*	492	B/D	
indomethacin, Indocin, Tivorbex	492	B/D	
Infergen, *interferon alfacon-1*	178	C	

Drug	Page Numbers	FDA Pregnancy Category	DEA Schedule
LoSeasonique, *ethinyl estradiol/ levonorgestrel*	485	X	
Lotemax, *loteprednol etabonate*	79, 238	C	
Lotensin, *benazepril*	205	D	
Lotensin HCT, *benazepril/ hydrochlorothiazide*	210	D	
loteprednol etabonate, **Alrex, Lotemax**	79, 136	C	
Lotrel, *amlodipine/benazepril*	213	D	
Lotrimin, *clotrimazole*	59, 116, 400, 402, 403, 405, 530	B	
Lotrisone, *clotrimazole/ betamethasone dipropionate*	117, 401, 404	C	
Lotronex, *alosetron*	240	B	
lovastatin, **Altoprev, Mevacor**	126, 219	X	
Lovaza, *omega 3-acid ethyl esters*	124, 217	C	
Lovenox, *enoxaparin*	516	B	
Lozol, *indapamide*	132, 171, 204	B	
Ludiomil, *maprotiline*	101	B	
Lufyllin GG, *dyphylline/ guaifenesin*	34	C	
luliconazole, Luzu Cream	400, 402, 404	C	
Lumigan, *bimatoprost*	151	C	
Lunesta, *eszopiclone*	140, 234	C	IV
Lupron Depot, *leuprolide acetate*	505	X	
lurasidone, **Latuda**	44, 508	B	
Luride, *fluoride*	142	NE	
Lucentis, ranibizumab	115	NE	
Lustra, Lustra AF, *hydroquinone*	200, 255	C	
Lutera, *ethinyl estradiol/ levonorgestrel*	480	X	

Drug	Page Numbers	FDA Pregnancy Category	DEA Schedule
Picato, *ingenol mebutate*	9	C	
Pilocar, *pilocarpine*	149	C	
pilocarpine, Isopto Carpine, Pilocar, Pilopine HS	149	C	
Pilopine HS, *pilocarpine*	149	C	
pimecrolimus, Elidel	105, 339, 352	C	
pindolol, Visken	202	B	
Pin-X, *pyrantel pamoate*	188, 327, 378, 399, 411, 451, 529	C	
pioglitazone, Actos	425	C	
piperacillin	537	B	
pirbuterol, Maxair, Maxair Autohaler	31	C	
piroxicam, Feldene	493, 494	C	
pitavastatin, Livalo	126	X	
Plan-B One Step, *levonorgestrel*	488	X	
Plaquenil, *hydroxychloroquine*	254, 366, 531	C	
Plavix, *clopidogrel*	519	B	
Plendil, *felodipine*	207	C	
Pliaglis Cream, *lidocaine/tetracaine*	489	B	
podofilox, Condylox	450	C	
polyethylene glycol, GlycoLax, MiraLax	88	C	
Poly-Pred Ophthalmic, *prednisolone acetate/neomycin sulfate/polymyxin b sulfate*	84	C	
Polysporin Ointment, Polysporin Ophthalmic Ointment, *polymyxin b/bacitracin zinc*	53, 83, 393	C	
polythiazide, Renese, Renese K	130, 170, 203	D	

Drug	Page Numbers	FDA Pregnancy Category	DEA Schedule
Qvar, *beclomethasone dipropionate*	501	C	
rabeprazole, Aciphex, Aciphex Sprinkle	147, 319, 455	B	
racepinephfine, Asthmanefrin	31	C	
Ragwitek, ambrosia artemisiifolia 12 amb a	371	C	
raloxifene, Evista	287	X	
raltegravir, Isentress	190, 195, 512	C	
ramelteon, Rozerem	234	C	
ramipril, Altace	169, 206	D	
Ranexa, *ranolazine*	17	C	
ranitidine, Zantac, Zantac Chewable Tablets, Zantac Efferdose	146, 318	B	
ranibizumab, Lucentis	115	NE	
ranolazine, Ranexa	17	C	
Rebetol, *ribavirin*	178	X	
Rebif, Rebif Rebidose, *interferon beta-1a*	260	C	
Reclast, *zoledronic acid*	287, 295	D	
Reglan, Reglan ODT, *metoclopramide*	148, 271	B	
Regranex Gel, *becaplermin*	434	C	
Relagard Therapeutic Vaginal Gel, *acetic acid/oxyquinolone*	39, 61	C	
Relpax, *eletriptan*	160	C	
Relenza, *zanamivir for inhalation*	233, 531	B	
Remeron, Remeron Soltab, *mirtazapine*	101, 346	C	
Remicade, *infliximab*	92, 94, 356, 359, 368, 437	C	

Drug	Page Numbers	FDA Pregnancy Category	DEA Schedule
Sular, *nisoldipine*	208	C	
sulconazole, Exelderm, Extina	401, 402, 404, 406	C	
sulfacetamide, Bleph-10, Cetamide, Isopto Cetamide, Klaron	4, 5, 53, 82, 393	C	
sulfasalazine, Azulfidine, Azulfidine EN-Tabs	93, 367, 436	B/D	
sulfinpyrazone, Anturane	155	C	
sulfisoxazole, Gantrisin	441, 537	B/D	
sulindac, Clinoril	493	C/D	
sumatriptan, Alsuma Injectable, Imitrex, Imitrex Injectable, Imitrex Nasal Spray, Onzetra Xsail, Sumavel DosePro, Zecuity Transdermal, Zembrace SymTouch	161	C	
Sumycin, *tetracycline*	6, 26, 54, 57, 187, 250, 253, 328, 336, 353, 377, 383, 390, 538, 574	D	
Suprax Oral Suspension, *cefixime*	56, 292, 325, 382, 384, 409, 433, 442, 534, 552	B	
Suprenza ODT, *phentermine*	273	C	IV
Surfak, *docusate calcium*	88	C	
Surmontil, *trimipramine*	22, 100, 115, 133, 164, 166, 238, 242, 276, 313, 339, 342, 346, 413	C	
Sustiva, *efavirenz*	192, 513	C	
Syeda, *ethinyl estradiol/ drospirenone*	483	X	
Symbicort, *budesonide/ formoterol*	32	C